Lipids and Lipidoses

Edited by G. Schettler

Contributors

R. M. Burton · D. G. Cornwell · W. Fuhrmann · W. Kahlke
L. W. Kinsell · D. Kritchevsky · R. J. Rossiter · G. Schettler
G. Schlierf · B. Shapiro · W. Stoffel · H. Wagener

With 146 Figures

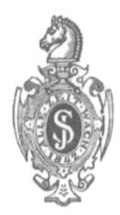

Springer-Verlag   Berlin · Heidelberg · New York 1967

The clinical chapters were translated into English by
Günter Schlierf

ISBN-13: 978-3-642-87369-0   e-ISBN-13: 978-3-642-87367-6
DOI: 10.1007/978-3-642-87367-6

Softcover reprint of the hardcover 1st edition 1967

Title-No. 1307

Preface

Advances which have been made in the field of lipid chemistry and bio-chemistry during the last ten years mainly are the results of progress in metho-dology. The introduction of isotopic and chromatographic techniques has not only enriched our knowledge of normal lipid metabolism but has also greatly enhanced the understanding of the various lipidoses. This is well illustrated by a comparison of the contents of the present monograph with those of my 1955 review in *Handbuch der Inneren Medizin* (Springer).

In addition to better information about the classic lipid thesaurismoses Nie-mann-Pick disease, Gaucher's disease and Tay-Sachs disease, the number of hereditary lipid storage diseases has increased considerably through the recogni-tion of new syndromes such as metachromatic leukodystrophy, Fabry's disease, Refsum's disease (heredopathia atactica polyneuritiformis), a-β-lipoproteinemia, and Tangier disease. Conversely, disorders such as Hand-Schüller-Christian disease which has been considered a lipidosis up to 1958 (THANNHAUSER) must now be differentiated from the hereditary disturbances of lipid metabolism.

Essential hyperlipemia which at one time seemed to be a well defined entity has now been recognized to consist of a number of subgroups, whose pathogeneses appear to be quite different, and whose classification is by no means definite. Similar problems exist for "essential hypercholesterolemia".

Since the knowledge of today is the key for the solutions of tomorrow, we are fortunate that the chapters on lipidoses are supplemented by a comprehensive account of lipid chemistry and biochemistry which has been coordinated by W. STOFFEL.

In accordance with our interpretation of the term lipidoses as hereditary disorders of lipid metabolism, a review of secondary hyperlipidemias has not been attempted here. Since they are considered as associated phenomena of disorders such as diabetic ketoacidosis, nephrosis or pancreatitis, their exclusion seems to be justifiable.

The book would not have been possible without the help of many coworkers. I would like to acknowledge gratefully the assistance of P. D. S. WOOD in the translation, the excellent secretarial work of Miss A. VAN OOSTEN, A. REINARTZ and M. KUCIAK, and the efforts of the Springer publishing company. Numerous colleagues have contributed valuable suggestions and criticisms. We shall ap-preciate any comments from the readers of this first English edition.

Heidelberg 1967   G. SCHETTLER

Contributors

R. M. Burton, Ph. D., Associate Professor, Department of Pharmacology and Beaumont-May Institute of Neurology, Washington University Medical School, Saint Louis, Missouri, 63110, U.S.A.

D. G. Cornwell, Ph. D., Professor and Chairman, Department of Physiological Chemistry, College of Medicine, The Ohio State University, Columbus, Ohio, 43210, U.S.A.

W. Fuhrmann, Dr. med., Dozent, Institut für Anthropologie und Humangenetik der Universität Heidelberg, 6900 Heidelberg, Germany.

W. Kahlke, Dr. med., Medizinische Klinik (Ludolf Krehl-Klinik) der Universität Heidelberg, 6900 Heidelberg, Germany.

L. W. Kinsell, M. D., D. Sc., Director, The Institute for Metabolic Research, Highland General Hospital, Oakland, California, 94606, U.S.A.

D. Kritchevsky, Ph. D., Member of The Wistar Institute of Anatomy and Biology, Professor of Biochemistry, Division of Animal Biology, School of Veterinary Medicine, University of Pennsylvania, Philadelphia, Pennsylvania, 19104, U.S.A.

R. J. Rossiter, Ph. D., Professor of Biochemistry, Department of Biochemistry, University of Western Ontario, London, Ontario, Canada.

G. Schettler, Dr. med., Professor für Innere Medizin, Direktor der Medizinischen Klinik (Ludolf Krehl-Klinik) der Universität Heidelberg, 6900 Heidelberg, Germany.

G. Schlierf, Dr. med., Medizinische Klinik (Ludolf Krehl-Klinik) der Universität Heidelberg, 6900 Heidelberg, Germany.

B. Shapiro, Ph. D., Professor, The Hebrew University, Hadassah Medical School, Department of Biochemistry, Jerusalem, Israel.

W. Stoffel, Dr. med., Dr. chem., Dozent, Physiologisch-chemisches Institut der Universität Köln, 5000 Köln, Germany.

H. Wagener, Dr. med., Dozent, Medizinische Klinik (Ludolf Krehl-Klinik) der Universität Heidelberg, 6900 Heidelberg, Germany.

Contents

Part I. Lipids

Biochemistry, Physiology, Methodology

The Chemistry of Mammalian Lipids. By W. Stoffel (With 11 Figures)

Biochemistry of Sphingosine Containing Lipids. By R. M. BURTON (With 11 Figures)

Lipoproteins. By D. G. CORNWELL

Methods for Separation and Determination of Lipids. By H. WAGENER (With 8 Figures)

Part II. Lipidoses

Clinic, Pathology, Pathophysiology, Genetics

Gangliosidoses. By G. SCHETTLER and W. KAHLKE (With 10 Figures)

Niemann-Pick Disease. By G. SCHETTLER and W. KAHLKE (With 6 Figures)

Metachromatic Leucodystrophy. By W. KAHLKE (With 3 Figures)

Contents   XI

A-β-Lipoproteinemia. By W. KAHLKE (With 6 Figures)

Tangier Disease. By W. KAHLKE (With 5 Figures)

Essential Hypercholesterolemia. By G. SCHETTLER, W. KAHLKE and G. SCHLIERF (With 6 Figures)

Essential Hyperlipemia. By L. W. KINSELL, G. SCHLIERF, W. KAHLKE and G. SCHETTLER (With 9 Figures)

Part I

Lipids

Biochemistry, Physiology, Methodology

The Chemistry of Mammalian Lipids

By

W. Stoffel

Introduction

Lipids differ significantly from carbohydrates, proteins and nucleic acids because of their molecular heterogeneity. Since the latter groups of compounds occur as oligo- or polymers of a limited number of constituent molecules, they are characterized within their respective group by close structural relationships. In contrary, common solubility properties rather than close structural relationships classify lipids as one group.

A very liberal system of classification permits a differentiation of the heterogeneous lipids into two groups:

A. Simple lipids

B. Complex lipids.

The *simple lipids* contain:

    I. glycerides

        1. monoglycerides,

        2. diglycerides,

        3. triglycerides,

    II. cholesterol and cholesterol esters.

    III. bile acids.

Glycerides, cholesterol and cholesterol esters are uncharged and, therefore, often called neutral lipids. Bile acids are chemically related to cholesterol and will be discussed in connection with the sterols.

The *complex lipids* contain, in addition to long chain fatty acids, a polyalcohol, phosphoric acid, a nitrogen base (choline, ethanolamine or serine) and/or hexoses. This large group may be subdivided into:

    I. glycerophospholipids,

    II. sphingolipids.

I. All glycerophospholipids share in common an L-α-glycerophosphoric acid skeleton, the structure and the Stuart-model is shown in the following figure:

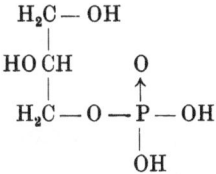

L-α-glycerophosphoric acid

Glycerophospholipids include the following:

    1. phosphatidic acids,

    2. phosphatidyl cholines (lecithins),

    3. phosphatidyl ethanolamines (colamine cephalins),

4. phosphatidyl serines (serine cephalins),
5. lyso-glycerophospholipids,
6. phosphatidyl glycerols,
7. cardiolipins,
8. phosphatidyl inositols (mono- and poly-phospho-inositides),
10. glyceryl ether phospholipids.

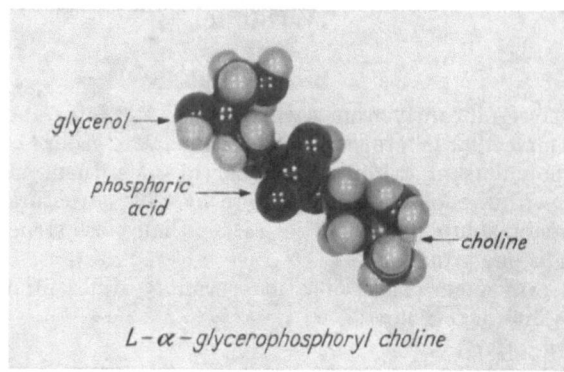

glycerol →

phosphoric acid →

← *choline*

$L-\alpha-glycerophosphoryl\ choline$

II. All *sphingolipids* contain the long chain aminoalcohol *sphingosine* and are comprised of:
1. sphingomyelin,
2. glycosphingolipids.

The latter include:
a) cerebrosides,
b) sulfatides,
c) ceramidepolyhexosides,
d) gangliosides.

The final chapter will discuss the chemistry of saturated and unsaturated fatty acids, which are integral constituents of all the molecules listed before, and also the chemistry of prostaglandins, which are derived from the polyunsaturated essential fatty acids.

A common feature of lipid chemistry is that there is not a single class of lipids which represent one distinct chemical moiety. Rather each class is characterized by its constituents, their molar ratios and their modes of linkages. The many different acyl-components (saturated and unsaturated fatty acids) e. g. in glycerophospholipids or the different fatty acids and different sphingosines (dihydro-, 18: and 20: sphingosines) of sphingolipids cause each well defined class to become an array of many different molecules with possibly different physico-chemical properties.

A. Simple Lipids

I. Glycerides

This group comprises the fatty acid esters of glycerol. Depending on the extent of esterification, usually with straight chain, even-numbered saturated and unsaturated fatty acids with 14 to 20 C-atoms, mono-, di- and triglycerides can be isolated from mammalian glycerides. Trace amounts of odd numbered or branched-chain fatty acids can also be detected by sensitive methods in any glyceride mixture. Mono- and diglycerides are minor portions of the glyceride fraction, except in intestinal mucosa, where particularly monoglycerides are absorbed as hydrolysis products of triglycerides. More than 95% of the adipose tissue, about 30% of the total liver lipids and only 10% of the total blood lipids in man consists of triglycerides.

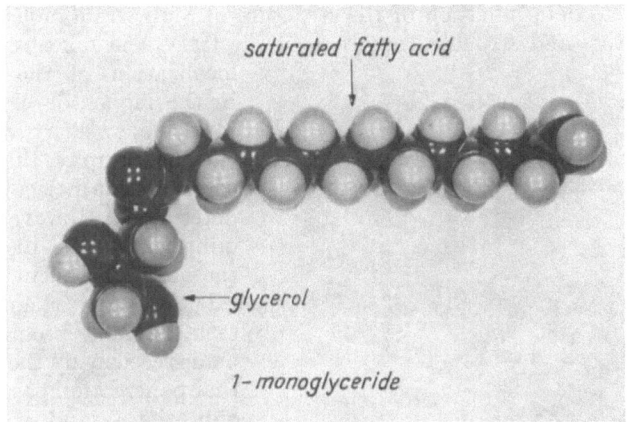

saturated fatty acid

←glycerol

1- monoglyceride

1. The acyl group in **monoglycerides** may be located at the α- or β-C-atom of glycerol:

$$
\begin{array}{cc}
\begin{array}{c}
\quad\quad\;\;\; O \\
\quad\quad\;\; \diagup\!\!\diagup \\
H_2C - OC - R \\
| \\
HO\,CH \\
| \\
H_2C\,OH
\end{array}
&
\begin{array}{c}
\quad\quad\quad H_2C\,OH \\
O \quad\quad\; | \\
\diagdown\!\!\diagdown \;\;\; | \\
R - CO\,CH \\
| \\
H_2C\,OH
\end{array}
\end{array}
$$

α-D-monoglyceride β-monoglyceride
(= 1-monoglyceride) (= 2-monoglyceride)

The β-monoglycerides are optically inactive; substitution on the α-C-atom results in an optically active monoglyceride. According to the Baer-Fischer rule (1939) this structure has α-D-configuration because oxidation of the molecule, barring hydrolysis of the substituent in α-position of the molecule, will yield a derivative of D-glyceraldehyde:

$$
\begin{array}{c}
H - C = O \\
| \\
HC\,OH \quad O \\
| \quad\quad \diagup\!\!\diagup \\
H_2C\,OC - R
\end{array}
$$

2. The **D-α,β-diglycerides** are the naturally occurring diglycerides, found as hydrolysis products of phosphatidyl choline acted upon by phospholipase C (chapter IV, 2) or as intermediates in the biosynthesis of a number of glycero-phospholipids and triglycerides.

$$
\begin{array}{c}
\quad\quad\quad\quad\quad\quad\quad O \\
\quad\quad\quad\quad\quad\quad\; \diagup\!\!\diagup \\
O \quad\; H_2C - O - C - R_1 \\
\| \quad\quad\quad | \\
R_2C - O - CH \\
\quad\quad\quad | \\
\quad\quad\; H_2C - OH
\end{array}
$$

D-α, β-diglyceride
(= 1,2-diglyceride)

3. Triglycerides are by far the most abundant glyceride group. Large depots are the subcutaneous, mesenteric and perinephric fat tissues. The α- and α'-acyl groups are largely saturated fatty acids, whereas the β-position contains an unsaturated fatty acid.

The complete determination of the structure of a glyceride molecule requires a) a quantitative and structural analysis of the fatty acid mixture, and b) the

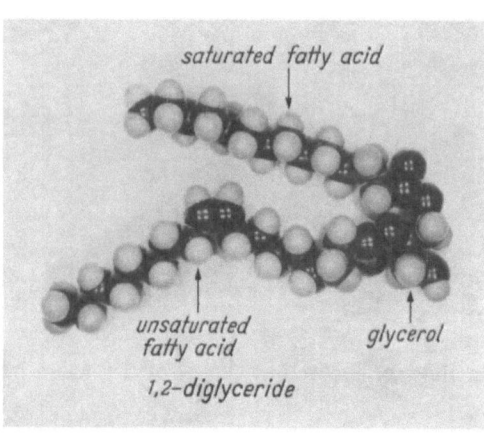

localization of the fatty acids in the mono-, di- or triglyceride molecule. Using vapour-phase chromatography, the fatty acids of a glyceride molecule are readily determined. However, the determination of the distribution of the acyl components in a glyceride molecule remains a difficult task. Valuable progress has been made recently by the observation that pancreatic lipase hydrolyses only the α- and α'-ester bonds (Mattson et al. 1961, 1962). In addition, oxidative cleavage of the unsaturated acyl groups without ester-hydrolysis leads to

dicarboxylic acid esters of glycerol instead of unsaturated fatty acid esters. These polar lipids may then be separated by column chromatography (Youngs 1961). Another very promising approach proves to be the separation of these oxidation products by thinlayer-chromatography (Privett et al. 1961).

Mono- and diglycerides tend to undergo positional isomerizations under the influence of elevated temperatures, acid treatment, and even under chromatography on acidic adsorbents. The separation of mono-, di- and triglycerides can be accomplished by a number of techniques: counter current distribution (Scholfield 1961), silicic acid chromatography (Borgström 1954, Hirsch et al. 1958) and thin-layer chromatography (Mangold 1961). Useful methods for the synthesis of mono-, di- and triglycerides and their properties have been reviewed in a recent article (Mattson et al. 1962).

The acyl groups can either be isolated as free fatty acids by alkaline hydrolysis or as their methyl esters by acid catalyzed transesterification. The most common, elegant and reliable method of fatty acid analysis is gas chromatography of the methyl esters (Lipsky et al. 1963).

II. Cholesterol and Cholesterol Esters

Cholesterol belongs to the large group of steroids characterized by the following tetracyclic ring system:

R_1 and R_2 = CH$_3$-groups
R_3 may vary considerably

The numbering of the steroid molecule (Fieser et al. 1959) generally used is that given in the figure. Counting is continued in the side chain R_3 as follows:

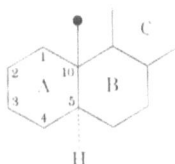

The juncture of ring A and B in the fully hydrogenated ring system gives rise to two isomers: a) the allo- (or trans-) series in which the hydrogen atom at C_5 and the methyl group at C_{10} are in trans position; b) the normal- (or *cis-*) serie in which the hydrogen atom and the methyl group are in the *cis* position:

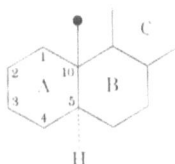
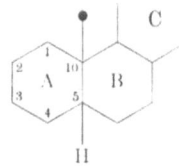

5α- or allo- or trans-series   5β- or normal- or cis-series

Substituents with α-orientation are projecting behind the plane, as indicated by broken lines, and those with β-orientation are projecting in front of the plane ond linked by solid lines. The prefix *allo* refers only to a change of the configuration af C_5 from 5 β to 5α; whereas *epi* refers to a change at C_3 from 3 β to 3α:

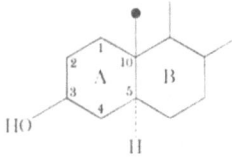
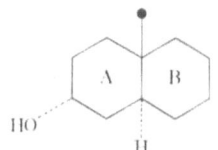

3β-cholestanol   3α-*(epi)*-cholestanol

The spatial arrangement of all steroids of the *allo-* and the *normal*-series puts the substituents in equatorial (e) or axial (a) positions:

-------- equatorial
———— axial

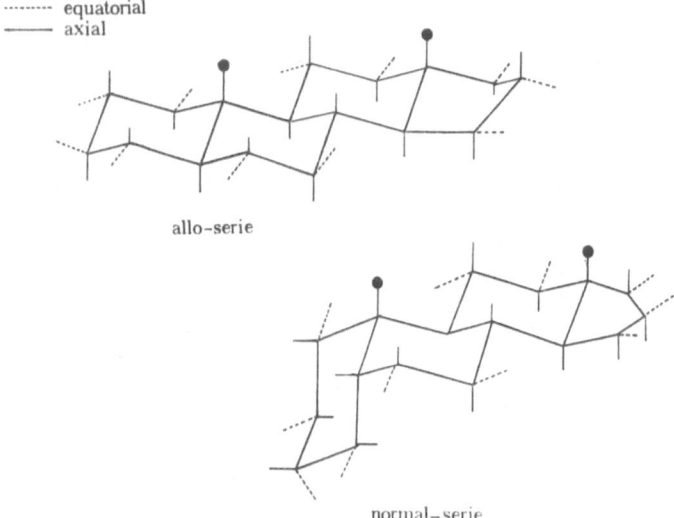

allo–serie

normal–serie

Table 1 gives some representative examples of the allo- and normal-series:

Table 1. *Representative members of the allo- and normal-series*

R	5 α (allo)	5 β (normal)
H	androstane	testane
CH₃CH₂	*allo*-pregnane	pregnane
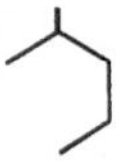	*allo*-cholane	cholane
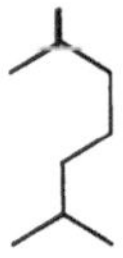	cholestane	coprostane

Cholesterol, cholest-5-en-3β-ol, has the following structure:

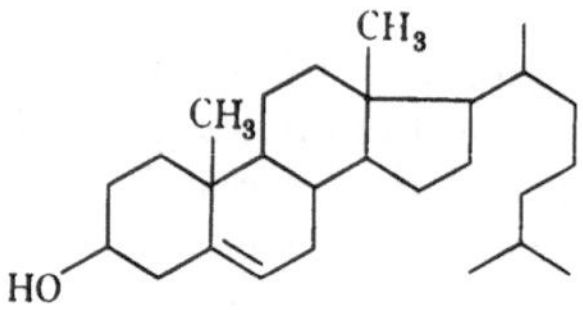

cholesterol

Hydrogenation produces the two isomers cholestanol (rings A/B *trans*) and coprostanol (rings A/B *cis*).

3β-hydroxysteroids can be separated selectively from 3α *(epi)*-isomers by precipitation with digitonin, the glycoside of the aglycon digitogenin (WINDAUS 1909). Cholesterol esters do not form digitonides, the addition compounds of digitonin (SPERRY 1963).

The total serum cholesterol amounts to about 150—200 mg %, more than three quarters of which is esterified predominantly with long chain unsaturated fatty acids (18:1, 18:2, 20:4) The structure of cholesteryl arachidonate is given in the next figure:

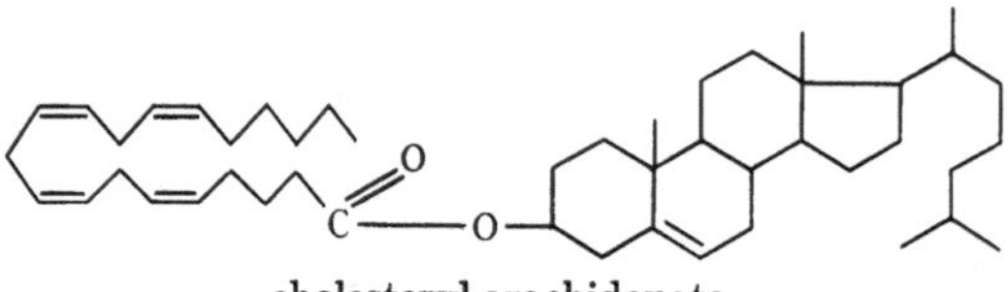

cholesteryl arachidonate

Isolation and separation methods of cholesterol and cholesterol esters are discussed in connection with those presented for complex lipids (HIRSCH et al. 1958, HORNING et al. 1960, CARROLL 1961).

An important intermediate in cholesterol biosynthesis is lanosterol, 4,4', 14α-trimethyl-$\Delta^{8,24}$-cholestadien-3β-ol (CLAYTON et al. 1956). The former is a major constituent of wool fat, but has also been isolated from liver.

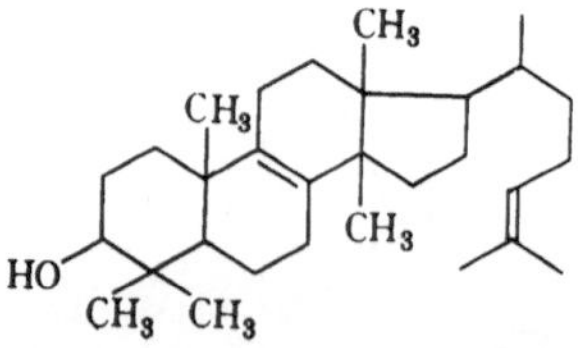

lanosterol

III. Bile Acids

The most important end products in mammalian cholesterol metabolism are the bile acids. The parent C_{24}-acid is cholanic acid with a ring structure identical to that of coprostanol (A/B cis). The bile acids are hydroxylated cholanic acids, all hydroxyl-groups have α-orientation. Consequently, they do not form digitonides. The principal acids are cholic acid (3α, 7α, 12α-trihydroxy-cholanic acid), chenodeoxycholic acid (3α,7α-dihydroxycholanic acid) and deoxy-cholic acid (3α, 12α-dihydroxycholanic acid). Lithocholic acid (3α-hydroxycholanic acid) also occurs in human bile, but only in small amounts.

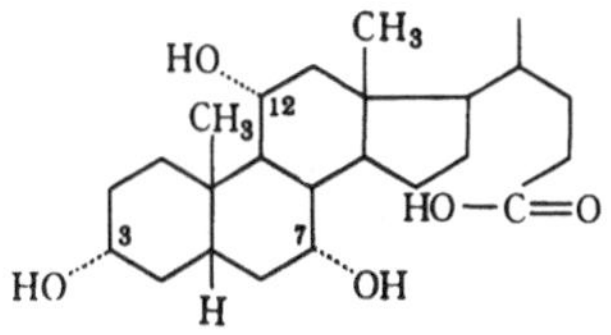

cholic acid

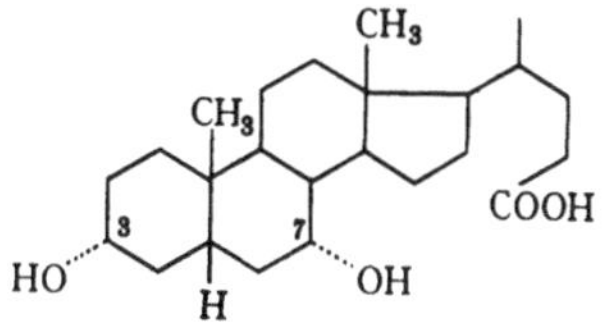

chenodeoxycholic acid

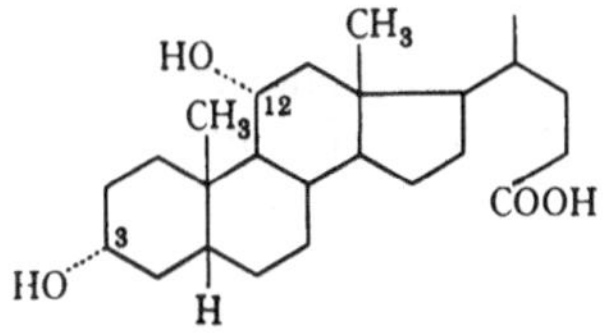

deoxycholic acid

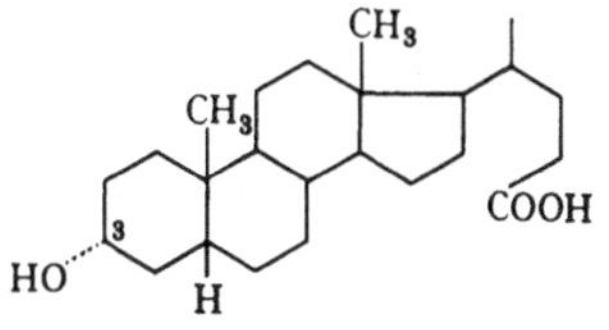

lithocholic acid

All bile acids are secreted in the bile exclusively as glycine and taurine conjugates, the glyco- and taurocholic acids (HASLEWOOD 1955, AHRENS et al. 1952). Amino acid and bile acid are linked by a peptide bond:

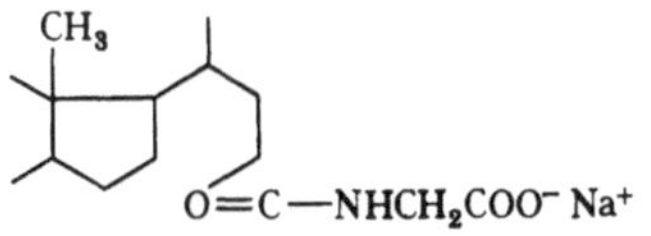

glycine conjugate

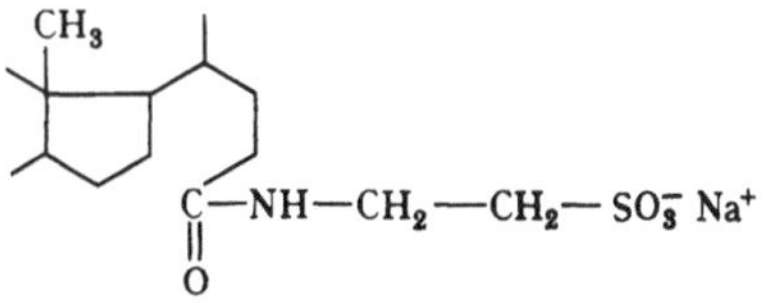

taurine conjugate

Thin-layer chromatography (ENEROTH 1963) and gas-liquid chromatography (SJÖVALL et al. 1961, VANDENHEUVEL et al. 1960, GRUNDY 1965) are the most rapid and reliable methods for identification of bile acids. The latter procedure is also used for quantitative estimation.

B. Complex Lipids

I. Glycerophospholipids

Common to all glycerophospholipids is the L-α-glycerophosphoric acid skeleton, the structure and molecular model are given in the next figures:

The alcoholic group of the β and α'-C-atom of glycerol may be either esterified with long chain fatty acids or one acyl group may be substituted by a long chain

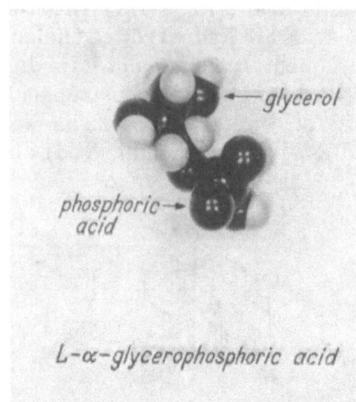

$$
\begin{array}{ll}
\alpha' & H_2C-OH \\
& \quad | \\
\beta & HOCH \quad O \\
& \quad | \qquad \uparrow \\
\alpha & H_2C-O-P-OH \\
& \qquad\qquad | \\
& \qquad\qquad OH
\end{array}
$$

L-α-glycerophosphoric acid
($=$ 3-glycerophosphoric acid)

L-α-glycerophosphoric acid

vinylalcohol or a saturated alcohol, thereby forming an ether linkage. Phosphoric acid is present in most of the glycerophospholipids as a diester, the second acid group being esterified with choline, ethanolamine, serine, inositol or glycerol. Only lysophosphatidic and phosphatidic acids occur as monoesters of phosphoric acid in animal tissues.

1. Phosphatidic Acids: They are present in very low concentration in many organs as intermediates in glycerophospholipid biosynthesis (chapter IV). These acids are diacyl-L-α-glycerophosphoric acids with the following structure:

$$
\begin{array}{l}
\qquad\qquad\qquad\quad O \\
\qquad\qquad\qquad\quad \| \\
\quad O \quad H_2C-OC-R_1 \\
\quad \| \qquad | \\
R_2-CO-CH \qquad O \\
\qquad\qquad | \qquad\quad \uparrow \\
\qquad\quad H_2C-O-P-OH \\
\qquad\qquad\qquad\quad | \\
\qquad\qquad\qquad\quad OH
\end{array}
$$

L-α-phosphatidic acid

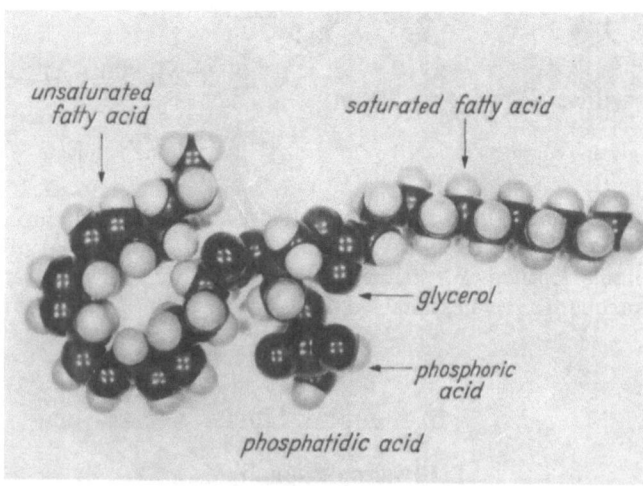

phosphatidic acid

Alkaline hydrolysis yields L-α-glycerophosphate (LONG et al. 1954). The alkali salts of phosphatidic acids are reasonably stable, whereas the free acids undergo intramolecular acid hydrolysis. The phosphate residue forms a cyclic phosphate by fission of the fatty acid ester bond.

The free acids are soluble in ether and ethanol; the sodium salt is soluble in ether but insoluble in ethanol (KATES 1955). Phosphatidic acids can be prepared enzymatically by the action of phospholipase D on phosphatidyl choline (HANAHAN 1957) with liberation of the nitrogen base. Phosphatidic acids with two identical acyl components have been prepared synthetically (BAER 1951; BAER et al. 1958). Isolation and purification may be accomplished using silicic acid or anion-exchange resins (KORNBERG et al. 1953). Nothing is known about the stability under the conditions of the chromatographic procedures.

Lysophosphatidic acids, the struc-ture of which is given in the next figure, have not yet been isolated from mammalian tissue. However, they are assumed to be intermediates in phosphatidic acid biosynthesis.

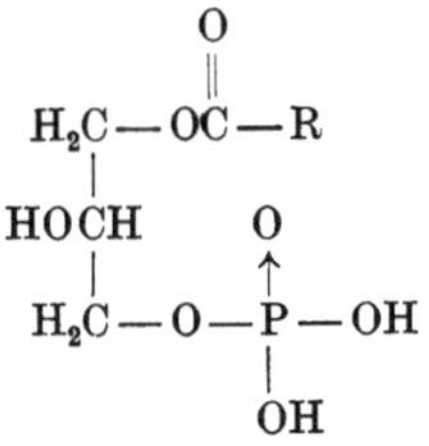

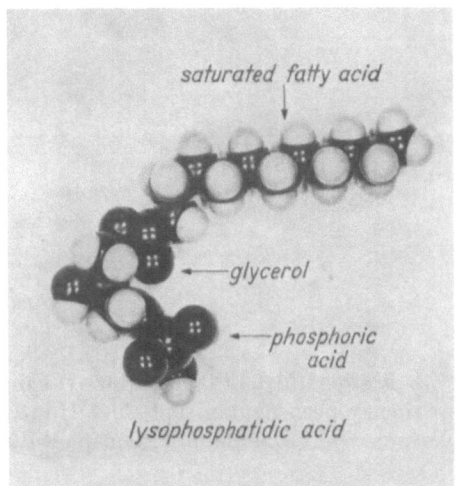

saturated fatty acid

—glycerol

—phosphoric acid

lysophosphatidic acid

$$\begin{array}{c} O \\ \parallel \\ H_2C-OC-R \\ | \\ HOCH \quad\quad O \\ | \quad\quad\quad \uparrow \\ H_2C-O-P-OH \\ | \\ OH \end{array}$$

L-α-lysophosphatidic acid

2. Phosphatidyl Cholines (Lecithins): One of the most abundant glycerophospho-lipids in any tissue is phosphatidyl choline:

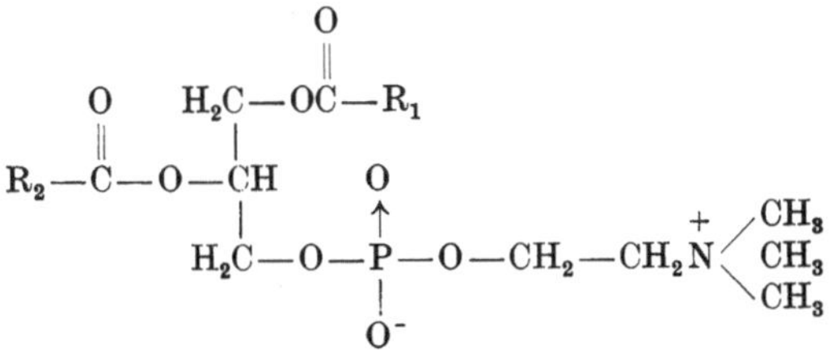

$$\begin{array}{c} O \\ \parallel \\ O \quad\quad H_2C-OC-R_1 \\ \parallel \quad\quad | \\ R_2-C-O-CH \quad\quad O \quad\quad\quad\quad\quad\quad\quad +\;\diagup CH_3 \\ | \quad\quad\quad\quad \uparrow \quad\quad\quad\quad\quad\quad\quad N{\Big\langle} CH_3 \\ H_2C-O-P-O-CH_2-CH_2\quad\quad \diagdown CH_3 \\ | \\ O^- \end{array}$$

L-α-phosphatidyl choline (lecithin)

The acyl groups in the α'- and β-positions of lecithins represent a mixture of a variety of saturated and unsaturated fatty acids. The β-position is esterified predominantly by unsaturated fatty acids of the C_{18}-, C_{20}-, and C_{22}-series, whereas the α'-position is esterified largely by saturated fatty acids. The unsaturated fatty acids of lecithins vary from one tissue to the other. The different cell organelles of the same tissue however have similar fatty acid patterns (MACFARLANE et al. 1960, GETZ et al. 1961).

Lecithins are soluble in ether, ethanol and chloroform and sparingly soluble in acetone. The separation of the choline and ethanolamine containing lipids can be achieved by aluminum oxide chromatography (HANAHAN et al. 1951, LONG et al. 1961). The most widely used method of separation and purification is silicic acid chromatography (HANAHAN et al. 1957). Analytical procedures have been compiled recently (ANSELL et al. 1964). The actions of different phospholipases on phosphatidyl choline have been described in chapter IV.

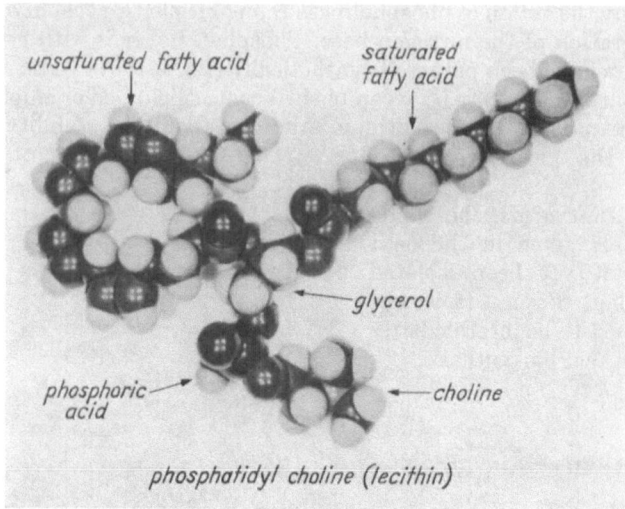

unsaturated fatty acid

saturated fatty acid

glycerol

phosphoric acid

choline

phosphatidyl choline (lecithin)

3. Phosphatidyl Ethanolamines (Cephalins): These glycerophospholipids have previously been named cephalins. However, it is now known that, in addition to phosphatidyl ethanolamine, phosphatidyl serine and phosphatidyl inositol also

$$
\begin{array}{c}
\quad\quad\quad\quad\quad O \\
\quad\quad\quad\quad\quad \parallel \\
\quad\quad O \quad\quad H_2C-OC-R_1 \\
\quad\quad \parallel \quad\quad\quad | \\
R_2-C-O-CH \quad\quad O \\
\quad\quad\quad\quad | \quad\quad \uparrow \quad\quad\quad\quad\quad + \\
\quad\quad H_2C-O-P-O-CH_2-CH_2-NH_3 \\
\quad\quad\quad\quad\quad | \\
\quad\quad\quad\quad\quad O^-
\end{array}
$$

L-α-phosphatidyl ethanolamine

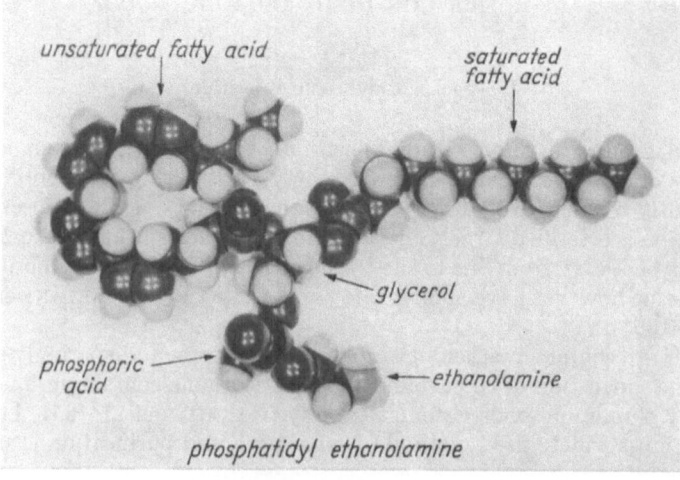

unsaturated fatty acid

saturated fatty acid

glycerol

phosphoric acid

ethanolamine

phosphatidyl ethanolamine

occur in the alcohol-insoluble cephalin fraction (FOLCH 1942, 1948). Phosphatidyl ethanolamine contains one mole of L-α-glycerophosphate, one mole ethanolamine and two moles fatty acids, saturated and unsaturated fatty acids in almost equal amounts (DEBUCH 1956). The unsaturated fatty acids, as in lecithins, are also located in the β-position. Because of their extreme sensitivity to light and oxygen, purification procedures are very elaborate.

4. Phosphatidyl Serines are widely distributed and were initially isolated from the cephalin fraction of brain (FOLCH 1948). Its positive ninhydrin reaction is due to L-serine. As compared to phosphatidyl choline and -ethanolamine, phosphatidyl serine represents a minor component of the glycerophospholipid mixture and generally occurs as the K^+-salt, other ions being Na^+, Mg^{++} and Ca^{++}. Its function in cation metabolism of erythrocytes has been discussed.

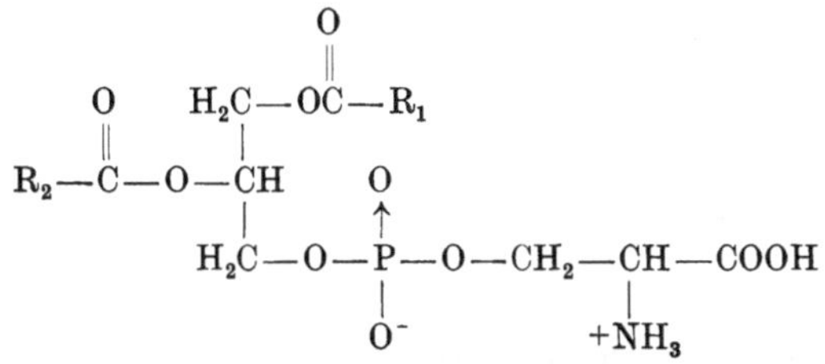

$$
\begin{array}{c}
\overset{O}{\overset{\|}{}} \\
\underset{}{H_2C-OC-R_1} \\
\end{array}
$$

$$
R_2-\overset{O}{\overset{\|}{C}}-O-\underset{}{CH}
$$

$$
H_2C-O-\overset{\uparrow}{P}-O-CH_2-CH-COOH
$$

$$
\underset{O^-}{} \qquad \underset{+NH_3}{}
$$

L-α-phosphatidyl L-serine

The chemical synthesis of saturated diacylglycerophosphorylserine has also established the L-configuration for this group of glycerophospholipids (BAER et al. 1955).

5. Lyso-glycerophospholipids: Another widely distributed class of lipids, which occurs only in small amounts, is comprised of the lyso-phosphatidyl cholines and lyso-phosphatidyl ethanolamines. These compounds are formed in normal tissue by the action of phospholipase A on phosphatidyl choline and phosphatidyl ethanolamine. The enzyme attacks the fatty acid ester bond in the β-position, splitting off a monoenoic or polyenoic fatty acid (TATTRIE 1959; HANAHAN 1960). The naturally occurring α'-acyl residues are predominantly saturated. The structures of lysophosphatidyl choline and lysophosphatidyl ethanolamine are given in the following figures:

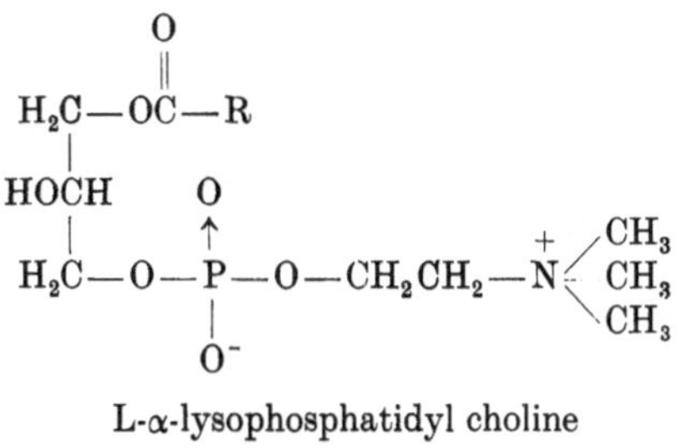

L-α-lysophosphatidyl choline 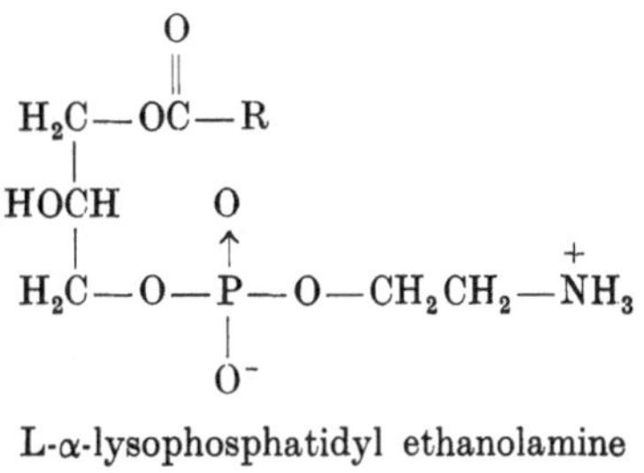   L-α-lysophosphatidyl ethanolamine

Lysolecithins are strongly haemolytic agents and have been shown to be formed in complement fixation reactions. A stimulating effect in phagocytosis has also been demonstrated (FISCHER et al. 1960, BURDZY et al. 1964).

The lyso-glycerophospholipids are insoluble in ether, petroleum ether and absolute acetone, but soluble in water, chloroform, and acetone-water mixtures.

Chromatography on silicic acid and recrystallization or reprecipitation from chloro-
form-ether are the most frequently used procedures for their isolation and purification.

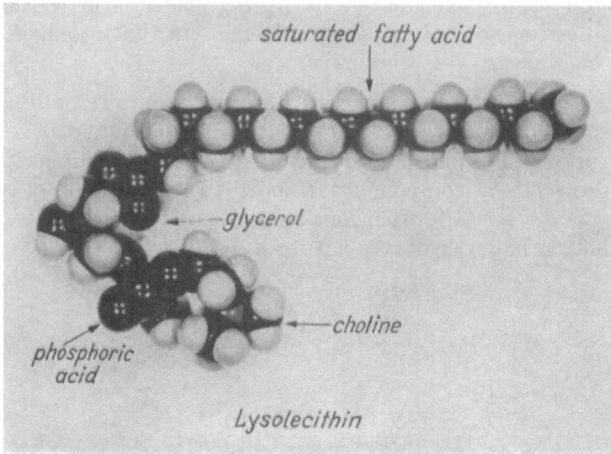

6. **Cardiolipin:** Cardiolipin was initially isolated from heart muscle and structurally it is closely related to phosphatidic acid (Pangborn 1941, 1942, 1947).
It has been recognized recently to be a component lipid of mitochondria (Strickland 1960). The chemical structure proposed on the basis of hydrolysis studies
(Macfarlane 1958) has been confirmed. The absolute configuration of cardiolipin
was determined in an elegant way (Le Cocq et al. 1964). After deacylation, an
optically active triglycerodiphosphate was isolated and identified which, on the
basis of its optical activity, must have the steric relationship which is comparable
to the lyxo-configuration. The structure of triglycerodiphosphate is given in the
following figure:

$$
\begin{array}{ccccc}
\text{HOCH}_2 & & & & \text{HOCH}_2 \\
| & & & & | \\
\text{HOCH} & \text{O} & & \text{O} & \text{HOCH} \\
| & \uparrow & & \uparrow & | \\
\text{H}_2\text{C}-\text{O}-\text{P}-\text{O}-\text{CH}_2-\text{CH}-\text{CH}_2-\text{O}-\text{P}-\text{O}-\text{CH}_2 \\
| & & | & & | \\
\text{O}^- & & \text{OH} & & \text{O}^-
\end{array}
$$

triglycerodiphosphate

This structure and its absolute configuration have been confirmed by chemical
synthesis (Plackett 1964). By analogy, cardiolipin may also be named diphosphatidyl glycerol. Thus cardiolipin has the following structure:

$$
\begin{array}{ccccc}
\text{O} & & & & \text{O} \\
\text{//} & & & & \text{//} \\
\text{R}_1-\text{CO}-\text{CH}_2 & & & & \text{R}_4-\text{C}-\text{O}-\text{CH}_2 \\
\text{O} & & & & \text{O} \\
\text{//} & & & & \text{//} \\
\text{R}_2-\text{CO}-\text{CH} & & & & \text{R}_3-\text{C}-\text{O}-\text{CH} \\
& \text{O} & & \text{O} & \\
& \uparrow & & \uparrow & \\
\text{H}_2\text{C}-\text{O}-\text{P}-\text{O}-\text{CH}_2-\text{CH}-\text{CH}_2-\text{O}-\text{P}--\text{O}\quad\text{CH}_2 \\
& | & | & | & \\
& \text{O}^- & \text{OH} & \text{O}^- &
\end{array}
$$

cardiolipin

The high content of mono-, di-, and trienoic fatty acids ((18:2[9,12] 72%, 18:1[9] 11%, 18:3[9,12,15] 5,2%) is characteristic for cardiolipin (MACFARLANE 1957).

Cardiolipin may function as a hapten and is the active principle of beef heart extracts in the complement fixation reaction with serum from syphilitic patients.

7. Phosphatidyl Glycerol: This class of lipids is chemically related to cardiolipin. It has been recognized in plant chloroplasts and recently in the mitochondria of animal cells. The following structure has been proposed (BENSON et al. 1958, 1961; HAVERKATE et al. 1964):

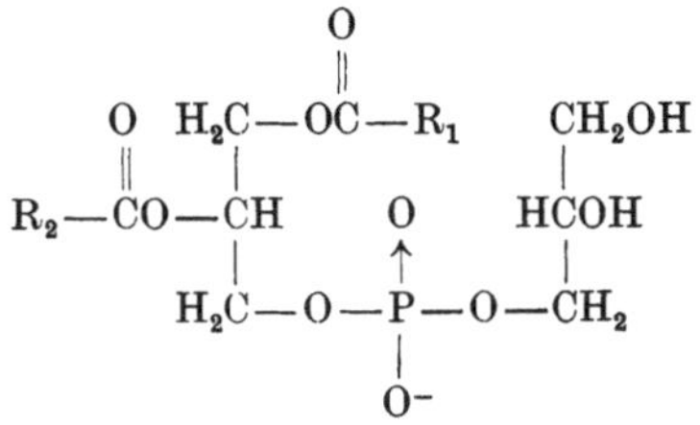

L-α-phosphatidyl D-glycerol

Interesting aspects concerning L-α-phosphatidyl glycerol have been obtained by the isolation of α'-O-amino acid esters of this compound. The lysine, ornithine and alanine esters of L-α-phosphatidyl glycerol have been isolated from gram positive bacteria (HOUTSMULLER et al. 1963). These activated amino acid esters, also named lipoamino acids, have not yet been demonstrated in animal tissues. As an example, the structure of the lysine ester is given in the next formula:

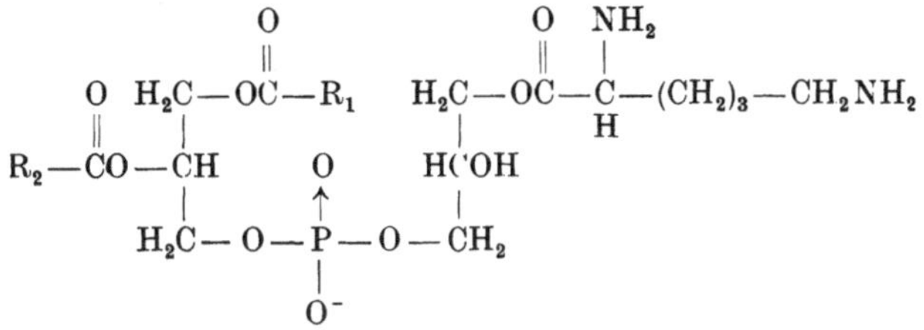

α'-O-L-lysyl-L-α-phosphatidyl D-glycerol

8. Phosphatidyl Inositols: Inositol has been found to be a constituent of tubercle bacillus phospholipids (ANDERSON 1930) and soybean phospholipids (KLENK et al. 1939). A hydrolysate of brain lipids has also yielded inositol (FOLCH et al. 1942). In all instances the optically inactive myo-inositol was the only isomer of inositol that has been isolated from lipids. Inositol is an integral constituent of a group of different types of phosphoinositides *a) monophosphoinositides, b) diphosphoinositides,* and *c) complex phosphoinositides.*

a) The structure of monophosphoinositides is shown in the following figure:

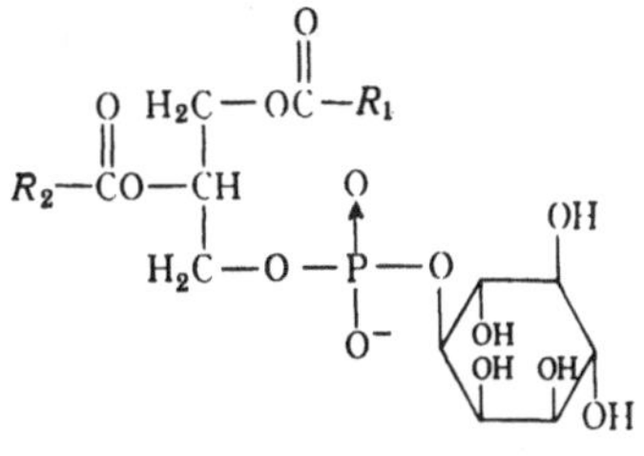

L-α-phosphatidyl monoinositol

Inositol is esterified in position 1 with phosphoric acid (Pizer et al. 1959). More than 50% of the total fatty acid mixture of heart and liver phosphoinositides is stearic acid. It is typical for this group of glycerophospholipids to have a high capacity for cations, namely Ca++ and Mg++ ions. Rich sources of this compound are heart muscle, liver (Hawthorne 1955) and brain (Hawthorne 1960; Hörhammer et al. 1960).

b) Another phosphoinositide with more than one molecule of phosphate has been isolated from brain (Folch 1949). It has recently been shown that this fraction contains a mixture of mono-, di- and triphosphoinositides (Grado et al. 1961; Tomlinson et al. 1961; Dawson 1960; Dittmer et al. 1962 a, b). After deacylation, 1-(α-glycerophosphoryl) L-myoinositol-4-phosphate and 1-(α-glycerophosphoryl)-L-myoinositol-4,5-diphosphate have been obtained (Brockerhoff et al. 1961; Dawson 1961):

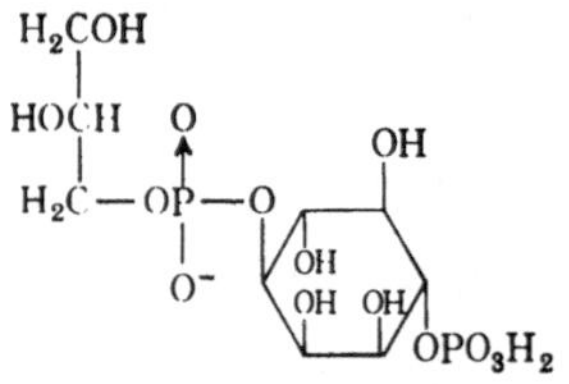

1-(α-glycerophosphoryl)-L-myoinositol-4-phosphate

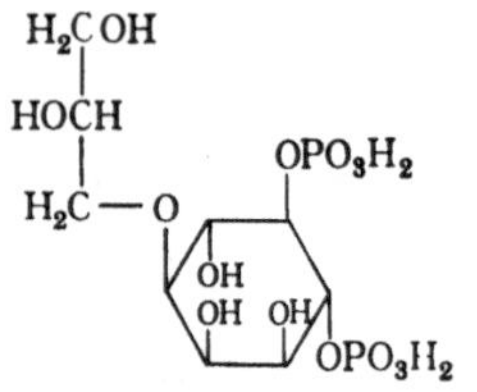

1-(α-glycerophosphoryl)-L-myoinositol-4,5-diphosphate

c) An even more complex glycerophosphoinositide has been isolated from brain (Klenk et al. 1961). Hydrolysis of this compound liberates, in addition to fatty acids and L-α-glycerophosphate, ethanolamine, inositol, batyl alcohol, mannose and N-acetyl-glucosamine. Three or four mannose residues and N-acetyl-glucosamine presumably are bound to inositol.

The most suitable isolation and purification procedures are repeated silicic acid chromatography (Hanahan 1958), aluminum oxide chromatography or the successive combined use of aluminium oxide and silicic acid chromatography (Hanahan 1960).

9. Choline and Ethanolamine Plasmalogens: Based on the early observation that the hydrolysis of glycerophospholipids of heart and brain tissues yielded a fatty aldehyde, the structure of an acetal phosphatide had been suggested (Feulgen et al. 1929; Thannhauser et al. 1951). However, catalytic hydrogenation followed by alkaline hydrolysis of a glycerophospholipid rich in plasmalogen yielded chimyl- and batylalcohol phosphate. This observation made a reevaluation of the structure of plasmalogens necessary.

In addition to a possible hemiacetal structure, a vinylether linkage of the aldehyde to the α'-carbon of glycerol analogous to batylalcohol was proposed (Klenk et al. 1954, 1955):

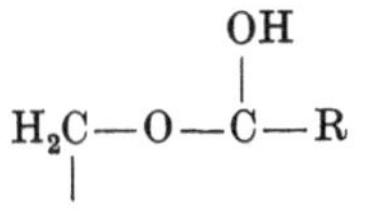

$$\text{OH}$$
$$| \quad \quad \quad \quad \quad \quad \quad \quad \quad \quad H \quad H$$
$$\text{H}_2\text{C}-\text{O}-\text{C}-\text{R} \quad \quad \quad \quad \text{H}_2\text{C}-\text{O}-\text{C}=\text{C}-\text{R}$$

hemiacetal structure 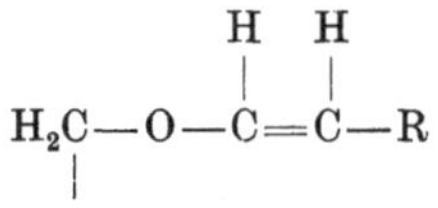   vinylether structure

Subsequent experimental results supported the proposed vinylether structure (RAPPORT et al. 1957, DEBUCH 1957, 1958). The olefinic bond in the vinylether was further shown to have a cis configuration (LANDS et al. 1962). Since the specific site of attack of phospholipase A is the β-position in phosphatidyl choline and ethanolamine, the position of the aldehyde must be at the α'-carbon of glycerol (MARINETTI et al. 1959). These results have provided conclusive evidence for the following structures:

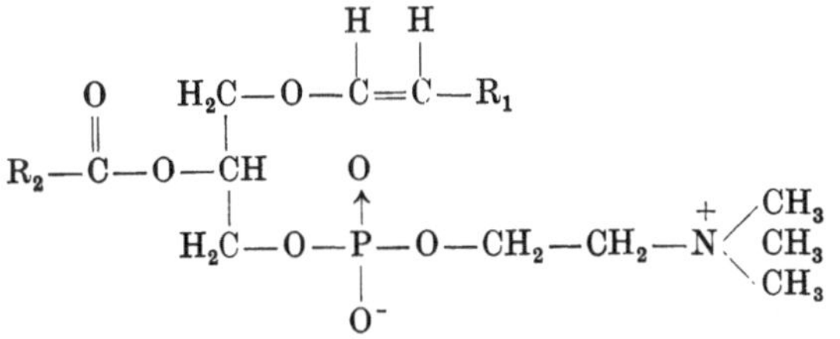

choline plasmalogen 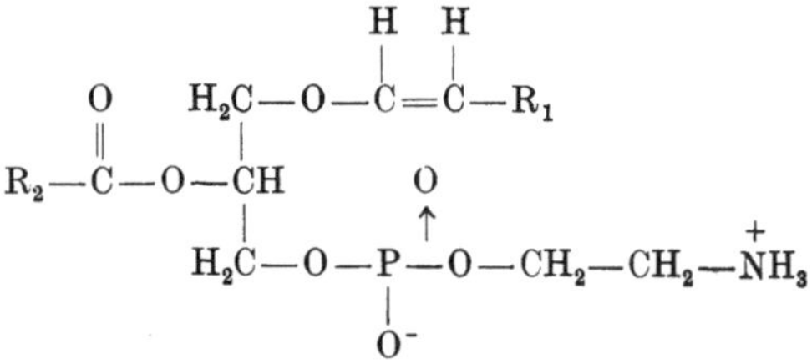   ethanolamine plasmalogen

The aldehydes, which have been isolated from these plasmalogens, are predominantly saturated and monounsaturated aldehydes (16:0, 18:0, $18:1^9$, $18:1^{11}$). In contrast, the fatty acids linked to the β-C-atom in choline plasmalogens are mostly C_{18}-unsaturated fatty acids, no C_{22}-polyenoic acids have been observed (KLENK et al. 1957; DEBUCH 1956). Heart muscle mainly contains choline plasmalogens, whereas brain tissue has ethanolamine and serine plasmalogens (KLENK et al. 1951; ANSELL et al. 1956). These are localized in brain white matter (WEBSTER 1960). Previous attempts to separate diacylglycerophosphoryl choline or -ethanolamine from the respective plasmalogens were unsuccessful.

10. Glyceryl Ether Phospholipids: A lipid similar to the ethanolamine plasmalogens has been isolated from egg yolk and recognized as a glyceryl ether phosphoethanolamine (CARTER et al. 1958). This molecule differs from the afore-mentioned plasmalogens in that the vinylether linkage is hydrogenated and that batylalcohol is liberated on alkaline hydrolysis. Small concentrations of glyceryl ether phospholipids also occur in bovine erythrocytes (HANAHAN et al. 1961, PIETRUSKO et al. 1960). Batylalcohol, which has been isolated from atheromata of human aorta (HARDEGGER et al. 1943), is a compound which may originate from this class of lipids.

The structure of a α'-alkoxy-β-acyl-L-α-glycerophosphorylethanolamine is given in the next figure:

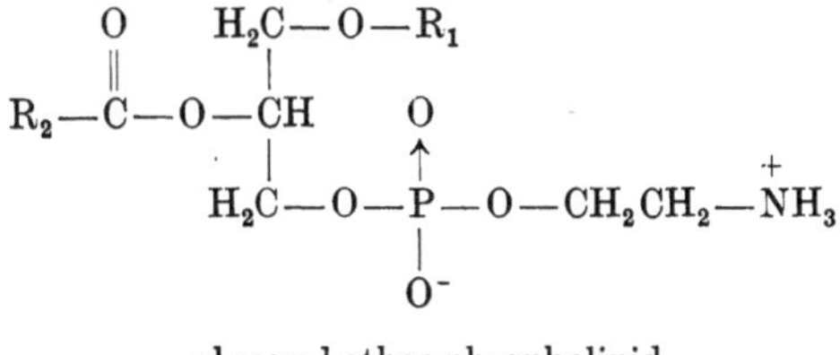

glyceryl ether phospholipid

II. Sphingolipids

Glycerol is the characteristic constituent of glycerides and glycerophospholipids. Another large class of lipids, the so-called sphingolipids, contains sphingosine as the characteristic polyalcohol.

The following subclasses of sphingolipids are known:

1. sphingomyelin or sphingophospholipids
2. glycosphingolipids, which are divided into
   a) cerebrosides
   b) sulfatides
   c) ceramide-polyhexosides (free of N-acetyl-neuraminic acid)
   d) gangliosides

Sphingosine is an unsaturated aminodiol, dihydroxyaminooctadecen (LEVENE 1913/14, KLENK 1929). The correct structure with the relative positions of the amino- and alcoholic groups and the stereochemistry corresponds to that given in the following formula (CARTER et al. 1942, 1947) and Stuart-model:

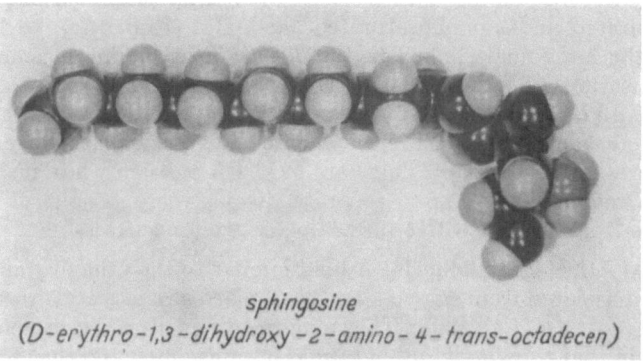

trans-D-erythro-1,3-dihydroxy-2-amino-4-octadecen

sphingosine
(D-erythro-1,3-dihydroxy-2-amino-4-trans-octadecen)

Carbon atom 2 has *D*-configuration (CARTER et al. 1951; KISS et al. 1954; KLENK et al. 1955) and the double bond *trans*-configuration (MISLOW 1952, MARINETTI et al. 1954). One of the most suitable derivatives of sphingosine is the crystalline triacetylsphingosine. Chemical syntheses of sphingosine and dihydrosphingosine support this structure (GROB et al. 1957; SHAPIRO et al. 1958). It has been shown recently that the C_{18}-sphingosine is always accompanied by a sphingosine with 20 C-atoms. Small amounts of dihydrosphingosine, which has also the D-erythro-configuration, always accompany the unsaturated sphingosines. Dihydrosphingosine is present in considerable concentration in cerebrosides of spinal cord (CARTER et al. 1947).

1. Sphingomyelin

Sphingomyelin was discovered by THUDICHUM (1884). After suitable methods for its isolation and purification had been devised (THIERFELDER et al.

1930), the chemical structure was established by hydrolysis studies. The isolation is largely facilitated by a preceeding mild alkaline hydrolysis (KLENK et al. 1941; DAWSON 1954). Acid hydrolysis yields a mixture of sphingosine phosphate, sphingosine phosphorylcholine and phosphorylcholine; alkaline hydrolysis liberates free sphingosine. By these hydrolysis studies (LEVENE 1916; RENNKAMP 1949; ROUSER et al. 1953; SWEELEY 1963) proof for the following structure was obtained:

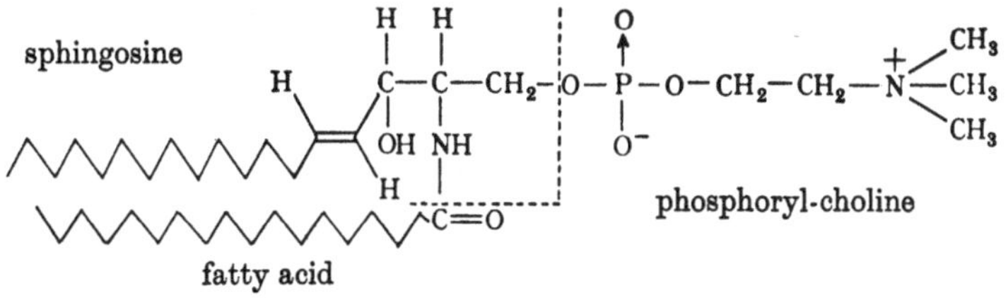

Chemical synthesis of the palmitoyl- and stearoyl-derivatives of dihydro-sphingomyelin confirmed this structure (SHAPIRO et al. 1958). Long chain saturated fatty acids, mono- and even diunsaturated fatty acids (predominantly stearic, lignoceric and nervonic acids) have been isolated from sphingomyelin, but no hydroxy fatty acids (SWEELEY 1963; KISHIMOTO et al. 1963; O'BRIEN et al. 1964).

The structure and configuration of sphingomyelin and the dihydro-derivative has been rigorously confirmed by the total synthesis (SHAPIRO et al. 1959, 1961).

Sphingomyelin is soluble in benzene, hot ethanol and ethylacetate; insoluble in acetone and ether. An approved method of the isolation and purification by chromatographic separation on silicic acid has been reported (HANAHAN 1961).

2. Glycosphingolipids

a) Cerebrosides

The constituents of a cerebroside molecule are a sphingosine or dihydrosphingosine base, a fatty acid and D-galactose. The fatty acid is linked by a peptide bond to the amino group of C-2, D-galactose galactosidically to the primary alcoholic group of sphingosine. The β-configuration of the natural cerebrosides, suggested by the susceptibility to hydrolysis by almond emulsin which is free of α-galactosidase activity (HELFERICH et al. 1933), was conclusively evidenced by these studies. Four different types of fatty acids give rise to four different types of cerebrosides:

cerasin, the acyl group of which are saturated fatty acids, particularly lignoceric acid:

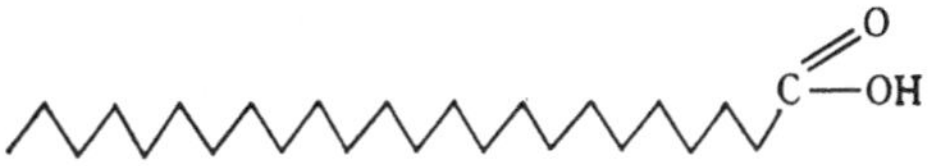

phrenosin or *cerebron*, with α-hydroxy saturated acids, mainly cerebronic acid:

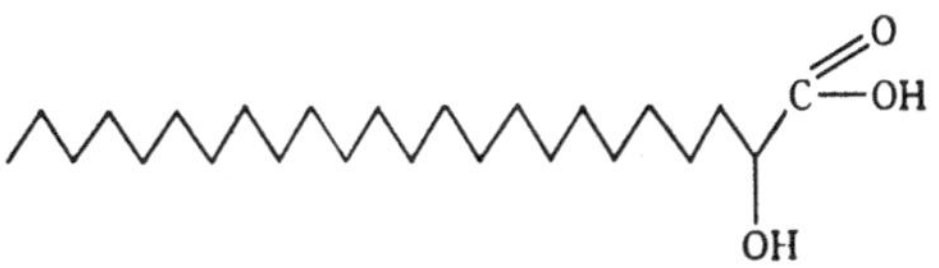

nervon, with the monounsaturated nervonic acid and

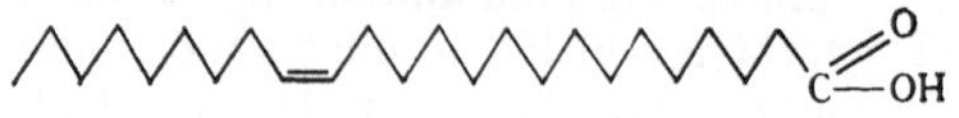

oxynervon, with a monounsaturated-α-hydroxy fatty acid as the main consti-tuent (KLENK 1926, 1930).

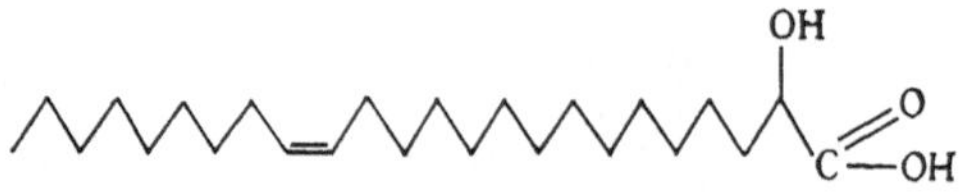

As a representative example the structure of phrenosine is shown in the next figure:

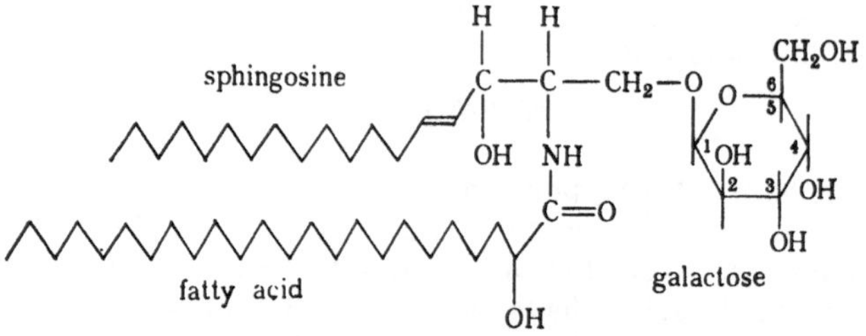

phrenosine (cerebron)

Vapour phase chromatography has shown that the fatty acids mentioned pre-viously are the main constituents, which are however accompanied by higher and lower homologues with 20 to 26 carbon atoms. The level of odd numbered homo-logous acids increases with age (KISHIMOTO et al. 1959). The α-hydroxy fatty acids possess the D-configuration.

Normal cerebrosides from brain are galactocerebrosides. An accumulation of glucocerebrosides has been found in Morbus Gaucher (KLENK 1940; RENNKAMP 1942).

Cerebrosides are soluble in hot ethanol, chloroform-methanol-mixtures; in-soluble in ether and cold ethanol. They can be purified by recrystallization from acetic acid or chloroform-methanol or by chromatography on activated magnesium silicate (Florisil) (RADIN et al. 1959). Alkaline hydrolysis of the peptide bond with barium hydroxide (KLENK 1926) results in the formation of psychosine; partial acid hydrolysis yields ceramide:

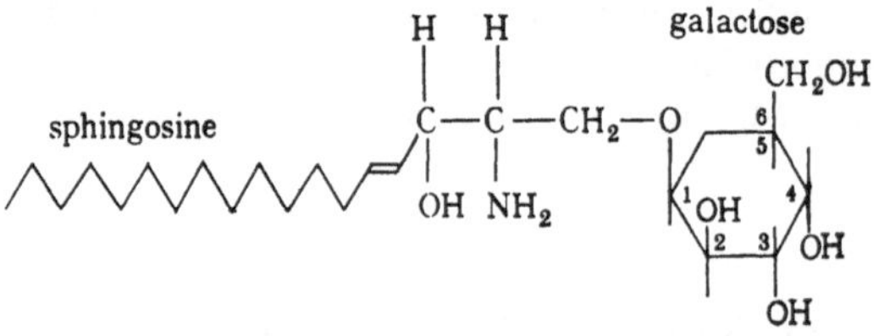

psychosine

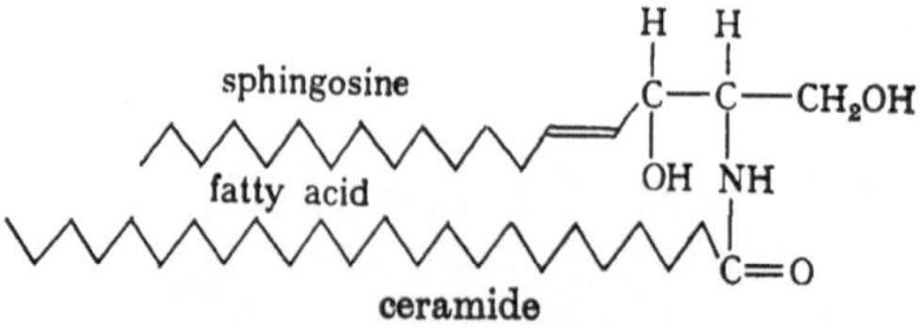

ceramide

Synthetic studies on psychosine (SHAPIRO et al. 1964), cerasine and phrenosine (SHAPIRO et al. 1961) confirmed the results of the earlier structural analyses.

b) Sulfatides

Sulfatides may be considered as sulfuric acid esters of cerebrosides. One cerebroside molecule contains one molecule of sulfuric acid. It had been widely accepted that the sulfuric acid group existed in ester linkage with C-6 of galactose (THANNHAUSER et al. 1953). However, recent studies have shown that sulfuric acid is linked to C-3 of galactose (YAMAKAWA et al. 1962, STOFFYN 1963), as shown in the next figure:

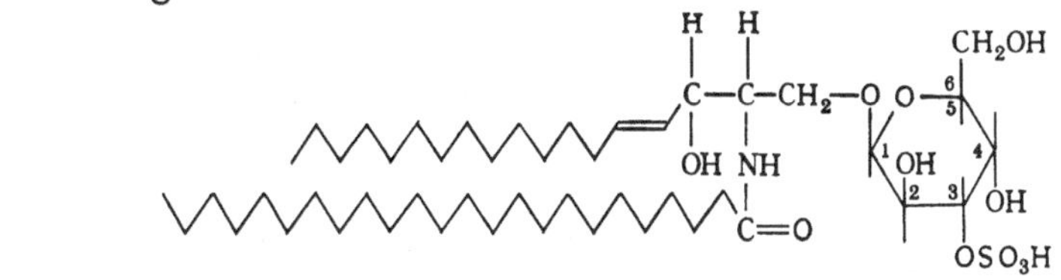

sulfatide

Usually sulfatides occur as alkali salts, predominantly the potassium salt. The sulfatides also contain the 18C- and 20C-homologous sphingosines and different fatty acids (O'BRIEN et al. 1964). Like cerebrosides, sulfatides are located in the white matter.

Improved isolation procedures have been described (RADIN 1957, JATZKEWITZ 1960, SVENNERHOLM et al. 1962).

Two lipoidoses are known in which sulfatides are involved:

1. Krabbe's leucodystrophy, characterized by an almost complete absence of sulfatides but with elevated cerebroside and glycerophosphatide levels in brain.

2. Scholz's metachromatic leucodystrophy, which is characterized by abnormal depositions of sulfatides in the central nervous system (JATZKEWITZ 1958, 1960, 1964).

c) Ceramide-polyhexosides

Ceramide dihexosides, mainly ceramide lactoside, have been isolated from spleen (KLENK 1942) and from erythrocytes (RAPPORT et al. 1962; MAKITA et al. 1962). A ceramide digalactoside accumulates in the kidney of patients with Fabry's disease (SWEELEY 1963); this is accompanied by a ceramide galactosyllactoside with the following structure expressed by short hand nomenclature:

$$\text{ceramide-}\beta\text{-gluc-}(4 \longleftarrow 1) \; \beta\text{-gal-}(4 \longleftarrow 1) \; \beta\text{-gal}$$

This *ceramide trihexoside* has also been isolated from normal kidney (MAKITA et al. 1964). Other ceramide trihexosides, which are present in liver, spleen and serum (SVENNERHOLM et al. 1963), contain, in addition to the ceramide lactoside, galactose or N-acetyl-galactosamine, linked to C-3 or C-4 of the terminal galactose:

$$\text{ceramide-gluc} \; (4 \longleftarrow 1) \; \text{gal} \; (4 \longleftarrow 1) \; \text{gal NHAc}$$

Ceramide tetrahexosides have been obtained from erythrocytes and designated as globosides (YAMAKAWA et al. 1952, 1960). Their structure has been elucidated:

$$\text{ceramide-gluc} \; (4 \longleftarrow 1) \; \text{gal} \; (4 \longleftarrow 1) \; \text{gal} \; (6 \longleftarrow 1) \; \text{gal NHAc}$$

Compared to the gangliotetraose, which is described in the next chapter, the difference is obvious: galNHAc is linked to the terminal and not to the central galactose moiety.

2*

Recently, glycolipids have found increasing interest in immunochemistry. Structurally related ceramide polyhexosides of erythrocytes are responsible for the antigenicity of blood group A and B (KLENK et al. 1951, 1960; KOSCIELAK 1963).

The structures of anti-A and anti-B, which can be rendered soluble by lipid extraction of erythrocyte stroma, have been elucidated recently (CHEESE et al. 1961, SCHIFFMAN et al. 1964). The structures of the determinant groups are:

anti-A   α-galNHAc (1 ⟶ 3) β-gal (1 ⟶ 4) galNHAc
                                  or (1 ⟶ 3)

anti-B   α-gal (1 ⟶ 3) β-gal (1 ⟶ 4) galNHAc
                                 or (1 ⟶ 3)

Ceramide itself is nonhaptogenic but the carbohydrate residues of glycolipids render them haptogenic. Ceramide lactose has been isolated from epidermoid carcinoma cultured in rats and has been named cytolipin H (RAPPORT et al. 1958, 1959).

When rabbits are injected with other animal tissue, the Forssman haptens are produced. These are able to lyse erythrocytes from sheep (FORSSMAN 1911). One of these FORSSMAN haptens is a ceramide linked to galactose and galactosamine (PAPIRMEISTER et al. 1955). The structure of these haptens leaves the question open whether they arise from ceramide polyhexosides, e.g. globosides, by degradation. It should be mentioned that the only noncarbohydrate lipid with haptogenic properties is cardiolipin. The question whether this haptogenic property is due to the free OH-group remains to be answered.

d) Gangliosides

The chemical analysis of brain lipids from a patient with Tay-Sachs' disease led to the discovery of a group of glycolipids, which were named gangliosides, because of its prevalent occurrence in brain gray matter (KLENK 1937). Gangliosides also occur in normal tissue and form a group of chemically closely-related compounds, differing from cerebrosides and ceramide polyhexosides by N-acetyl-neuraminic acid the typical and, for the group of the gangliosides, characteristic additional constituent. Gangliosides are water soluble and react acidically due to one or more N-acetyl-neuraminic acid residues. These are linked to one, two, three or four hexose moieties by a ketosidic linkage. The glycosidic linkages of the carbohydrate part have β-configuration. This hydrophilic group of the molecule is linked by a glycosidic linkage to the lipophilic part, a ceramide, which in general consists of stearic acid and trace amounts of higher and lower homologues linked by a peptide bond to 18: and 20: sphingosine. The concentration of the 20: sphingosine increases with age (SAMBASIVARAO et al. 1964). Modern analytical methods such as column-, thin-layer chromatography and counter current distribution permit the separation of the rather complex mixture of this group of different but closely-related gangliosides, the structures of which have been elucidated recently (KLENK et al. 1960, 1961, 1962, 1963, 1964, 1965; KUHN et al. 1963, 1964). Although there is now a general agreement about the chemical structures of the main components, their nomenclature is rather confusing. The nomenclatures of the two pioneers in this field, KLENK and KUHN, and a third one introduced in a recent review article (SVENNERHOLM 1964) are given in the following table, which summarizes those gangliosides the structures of which have been elucidated to date (p. 22). A very suitable numbering system by B. BURTON has also been introduced and will be used in chapter V. This scheme easily permits a further expansion as new gangliosides are discovered. No doubt, the most fruitful and clear designation is the chemical one, given in the table as short hand designation.

The methods of choice applied in the structural studies of these complex molecules were partial hydrolysis and permethylation methods (KLENK et al. 1961, 1964), and the method of acetolysis (KUHN et al. 1963) and ozonolysis followed by alkali fragmentation. The latter method leaves the carbohydrate moiety unimpaired, whereas the lipid residue, the N-acyl-sphingosine-residue, is cleaved off (WIEGANDT et al. 1965). This analytical work led to the concept that all major gangliosides possess one basic structure, namely that of ganglioside $B_3(=A_2=G_{GNTI}=G_{M\,1})$, which is given in the following figure:

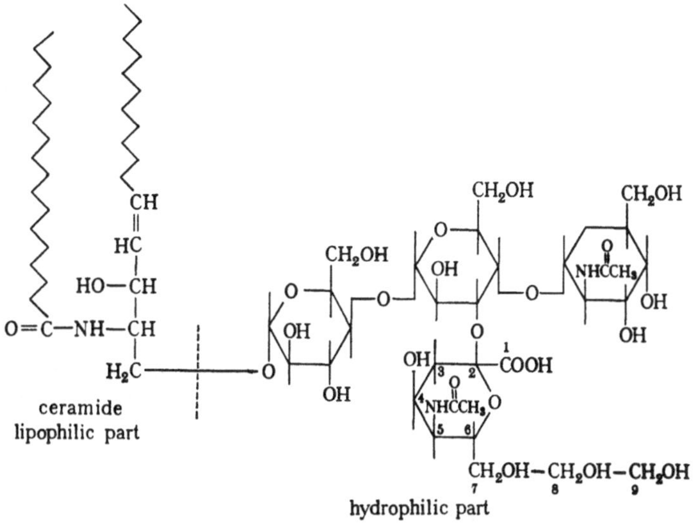

CH
‖
HC
|
HO—CH
|
O=C—NH—CH
|
H₂C

ceramide
lipophilic part

CH₂OH CH₂OH

CH₂OH

OH

OH

NHCCH₃

OH

OH

OH COOH

NHCCH₃

CH₂OH—CH₂OH—CH₂OH

hydrophilic part

ganglioside B_3 $(A_2 = G_{GNTI} = G_{M1})$

The ganglioside $B_2 (A_1 = G_{GNTII} = G_{M\,2})$, predominantly occurring in Tay-Sachs disease, lacks the terminal galactose residue of ganglioside B_3 and can be described by the following short hand designation:

$$cer \longleftarrow gluc(4 \longleftarrow 1)\ gal(4 \longleftarrow 1)\ galNAc$$
$$\begin{pmatrix} 3 \\ \uparrow \\ 2 \end{pmatrix}$$
$$neur\ NAc$$

In ganglioside $B_4 (= B_1 = G_{GNTII} = G_{D1\,a})$ an additional N-acetyl-neuraminic acid molecule is linked by a ketosidic linkage to the C 3 of the terminal galactose of ganglioside B_3:

$$cer \longleftarrow gluc(4 \longleftarrow 1)\ gal\ (4 \longleftarrow 1)\ gal\ NAc\ (3 \longleftarrow 1)\ gal\ (3 \longleftarrow 2)\ neurNAc$$
$$\begin{pmatrix} 3 \\ \uparrow \\ 2 \end{pmatrix}$$
$$neurNAc$$

The N-acetyl-neuraminic acid linked to the terminal galactose is susceptible to enzymatic hydrolysis by neuraminidase, whereas the N-acetyl-neuraminic acid bonded to the central galactose residue is resistant to enzymatic cleavage.

Another major constituent of the brain ganglioside mixture is ganglioside $C_3 (= C_3 = G_{GNTIII})$. This molecule has the basic structure of B_3, but has one additional neuraminic acid residue linked by a 2→8-bond to the N-acetyl-neuraminic

Gangliosides

Structure (short hand designation)	KLENK (1963, 1964, 1965)	KUHN (1963, 1964)	SVENNERHOLM (1964)	BURTON
neurNAc(2 → 3)gal → cer gal(1 → 3)[neurNAc(2 → 3)]gal → cer	D	Ggal		A₁
neurNAc(2 → 3)gal(1 → 4)glu → cer	B₂	Glact	GM3	B₁
galNAc(1 → 4)[neurNAc(2 → 3)]gal(1 → 4)glu → cer	A₁	GGNTrII	GM2	B₂
gal(1 → 3)galNAc(1 → 4)[neurNAc(2 → 3)]gal(1 → 4)glu → cer	A₂	GGNTI	GM1	B₃
neurNAc(2 → 3)gal(1 → 3)galNAc(1 → 4)[neurNAc(2 → 3)]gal(1 → 4)glu → cer	B₁	GGNTII	GD1a	B₄
neuNAc(2 → 8)neurNAc(2 → 3)gal(1 → 4)glu → cer	A₃	G'lact		C₁
galNAc(1 → 4)[neurNAc(2 → 8)neurNAc(2 → 3)]gal(1 → 4)glu → cer	C₁	GGNTIII		C₂
gal(1 → 3)galNAc(1 → 4)[neurNAc(2 → 8)neurNAc(2 → 3)]gal(1 → 4)glu → cer	C₃	GGNTIV	GT1	C₃
neurNAc(2 → 3)gal(1 → 3)galNAc(1 → 4)[neurNAc(2 → 8)neurNAc(2 → 3)]gal(1 → 4)glu → cer				C₄

acid which is bonded to the central galactose. Neuraminidase can also split this ketosidic bond between the two N-acetyl-neuraminic acids yielding ganglioside B_3:

$$\text{cer} \longleftarrow \text{gluc (4} \longleftarrow \text{1) gal (4} \longleftarrow \text{1) galNAc (3} \longleftarrow \text{1)}$$
$$\binom{3}{\uparrow\;2} \qquad \text{gal (3} \longleftarrow \text{2) neurNAc}$$
$$\text{neurNAc (8} \longleftarrow \text{2) neurNAc}$$

The other gangliosides listed in the table are minor components of the total ganglioside mixture. They differ in the size of the hydrophilic carbohydrate part and in the number of N-acetyl-neuraminic acid molecules. The different chromatographic behaviour, particularly in thin-layer chromatography allows their easy detection. A ganglioside with a simple structure has been isolated from horse erythrocytes (Yamakawa 1951; Klenk et al. 1952). It has been named haematoside and its exact structure determined. N-acetyl-neuraminic acid is substituted by N-glycolyl-neuraminic acid:

$$\text{cer} \longleftarrow \text{gluc (4} \longleftarrow \text{1) gal (3} \longleftarrow \text{2) neurNGlyc}$$

The predominant fatty acid of the ceramide part is lignoceric acid. Whereas haematoside is free of hexosamine, a ganglioside isolated from bovine erythrocytes and spleen contains N-acetyl-glucosamine and an additional galactose molecule. The exact structure of this ganglioside is shown below:

$$\text{cer} \longleftarrow \text{glu (4} \longleftarrow \text{1) gal (3} \longleftarrow \text{1) gluNAc (4} \longleftarrow \text{1)}$$
$$\binom{3}{\uparrow\;2}$$
$$\text{neurNGlyc}$$

A similar trisaccharide with N-acetyl-neuraminic acid instead of N-glycolyl-neuraminic acid has been isolated from mammary gland and milk (Caputto et al. 1954; Kuhn et al. 1959).

Gangliosides tend to aggregate in water solution, wheras organic solvents such as dimethylformamide prevent this association of molecules (Klenk et al. 1960; Howard et al. 1964). Strandin (Folch 1954) isolated from brain gray matter proved to be a ganglioside mixture the high molecular weight of which results from a micellar arrangement in aqueous solutions (DAUN 1952). The name mucolipid (ROSENBERG et al. 1956) for ganglioside is less definitive than the well defined and accepted name ganglioside, and should be avoided.

III. Fatty Acids and Fatty Aldehydes

Only those fatty acids, which are relevant to the lipid classes described in the previous sections and to mammalian metabolism, will be discussed.

It is very striking that saturated and unsaturated *fatty acids* are present in glycerophospholipids in approximately equal amounts. In plasmalogens, the aldehydes stand for the saturated fatty acids. Using sensitive methods, only trace amounts of lauric (12:0), myristic (14:0), odd-numbered, and branched saturated fatty acids can be detected in the total fatty acid mixtures of glycerides and glycerophospholipids of different origin. The component saturated fatty acids of these lipids are palmitic (16:0) and stearic acid (18:0). The homologous long chain saturated acids between 20:0 and 26:0 and their α-hydroxy-derivatives occur in cerebrosides. These acids have been mentioned in section B II, 2a.

The presence of mono- and polyunsaturated fatty acids is of particular importance for the structure and function of phospholipids. All polyenoic fatty acids of mammalian origin are characterized by the positional arrangement of the double bonds, the *cis*-configuration of the olefinic bonds, and the *polyallyl-structure* of the double bond system, in which the double bonds are separated by one CH_2-group.

Depending on the first double bond counted from the terminal CH_3-group, four families of polyenoic acids can be differentiated with regard to the parent fatty acids:

1. the palmitoleic acid family,
2. the oleic acid family,
3. the linoleic acid family,
4. the linolenic acid family.

The most common acids are listed below:

1. *Palmitoleic acid* (cis hexadec-9-enoic-acid)

    cis octadec-11-enoic acid (vaccenic acid)

2. *Oleic acid* (cis octadec-9-enoic acid)

    cis eicos-11-enoic acid
    all cis eicosa-5,8,11-trienoic acid

3. *Linoleic acid*
  (all cis octadeca-9,12-dienoic acid)

    all cis octadeca-6,9,12-trienoic acid (γ-linolenic acid)
    all cis eicosa-11,14-dienoic acid
    all cis eicosa-8,11,14-trienoic acid (homo-γ-linolenic acid)
    all cis eicosa-5,8,11,14-tetraenoic acid (arachidonic acid)
    all cis docosa-10,13,16-trienoic acid
    all cis docosa-7,10,13,16-tetraenoic acid
    all cis docosa-4,7,10,13,16-pentaenoic acid

4. *Linolenic acid*
  (all cis octadeca-9,12,15-trienoic acid)

    all cis octadeca-6,9,12,15-tetraenoic acid
    all cis eicosa-5,8,11,14,17-pentaenoic acid
    all cis docosa-7,10,13,16,19-pentaenoic acid
    all cis docosa-4,7,10,13,16,19-hexaenoic acid

The distribution of these polyenoic acids is specific for each organ and characteristic for each lipid class. The common procedure for the isolation of fatty acids from different lipid classes is: transesterification ⟶ saponification and separation of the unsaponifiable material ⟶ esterification, followed by vapor-phase chromatography (gas chromatography) of the methylester mixture. The complete characterization of the structure of any unsaturated fatty acid includes the determination of:

1. the *chain length* based on the retention time or carbon number (WOODFORD 1960) after catalytic hydrogenation,

2. the *number of double bonds* (UV-spectroscopy before and after alkali isomerization, relative retention time or carbon number),

3. the *location of the double bonds* (by oxidative and reductive ozonolysis),

4. the *geometric configuration* of the double bonds (IR-spectroscopy).

Thin-layer chromatography on silver nitrate impregnated silicic acid plates is a suitable method for preparative and semi-preparative separation according to the number of double bonds of the unsaturated fatty acid methylesters. Separation can also be achieved by preparative gas chromatography, on the basis of chain length and degree of unsaturation; this method however is less satisfactory. The main *fatty aldehydes*, which have been isolated from plasmalogens, are: n-hexadecanal, n-octadecanal, *cis* octadec-9-enal, octadec-11-enal.

VI. Prostaglandins

A group of lipid soluble 20C-acids, called prostaglandins, are chemically and biogenetically closely related to the polyenoic acids. These acids with a five-membered ring, a keto group, two hydroxy groups and one to three double bonds are formed from essential fatty acids. The first report on smooth muscle stimulating compounds in human seminal fluid and sheep vesicular glands (GOLDBLATT 1933, 1935; v. EULER 1934, 1936) was followed by their isolation (BERGSTRÖM 1957) and structural elucidation (BERGSTRÖM et al. 1962, 1963). Three prostaglandins, namely PGE_1, PGE_2 and PGE_3, isolated from different animals and organs such as lung, thymus, brain and iris, originate from eicosa-8,11,14-trienoic acid, arachidonic acid and eicosa-5,8,11,14,17-pentaenoic acid. The chemical relationship is obvious from a comparison of their chemical structures:

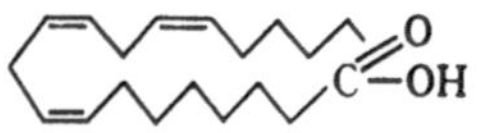

eicosa-8,11,14-trienoic acid

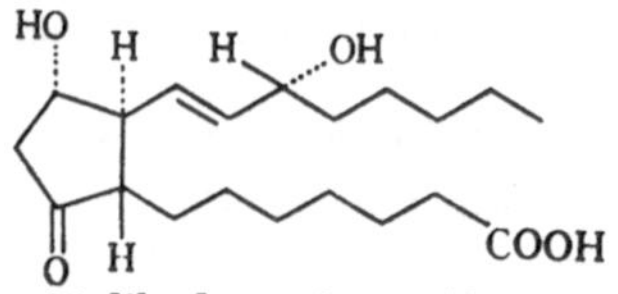

PGE_1 (11α,15-dihydroxy-9-oxo-13-prostenoic acid)

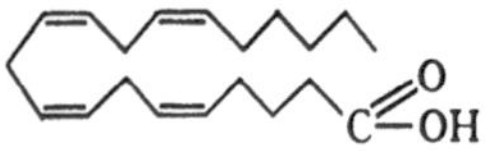

arachidonic acid

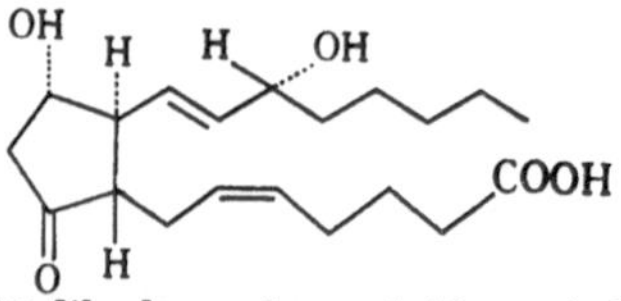

PGE_2 (11α,15-dihydroxy-9-oxo-5,13-prostadienoic acid)

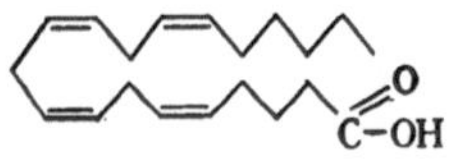

eicosa-5,8,11,14,17-pentaenoic acid

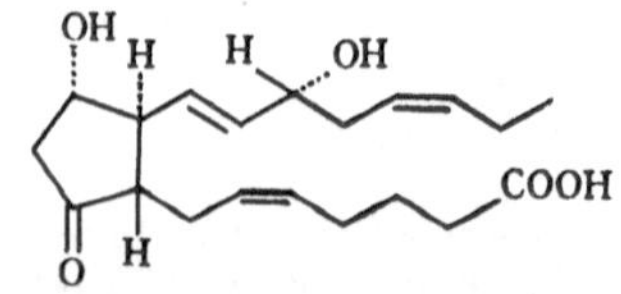

PGE_3 (11α,15-dihydroxy-9-oxo-5,13,17-prostatrienoic acid)

The double bond between C-13 and C-14 ha. *trans*-configuration. All prostaglandins may be regarded as derivatives of the parent prostanoic acid, the unsubstituted acid, with the following structure:

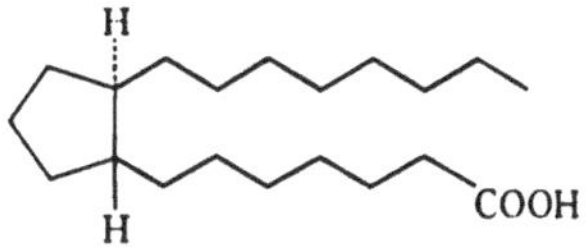

prostanoic acid

The reduction of the carbonyl group leads to the trihydroxy compounds named $PGF_{1\alpha}$, $PGF_{2\alpha}$ and $PGF_{3\alpha}$.

The structures have been established by degradative and mass-spectrometric analyses. The prostaglandins are crystalline compounds.

The direct precursorship of the polyenoic acids in the biosynthesis has been shown recently (VAN DORP et al. 1964; BERGSTRÖM et al. 1964). The biological function of the prostaglandins is only poorly understood. They act as vasodepressors, stimulate smooth muscles and depress the norepinephrine stimulated release of free fatty acids (STEINBERG et al. 1963). PGE_1, injected intravenously, however elevates the free fatty acid level and glycerol concentration of blood plasma in the absence of norepinephrine (BERGSTRÖM et al. 1964). A comprehensive review has recently been published by SAMUELSSON (1965).

References

AHRENS jr., E. H., and L. C. CRAIG: The extraction and separation of bile acids. J. biol. Chem. **195**, 763 (1952).

ANDERSON, R. J.: The chemistry of the lipoids of tubercle bacilli. XIV. The occurrence of inosite in the phosphatide from human tubercle bacilli. J. Amer. chem. Soc. **52**, 1607 (1930).

ANSELL, G. B., and J. N. HAWTHORNE: Phospholipids, p. 40. Amsterdam: Elsevier Publ. Comp., 1964.

— and J. M. NORMAN: Observations on the acetalphospholipids of brain tissue. J. Neurochem. **1**, 32 (1956).

AUSTIN, J. H.: Studies on globoid (Krabbe) Leucodystrophy II. J. Neurochem. **10**, 921 (1963).

BAER, E.: Synthesis of enantiomeric α-phosphatidic acids. J. biol. Chem. **189**, 235 (1951).

— and D. BUCHNEA: Synthesis of unsaturated α-phosphatidic acids and α-bis-phosphatidic acids. Cardiolipin substituents, IV. Arch. Biochem. **78**, 294 (1958).

— and H. O. L. FISCHER: Studies on acetone-glyceraldehyde. V. Synthesis of optically active glycerides from d(+) acetone glycerol. J. biol. Chem. **128**, 475 (1939).

BENSON, A. A., and B. MARUO: Plant phospholipids. I. Identification of the phosphatidyl glycerols. Biochem. biophys. Acta (Amst.) **27**, 189 (1958).

— and M.MIYANO: The phosphatidyl glycerol and sulfolipid of plants. Biochem. J.**81**,31 P(1961).

BERGSTRÖM, S., and J. SJÖVALL: The isolation of prostaglandin. Acta chem. scand. **11**, 1086 (1957).

— L. A. CARLSSON, and L. ORÖ: Effect of prostaglandins on catecholamine induced changes in the free fatty acids of plasma and in blood pressure in the dog. Acta physiol. scand. **60**, 170 (1964).

— H. DANIELSSON, and B. SAMUELSSON: The enzymatic formation of prostaglandin E_2 from arachidonic acid. Prostaglandins and related factors 32. Biochim. biophys. Acta (Amst.) **90**, 207 (1964).

— R. RYHAGE, B. SAMUELSSON, and J. SJÖVALL: The structure of prostaglandins E_1, $F_{1}\alpha$ and $F_1\beta$. J. biol. Chem. **238**, 3555 (1963).

— — — — The structure of prostaglandin E, F_1 and F_2. Acta chem. scand. **16**, 501 (1962).

BOGOCH, S.: Studies on the structure of brain ganglioside. Biochem. J. **68**, 319 (1958).

BORGSTRÖM, B.: Separation of mono-, di- and triglycerides. Acta physiol. scand. **30**, 231 (1954).

BROCKERHOFF, H., and C. E. BALLOU: The structure of the phosphoinositide complex of beef brain. J. biol. Chem. **236**, 1907 (1961).

BURDZY, K., P. G. MUNDER, H. FISCHER u. O. WESTPHAL: Steigerung der Phagocytose von Peritonealmacrophagen durch Lysolecithin. Z. Naturforsch. **19 b**, 1118 (1964).

Carroll, K. K.: Separation of lipid classes by chromatography on florisil. J. Lipid. Res. **2**, 135 (1961).

Carter, H. E., and F. L. Greenwood: Biochemistry of sphingolipides, VII. Structure of cerebrosides. J. biol. Chem. **199**, 283 (1952).

— F. J. Glick, W. P. Norris, and G. E. Phillips: Biochemistry of sphingolipides. III. Structure of sphingosine. J. biol. Chem. **170**, 285 (1947).

— and C. G. Humiston: Biochemistry of sphingolipides, V. The structure of sphingine. J. biol. Chem. **191**, 727 (1951).

— W. P. Norris, F. J. Glick, G. E. Phillips, and R. Harris: Biochemistry of sphingolipides, II. Isolation of dihydrosphingosine from the cerebroside fractions of beef brain and spinal cord. J. biol. Chem. **170**, 269 (1947).

Cheese, I. A. F. L., and W. T. J. Morgan: Two serologically active trisaccharides isolated from human blood group A substances. Nature (Lond.) **191**, 149 (1961).

Clayton, R. B., and K. Bloch: Biological synthesis of lanosterol and agnosterol. J. biol. Chem. **218**, 305 (1956).

Daun, H.: Zur Kenntnis des Folch'schen Strandins. Dissertation Köln, 1952.

Dawson, R. M. C.: The measurement of ^{32}P-labelling of individual cephalins and lecithins in a small sample of tissue. Biochim. biophysic. Acta (Amst.) **14**, 374 (1954).

— A hydrolytic procedure for the identification and estimation of individual phospholipids in biological samples. Biochem. J. **75**, 45 (1960).

— and J. C. Dittmer: Evidence for the structure of brain triphosphoinositide from hydrolytic degradation studies. Biochem. J. **81**, 540 (1961).

Debuch, H.: Beitrag zur chemischen Konstitution der Acetalphosphatide und zur Frage des Vorkommens des Colamin-Kephalins im Gehirn. Hoppe-Seylers Z. physiol. Chem. **304**, 109 (1956).

— Nature of the linkage of the aldehyde residue in natural plasmalogens. Biochem. J. **67**, 27 P (1957).

— Nature of the linkage of the aldehyde residue in natural plasmalogens. J. Neurochem. **2**, 243 (1958).

Dorp, D. A. v., R. K. Beerthuis, D. H. Nugteren, and H. Vonkeman: The biosynthesis of prostaglandins. Biochim. biophys. Acta (Amst.) **90**, 204 (1964).

Eneroth, P.: Thin-layer chromatography of bile acids. J. Lipid Res. **4**, 11 (1963).

Euler, U. S. v.: Zur Kenntnis der pharmakologischen Wirkungen von Nativsekreten und Extrakten männlicher accessorischer Geschlechtsdrüsen. Naunyn-Schmiedebergs Arch. exp. Path. Pharmak. **175**, 78 (1934).

— Über die spezifische blutdrucksenkende Substanz des menschlichen Prostata- und Samenblasensekrets. Klin. Wschr. **33**, 1182 (1935).

— On the specific vaso-dilating and plain muscle stimulating substances from accessory genital glands in man and certain animals (prostaglandin and vesiglandin). J. Physiol. (Lond.) **88**, 213 (1936).

Feulgen, R., K. Imhäuser u. M. Behrens: Zur Kenntnis des Plasmalogens. Hoppe-Seylers Z. physiol. Chem. **180**, 161 (1929).

Fieser, L., u. M. Fieser: Steroide, p. 1—96. Verlag Chemie: Weinheim, Bergstraße 1961.

Fischer, H., u. I. Haupt: Über das cytolysierende Prinzip von Serum-Komplement. Naturwissenschaften **47**, 137 (1960).

Folch, J.: Brain cephalin, a mixture of phosphatides. Separation from it of phosphatidyl serine, phosphatidyl ethanolamine, and a fraction containing an inositol phosphatide. J. biol. Chem. **146**, 35 (1942).

— The chemical structure of phosphatidyl serine. J. biol. Chem. **174**, 439 (1948).

— Complete fractionation of brain cephalin: Isolation from it of phosphatidyl serine, phosphatidyl ethanolamine, and diphosphoinositide. J. biol. Chem. **177**, 497 (1949).

— Brain diphosphoinositide, a new phosphatide having inositol metadiphosphate as a constituent. J. biol. Chem. **177**, 505 (1949).

— S. Arsove, and J. A. Meath: Isolation of brain strandin, a new type of large molecule tissue component. J. biol. Chem. **191**, 819 (1954).

— and D. W. Wooley: Inositol, a constituent of a brain phosphatide. J. biol. Chem. **142**, 963 (1942).

Forssman, J.: Die Herstellung hochwertiger spezifischer Schafhaemolysine ohne Verwendung von Schafblut. Biochem. Z. **37**, 78 (1911).

Getz, G. S., and W. Bartley: The intracellular distribution of fatty acids in rat liver. Biochem. J. **78**, 307 (1961).

Goldblatt, M. W.: Chem. and Industry **52**, 1056 (1933).

— Properties of human seminal plasma. J. Physiol. (Lond.) **84**, 208 (1935).

Grado, C., and C. E. Ballou: Myo-inositol phosphates obtained by alkaline hydrolysis of beef brain phosphoinositide. J. biol. Chem. **236**, 54 (1961).

GRAF, L., P. SKIPSKI, and N. F. ALONZO: Immunochemical studies of organ and tumor lipids. VI. Isolation and properties of cytolipin H. Cancer 12, 438 (1959).

GRAY, G. M., and M. G. MACFARLANE: Separation and composition of the phospholipids of ox heart. Biochem. J. 70, 409 (1958).

GROB, C. A., u. F. GADIENT: Die Synthese des Sphingosins und seiner Stereoisomeren. Helv. chim. Acta 40, 1145 (1957).

GRUNDY, S. M., E. H. AHRENS Jr., and T. A. MIETTINEN: Quantitative isolation and gas-liquid chromatographic analysis of total fecal bile acids. J. Lipid Res. 6, 397 (1965).

HANAHAN, D. J.: The Lecithinases. Prog. Chem. Fats Lipids 4, 141—176 (1957).
— Lipide Chemistry, p. 114. New York: Wiley and Sons 1960.
— H. BROCKERHOFF, and E. J. BARRON: The site of attack of phospholipase (lecithinase) A on lecithin: a reevaluation. J. biol. Chem. 235, 1917 (1960).
— J. C. DITTMER, and E. WARASHINA: A column chromatographic separation of classes of phospholipides. J. biol. Chem. 228, 685 (1957).
— and J. N. OLLEY: Chemical nature of monophosphoinositides. J. biol. Chem. 231, 813 (1958).
— M. B. TURNER, and M. E. YAYKO: The isolation of egg phosphatidylcholine by adsorption column technique. J. biol. Chem. 192, 623 (1951).
— and R. WATTS: The isolation of an α'-alkoxy-β-acyl-L-α-glycerophosphorylethanolamine from bovine erythrocytes. J. biol. Chem. 236, PC 59 (1961).

HARDEGGER, E., L. RUZICKA u. E. TAGMANN. 202. Untersuchungen über Organextrakte. Zur Kenntnis der unverseifbaren Lipoide aus arteriosklerotischen Aorten. Helv. chim. Acta 26, 2205 (1943).

HASLEWOOD, G. A. D.: Recent development in our knowledge of bile salts. Physiol. Rev. 35, 178 (1955).

HAVERKATE, F., and L. L. M. VAN DEENEN: The stereochemical configuration of phosphatidyl glycerol. Biochim. biophys. Acta (Amst.) 84, 106 (1964).

HAWTHORNE, J. N.: The ethanol-insoluble phosphatides of mammalian liver. Biochem. J. 59, II (1955).
— The inositol phospholipids. J. Lipid Res. 1, 255 (1960).

HELFERICH, B., H. APPEL u. R. GOOTZ: Über Emulsin. X. Z. physiol. Chem. 215, 277 (1933).

HIRSCH, J., and E. H. AHRENS jr.: The separation of complex lipid mixtures by the use of silicic acid chromatography. J. biol. Chem. 233, 311 (1958).

HÖRHAMMER, L., H. WAGNER u. J. HÖLZL: Über die Inositphosphatide des Rinderhirns. Biochem. Z. 332, 269 (1960).

HORNING, M. G., E. A. WILLIAMS, and E. C. HORNING: Separation of tissue cholesterol esters and triglycerides by silicic acid chromatography. J. Lipid. Res 1, 482 (1960).

HOUTSMULLER, U. M. T., and L. L. M. VAN DEENEN: Identification of a bacterial phospholipid as an O-ornithine ester of phosphatidyl glycerol. Biochim. biophys. Acta (Amst.) 70, 211 (1963).

JATZKEWITZ, H.: Zwei Typen von Cerebrosid-Schwefelsäureestern als sog. „Prä"-Lipoide und Speichersubstanzen bei der Leucodystrophie, Typ Scholz (Metachromatische Form der diffusen Sklerose). Hoppe-Seylers Z. physiol. Chem. 311, 279 (1958).
— Die Leucodystrophie, Typ Scholz (metachromatische Form der diffusen Sklerose) als Sphingolipoidose (Cerebrosid-Schwefelsäureester-Speicherkrankheit). Hoppe-Seylers Z. physiol. Chem. 318, 265 (1960).

KATES, M.: Hydrolysis of lecithin by plant plastid enzymes. Canad. J. Biochem. 33, 575 (1955).

KISHIMOTO, Y., and N. S. RADIN: Structures of the normal unsaturated fatty acids of brain sphingolipids. J. Lipid Res. 4, 437 (1963).

KISS, J., G. FODOR u. D. BANFI: Zurückführung der Konfiguration des (natürlichen) Sphingosins auf die der D-erythro-2-Amino-3, 4-dioxybuttersäure. Helv. chim. Acta 37, 1471 (1954).

KLENK, E.: Über die partiellen Spaltprodukte von Cerebron. Hoppe-Seylers Z. physiol. Chem. 153, 74 (1926).
— Über Sphingosin. Hoppe-Seylers Z. physiol. Chem. 185, 169 (1929).
— Beiträge zur Chemie der Lipoidosen. Hoppe-Seylers Z. physiol. Chem. 267, 128 (1948).
— Zur Biochemie der Haemagglutination. Angew. Chem. 72, 482 (1960).
— u. P. BÖHM: Zur Kenntnis der Kephalinfraktion des Gehirns. Hoppe-Seylers Z. physiol. Chem. 288, 98 (1951).
— u. H. DEBUCH: Zur Kenntnis der cholinhaltigen Plasmalogene (Acetalphosphatide des Rinderherzmuskels). Hoppe-Seylers Z. physiol. Chem. 299, 66 (1955).
— — The Lipides. Ann. Rev. Biochem. 28, 39 (1959).
— u. H. FAILLARD: Über Sphingosin. Hoppe-Seylers Z. physiol. Chem. 299, 48 (1955).
— u. W. GIELEN: Zur Kenntnis der Ganglioside des Gehirns. Hoppe-Seylers Z. physiol. Chem. 319, 283 (1960).
— — Untersuchungen über die Konstitution der Ganglioside aus Menschengehirn und die Trennung des Gemisches in die Komponenten. Hoppe-Seylers Z. physiol. Chem. 326, 144 (1961).

28 W. STOFFEL:

KLENK, E., u. W. GIELEN: Über ein zweites hexosaminhaltiges Gangliosid aus Menschengehirn Hoppe-Seylers Z. physiol. Chem. **330**, 218 (1963).
— — Über ein chromatographisch einheitliches, hexosaminfreies Gangliosid aus Menschengehirn. Hoppe Seylers Z. physiol. Chem. **333**, 162 (1963).
— — Gangliosid A_3. Hoppe-Seylers Z. physiol. Chem. (in Vorbereitung).
— — and G. PADBERG: The structure of gangliosides in cerebral Sphingolipoidoses. Symposium on Tay-Sachs Disease and allied Disorders. 1962, p. 301.
— u. U. W. HENDRICKS: An inositol phosphatide containing carbohydrate, isolated from human brain. Biochim. biophys. Acta (Amst.) **50**, 602 (1961).
— and L. HOF: Über die Struktur zweier hexosaminhaltiger Ganglioside des menschlichen Gehirns. Dissertation L. HOF, 1965, Cologne. Unpublished.
— u. G. KRICKAU: Über die Fettsäuren der cholinhaltigen Acetalphosphatide und des Lecithins vom Rinderherzmuskel. Hoppe-Seylers Z. physiol. Chem. **308**, 98 (1957).
— u. W. KUNAU: Beitrag zur Konstitution der Ganglioside. Hoppe-Seylers Z. physiol. Chem. **335**, 275 (1964a).
— u. K. LAUENSTEIN: Über die zuckerhaltigen Lipoide der Formbestandteile des menschlichen Blutes. Hoppe-Seylers Z. physiol. Chem. **288**, 220 (1951).
— — Über die zuckerhaltigen Lipoide des Erythrocytenstromas von Mensch und Rind. Hoppe-Seylers Z. physiol. Chem. **291**, 249 (1952).
— U. LIEDTKE u. W. GIELEN: Das Gangliosid bei der infantilen amaurotischen Idiotie vom Typ Tay-Sachs. Hoppe-Seylers Z. physiol. Chem. **334**, 186 (1963).
— u. G. PADBERG: Über die Ganglioside von Pferdeerythrocyten. Hoppe-Seylers Z. physiol. Chem. **327**, 249 (1962).
— u. F. RENNKAMP: Über die Reindarstellung von Sphingomyelin aus Gehirn. Hoppe-Seylers Z. physiol. Chem. **267**, 145 (1940).
— — Über die Ganglioside und Cerebroside der Rindermilz. Hoppe-Seylers Z. physiol. Chem. **273**, 253 (1942).
— u. R. SAKAI: Inositmonophosphorsäure, ein Spaltprodukt der Sojabohnenphosphatide. Hoppe-Seylers Z. physiol. Chem. **258**, 33 (1939).
— u. H. WOLTER: Über die zuckerhaltigen Lipoide des Erythrocytenstromas vom Pferde. Hoppe-Seylers Z. physiol. Chem. **291**, 259 (1952).
KORNBERG, A., and W. E. PRICER: Enzymatic esterification of α-glycerophosphate by long chain fatty acids. J. biol. Chem. **204**, 345 (1953).
KOSCIELAK, J.: Bloodgroup A specific glycolipids from human erythrocytes. Biochim. biophys. Acta (Amst.) **78**, 313 (1963).
KUHN, R., u. R. BROSSMER: Über das durch Viren der Influenza-Gruppe spaltbare Trisaccharid der Milch. Chem. Ber. **92**, 1667 (1959).
— u. H. EGGE: Über Ergebnisse der Permethylierung der Ganglioside G_I und G_{II}. Chem. Ber. **96**, 3338 (1963b).
— u. H. WIEGANDT: Die Konstitution der Ganglio-N-tetraose und des Gangliosids G_I. Chem. Ber. **96**, 866 (1963a).
— — Die Konstitution der Ganglioside G_{II}, G_{III} und G_{IV}. Z. Naturforsch.18b, 541 (1963c).
— — Weitere Ganglioside aus Menschenhirn. Z. Naturforsch. **19b**, 256 (1964a).
LEVENE, P. A.: Sphingomyelin. III. J. biol. Chem. **24**, 69 (1916).
— and W. A. JACOBS: On sphingosine. J. biol. Chem. **11**, 547 (1912).
— and C. J. WEST: On sphingosine. The oxidation of sphingosine and dihydrosphingosine. J. biol. Chem. **16**, 549 (1913/14).
— — On sphingosine. The oxidation of sphingosine and dihydrosphingosine. J. biol. Chem. **18**, 481 (1914).
— — Sphingosine. Some derivatives of sphingosine and dihydrosphingosine. J. biol. Chem. **24**, 63 (1916).
LE COQ, J., and C. E. BALLOU: On the structure of cardiolipin. Biochemistry **3**, 976 (1964).
LIPSKY, S. R., and R. A. LANDOWE: The identification of fatty acids by gas chromatography, in Methods in Enzymology, Vol. VI, p. 513. New York: Academic Press 1963.
LONG, C., and M. F. MAGUIRE: The structure of naturally occurring phosphoglycerides. Biochem. J. **57**, 223 (1954).
— and D. A. STAPLES: Chromatographic separation of brain lipids. Biochem. J. **80**, 557 (1961).
MACFARLANE, M. G.: The biochemistry of bacterial toxins. Biochem. J. **42**, 587 (1948).
— Characterisation of lipoamino-acids as O-amino-acid esters of phosphatidyl-glycerol. Nature (Lond.) **196**, 136 (1962).
— The structure of cardiolipin. Biochem. J. **92**, 12C (1964).
— and G. M. GRAY: Composition of cardiolipin. Biochem. J. **67**, 25P (1957).
— — and L. W. WHEELDON: Fatty acid composition of phospholipids from subcellular particles of rat liver. Biochem. J. **77**, 626 (1960).
— and L. W. WHEELDON: Position of fatty acids in Cardiolipin. Nature (Lond.) **183**, 1808 (1955).

MAKITA, A.: Biochemistry of organ glycolipids. II. Isolation of human kidney glycolipids. J. Biochem. (Tokyo) 55, 269 (1964).
— M. IWANAGA, and T. YAMAKAWA: The chemical structure of human kidney globosides. Biochem. J. (Tokyo) 55, 202 (1964).
— and T. YAMAKAWA: Biochemistry of organ glycolypids. Ceramide oligohexosides of human, equine and bovine spleen. J. Biochem. (Tokyo) 51, 124 (1962).
— — Biochemistry of organ glycolipids. III. The structures of human kidney cerebroside sulfuric ester, ceramide dihexoside and ceramide trihexoside. J. Biochem. (Tokyo) 55, 365 (1964).
MANGOLD, H. K., in E. STAHL: Dünnschichtchromatographie. Berlin-Göttingen-Heidelberg: Springer 1960.
MARINETTI, G. V., J. ERBLAND, and E. STOTZ: The hydrolysis of lecithins by snake venom phospholipase A. Biochim. biophys. Acta (Amst.) 33, 403 (1959).
— and E. STOTZ: Studies on the structure of sphingomyelin. IV. Configuration of the double bond in sphingomyelin and related lipids and a study of their infrared spectra. J. Amer. chem. Soc. 76, 1347 (1954).
MATTSON, F. H., and R. A. VOLPENHEIN: Synthesis and properties of glycerides. J. Lipid Res. 3, 281 (1962).
— — The use of pancreatic lipase for determining the distribution of fatty acids in partial and complete glycerides. J. Lipid Res. 2, 58 (1961).
MIETTINEN, T. A., E. H. AHRENS Jr., and S. M. GRUNDY: Quantitative isolation and gasliquid chromatographic analysis of total dietary and fecal neutral steroids. J. Lipid Res. 6, 411 (1965).
MISLOW, K.: The geometry of sphingosine. J. Amer. chem. Soc. 74, 5155 (1952).
NAKAYAMA, T.: Studies on the conjugated lipids. 1. On the configuration of cerebrosides. J. Biochem. (Tokyo) 37, 309 (1950).
O'BRIEN, J. S., and G. ROUSER: The fatty acid composition of brain sphingolipids: sphingomyelin, ceramide, cerebroside and cerebroside sulfate. J. Lipid Res. 5, 339 (1964).
PANGBORN, M. C.: A new serologically active phospholipid from beef heart. Proc. Soc. exp. Biol. (N. Y.) 48, 484 (1941).
— The composition of cardiolipin. J. biol. Chem. 168, 351 (1947).
PAPIRMEISTER, B., and M. F. MALLETTE: The isolation and some properties of the Forssman hapten from sheep erythrocytes. Arch. Biochem. 57, 94 (1955).
PIETRUSZKO, R., and G. M. GRAY: Formation of the cyclic acetal phospholipid during alkaline and enzym hydrolysis of choline plasmalogen. Biochem. biophys. Acta (Amst.) 44, 197 (1960).
PLACKETT, P.: A synthesis of 1,3-Di-O-(glycerol-3'-phosphoryl-) glycerol. Austr. J. Chem. 17, 101 (1964).
PIZER, F. L., and C. E. BALLOU: Studies on myo-inositol phosphates of natural origin. J. Amer. chem. Soc. 81, 915 (1959).
PRIVETT, O. S., and M. L. BLANK: A new method for the analysis of component mono-, di- and triglycerides. J. Lipid Res. 2, 37 (1961).
PROSTENIK, M., and B. MAJHOFER-ORESCANTIN: Occurrence of a new sphingolipid base C_{20}-sphingosine in horse and beef brain. Naturwissenschaften 47, 399 (1960).
— u. N. Z. STANACEV: Studien in der Reihe der Sphingolipoide über die Struktur der Cerebrin-Base aus Hefe. Chem. Ber. 91, 961 (1958).
RADIN, N. S., and J. R. BROWN: Cerebrosides. Biochem. Preparations 7, 31 (1959).
RAPPORT, M. M., L. GRAF, and N. F. ALONZO: Immunochemical structures of organ and tumor lipids. V. Lipid hapten of a human epidermoid carcinoma grown in rats. Cancer 11, 1136 (1958).
— B. LERNER, N. ALONZO, and R. E. FRANZL: The structure of plasmalogens. II. Crystalline lysophosphatidal ethanolamine (Acetalphospholipide). J. biol. Chem. 225, 859 (1957).
— H. SCHNEIDER, and L. GRAF: Immunochemical studies of organ and tumor lipids. J. biol. Chem. 237, 1056 (1962).
RENNKAMP, F.: Untersuchungen über das Sphingomyelin und die ätherunlöslichen Glycerinphosphatide des Gehirns. Hoppe-Seylers Z. physiol. Chem. 284, 215 (1949).
ROSENBERG, A., and E. CHARGAFF: Inhibition of influenza virus haemagglutination by a brain lipid fraction. Nature (Lond.) 177, 234 (1956).
— — Nitrogenous constituents of an ox brain mucolipid. Biochem. biophys. Acta (Amst.) 21, 588 (1956).
ROUSER, G., J. F. BERRY, G. MARINETTI, and E. STOTZ: Studies on the structure of sphingomyelin. I. Oxidation of products of partial hydrolysis. J. Amer. chem. Soc. 75, 310 (1953).
SAMBASIVARAO, K., and R. H. McCLUER: Lipid components of gangliosides. J. Lipid Res. 5, 103 (1964).
SAMUELSSON, B.: Die Prostaglandine. Angew. Chemie 77, 445 (1965).
SCHIFFMAN, G., E. A. KABAT, and W. THOMPSON: Immunochemical studies on blood groups XXXII. Immunochemical properties of and possible partial structure for the blood group A, B and H antigenic determinants. Biochemistry 3, 587 (1964).

SCHOLFIELD, C. R.: Counter current distribution. J. Amer. Oil Chem. Soc. 38, 562 (1961).
SHAPIRO, D., and H. M. FLOWERS: Synthetic studies on sphingolipids. VI. The total syntheses of cerasine and phrenosine. J. Amer. chem. Soc. 83, 3327 (1961).
— — Studies on sphingolipids. VII. Synthesis and configuration of natural sphingomyelins. J. Amer. chem. Soc. 84, 1047 (1961).
— — and S. SPECTOR-SHEFER: Synthetic studies on sphingolipids. III. The synthesis of dihydrosphingomyelin. J. Amer. chem. Soc. 81, 3743 (1959).
— — — Synthetic studies on sphingolipids. IV. The synthesis of sphingomyelin. J. Amer. chem. Soc. 81, 4360 (1959).
— — — The synthesis of dihydrosphingomyelin. J. Amer. chem. Soc. 80, 2339 (1964).
— E. S. RACHAMAN, and T. SHERADSKY: Synthetic studies on sphingolipids. X. Synthesis of psychosine. J. Amer. chem. Soc. 86, 4472 (1964).
SJÖVALL, J., C. R. MELONI, and D. A. TURNER: A study of the separation of substituted cholanic acids by gas-liquid chromatography. J. Lipid Res. 2, 317 (1961).
SPERRY, W. M.: Quantitative isolation of sterols. J. Lipid Res. 4, 221 (1963).
STEINBERG, D., M. VAUGHAN, P. J. NESTEL, and S. BERGSTRÖM: Effects of prostaglandin E opposing those of catecholamines on blood pressure and on triglyceride breakdown in adipose tissue. Biochem. Pharm. 12, 764 (1963).
SVENNERHOLM, E., and L. SVENNERHOLM: Isolation of blood serum glycolipids. Acta chem. scand. 16, 1282 (1962).
— — The separation of neutral blood-serum glycolipids by thin-layer chromatography. Biochim biophys. Acta 70, 432 (1963).
— — Neutral glycolipids of human blood serum, spleen and liver. Nature (Lond.) 198, 688 (1963).
SVENNERHOLM, L.: On sialic acid in brain tissue. Acta chem. scand. 10, 694 (1956).
— The gangliosides. J. Lipid Res. 5, 145 (1964).
— and H. THORIN: Quantitative isolation of brain sulfatides. J. Lipid Res. 3, 483 (1962).
SWEELEY, C. C.: Purification and partial characterization of sphingomyelin from human plasma. J. Lipid Res. 4, 402 (1963).
— and B. KLIONSKY: Fabry's disease: Classification as a sphingolipoidosis and partial characterization of a novel glycolipid. J. biol. Chem. 238, PC 3148 (1963).
TATTRIE, N. H.: Positional distribution of saturated and unsaturated fatty acids on egg lecithin. J. Lipid Res. 1, 60 (1959).
THANNHAUSER, S. J., N. F. BONCODDO, and G. SCHMIDT: Studies of acetal phospholipides of brain. J. biol. Chem. 188, 417, 423, 427 (1951).
THIERFELDER, H., u. E. KLENK: Die Chemie der Cerebroside und Phosphatide. S. 128. Berlin: Springer, 1930.
THUDICHUM, J. L. W.: The chemical constitution of the brain. p. 105. London 1884.
TOMLINSON, R. V., and C. E. BALLOU: Complete characterization of myo-inositol polyphosphates from beef brain phosphoinositide. J. biol. Chem. 236, 1902 (1961).
TRUCCO, R. E., and R. CAPUTTO: Neuramin-lactose, a new compound isolated from the mammary gland of rats. J. biol. Chem. 206, 901 (1954).
VANDENHEUVEL, W. J. A., C. C. SWEELEY, and E. C. HORNING: Microanalytical separations by gas chromatography in the sex hormone and bile acid series. Biochem. biophys. Res. Commun. 3, 33 (1960).
WAGNER, H., L. HÖRHAMMER u. P. WOLFF: Dünnschichtchromatographie von Phosphatiden und Glycolipiden. Biochem. Z. 334, 175 (1961).
WARNER, H. R., and W. E. M. LANDS: The configuration of the double bond in naturally occurring alkenyl-ethers. J. Amer. chem. Soc. 85, 60 (1963).
WEBSTER, G. R.: Studies on the plasmalogens of nervous tissue. Biochim. biophys. Acta (Amst.) 44, 109 (1960).
WINDAUS, A.: Über die Entgiftung der Saponine durch Cholesterin. Chem. Ber. 42, 238 (1909).
WOODFORD, F. P., and C. M. VAN GENT: Gas-liquid chromatography of fatty acid methyl esters: The "carbon-number" as a parameter for comparison of columns. J. Lipid Res. 1, 188 (1960).
YAMAKAWA, T., and S. SUZUKI: The chemistry of the lipids of posthemolytic residue or stroma of erythrocytes. I. Concerning the ether-insoluble lipids of lyophilized horse blood stroma. J. Biochem. (Tokyo) 38, 199 (1951).
— — The chemistry of the lipids of posthemolytic residue or stroma of erythrocytes. II. On the structure of haemataminic acid. J. Biochem. (Tokyo) 39, 175 (1952).
— — The chemistry of the lipids of posthemolytic residue or stroma of erythrocytes. III. Globoside, the sugar containing lipid of human blood stroma. J. Biochem. (Tokyo) 39, 393 (1952).
— S. YOKOYAMA, and N. HANDA: Chemistry of lipids of posthemolytic residue or stroma of erythrocytes. XI. Structure of globoside, the main mucolipid of human erythrocytes. Biochem. J. (Tokyo) 53, 28 (1963).

C. Fatty Acid Oxidation

The complete combustion of fatty acids to CO_2 and H_2O releases high energies. In general, such oxidative reactions proceed in the mitochondrion of the cell and the high energy which is produced will be stored as high energy compounds such as adenosinetriphosphate. The basic underlying enzymatic reactions of fatty acid oxidation are universal in nature. The reaction sequence by which fatty acids are oxidized in a way such that acetate units are split off successively, is known as the β-oxidation cycle (KNOOP 1904).

I. β-Oxidation of Saturated Fatty Acids

The oxidation of saturated fatty acids which are chemically relatively inert, is initiated by

a) *the formation of the coenzyme A thioester*. These thioesters possess a high group transfer potential because of the high energy ester bond. This activation reaction is catalyzed in the following way by the enzyme thiokinase:

$$\text{fatty acid} + \text{CoASH} + \text{ATP} \xrightarrow[\text{Mg}^{++}]{\text{thiokinase}} \text{fatty acyl-CoA} + \text{AMP} + \text{PP}$$

Three thiokinases occur in the cell according to the chain length of fatty acids: one for acetic acid (acetokinase) (LIPMANN 1952), one for fatty acids from C_4-C_{12} (MAHLER et al. 1952) and one for long chain fatty acids C_8-C_{18} (KORNBERG et al. 1953). The former two have been isolated from mitochondria and the latter from microsomal particles.

b) The second step of β-oxidation is an α-β-*dehydrogenation of the acyl-CoA* which is catalyzed by acyldehydrogenases. Three different enzymes specific for certain chain lengths, C_4-C_8, C_8-C_{12} and C_8-C_{16}, have been isolated from mitochondria. These enzymes contain a flavoadenine dinucleotide (FAD) as the prosthetic group. The electrons are transferred to another flavoprotein, the electron transferring flavoprotein (CRANE et al. 1956), which is directly linked to the respiratory chain of the mitochondria. The reaction product of this dehydrogenation reaction is the a, β-trans-unsaturated acyl-CoA thioester (WAKIL 1956).

$$\text{RCH}_2\text{CH}_2\text{CO} \sim \text{SCoA} \xrightarrow{-2\text{H}} \overset{\displaystyle \text{H}}{\underset{\displaystyle \text{H}}{\text{R}\overset{|}{\text{C}}} = \text{C}\overset{|}{\text{CO}} \sim \text{SCoAH}}$$

c) The trans-a, β-unsaturated acyl-CoA esters from C_4 to C_{18} are subsequently *hydrated by one enzyme, the enoyl-CoA-hydrase* (crotonase) to the $L(+)$ hydroxyacyl-CoA derivative (WAKIL et al. 1954, STERN et al. 1956). This enzyme has been crystallized (STERN 1956).

d) The β-hydroxyacyl-CoA compound is then *oxidized by a β-hydroxyacyl-CoA dehydrogenase* to β-ketoacyl-CoA. The electrons are transferred to NAD^+:

$$\text{L}(+)\,\text{RCHOHCH}_2\text{COSCoA} + \text{NAD}^+ \rightleftharpoons \underset{\displaystyle \text{O}}{\text{RC}\overset{\|}{}\text{—CH}_2\text{COSCoA}} + \text{NADH} + \text{H}^+$$

This enzyme, which also has been crystallized, is specific for the $L(+)$ form of the β-hydroxyacyl-CoA ester (LYNEN et al. 1953).

e) In the last step, the β-keto-CoA ester is *cleaved thiolytically* (LYNEN 1952) according to the following reaction:

$$\underset{\displaystyle \text{O}}{\text{RCCH}_2\text{CO}\overset{\|}{}\sim\text{SCoA}} + \text{CoASH} \rightleftharpoons \underset{\displaystyle \text{O}}{\text{RC}\overset{\|}{}\sim\text{SCoA}} + \text{CH}_3\text{CO}\sim\text{SCoA}$$

As an example of the foregoing oxidation cycle the complete oxidation of palmitic acid would require seven passages through the β-oxidation cycle and release ultimately 2500 kcal (KREBS et al. 1960).

$$\text{palmitic acid} + 23\,O_2 \rightarrow 16\,CO_2 + 16\,H_2O + 2500\,\text{kcal}$$

II. β-Oxidation of Unsaturated Fatty Acids

Two chemical features are characteristic for the naturally occurring mono- and polyunsaturated fatty acids: a) the double bonds possess *all-cis* configuration, b) the double bonds are isolated by one CH_2-group. It is a reasonable assumption that the saturated carboxylic and terminal methyl end of unsaturated acids are degraded by the reaction sequence described in the preceeding chapter. However, oxidation of the cis-β, γ- and cis-α, β-unsaturated acyl-CoA intermediates requires two additional enzymes: a) cis-β, γ-trans-α, β-enoyl-CoA-isomerase and b) $D(-)$ hydroxyacyl-CoA epimerase. The isomerase catalyzes the following reaction:

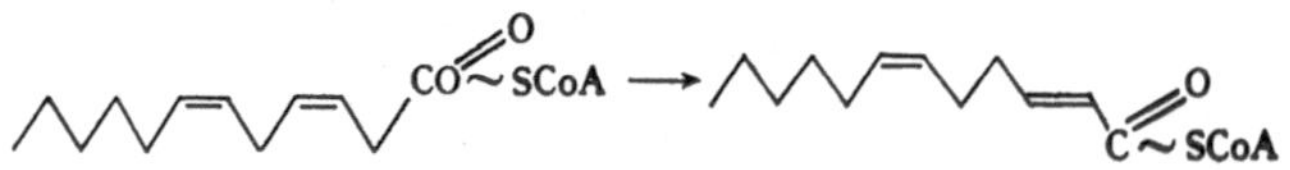

The reaction product can then be hydrated by enoyl-CoA hydrase to $L(+)$ β-hydroxyacyl CoA and enters the β-oxidation spiral. α,β-cis unsaturated acyl-CoA esters are hydrated by enoyl-CoA hydrase to the $D(-)$ enantiomeric form similar to isocrotonyl-CoA which is hydrated to $D(-)$ β-hydroxybutyryl-CoA (WAKIL 1957). This $D(-)$ form is epimerized by the $D(-)$ β-hydroxyacyl-CoA epimerase to the $L(+)$ antipode which is the specific substrate for β-hydroxyacyl-CoA dehydrogenase. Both enzymes have been isolated from mitochondria of rat liver and shown to be present in all organs, the concentration in brain however being very low. The two enzymes exhibit no specificity for different chain lengths. As an example the reaction sequence in the β-oxidation of linolyl-CoA is summarized in the next figure (STOFFEL et al. 1965 a, b):

1-[14] C-labeled di-, tri- and tetraenoic fatty acids are oxidized by isolated mitochondria at nearly the same rate as palmitic acid (STOFFEL et al. 1965).

Recently the stimulating effect of carnitine (β-hydroxy-γ-trimethylammonium-butyrate)

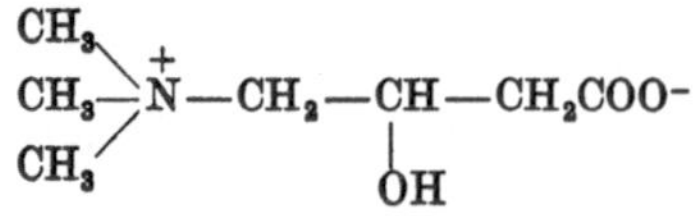

on fatty acid oxidation has been reported. It has been suggested that the transport of long chain fatty acid groups from the extra- into the intramitochondrial compartment is facilitated by a transacylation from coenzyme A to carnitine (FRITZ et al. 1963 a, 1963 b; BREMER 1962 a, b and 1963).

This stimulation has also been observed for the oxidation of unsaturated fatty acids (STOFFEL et al. 1965).

III. α-Oxidation

A large group of even- and odd-numbered α-hydroxy fatty acids with 20 to 26 C-atoms occurs in brain cerebrosides (see chapter BII, 2a). These acids are formed by a direct α-hydroxylation in the cytoplasmic reticulum. The loss of one C-atom of the α-hydroxy acids leads to the odd-numbered fatty acids (FULCO et al. 1961).

β-oxidation gives rise to an elevated concentration of acetoacetate. It has been assumed that hydrolytic cleavage of the acetoacetyl-CoA ester by a deacylase produces this ketone body. Experiments with liver mitochondria have recently shown that acetoacetate is formed exclusively in the liver by a deacylation of acetoacetyl-CoA (SEGAL 1960). These results are at variance with a mechanism by which acetoacetyl-CoA is not hydrolyzed but condensed with acetyl-CoA forming β-hydroxy-β-methylglutaryl-CoA (LYNEN 1959):

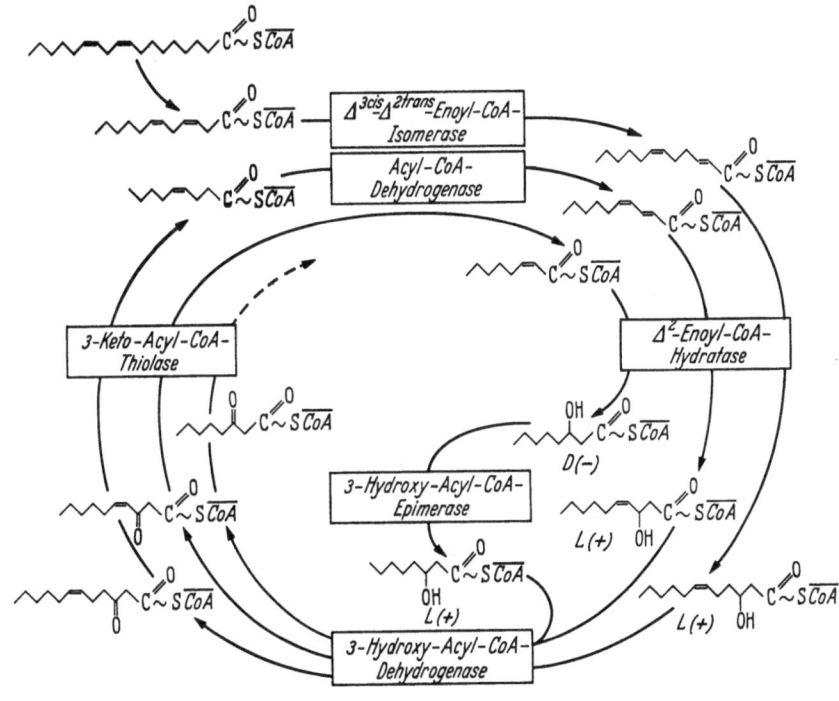

The condensing enzyme for this reaction has been isolated (RUDNEY 1957). β-hydroxy-β-methylglutaryl-CoA can then either be used for the terpene and cholesterol synthesis or cleaved to yield acetoacetate and acetyl-CoA. The cleaving enzyme has also been purified (BACHAWAT et al. 1955, 1956).

D. Biosynthesis of Fatty Acids

I. Biosynthesis of Saturated Fatty Acids

It has been known for more than 100 years that carbohydrates can be transformed into fatty acids. These and other food stuffs form metabolites which ultimately yield acetate. Isotope experiments (RITTENBERG et al. 1936) indicated that the total carbon chain of saturated long chain fatty acids is built up from acetate units in a head-to-tail connection. Liver is the main organ of fatty acid synthesis.

After the enzymatic mechanism of β-oxidation was elucidated, it has been assumed, that the biosynthesis of saturated fatty acids may proceed by a reversal of the β-oxidation starting from acetate.

It was possible to synthesize medium chain length fatty acids through a proper combination of β-oxidation enzymes (Seubert et al. 1957). However, alloxan diabetic rats with an intact β-oxidation in liver have an extremely depressed fatty acid synthesis (Brady et al. 1956). Also the unfavorable equilibrium of the β-ketothiolase reaction, which is far on the side of cleavage, made the synthesis by reversal of the β-oxidation steps appear very unlikely (Lynen et al. 1957).

Evidence was obtained that fatty acid synthesis proceeds in the cytoplasmic fraction rather than in the mitochondria. A supernatant enzyme system was able to synthesize palmitic acid starting from acetyl-CoA in the presence of NADPH, Mn^{++}, HCO_3^- and ATP. The purified enzyme system was free of oxidation enzymes. HCO_3^- was not incorporated into the fatty acid but had a cofactor role. Subsequent experiments showed that acetyl-CoA is carboxylated to malonyl-CoA by acetyl-CoA-carboxylase, which contains d-biotin as coenzyme. Early investigations gave strong evidence for the participation of biotin in a number of carboxylation (CO_2-fixation) reactions (Lardy et al. 1956). The enzyme acetyl-CoA-carboxylase has been isolated (Brady et al. 1958, Lynen et al. 1959, Wakil et al. 1958). CO_2 forms the free carboxy-group of malonyl-CoA. The equation of the malonyl-CoA synthesis is:

$$CH_3CO \sim SCoA + ATP + HCO_3^- \rightleftharpoons HOOCCH_2CO \sim SCoA + ADP + P_i$$

The general basic mechanism of the carboxylation reactions (acetyl-, propionyl-, butyryl-CoA and pyruvate) is the fixation of HCO_3^- in an ATP dependent reaction to the 1'-N of the biotin molecule:

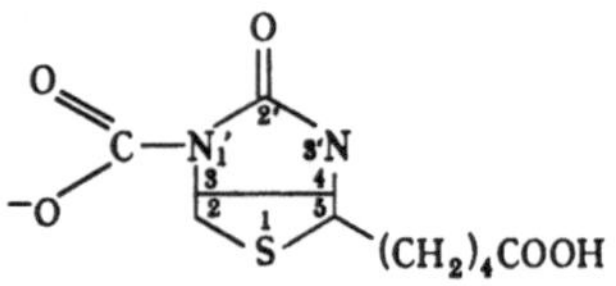

1'-N-carboxy-d-biotin

Saturated fatty acid biosynthesis includes the following reaction sequence: The first step is the condensation of acetyl-CoA and malonyl-CoA with simultaneous decarboxylation. The two thioesters first are transacylated from CoA to SH-groups of the fatty acid synthetase. The condensation reaction proceeds between the enzyme-bound substrates forming acetoacetyl-S-enzyme. The intermediates remain covalently bound to the protein by thioester linkages. Acetoacetyl-S-enzyme is then reduced by NADPH to D(—) β-hydroxybutyryl-S-enzyme, dehydrated to trans-2-butenoyl-S-enzyme. The resulting α, β-unsaturated fatty acyl-S-enzyme is reduced by a second NADPH. $FMNH_2$ mediates the electron transfer from NADPH. Palmitic acid is synthesized by seven passages of this reaction sequence according to the following equation:

$$CH_3CO \sim SCoA + 7\,HOOCCH_2CO \sim SCoA + 14\,NADPH + H^+ \longrightarrow CH_3(CH_2)_{14}COOH$$
$$+ 7\,CO_2 + 8\,CoASH + 14\,NAD^+ + 6\,H_2O$$

The sequence of reactions leading to the de novo synthesis of saturated fatty acids in E. coli occurs with the substrates bound to an acyl carrier protein (ACP) as thioesters (Goldman et al. 1963, 1964; Majerus et al. 1964, 1965, Wakil et al. 1964). This substrate binding site of ACP has been shown to be the SH-group of a prosthetic group, 4'-phosphopantetheine, which again is linked to the hydroxyl group of serine through a phosphodiester linkage (MAJERUS et al. 1965). Mammalian fatty acid synthetase also contains protein-bound 4'-phosphopantetheine, which strongly suggests that a protein similar to ACP is present in the mammalian multi-enzyme complex (LARRABEE et al. 1965).

Both acetyl-CoA-carboxylase and fatty acid synthetase have been isolated from the cytoplasma of mammalian liver cells (WAKIL et al. 1959) and brain tissue (BRADY 1960).

II. Biosynthesis of Mono- and Polyunsaturated Fatty Acids

a) Monoenoic Acids: Strong indications were obtained by experiments with deuterated saturated fatty acids that dehydrogenation of these fatty acids, mainly stearic and palmitic acid, could lead to monoenoic acids. If animals were raised to maximal body D_2O levels, saturated fatty acids with a deuterium content higher than that of the monoenoic acids were isolated, which must originate from de-hydrogenated saturated fatty acids (SCHOENHEIMER et al. 1936a, b). Experiments with 1-^{14}C-myristic acid (ANKER 1952), palmitic and stearic acid (DAUBEN et al. 1953) supported this concept.

Early *in vitro* studies using the discoloration of methyleneblue for a quanti-fication of the dehydrogenation reaction of long chain saturated fatty acids were inconclusive because of insufficient analytical proof for a monounsaturated reaction product with a central olefinic bond (LANG 1939a; LANG et al. 1939b; ANNAU et al. 1942, LE BRETON et al. 1948, JACOB et al. 1953a, b, 1956). Conclusive evidence for the direct transformation of 1-^{14}C-stearic acid to oleic acid in the presence of ATP has been shown with the 10,000 × g supernatant of rat liver. Oleic acid has been characterized by degradation (BERNHARD et al. 1958).

Recent studies have revealed insight into the dehydrogenation reaction of palmitoyl-CoA (BLOOMFIELD et al. 1958). The reaction appears to be a mixed function oxidase reaction. The only cofactors required are molecular oxygen and reduced NADP+. This enzyme introduces the isolated double bond with high stereo-, geometrical and positional specificity as shown with 9-D and 9-L-^{3}H-stearic acid. Only the 9-D hydrogen is lost (SCHROEPFER et al. 1964).

In conclusion it may be stated that long chain monounsaturated fatty acids are formed in mammalian organisms by direct dehydrogenation of the fully saturated precursor:

$$\text{stearoyl-CoA} \xrightarrow{\text{O}_2, \text{NADPH}} \text{oleyl-CoA}$$

b) Polyunsaturated Fatty Acids: In view of our present knowledge, the bio-synthesis of polyunsaturated fatty acids in mammals must clearly be distinguished from that of monounsaturated fatty acids. Polyunsaturated fatty acids belonging to the linoleic and linolenic acid families are derived by chain elongation and de-saturation from the parent dienoic and trienoic acid, respectively. These two acids cannot be synthesized by the animal cell; they are essential dietary components (BURR 1929). Experiments with D_2O (BERNHARD et al. 1940, 1942) showed that linoleic acid and linolenic acid were not labeled. The administration of 1-^{14}C-acetate to rats yielded eicosatetraenoic acid (arachidonic acid) (MEAD 1953) and docosa-polyunsaturated fatty acids (KLENK 1954, 1955) carrying the label in the carboxylic end. This indicated that only chain elongation and introduction of additional double bonds have occurred. The following sequence of arachidonic acid synthesis has been concluded from the precursor relationship of linoleic (STEINBERG 1956) and γ-linolenic acid (MEAD et al. 1957): linoleic acid $\xrightarrow{-2\,H}$ γ-linolenic acid $\xrightarrow{+C_2}$ eicosatrienoic acid $\xrightarrow{-2\,H}$ arachidonic acid. Subsequent dehydrogenation and chain elongation transforms α-linolenic into eicosa-5,8,11,14,17-pentaenoic and docosa-4,7,10,13,16,19-hexaenoic acid (MEAD 1957). On the basis of these experiments *in vivo* the interconversion of linoleic and linolenic acid into 20C and 22C-poly-unsaturated fatty acids appeared to consist of two reactions: a) chain elongation and b) desaturation.

Studies in vitro showed that the chain elongation mechanism of polyunsaturated fatty acids proceeds in an analogous manner to saturated fatty acid synthesis: malonyl-CoA is the activated C_2-unit and NADPH provides the reduction equivalents. Instead of acetyl-CoA the polyunsaturated fatty acyl-CoA is the primer. Also the cell compartment of the synthesis is different: saturated fatty acid synthesis proceeds in the cytoplasm, whereas the chain elongation enzyme system is bound to the cytoplasmic reticulum. It has been partially purified and appears to be a lipoprotein. The enzyme exhibits no specificity for the methyl end of the substrates. However the length of the carboxy-end determines the affinity for the enzyme. Rapid chain elongation occurs with acids having a carboxy-end with less than 7C atoms, those with more than 8 C atoms are first desaturated and then elongated. The enzyme responsible for the introduction of these *all cis* double bonds in a polyallyl-rhythm is also bound to the cytoplasmic reticulum. The mechanism by which the CoA-esters are desaturated in the presence of molecular oxygen and NADPH is still unknown (STOFFEL 1961). The experiments *in vitro* confirm the pathway for arachidonic acid biosynthesis suggested before from feeding experiments (MEAD et al. 1957) and support the following additional sequence:

$$\text{linoleic} \longrightarrow \text{eicosa-11,14-dienoic} \longrightarrow \text{arachidonic acid}$$

In mammals the introduction of new double bonds into mono- and poly-unsaturated fatty acids exclusively occurs in the carboxyl end and is never directed toward the terminal methyl-group. Therefore no transition of fatty acids belonging to the linoleic acid family into those of the linolenic acid type has been observed. This has been shown by means of terminally labeled synthetic polyunsaturated fatty acids (STOFFEL 1961, KLENK 1964). The complete enzyme system for poly-unsaturated fatty acid synthesis is arranged on the cytoplasmic membranes. In view of the importance of polyunsaturated fatty acids for the structure of glycero-phospholipids, it is interesting to mention the acyl-transferases catalyzing the acylation of the β-position of lysolecithin, lysophosphatidic acid and L-α-glycero-phosphate. These and other enzymes of phospholipid biosynthesis are located in the cytoplasmic reticulum, which therefore appears to be the main site of lipid synthesis of the cell.

Experiments with specifically labeled synthetic fatty acids have given conclusive evidence that no biohydrogenation of mono- and polyunsaturated fatty acids occurs in the mammalian liver (STOFFEL et al. 1964). Feeding experiments with doubly-labeled linoleic, arachidonic and stearic acid disprove the often suggested hypothesis of a partial degradation and elongation of the carboxyl end of fatty acids. From these experiments, the conclusion has been drawn that a fatty acid molecule is completely degraded on contact with the β-oxidation multi-enzyme of the mitochondrion.

c) **Control mechanisms of fatty acid synthesis:** Fatty acid synthesis is severely impaired in diabetic liver and on starvation (DRURY et al. 1940, STETTEN et al. 1944). NADPH has been suggested to be the limiting factor (LANGDON 1957,

SIPERSTEIN 1959) and the stimulation by acids of the tricarboxylic acid cycle has been interpreted in this sense (ABRAHAM et al. 1960). On the other hand, the activation by tricarboxylic acids, particularly citric acid, of acetyl-CoA carboxylase has been explained by a favorable change of the protein conformation (VAGELOS et al. 1963). Also it has been shown that the stimulation of fatty acid synthesis is caused by an incorporation of acetyl-CoA after fission of citrate according to the following equation (SPENCER et al. 1962):

$$\text{Citrate} + \text{CoASH} + \text{ATP} \longrightarrow \text{Acetyl-CoA} + \text{oxaloacetate} + \text{ADP} + \text{Pi}$$

Long chain acyl-CoA esters cause a competitive inhibition of acetyl-CoA-carboxylase. The elevated levels of long chain fatty acid Co-A esters in diabetes and on starvation may be the basis of the keto-acidosis (BORTZ et al. 1963). Citrate synthase (condensing enzyme) is also inhibited by long chain acyl-CoA esters (WIELAND et al. 1963a, b). It appears therefore that the product of fatty acid synthesis is able to regulate the synthesis by means of a feed back mechanism.

References

ABRAHAM, S., E. LORCH, and I. L. CHAIKOFF: Localization of the stimulating effect of isocitrate on fatty acid synthesis by rat liver. Biochem. biophys. Res. Commun. 7, 190 (1960).
— K. J. MATTHES, and I. L. CHAIKOFF: Fatty acid synthesis from acetate by normal and diabetic rat liver homogenate fractions. J. biol. Chem. 235, 2551 (1960).
ALBERTS, A. W., P. W. MAJERUS, B. TALAMO, and P. R. VAGELOS: Acyl-Carrier Protein II. Intermediary Reactions of fatty acid synthesis. Biochemistry 3, 1563 (1964).
ANKER, H. S.: On the mechanism of fatty acid synthesis in vivo. J. biol. Chem. 194, 177 (1952).
ANNAU, E., A. EPERJESSY u. O. FELSZEGLY: Biologische Dehydrierung der Lecithine und der Fettsäuren. Hoppe Seylers Z. physiol. Chem. 277, 58 (1942).
BACHHAWAT, B. K., W. G. ROBINSON, and M. J. COON: The enzymatic cleavage of β-hydroxy-β-methylglutaryl coenzyme A to acetoacetate and acetyl-CoA. J. biol. Chem. 216, 727 (1955).
— — — Enzymatic carboxylation of β-hydroxyisovaleryl-coenzyme A. J. biol. Chem. 219, 539 (1956).
BERNHARD, K., J. v. BÜLOW-KÖSTER u. H. WAGNER: Die enzymatische Dehydrierung der Stearinsäure zu Ölsäure. Helv. chim. Acta 42, 152 (1959).
— M. ROTHLIN u. H. WAGNER: Zur Frage der Hydrierung ungesättigter Fettsäuren im Tierkörper. Helv. chim. Acta 41, 1155 (1958).
— and R. SCHOENHEIMER: The inertia of highly unsaturated fatty acids in the animal, investigated with deuterium. J. biol. Chem. 133, 707 (1940).
— H. STEINHAUSER u. F. BULLET: Fettstoffwechsel-Untersuchungen mit Hilfe von Deuterium als Indikator. I. Zur Frage der lebensnotwendigen Fettsäuren. Helv. chim. Acta 25, 1313 (1942).
BLOOMFIELD, D. K., and K. BLOCH: The role of oxygen in the biosynthesis of unsaturated fatty acids. Biochim. biophys. Acta (Amst.) 30, 220 (1958).
— — The formation of △⁹-unsaturated fatty acids. J. biol. Chem. 235, 337 (1960).
BORTZ, W. M., and F. LYNEN: The inhibition of acetyl CoA carboxylase by long chain acyl CoA derivatives. Biochem. Z. 337, 505 (1963a).
— — Elevation of long chain acyl CoA derivatives in livers of fasted rats. Biochem. Z. 339, 77 (1963b).
BRADY, R. O.: The enzymatic synthesis of fatty acids by aldol condensation. Proc. nat. Acad. Sci. (Wash.) 44, 993 (1958).
— Biosynthesis of fatty acids. J. biol. Chem. 235, 3099 (1960).
— A. M. MAMOON, and E. R. STADTMAN: The effect of citrate and coenzyme A on fatty acid metabolism. J. biol. Chem. 222, 795 (1956).
BREMER, J.: Carnitine in intermediary metabolism. The metabolism of fatty acid esters of carnitine by mitochondria. J. biol. Chem. 237, 3628 (1962).
— Carnitine in intermediary metabolism. The biosynthesis of palmityl-carnitine by cell subfractions. J. biol. Chem. 238, 2774 (1963).
BURR, G. O., and M. M. BURR: A new deficiency disease produced by the rigid exclusion of fat from the diet. J. biol. Chem. 82, 345 (1929).
CRANE, F. L., and H. BEINERT: On the mechanism of dehydrogenation of fatty acyl derivatives of coenzyme A. II. The electron-transferring flavoprotein. J. biol. Chem. 218, 717 (1956).

Dauben, W. G., E. Hoerger, and J. W. Petersen: Distribution of acetic acid carbon in high fatty acids synthesized from acetic acid by the intact mouse. J. Amer. chem. Soc. **75**, 2347 (1953).

Drury, D. R.: The role of insulin in carbohydrate metabolism. Amer. J. Physiol. **131**, 536 (1940).

Fritz, I. B., S. K. Schultz, and P. A. Srere: Properties of partially purified carnitine acetyl-transferase. J. biol. Chem. **238**, 2509 (1963).

— and K. T. N. Yue: Long-chain carnitine acyltransferase and the role of acylcarnitine derivatives in the catalytic increase of fatty acid oxidation induced by carnitine. J. Lipid Res. **4**, 279 (1963).

Fulco, A. J., and J. F. Mead: The biosynthesis of lignoceric, cerebronic and nervonic acids. J. biol. Chem. **236**, 2416 (1961).

Goldman, P.: Acyl-bound intermediates in fatty acid synthesis. J. biol. Chem. **239**, 3663 (1964).

— A. W. Alberts, and P. R. Vagelos: The condensation reaction of fatty acid synthesis. J. biol. Chem. **238**, 3579 (1963).

Jacob, A.: Décomposition en ses divers constituants du système enzymatique de désaturation des acides gras supérieurs. C. R. Soc. Biol. (Paris) **147**, 1044 (1953).

— Rôle de l'hypoxanthine dans la désaturation des acides gras supérieurs. C. R. Acad. Sci. (Paris) **242**, 2180 (1956).

Kallen, R. G., and J. M. Lowenstein: The stimulation of fatty acid synthesis by isocitrate and malonate. Arch. Biochem. **96**, 188 (1962).

Klenk, E.: Über die Bildung der C_{20}- und C_{22}-Polyenfettsäuren im Tierkörper. Naturwissenschaften **41**, 68 (1954).

— Über die Biogenese der C_{20}- und C_{22}-Polyenfettsäuren in der Säugertierleber. Hoppe-Seylers Z. physiol. Chem. **302**, 268 (1955).

— Metabolism of polyunsaturated fatty acids. VI. International Congress of Biochemistry, New York 1964.

Kornberg, A., and W. E. Pricer: Enzymatic synthesis of the coenzyme A derivatives of long chain fatty acids. J. biol. Chem. **204**, 329 (1953).

Krebs, H. A., and J. M. Lowenstein: in Metabolic Pathways I, p. 129, edit. by D. M. Greenberg. New York: Academic Press 1960.

Lang, K.: Über die tierische Fettsäuredehydrase und ihre Codehydrase. Hoppe-Seylers Z. physiol. Chem. **261**, 240 (1939a).

— u. F. Adickes: Über die tierische Fettsäuredehydrase. Hoppe-Seylers Z. physiol. Chem. **262**, 123 (1939).

— u. H. Mayer: Über die tierische Fettsäuredehydrase und ihre Codehydrase. Hoppe-Seylers Z. physiol. Chem. **261**, 249 (1939b).

Langdon, R. G.: The biosynthesis of fatty acids in rat liver. J. biol. Chem. **226**, 615 (1959).

Lardy, H. A., and J. Adler: Synthesis of succinate from propionate and ticcubonate by soluble enzymes from liver mitochondria. J. biol. Chem. **219**, 933 (1956).

Larrabee, A. L., E. G. Mc Daniel, H. A. Bakerman, P. R. Vagelos: Acylcarrier protein, V. Identification of 4'-phosphopantetheine bound to a mammalian fatty acid synthetase preparation. Proc. Nat. Acad. Sci. (Wash.) **54**, 267 (1965).

Le Breton, E., and J. Champougny-Clement: La désaturase des acides gras supérieurs. Arch. sci. physiol. **2**, 243 (1948).

Lipmann, F., M. E. Jones, S. Black, and R. M. Flynn: Enzymatic pyrophosphorylation of coenzyme A by adenosine triphosphat. J. Amer. chem. Soc. **74**, 2384 (1952).

Lynen, F.: Proc. Intern. Symposium on Enzyme Chemistry (Tokyo and Kyoto) **2**, 57 (1957).

— Participation of acyl-CoA in carbon chain biosynthesis. J. cell comp. Physiol. **54**, 33 (1959).

— U. Henning, C. Bublitz, B. Sörbo u. L. Kröplin-Rueff: Der chemische Mechanismus der Acetessigsäurebildung in der Leber. Biochem. Z. **330**, 269 (1958).

— J. Knappe, E. Lorch, G. Jütting u. E. Ringelmann: Die biochemische Funktion des Biotins. Angew. Chem. **71**, 481 (1959).

— and S. Ochoa: Enzymes of fatty acid metabolism. Biochim. biophys. Acta (Amst.) **12**, 299 (1953).

— L. Wessely, O. Wieland u. L. Rueff: Zur β-Oxydation der Fettsäuren. Angew. Chem. **64**, 687 (1952).

Mahler, H. R., S. Wakil, and R. M. Bock: Studies on fatty acid oxidation. I. Enzymatic activation of fatty acids. J. biol. Chem. **204**, 453 (1953).

Majerus, P. W., A. W. Alberts, and P. R. Vagelos: Acyl-carrier-protein, III. An enoyl-hydrase specific for acyl-carrier protein thioesters. J. biol. Chem. **240**, 618 (1965).

— — — The acyl-carrier protein of the fatty acid synthesis. Purification, physical properties, and substrate binding site. Proc. Nat. Acad. Sci. (Wash.) **51**, 1231 (1964).

— — — Acyl-carrier-protein, IV., The identification of 4'-phosphopantetheine as the prosthetic group of the acyl carrier protein. Proc. Nat. Acad. Sci. (Wash.) **53**, 410 (1965).

MEAD, J. F.: The metabolism of the essential fatty acids. Distribution of unsaturated fatty acids in rats on fat-free and supplemented diets. J. biol. Chem. 227, 1025 (1957).
— and D. R. HOWTON: Metabolism of essential fatty acids. VII. Conversion of γ-linolenic acid to arachidonic acid. J. biol. Chem. 229, 575 (1957).
— G. STEINBERG, and D. R. HOWTON: Metabolism of essential fatty acids. Incorporation of acetate into arachidonic acid. J. biol. Chem. 205, 683 (1953).
PARDEE, A. B., and L. L. INGRAHAM: in Metabolic Pathways I, p. 1, edit. by D. M. GREENBERG. New York: Academic Press 1960.
RUDNEY, H.: The biosynthesis of β-hydroxy-β-methylglutaric acid. J.biol.Chem.227,363(1957).
SCHOENHEIMER, R., and D. RITTENBERG: Deuterium as an indicator in the study of intermediary metabolism. V. The desaturation of fatty acids in the organisms. J. biol. Chem. 113, 505 (1936).
SCHROEPFER, G. J., and K. BLOCH: Enzyme is stereospecific. D-hydrogen removed from C-9 during conversion of stearic to oleic acid. Chem. Engng. News 42, 44 (1964).
— — The stereospecific conversion of stearic to oleic acid. J. biol. Chem. 240, 54 (1965).
SEGAL, H. L., and G. K. K. MENON: Evidence for the formation of acetoacetate by direct deacylation of acetoacetyl-CoA in liver mitochondria. Biochem. biophys. Res. Commun. 3, 406 (1960).
SEUBERT, W., G. GREULL, u. F. LYNEN: Die Synthese von Fettsäuren mit gereinigten Enzymen des Fettsäurecyclus. Angew. Chem. 69, 359 (1957).
SIPERSTEIN, M. D.: Interrelationships of glucose and lipid metabolism. Amer. J. Med. 26, 685 (1959).
SPENCER, A. F., and J. M. LOWENSTEIN: The supply of precursors for the synthesis of fatty acids. J. biol. Chem. 237, 3640 (1962).
STEINBERG, G., W. H. SLATON jr., D. R. HOWTON, and J. F. MEAD: Metabolism of essential fatty acids. IV. Incorporation of linoleate into arachidonic acid. J. biol. Chem. 220, 257 (1956).
STERN, J. R., A. DEL CAMPILLO, and I. RAW: Enzymes of fatty acid metabolism. J. biol. Chem. 218, 971, 985 (1956).
STETTEN, D., and G. E. BOXER: Studies in carbohydrate metabolism. III. Metabolic defects in alloxan diabetes. J. biol. Chem. 156, 271 (1940).
STOFFEL, W.: Biosynthesis of polyenoic fatty acids. Biochem. biophys. Res. Commun. 6, 270 (1961).
— u. K. L. ACH: Der Stoffwechsel der ungesättigten Fettsäuren. II. Eigenschaften des kettenverlängernden Enzyms. Zur Frage der Biohydrogenierung der ungesättigten Fettsäuren. Hoppe-Seylers Z. physiol. Chem. 337, 123 (1964).
— u. H. CAESAR: Der Stoffwechsel der ungesättigten Fettsäuren. V. Zur β-Oxydation der Mono- und Polyenfettsäuren. Der Mechanismus der enzymatischen Reaktionen an cis-α, β-Enoyl-CoA-Verbindungen. Hoppe-Seylers Z. physiol. Chem. 341, 76 (1965).
— R. DITZER u. H. CAESAR: Der Stoffwechsel der ungesättigten Fettsäuren. III. Zur β-Oxydation der Mono- und Polyenfettsäuren. Der Mechanismus der enzymatischen Reaktionen an cis β, γ-Enoyl-CoA-Verbindungen. Hoppe-Seylers Z. physiol. Chem. 339, 167 (1964).
— and H. G. SCHIEFER: Der Stoffwechsel der ungesättigten Fettsäuren. IV. Zur β-Oxydation der Mono- und Polyenfettsäuren. Untersuchungen in vivo und in vitro mit doppelt (3H,14C)- und 1-14C-markierten Mono- und Polyenfettsäuren. Hoppe-Seylers Z. physiol. Chem. 341, 84 (1965).
VAGELOS, P. R., A. W. ALBERTS, and D. B. MARTIN: Activation of acetyl-CoA carboxylase and associated alteration of sedimentation characteristics of the enzyme. Biochem. biophys. Res. Commun. 8, 4 (1962).
— — — Studies on the mechanism of activation of acetyl-coenzyme A carboxylase by citrate. J. biol. Chem. 238, 533 (1963).
WAKIL, S. J.: Studies on the fatty acid oxidizing system of animal tissues. IX. Stereospecificity of unsaturated acyl CoA hydrase. Biochim. biophys. Acta (Amst.) 19, 497 (1956).
— and H. R. MAHLER: Studies on the fatty oxidizing system of animal tissues. V. Unsaturated fatty acyl-coenzyme A hydrase. J. biol. Chem. 207, 125 (1954).
— E. L. PUGH, and F. SAUER: The mechanism of fatty acid synthesis. Proc. Nat. Acad. Sci. (Wash.) 52, 106 (1964).
— E. B. TITCHENER, and D. M. GIBSON: Evidence for the participitation of biotin in the enzymic synthesis of fatty acids. Biochim. biophys. Acta (Amst.) 29, 225 (1958).
— — — Studies on the mechanism of fatty acid synthesis. Biochim. biophys. Acta (Amst.) 34, 227 (1959).
WIELAND, O., and L. WEISS: Increase in liver acetyl-coenzyme A during ketosis. Biochem. biophys. Res. Commun. 10, 333 (1963a).
— — Inhibition of citrate-synthase by palmityl-coenzyme A. Biochem. biophys. Res. Commun. 13, 26 (1963b).

Biochemistry of Triglycerides

By

B. Shapiro

Introduction

Triglycerides are the main energy storage material of the animal body and make up a large part of its caloric intake. Being a comparatively inert group of substances, they can be stored in large amounts. As water insoluble materials they are deposited as droplets of concentrated energy reserve, lacking osmotic activity and not requiring the concomitant deposition of large amounts of water. On the other hand, their insolubility in water makes it necessary for the organism to devise special methods and vehicles of transport in the aqueous medium of the animal body.

This mechanism of transport is the main topic of the following discussion, as it is in this aspect that the specific metabolism of triglycerides is involved. The total combustion of these substances, as well as their biosynthesis from sugar is common with that of other lipids and free fatty acids and is dealt with in the chapter by STOFFEL.

I. Absorption from the Intestine

Two basic facts, concerning the absorption of fat from the intestine and about the factors involved in enabling these water insoluble substances to penetrate the intestinal barrier, have been known from the earliest days of physiological science. The first, the importance of pancreatic juice and of bile for the digestion and absorption of fat, was recognized already by CLAUDE BERNARD (1856). The second fact was that absorbed fat, after penetration across the intestinal barrier, appears in the lymph ducts as triglycerides. Collection of intestinal lymph was performed as early as 1880 by MUNK on a patient with a spontaneous lymph fistula and also on anaesthetized dogs with thoracic duct fistulas (MUNK and ROSENSTEIN (1891). However, only when a technique became available for the collection of lymph from the intestinal and thoracic duct of non-anaesthesized rats (BOLLMAN et al. 1948), yields of up to 90% of the absorbed fat could be obtained and conclusive proof became available to show that the absorbed fat is transported practically completely via the lymphatics and is made up predominantly of triglycerides (see review by BERGSTRÖM and BORGSTÖM 1955).

1. Lipolysis in the Lumen

These observations were the basis of two competing theories.

PFLÜGER (1901), put forward the hypothesis that the complete hydrolysis of glycerides by pancreatic lipase was an essential step in triglyceride absorption. The "lipolytic theory", was further advanced by VERZAR and McDOUGAL (1936), who also demonstrated the hydrotropic action of bile salts, which causes the solubilization of fatty acids and enables them to cross the intestinal barrier. This theory requires also the resynthesis of the triglycerides in the intestinal cells, to account for the composition of the fat in the lymphatics. FRAZER (1946), on the other hand, claimed that conditions in the intestinal tract do not lead to complete hydrolysis of triglycerides by pancreatic lipase, and partial glycerides are formed. According to the "Particulate absorption theory" it is the function of these partial glycerides in conjunction with bile salts and fatty acids to provide an effective system for the fine dispersion of fat. The micelles formed can now penetrate the intestinal mucosa. In this way considerable amounts of the original, unhydrolyzed fat can find their way into the thoracic duct. As will be seen in the following discussion present opinion is somewhere between these two theories.

a) **Pancreatic Lipase:** The properties and methods of purification have recently been reviewed (KATES 1960; DESNUELLE 1961). The enzyme hydrolyzes preferentially the α-positions of the triglyceride molecules and is specific for long chain fatty acid esters in emulsified form. β-monoglycerides are formed during digestion of triglycerides by pancreatic lipase (MATTSON et al. 1952), as well as in the intestinal content, following a meal rich in triglycerides. For complete hydrolysis a shift to the α-position seems to be necessary (BORGSTRÖM and HOFMANN 1963). Lipolysis is activated by bile salts. These activators aid in the emulsification of fats, but also displace the pH optimum from pH 8.0 to 6.0 (BORGSTRÖM 1954) and increase lipolysis to a degree which could not be explained simply by the enlargement of interface area (DESNUELLE 1961). The positional specificity of pancreatic lipase has been used as an analytical tool for the determination of the arrangement of the fatty acids in the triglyceride molecule (SAVARY et al. 1956; MATTSON and BECK 1956).

b) **The Extent of Hydrolysis:** The extent to which hydrolysis actually progresses is not easy to establish from observations on the intestinal contents of animals during fat absorption. The formation of breakdown products goes on concurrently with their absorption, and the contents of the intestinal lumen is the result of two competing processes, i. e. lipolysis and resorption.

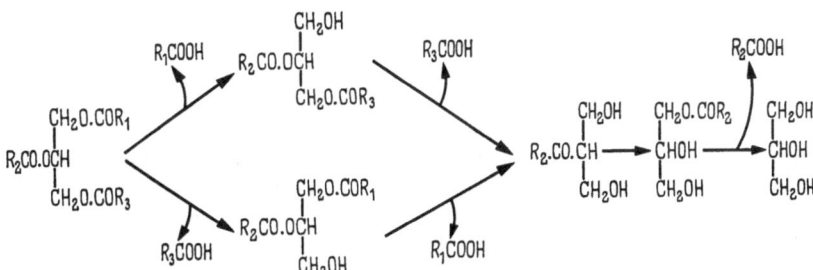

Figure 1. Specificity of pancreatic lipase

Observations on the composition of the resorbed fat, i. e. that transported in the lymphatics, leads to the uniform result that almost all the fatty acids of the diet are recovered in the lymphatics as triglycerides, irrespective of whether fed as triglycerides, other esters or as free fatty acids (see BERGSTRÖM and BORGSTRÖM 1955). A mechanism must be present in the intestinal cells for the esterification of free fatty acids (see chapter b). The presence of triglycerides in the lymphatics, therefore, does not provide any information on the form of the absorbed lipid mixture and on the extent of lipolysis.

A means of estimating the extent of total hydrolysis was proposed, using glycerol labelled triglycerides. This method is based on the finding that free glycerol is used only to a very limited extent for the formation of lymphatic and intestinal wall triglycerides (Favarger et al. 1951; Bernhard et al. 1952) and therefore any glycerol set free in the hydrolysis of triglycerides is not reutilized for triglyceride synthesis in the intestine. The fatty acids which are reconverted into triglycerides, on their way to the lymphatics, must have combined with a glycerol source other than the free glycerol formed. Examining the lymph of animals fed triolein labelled in both the glycerol and the fatty acid part, the loss of labelled glycerol relative to that of the fatty acids would, therefore, serve as a measure of total hydrolysis. Experiments of this type led to estimates of 25—50% total hydrolysis (Bernhard et al. 1952; Reiser et al. 1952; Borgström 1952). Contrary to previous assumptions, recent findings indicate that some glycerol may be incorporated into glyceride glycerol by the intestine (Saunders and Dawson 1962; Clark and Hübscher 1962; Hässler and Isselbacher 1962). This would put the above estimates somewhat too low.

The fate of the rest of the fat is more difficult to ascertain. Since glycerol absorbed as mono- and diglycerides is reutilized and reconverted into triglycerides (see 2b), the above method cannot distinguish between the resorption of unsplit triglycerides and that of partial glycerides. The estimate as to the part of these partial glycerides in the absorbed fat mixture has been based on the examination of the degree of redistribution of fatty acids in the newly synthesized triglycerides. By feeding glycerides containing known fatty acids in their inner chains (β-position) or by feeding triglycerides together with labelled free fatty acids and examining the configuration of the lymph triglycerides, it could be established that most of the fatty acids in the β-position remained attached to their original glycerol. The part of the fatty acids replaced in this position did not exceed that which might correspond to the totally hydrolyzed triglycerides, as estimated above (Reiser et al. 1952; Borgström 1955a; Savary et al. 1961; Mattson and Volpenhein 1962). These results indicate that a considerable part of the triglyceride may be absorbed without hydrolysis beyond the monoglyceride stage. They do not answer the question, how much may be resorbed as di-and triglycerides.

In experiments of the type mentioned above the fatty acids in the α-position had been almost completely exchanged with other fatty acids supplied, while those in the β-position remained largely attached to its original glycerol. This led Reiser et al. (1952), to the conclusion that the part of the triglycerides which are not completely hydrolyzed, are largely degraded to mono-glycerides.

This conclusion is, however, open to criticism since it was shown by Bergström et al. (1952) that fatty acids in the α-position exchange with triglyceride fatty acids already in the intestinal lumen. This exchange is catalyzed by pancreatic lipase. In order to overcome this difficulty, Borgström et al. (1957b) fed triglycerides containing 2,2′ dimethyl-fatty acids. These esters are resistant to the action of pancreatic lipase and have to be absorbed without hydrolysis. From their concentration in the glycerides of the intestinal contents it was calculated that a hydrolysis of about 60% of the fatty acids took place during the absorption process. All these results lead to the conclusion, that the lipid mixture taken up from the intestinal lumen is mainly a mixture of monoglycerides and free fatty acid, with limited amounts of di-and triglycerides. This is also in harmony with deductions arrived at from the more detailed investigations on the fate of triglycerides in the intestinal lumen as described in the next chapter.

c) **Emulsification:** During recent years interest hast been focused on the physicochemical processes occuring in the intestinal contents during lipid digestion and their importance for the absorption of lipids. This aspect has been recently reviewed by Borgström (1964) and the following is the sequence of events described: Lipid digestion may start to some extent in the stomach. 10—20% free fatty acids were found in stomach contents of humans being fed triglycerides (BORGSTRÖM et al. 1957a). The main absorption of dietary fat in the human starts in the distal duodenum and is completed in the proximal jejunum. The length of time that the chyme is exposed to the pancreatic juice and bile, before absorption of the fat, is comparatively short. It has a pH around 6 and contains bile salts in a concentration of 4—10 m Equ/1. In addition the bile adds to it lecithin, cholesterol and mucopolysaccharides.

Bile salts have most of the properties of an anionic detergent, forming micellar solutions above their critical micellar concentrations. They possess a low capacity for the solubilisation of non-polar substances but a high one for polar ones. The triglycerides of the dietary fats would thus be expected to be emulsified to a limited extent in the duodenum by bile salts, aided by the free fatty acids formed in the stomach and the other bile constituents.

The pancreatic lipase which is active mainly in an oil phase now attacks the triglycerides, hydrolyzing the primary hydroxyl groups and forming β-monoglyce-rides. The hydrolysis of these compounds seems to require isomerization to the α-monoglyceride, which is a relatively slow-process under the conditions prevailing in the intestinal content during fat absorption. The products of lipolysis, fatty acids and monoglycerides, are very effectively solubilized by the bile salts. These processes result in the formation of two phases (HOFMANN 1963; HOFMANN and BORGSTRÖM 1964), a micellar phase composed of bile salts, monoglyceride and fatty acids with little tri-and diglycerides and an oil phase containing the tri-and diglycerides. Monoglycerides and fatty acids are continuously generated from the oil phase and transferred to the micellar one. It is from these latter particles that material is absorbed by the intestinal cells (see following chapter).

2. Uptake and Metabolism in the Intestinal Cells

a) **Uptake:** Experiments with intestinal preparations of the rat and hamster in vitro, conducted by JOHNSTON and BORGSTRÖM (1963), demonstrated the capa-bility of this tissue to extract monoglycerides and fatty acids from their bile salt micelles, but take up emulsified triglycerides to a very limited extent. The uptake seems to be an energy-independent process and is directly proportional to the concentration. It is effected to the same extent by different parts of the intestine, and even by boiled preparations.

This initial uptake is followed by an enzymatic process, i.e. resynthesis of triglycerides from the monoglycerides and fatty acids, which is the rate limiting step, reestablishing the concentration gradient between the intestinal cells and the lumen, resulting in continuous absorption of lipids.

This picture of the mechanism of uptake by the intestine is not easily recon-ciled with that obtained by morphological observations. This aspect has recently been reviewed by PALAY and REVEL (1964). Particulate fat in the intestinal lumen was shown to penetrate between the microvilli of the striated border and was then absorbed into the intestinal epithelial cells by passing into pinocytotic vesicles. These vesicles traverse the terminal web and the fat droplets were deposited within the lumen of the endoplasmic reticulum. They are transported in the Golgi apparatus and finally out of the cell along its lateral border.

There is however, still some doubt about this interpretation of the morpholo-gical observations and it is difficult to estimate what the quantitative importance of this type of transport is (LACY and TAYLOR 1962; MILLINGTON and FINEAN 1962). It is quite possible that the pinocytotic mechanism is relevant mainly to the uptake of the droplets from the oil phase, described above. The micellar

monoglycerides and free fatty acids are absorbed by the brush border without
any physiological activity. Only subsequently, for the resynthesis of triglycerides,
active metabolism is required. This synthesis takes place presumably by enzymes
in the endoplasmic reticulum (see chapter 2b) and part of the fat droplets found
in this structure may result from these synthetic processes.

b) **Resynthesis of Triglycerides in Mucosal Cells:** Evidence for the capacity of the
intestinal mucosa to esterify fatty acids was obtained by JOHNSTON (1958, 1959)
who incubated everted segments of the small intestine with labelled free fatty
acids and demonstrated their appearance as glycerol esters on the serosal side.

The formation of triglycerides from free fatty acids in subcellular preparations
of intestinal mucosa was shown to require the presence of ATP, Coenzyme A and
Mg^{++}. Addition of L-α-glycerophosphate to the incubation mixture increased the
synthesis manyfold (DAWSON and ISSELBACHER 1960; CLARK and HÜBSCHER
1960, 1961). These requirements are similar to those found for triglyceride synthesis in liver particles (see chapter III 2) and it was therefore considered likely
that triglyceride synthesis in the intestine proceeds by the same reaction steps as
in liver.

Furthermore it was possible to demonstrate the presence in the intestine of all
the enzymes required for these steps. Fatty acid-coenzyme A synthesis was
demonstrated by AILHAUD et al. (1962) and by CLARK and HÜBSCHER (1960).
The involvement of phosphatidic acid could be demonstrated by isolation of
radioactive phosphatidic acid in intestinal preparations incubated with radioactive fatty acids or phosphoric acid (JOHNSTON and BEARDEN 1960). Furthermore,
a significant dilution effect in the synthesis of glycerides from ^{14}C-fatty acids
occurred by the addition of phosphatidic acid (CLARK and HÜBSCHER 1961).
Phosphatidic acid phosphatase activity in the intestine was reported by COLE-
MAN and HÜBSCHER (1962) and by JOHNSTON and BEARDEN (1962). Finally,
the conversion of diglyceride into triglycerides by the addition of a fatty
acid — CoA was shown to take place in the intestine by CLARK and HÜBSCHER
(1961).

In addition to the pathway employing α-glycerophosphate as fatty acids acceptor, a second one was discovered in intestinal mucosa esterifying monoglycerides
without the intermediate formation of phosphatidic acid (CLARK and HÜBSCHER
1960; SENIOR and ISSELBACHER 1962; JOHNSTON and BROWN 1962). This latter
enzyme system is of considerable importance in intestinal cell metabolism, since
substantial amounts of monoglycerides seem to be absorbed from the digestive
tract. The enzymes catalyzing triglyceride synthesis from monoglycerides reside
primarily in the microsome fraction of the mucosal homogenate (HÜBSCHER et al.
1963; BROWN and JOHNSTON 1964). Both α- and β-monoglycerides are utilized.
However, the β-isomere seems to be preferred.

c) **Phospholipids:** During the absorption of fat, considerable changes occur also
in the fatty acids of the phospholipids of the intestinal mucosa, although the total
amount of the phospholipids remains constant (SINCLAIR 1929). In addition to the
increased fatty acid turnover in the phospholipids, an increased turnover was
also found in the phosphorus part of these molecules (ARTOM et al. 1937). It
was postulated by SCHMIDT-NIELSEN (1946) that this increased turnover of phospholipids is a process of much importance to fatty acid uptake. However, the
evidence so far available, concerning the role and the quantitative significance
of the changes observed in the phospholipids of the intestinal mucosa is still
not clear.

d) **Fate of Short Chain Fatty Acids:** Only long chain fatty acids appear in the
thoracic duct as glycerides, while fatty acid molecules with chain length of ten or

less carbon are transported unesterified in the portal blood stream (BLOOM et al. 1951; KYASU et al. 1952; BORGSTRÖM 1956 b; BLOOMSTRAND et al. 1958).

Differences in the behaviour of fatty acids during absorption are probably due partly to their physical properties and partly to variations in their intramucosal metabolism. The different fate of the medium length fatty acid may be ascribed to the low activity of esterifying enzymes towards them (DAWSON and ISSEL-BACHER 1960), as well as to extensive hydrolysis of their glycerides by a specific lipase present in the microsomal fraction of intestinal mucosa. ^{14}C-trioctanoin was shown to enter mucosal cells without prior hydrolysis in the lumen (PLAYOUST and ISSELBACHER 1964). These fats seem to be hydrolysed in the mucosa cells. The presence of a specific monoglyceride lipase has been demonstrated in epithelial subcellular fragments (SENIOR and ISSELBACHER 1963). This enzyme may be of possible role in the intracellular completion of fat digestion, especially in the absorption of glycerides with medium chain fatty acids, which have to be liberated and transported via the portal blood as free acids.

Studies in a patient with chyluria (BLOOMSTRAND et al. 1958) and with chylo-thorax (FERNANDES et al. 1955), indicate that the route of absorption in man is the same as in animals. In patients with celiac disease and cystic fibrosis of the pancreas, medium chain triglycerides seem to be more completely absorbed than those containing fatty acids of higher molecular weight (VAN DE KAMER and WEIJERS 1961; FERNANDEZ et al. 1962). Eight and ten carbon fatty acids in neutral fat have been used in the management of pancreatogenous steatorrhea (BORGSTRÖM 1960).

The processes involved in triglyceride absorption may be summarized in the following scheme.

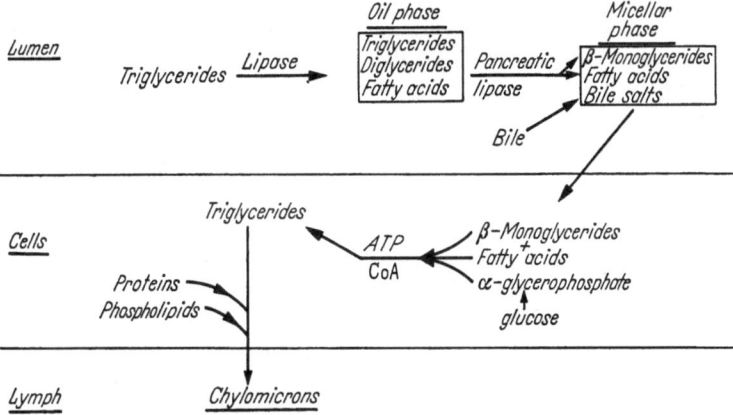

Figure 2. Triglyceride absorption by the intestine

II. Metabolism of Lymph and Blood Chylomicra

1. Rate and Site of Removal

The triglycerides, after leaving the intestinal cells, enter the lymphatics draining the small intestine. Here, they are present as small, light scattering particles known as chylomicra. These particles are composed of a triglyceride core, comprising 85—90% of the lipids, and of phospholipids, cholesterol and protein, which stabilize the fat particles. The amount of phospholipids present is more than enough to form a monomolecular surface layer on the particles. Treatment of chylomicra with lecithinase causes flocculation (Robinson 1955). A detailed review on the metabolism of chylomicra has been presented by Dole and Hamlin (1962).

The chylomicra enter the systemic blood circulation by way of the jugular vene. They can be seen in the blood, following a fatty meal, by a dark field microscope (Gage and Fish 1924). They gradually disappear from the circulation at a rate varying with the species. In the human, the rate of entry into the blood after a fat rich meal may exceed the rate of removal and the blood becomes turbid. In the rat removal is much more rapid and turbidity of plasma is rarely encountered.

The rate of disappearance of chylomicra from the blood circulation has been the object of many investigations. The method of estimation is based generally on the injection of radioactive chylomicra. These may be produced either by artificial emulsification in blood serum of labelled triglycerides or by feeding a donor animal with labelled fat or fatty acids and collecting the thoracic chyle, containing the labelled chylomicra. With such labelled material the half time of disappearance of chylomicra from the blood was 4—14 minutes in the rat (French and Morris 1957) and 15—24 minutes in the dog (Havel and Fredrickson 1956). The half life time increases with the dose injected. The disappearance curve follows a singly exponential function only during the first part and then becomes more complex. This complexity seems to be due to several causes, i. e. to a slower clearance rate of the labelled phospholipids present in the chylomicra (Olivecrona et al. 1961) and to the recirculation of the absorbed fatty acids in the blood in the form of β-lipoproteins (Bierman and Hamlin 1962; Nestel et al. 1962).

A large part of the injected triglycerides removed from the circulation is initially taken up by the liver (Bragdon and Gordon 1958; French and Morris 1958; Borgström and Jordan 1959; Stein and Shapiro 1960). The rest is converted to carbon dioxide and is taken up by adipose tissue, skeletal and cardiac muscle. The nutritional state of the animal has considerable effect on this distribution (Bragdon and Gordon 1958). While in the starved rat very little triglyceride appears initially in adipose tissue and the bulk is in the liver and as respiratory CO_2, in the carbohydrate fed animal, 25—30% can be found in adipose tissue several minutes after the injection and very little is burned to CO_2. After longer periods, part of the chylomicron fatty acids can be found in various serum lipoprotein fractions and in adipose tissue.

The uptake of particles has previously been thought to be the task of the reticuloendothelial cells. It could actually be shown that exogenous cholesterol enters Kupffer cells (Friedman et al. 1954) but this process does not seem to be essential for the assimilation of triglycerides nor is it quantitatively important (van den Bosch et al. 1961). Blocking the Kupffer cells by injections of colloidal carbon did not interfere with the removal of fat and its deposition in the parenchymal cells of the liver (Waddell et al. 1954). It seems to be mainly the function of the parenchymal cells to assimilate and metabolize chylomicron triglycerides (DiLuzio 1960) whereas artifical fat emulsions are also taken up by the reticuloendothelial cells of the liver.

2. Clearing Factor and the Mechanism of Uptake by the Tissues

Considerable interest has been aroused by the discovery of Hahn (1943) that heparin, in addition to its well known action as anticoagulant, will also accelerate the clearing of turbid plasma. When injected intravenously to an animal, which is absorbing fat and has a visible lipemia, the plasma will clear in a few minutes.

The relation of this phenomenon to the metabolism of blood triglycerides has been reviewed by Robinson and French (1960). It is not heparin itself which acts on the plasma chylomicra, since addition of heparin to a lipemic plasma in vitro does not cause clearing. On the other hand, the plasma of animals, to which heparin had been injected, contains a factor which will cause clearing when added to lipemic plasma in vitro. This factor has been named "clearing factor". Its nature and activity has been investigated extensively and comprehensive reviews are available (ROBINSON and FRENCH 1957; LEVY 1958). It is generally accepted that the clearing factor is a lipase, which hydrolyzes the triglycerides of chylomicra. It is relatively inactive towards triglyceride emulsions, but these become effective substrates when coated with small amounts of a serum protein. The factor was therefore named "Lipoprotein lipase" (KORN 1955a, b). In addition to this protein, serum albumin is required for the activity of the clearing factor. Its function seems to be that of an acceptor for the fatty acids, formed by the action of the enzyme on the triglycerides. Clearing is brought about by complete or partial lipolysis, the fatty acid-albumin complex serving as dispersing agents for the residual glycerides. These smaller particles formed may be more easily assimilated by the tissues. Fatty acid-albumin complexes injected into the circulation are removed very rapidly, with a half life time of less than 2 minutes (LAURELL 1957; FREDRICKSON et al. 1958a, b).

The lipolytic action of the clearing factor appears, therefore, to be an adequate explanation of the clearing of lipemic plasma following injection of heparin. The importance of this factor in the removal of chylomicra from the blood during normal conditions is however still problematical. The case for the assumption, that triglyceride lipolysis in the blood by the heparin lipoprotein lipase is a major pathway for the clearance of alimentary neutral fat from the blood stream, has been summarized by ENGELBERG (1960). Some of the arguments in favour of this concept are: a) Rapid changes take place in the state of dispersion of triglycerides in blood plasma. Following the ingestion of a fat meal or the injection of chylomicra, a rapid conversion into smaller lipoprotein species has been described in man and in animals (JONES et al. 1951; GITLIN and CORNWELL 1956; PIERCE 1954). b) The concentration of unesterified fatty acids in the plasma rises after the injection of fat emulsions (GROSSMAN et al. 1955; HAVEL and FREDRICKSON 1956). Mono and diglycerides appear in the plasma at the same time (CARLSON and WADSTROEM 1957; MEAD and FILLERUP 1957). These data suggest an intimate relationship between the removal of chylomicra from the blood and the lipolysis of their triglyceride component, although the site at which this occurred was not established. c) The disappearance from the blood of labelled triglycerides of chylomicra was found to be more rapid than that of the labelled phospholipids of these particles (McCANDLESS and ZILVERSMIT 1958). This argues against the particulate removal of intact chylomicra by pinocytosis or similar mechanisms. d) The injection of protamine or toluidine blue, substances which inhibit heparin, causes increases in lipemia in animals (BROWN 1952; SPITZER 1953; BRAGDON and HAVEL 1954) and in man (GRUNER et al. 1953). This may serve as indirect evidence for the participation of heparin in the normal removal of chylomicra. However, the possibility must also be considered that these agents may act by changing the surface properties of chylomicra and so hamper their removal, rather than by their inhibition of heparin action. e) A lipase, resembling in its properties that of the heparin clearing factor, has frequently, though not always, been found in the plasma of humans (ENGELBERG 1958b) and an inverse correlation was established between its activity and that of the level of larger fat particles (low density lipoproteins). At the same time, blood heparin levels were also related with the activity of clearing factor lipase and with lipemia (ENGELBERG 1955). f) Lipemia provides a stimulus for increasing the levels of heparin and of lipoprotein lipase activity in plasma (Engelberg 1958a, 1957). This seems to represent a normal response to a physiological demand, by which the body adapts to the large influx of fat by the release of endogenous heparin. This, in turn, activates the clearing factor lipase and promotes the elimination of alimentary triglycerides from the blood circulation. g) An association has been found between essential hyperlipemia and the interference with the triglyceride lipolytic mechanism. The defect in this mechanism may be of several types. The source of hyperlipemia may be a decreased response to heparin to form clearing factor (Havel 1956). In other cases, a lack of sufficient endogenous heparin was apparently the cause of the hyperlipemia (Engelberg 1960). Low levels of heparin were found and clearing factor formation became normal after the injection of exogenous heparin. In patients with nephrotic syndrome, the cause of hyperlipemia may be attributed to the low levels of plasma albumin, which is part of the clearing mechanism. In accordance with this it has been shown that when plasma albumin is elevated, a decrease in the lipid level results (Rosenman et al. 1956; Burack et al. 1958).

The case for the participation of intravascular lipolysis by lipoprotein lipase seems to be quite impressive. The quantitative importance of this process for chylomicron removal is, however, less clear. An attempt to arrive at a quantitative estimate has been based on the infusion into a dog, at constant rate over a two hour period, of fatty acid labelled chylomicra. The specific activity of the free fatty acid fraction reached a constant level of around 10% of the infused chylomicron glyceride fatty acids (Fredrickson et al. 1958b). This finding indicates that at most one tenth of the free fatty acids in the plasma are derived from intravascular splitting of chylomicra. If free fatty acids were the sole lipid substance available to the tissues, one would expect that $^{14}CO_2$ formation from radioactive triglycerides would be only about one tenth that obtained when the same amount is injected in the form of radioactive free fatty acids. This, however, was not the case and $^{14}CO_2$ formation was similar whether fat was injected as free fatty acid or as chylomicron glycerides. A large fraction of the latter must therefore have been removed from the circulation and utilized by the tissues as glycerides. A similar conclusion has been drawn from experiments which show that the distribution of radioactive fatty acids in the various tissues differs when injected as free acids or as chylomicra (Bragdon and Gordon 1958). More conclusive evidence for the ability of the liver to take up unhydrolyzed triglycerides was obtained by injecting emulsions of triglycerides labelled in both the glycerol and the fatty acid moieties. The labelled triglycerides recovered from the liver 5—10 minutes after the injection had preserved the ratio of label in the glycerol to that of the fatty acid of the injected material (Borgström and Jordan 1959; Stein and Shapiro 1960; Olivecrona 1962a). These experiments indicate that intravascular lipolysis is not absolutely required for clearance from the blood, at least as far as the liver is concerned.

Electron microscopic studies have shown that in the liver of the rat the sinusoids are lined by a discontinuous endothelium. The cells have no well defined basement membrane and may be separated from each other by gaps of several thousand Ångström units. When particles of smaller diameter than these gaps are introduced into the circulation they can enter the subendothelial space of Disse and come into direct contact with the microvilli on the surface of the hepatic parenchymal cells (Bennet et al. 1959). Following the intravenous injection of chyle, chylomicrons could be seen within the lumen of hepatic sinusoids, within gaps of their endothelial lining and within the subendothelial space (French 1963).

With other tissues, like heart muscle and adipose tissue, the capillaries are of the unfenestrated type. They possess a continuous endothelium with individual cells closely applied to each other at their borders, and an uninterrupted basement membrane. There exists a potential structural barrier in these tissues between the parenchymal cells and the chylomicra in the circulation. One would therefore expect different requirements for the penetration of chylomicra into liver and into one of these tissues.

An alternative viewpoint assigns to clearing factor lipase a function in fat transport not related to intravascular lipolysis. According to this view (ROBINSON and FRENCH 1960), this factor is not normally active in the blood and its appearance there in high concentration is an artificial consequence of heparin injection. The rapidity of its appearance in the blood is due to its location at a site readily accessible to the circulation, i.e. the vessel walls. It is here that its hydrolytic activity is thought to promote the passage of triglycerides. This may be done either by complete hydrolysis to fatty acids or by partial splitting and the formation of smaller particles which can penetrate the vessel walls. The problem, thus is similar to that arising about absorption in the intestine and still awaits clarification.

An enzyme with properties resembling those of the heparin-clearing factor lipase has been found in extracts of heart, adipose and other tissues (KORN 1955a; KORN and QUIGLEY 1957; ISELIN and SCHULER 1957). Perfusion of heparin through the circulation of many organs causes the liberation of clearing factor into the perfusate (JEFFRIES 1954; ROBINSON and HARRIS 1959; SWANK and LEVY 1952) while no activity is released from liver or brain.

Within twenty seconds of injecting heparin into the femoral artery of a rabbit, blood samples of the femoral vein contained lipolytic activity. As this time is no greater than that required for the heparin to traverse the capillary bed of the hind limb, this result indicates that the enzyme is readily accessible to heparin in the circulating blood (ROBINSON and HARRIS 1959). The enzyme is also found in the perfusate, when a heparin-serum albumin solution is perfused through an isolated hind limb. These findings led to the conclusion that the clearing factor is not present in the blood but is released into it by excessive doses of heparin. It is located in the capillary epithelium or on cell surfaces and its normal function is to act at these sites to facilitate transport of fat across the barriers. In accord with this concept is the distribution of lipoprotein lipase in the extrahepatic tissues, where an uninterrupted capillary epithelium exists and a special mechanism for fat transport is required.

III. Metabolism of Triglycerides in the Liver

1. Uptake and Release

Evidence discussed in the previous chapter suggests that the liver assimilates plasma triglycerides without prior hydrolysis. In addition, the liver can also form triglycerides from free fatty acids, supplied by the blood as well as from those synthesized in the liver from carbohydrates. Very little free fatty acid is stored by the liver and free acids coming in from any source are rapidly esterified. Five minutes after C^{14}-palmitic acid is injected into the blood circulation more than 50% can be recovered in the liver in the esterified form, mainly as triglycerides (STEIN and SHAPIRO 1959; LAURELL 1959a; OLIVECRONA 1962b). The newly formed triglycerides are not mixed with the bulk of the liver triglycerides but are located on the tissue particles, mitochondria and microsomes, i.e. at the sites of their esterification (see Chapter III, 2). A similar localization was found for the preformed triglycerides taken up from the blood (STEIN and SHAPIRO 1960).

Following this initial deposition, the triglycerides are rapidly metabolized. The fatty acids are transferred to phospholipids and to other triglycerides. A large part of the assimilated radioactive fatty acids disappear from the liver. This disappearance can be accounted for by partial combustion to $^{14}CO_2$ and to re-excretion into the blood in the form of lipoproteins. The formation of serum lipoproteins from free fatty acids or from triglycerides could be demonstrated in the intact animal injected with ^{14}C-palmitic acid. Maximal labelling of the plasma triglycerides occurred 30—50 minutes after the injection. Most of these triglycerides were associated with the plasma low density lipoproteins (LAURELL 1959 b).

When livers, in which the triglycerides had been labelled by injection of ^{14}C-palmitic acid, were perfused with a serum albumin solution, triglycerides were released by the liver into the perfusate. The specific activity of the released triglycerides was greater than that of the bulk of the liver triglycerides, but less than that of the triglycerides associated with the particles of the liver cell (STEIN and SHAPIRO 1959). This indicates that the triglycerides assimilated on the particles are metabolized there to form plasma lipoproteins.

A convenient method to study triglyceride release is the use of liver slices from rats which had previously been treated with ^{14}C-palmitic acid. Such slices release triglycerides into the medium of incubation. Maximal release was found when the medium contained lipoproteins (HAMOSH and SHAPIRO 1961). Several investigators have used the perfused isolated liver for the study of glyceride uptake and release (HEIMBERG et al. 1958 a, b; MORRIS and FRENCH 1958; HILLYARD et al. 1959). In such a preparation it was possible to measure the rate of uptake and release of triglycerides. The uptake was more rapid in the livers from starved rats than from normally fed animals. With livers from fed but not from fasted animals a net increase in perfusate triglycerides was observed (HEIMBERG et al. 1962 b). This increase was associated with an increase in the plasma lipoprotein fraction of density below 1.006 (KAY and ENTENMAN 1961). In perfusion experiments in which an artificial perfusion fluid was used in place of blood, somatotropin increased the rate of uptake of esterified fatty acids from fed animals whereas hydrocortisone decreased the rapid uptake by livers of fasted rats to that of livers from normally fed male rats (HEIMBERG et al. 1958 b).

As stated before, the metabolism of triglycerides in the liver, leading to the secretion into the blood of lipoproteins, is accompanied by a reshuffle of the fatty acids in the triglycerides. This was established by the use of ^{14}C-glycerol-H^3-fatty acid labelled triglycerides. Following their uptake as unsplit triglycerides the ^{14}C-glycerol part becomes gradually smaller, indicating a complete degradation of the triglyceride and resynthesis of new molecules from the H^3-fatty acid and unlabelled glycerol, supplied by the liver. Part of the H^3-fatty acid also turn up in the phospholipids (BORGSTRÖM and JORDAN 1959; STEIN and SHAPIRO 1960). Similar results were obtained by the use of glyceryl tripalmitin-1-^{14}C in the perfused liver (RODBELL et al. 1964). Tripalmitin can be readily separated from triglycerides containing unsaturated fatty acids and since the liver forms mixed triglycerides, it was possible to differentiate between unmetabolized and newly formed triglycerides in the hepatic cells and in blood. It was found that the amount of unmetabolized tripalmitin was essentially the same at all time points between 5 and 60 minutes of perfusion. During this time the "metabolized" triglycerides and phospholipids steadily increased. This suggested that the tripalmitin was initially taken up at an "entry site", which becomes rapidly saturated. Further uptake was now slower, depending on the metabolism, (i.e. the reshuffle of the fatty acids as stated above), which moves tripalmitin from the "entry site" to other parts of the cell and makes place for additional amounts of blood triglyceride.

This would also explain the finding that clearance of triglyceride from the blood is in inverse relationship to the blood triglyceride concentration. With low concentrations, most of the triglycerides are taken up by the "entry site", i.e. rapidly. With higher concentration this site becomes saturated and further uptake depends on the slower process of shifting the triglycerides from this site.

It seems likely that the reshuffle of triglycerides observed, which appears to have little to do with the metabolism of fatty acids and do not bring about any changes in the overall composition of the liver lipids, is related to the transport of these molecules from one site of the liver to another (from "entry site" to the site of synthesis of lipoproteins).

2. Synthesis of Triglycerides

The pathway of fatty acids esterification to triglycerides has been initially worked out with homogenates of liver, but has later been found to proceed on similar lines in all other tissues examined (see chapter I and IV). The incorporation of radiopalmitate into triglycerides by rat liver homogenates was found to depend on the presence of ATP (TIETZ and SHAPIRO 1956). This finding made it apparent that triglyceride synthesis is not brought above by the reversal of its degradation by lipolytic enzymes. It rather pointed to the necessity for an ATP dependent activation of the fatty acid to form fatty acyl — CoA. Such on activation has previously been shown by KORNBERG and PRICER (1953) to be necessary for esterification. They also showed that the acceptor for the fatty acid moiety is not free glycerol but L-α-glycerophosphate, giving as product phosphatidic acid. Glycerol can serve as precursor only when converted to α-glycerophate by a glycerokinase, present in liver, again requiring ATP (BUBLITZ and KENNEDY 1954). α-glycerophosphate can also be formed by the reduction of dihydroxy-acetone-phosphate, an intermediate of the glycolytic breakdown of sugars.

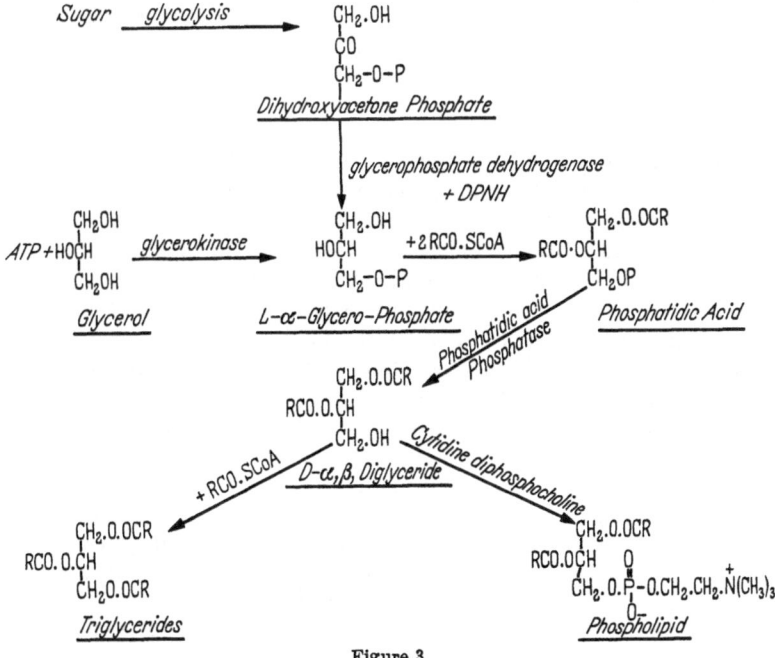

Figure 3.

α-glycerophosphate is also required in the synthesis of lipids which contain no phosphorus. It was shown to be essential for the formation of triglycerides by liver microsomes and mitochondria (Stein and Shapiro 1957, 1958; Stein, Tietz and Shapiro 1957; Tzur, Tal and Shapiro 1964).

These finding brought triglyceride synthesis in line with the synthesis of phospholipids, which was shown by Smith et al. (1957) to proceed by removal of the phosphate from phosphatidic acid, with the formation of an α : β-diglyceride. Diglyceride can now be converted into phospholipid, by cytidine-diphosphate-choline or ethanolamine (Kennedy and Weiss 1956) or into neutral triglycerides by the addition of one more fatty acid, derived from fatty acyl-coenzyme A. (Weiss and Kennedy 1956, 1960).

These results are summarized in figure 3.

3. Fatty Livers

Triglyceride accumulation in the liver (i.e. fatty livers) can be brought about by agents which will cause an increased synthesis of triglycerides, decreased oxidation, increased uptake of triglycerides or fatty acids from the blood, decreased secretion of triglycerides by the liver, or a combination of any of these factors.

It seems well established that fatty livers produced by starvation, diabetes or the administration of anterior pituitary hormones are primarily due to an increased mobilization of fatty acids from adipose tissue (see chapter III 2) (Barrett et al. 1938; Stetten and Salcedo 1944). The rate of hepatic triglyceride synthesis is directly proportional to the level of free fatty acids in the blood (Feigelson et al. 1961), and increased mobilization will therefore result in accelerated triglyceride synthesis.

The source of fatty livers due to deficiency of choline in the diet is much less clear. Choline is a constituent of lecithin and as such might be supposed to aid in phospholipid synthesis. It has actually been shown to increase the turnover rate of phospholipids in the liver, but did not cause any net increase in plasma and liver phospholipids. No increased secretion of phospholipids into the blood could be found, following choline administration to deficient rats (Entenman et al. 1946; Zilversmit and Diluzio 1958). The relationship between increased synthesis of phospholipids in the liver and the action of choline on the prevention and cure of fatty livers ("lipotropic action") is not at all clear.

In addition to this effect choline seems to have an accelerating effect on fatty acid oxidation (Artom 1958). The mechanism of this action is unknown, nor is it clear whether the quantitative effect on fatty acid oxidation could explain the accumulation of fat in the liver of choline deficient animals.

Choline can be replaced by other substances capable of donating methyl groups, such as methionine or betaine. Similarly vitamin B_{12}, a factor in the synthesis of methyl groups, also has a lipotropic effect when administered together with homocysteine (Bennett et al. 1951).

Fatty livers are also formed, in the presence of adequate choline, by diets deficient in amino acids other than methionine. This has been shown for threonine (Singal et al. 1954) lysine and tryptophan (Vennart et al. 1958). Threonine deficiency, like choline deficiency, also leads to an increased synthesis of fatty acid from acetate (Yoshida and Harper 1960). An increase in synthesis has also been observed when cystine is added to a low protein diet. The relative importance of these effects for the formation of fatty livers is still uncertain.

Fatty livers can be induced by the administration of ethionine (Farber et al. 1950; Wells 1958). This effect can be counteracted by the simultaneous administration of methionine but not of choline. Ethionine feeding caused reduction of the plasma lipid and lipoprotein levels (FEINBERG et al. 1954). This led to the assumption that ethionine interferes with the synthesis of lipoproteins which are required for the secretion of the triglycerides by the liver. In agreement with this it could be shown that protein as well as phospholipid synthesis was inhibited (HARRIS and ROBINSON 1961). As the livers of ethionine treated animals readily take up chylomicra and esterify free fatty acids normally, ethionine seems to produce a congested liver, which cannot synthesize lipoproteins and is unable to secrete the fat into the circulation (BORGSTRÖM et al. 1961; OLIVECRONA 1962c).

According to recent papers, the action of liver poisons like carbon tetrachloride and white phosphorus in the induction of fatty livers is similar to that indicated for ethionine. Here too the fatty liver is associated with low plasma lipid levels. A short time after the injection of carbon tetrachloride into the animal, marked dilatations of the cysternae of the endoplasmic reticulum are discernable (SMUCKLER and BENDITT 1963). This is the site of protein and lipoprotein synthesis and of the presumed triglyceride secretory mechanism (BYERS and FRIEDMAN 1960). RECKNAGEL and LOMBARDI (1961) have suggested that this structure is the key focus of carbon tetrachloride action and its destruction the cause of fat accumulation.

This hypothesis is in accord with the findings of MALING et al. (1962) that upon injection of $1-^{14}C$-palmitate to a carbon tetrachloride treated rat, the labelled triglycerides appearing in the blood are much less radioactive than in normal rats. Using an isolated perfused liver, HEIMBERG et al. (1962a) found a decrease in the triglyceride release into the perfusate, when CCl_4 is added. A block in lipoprotein synthesis in livers of carbon tetrachloride treated rats has been demonstrated by SEAKINS and ROBINSON (1963) and by AIYAR et al. (1964).

In this connection it is of interest that several other substances, known to interfere with protein synthesis, also cause fatty livers. Thus, administration of puromycin produces a fatty liver together with a decreased plasma lipoprotein level (ROBINSON and SEAKINS 1962). Orotic acid, which interferes with the normal formation of hepatic nucleotides and thus may affect protein synthesis, also causes fatty livers with low plasma lipoproteins (STANDERFER and HANDLER 1955; CREASEY et al. 1961).

On the other hand, the ethiology of fatty livers caused by alcohol is still debated and manifold effects of alcohol have been reported. In man a fatty liver can result from acute or chronic ethanol ingestion. In the rat a single dose of ethanol or the chronic administration causes an increase in liver lipids (DILUZIO 1958; MALLOV 1955). MALLOV (1961) demonstrated an increased mobilization of free fatty acids from the depots, caused by alcohol administration. On the other hand, SCHAPIRO et al. (1964) showed in the perfused liver, that addition of ethanol to the perfusate decreased the secretion of neutral glycerides by the liver. However, with ethanol no decrease in protein synthesis could be shown (SEAKINS and ROBINSON 1964), and normal or elevated plasma lipids were found.

A case of increased release of triglycerides from the liver and a rise in plasma lipoprotein levels is found in the nephrotic syndrome. This seems to be brought about by increased lipoprotein formation in the liver (MARSH and DRABKIN 1960).

IV. Metabolism of Triglycerides in Adipose Tissue

1. Deposition of Triglycerides

The final site of deposition of dietary fatty acids, as well as the quantitatively major source of triglyceride reserves in the body is adipose tissue. It is by now well established that this tissue is not merely an inert pool of stored fat, but is one of the major centers of activity, as far as fat metabolism, synthesis, storage and mobilization is concerned. Most metabolic functions found in other body tissues can also be shown to occur in adipose tissue, but the enzymatic systems involved in fatty acid metabolism are especially active. This enzymatic outfit is in line with the adaptation of adipose tissue to perform its specific physiological function of store and source of fatty acids (see Kinsell 1962 and Rohdall 1963).

A considerable part of the fat ingested is deposited in adipose tissue. Using fat with labelled fatty acids, this was found to be true even when the animal is in caloric deficit and a net decrease in stored fatty acids takes place. Inflow and outflow go on continuously (Schönheimer and Rittenberg 1935; Bernhard and Steinhauser 1943).

As stated before, fatty acids from the digestive tract appear in the blood circulation as triglycerides in chylomicra. Although these are primarily taken up by the liver, a considerable part ends up in adipose tissue. Thus, Reiser et al. (1960) found that 6 hours following oral ingestion of tripalmitin, labelled both in the glycerol and in the fatty acid part, adipose tissue contained ten times more labelled palmitic acid than the liver. However, very little of the glycerol part of the ingested tripalmitin appeared in adipose tissue and had presumably been removed by the liver during the reshuffle of the triglycerides and formation of the lipoprotein (see III_1). It is from the serum lipoproteins that adipose tissue must have taken up most of its fatty acids.

Not all of the chylomicron triglycerides have to pass through the liver and recycle in the blood as lipoproteins, in order to be incorporated in adipose tissue. A part of the chylomicron triglycerides may be taken up directly. This depends on the nutritional state of the animal. When fatty acid labelled chylomicra are injected into a fasting animal only small amounts can be discovered in adipose tissue, short intervals after the injection. However, if this experiment is performed with a carbohydrate fed animal, as much as 25% can be found in adipose tissue after short periods (Bragdon and Gordon 1958).

The mechanism of penetration of chylomicron or of lipoprotein triglycerides into adipose tissue has been the subject of many investigations. It seems established that partial or complete hydrolysis of the triglycerides and resynthesis of new triglycerides takes place prior to their final deposition in the fat droplet of the adipose cells. This process of hydrolysis and synthesis most likely facilitates the transport of the triglycerides from the blood to the fat droplets. It is, however, still debated where this hydrolysis takes place. Is it outside the adipose cells, in the vascular space or at the capillary endothelium, or in a special part of the adipose cell from which it is transported by reshuffling of the triglyceride fatty acids, as seems to be the case in the liver ?

Experiments, performed to solve this problem, in which triglycerides are injected in vivo are difficult to interpret, as the exchange of triglyceride fatty acids of the plasma with those of the liver is much more rapid than any net uptake by adipose tissue. (Carlson and Ekeland 1963). As a result, most of the triglycerides appearing in adipose tissue have previously gone through the reshuffle of fatty acids in the liver, and have lost most of their original glycerol moiety. When triglycerides labelled in both their glycerol and their fatty acid were injected (Borgström and Jordan 1959), three times as much fatty acid appeared in adipose tissue than glycerol. This may be interpreted that at least one third of the triglycerides were taken up directly by adipose tissue without going through the liver and without prior total hydrolysis, since any free glycerol formed would not be reincorporated into adipose tissue triglycerides (see chapter 4b). In a similar set of experiments, but analyzing the tissues short times after the injection of doubly labelled triglycerides, OLIVECRONA (1962a), found 10% of the fatty acids with equivalent amounts of glycerol in the adipose tissue triglycerides. Only later did the radioglycerol content of the triglycerides decrease in comparison with the radiofatty acids. This behaviour, which is similar to that occurring in the liver (see chapter 3a), points to the conclusion that here too a reshuffling of the triglycerides in the tissue takes place prior to the final deposition in the fat droplets.

Studies in vitro with pieces of adipose tissue incubated in saline solution containing triglyceride emulsions or in serum corroberate the above assumption. Only triglycerides or free fatty acids are taken up from lipid mixtures, while phospholipids cholesterol are left in the medium (STERN and SHAPIRO 1954). The process of triglyceride uptake was dependant on metabolic processes of the tissue. It was abolished by heating the tissue to 60° C, decelerated by lowering the temperature of incubation and by poisoning with cyanide or fluoride (SHAPIRO, WEISSMANN, BENTOR and WERTHEIMER 1948, 1952). Free fatty acids can also be taken up. This uptake is followed by rapid esterification to triglycerides (SHAPIRO, CHOWERS and ROSE 1957).

These findings make it probable that disruption and resynthesis of the ester bonds play a role at some phase of the facilitated transport of triglycerides into the adipose tissue cells. It is, however, not yet settled where these processes take place. Lipoprotein lipase has been implicated in this process. A lipoprotein lipase, similar to that appearing in blood following heparin injection, has been extracted from adipose tissue (KORN 1955a) and is released into the medium when adipose tissue is incubated in a solution containing heparin (HOLLENBERG 1959; CHERKES and GORDON 1959; ROBINSON 1960).

The nutritional conditions inducing activity of the lipoprotein lipase released by the tissue coincide with those increasing triglyceride uptake (BRAGDON and GORDON 1958; HAVEL, FELTS and VAN DUYNE 1962; BEZMAN, FELTS and HAVEL 1962). However, this correlation is far from complete. Poisons which are effective lipoprotein lipase inhibitors did not interfere with the uptake of triglycerides, while others which have no effect on the enzyme caused substantial reduction of uptake (MARKSCHEID and SHAFRIR 1963).

Even if we accept the evidence that lipoprotein lipase participates in triglyceride uptake, it is not yet established where the site of the lipolytic process is. Is it the intravascular space where the enzyme was first discovered, at the capillary membrane as suggested by (ROBINSON and FRENCH 1960) or in the adipose cell itself, where most of the enzyme was shown to be located (RODBELL 1964).

Experiments with isolated adipose tissue which is incubated with labelled triglycerides point to the conclusion that the process of assimilation of triglycerides proceeds in two phases. An initial rapid uptake, insensitive to poisons of lipoprotein lipase, is followed by a slower, sensitive phase. It is this second phase in which hydrolysis and resynthesis takes place, as indicated by changes in the triglyceride fatty acids (RODBELL 1960) in the glycerol to fatty acid ratios of radioactivity (ROSE and SHAPIRO 1960) and by shift of the labelled triglycerides from one compartment to another (MARKSCHEID and SHAFRIR 1964). If lipoprotein lipase participates in the uptake, it is presumably at a site not accessible to the poisons in the medium.

As in the other tissues, so far discussed, triglyceride assimilation by adipose tissue is carried out by initial uptake at a site in the tissue, followed by a facilitated transfer of the fat to other parts of the cells. This latter process involves hydrolysis and resynthesis of the triglycerides.

2. Mobilization of Triglycerides

Adipose tissue triglycerides are mobilized as their split products — fatty acids and glycerol. The identification of free fatty acids as the main form of transport of fat from adipose tissue has opened a completely new scope to our understanding of energy metabolism. The elevation of this minor plasma constituent to the rank of a major metabolite was made acceptable by the detection of its extremely rapid turnover. Half life times of approximately two minutes were reported for plasma free fatty acids. Free fatty acids are burnt in many organs and can supply a considerable portion of the metabolic energy of heart and skeletal muscle. A detailed discussion on the metabolism of free fatty acids has been published (FREDRICKSON and GORDON 1958).

The rate of release of free fatty acids from the tissue is regulated by the nutrional state of the animal and by hormones. Starvation and injection of epinephrine increases fatty acid contration in the blood, whereas glucose and insulin have the opposite effect (DOLE 1956; GORDON and CHERKES 1957).

Evidence that adipose tissue is the source of the plasma free fatty acids has been obtained. Blood irrigating areas rich in adipose tissue become enriched with free fatty acids (GORDON and CHERKES 1957) while blood draining liver and cardiac muscle loose free fatty acids. The release of fatty acids from adipose tissue can be demonstrated by incubating pieces of the tissue in media containing serum albumin (RESHEF, SHAFRIR and SHAPIRO 1957, 1958; SHAPIRO 1957; GORDON and CHERKES 1958; WHITE and ENGEL 1958a).

The discharge of fatty acid from isolated tissue is stimulated by epinephrine and norepinephrine (GORDON and CHERKES 1957; WHITE and ENGEL 1958a), by ACTH and TSH (WHITE and ENGEL 1958b), by growth hormone (LEBOEUF and CAHILL 1961) and by glucagon (HAGEN 1961; VAUGHAN 1960). Detailed reviews on this aspect have recently appeared (WINEGRAD 1962; WERTHEIMER and SHAFRIR 1960; VAUGHAN 1961).

All the factors which increase free fatty acid concentrations in blood in vivo have also been shown to increase the release of the acid from the tissue into an albumin medium in vitro. These factors therefore, must exert their regulatory effect by direct action on adipose tissue.

Epinephrine, injected in vivo, exerts an effect on adipose tissue, which can still be revealed by the increased fatty acid mobilizing activity of the tissue, examined in vitro (RESHEF and SHAPIRO 1960). No increased release could be demonstrated in tissues of adrenalectomized animals, injected with epinephrine. Cortisone was also required to obtain this effect. The interdependance of epinephrine and cortical hormones was also shown in experiments in vivo. The elevation of plasma free fatty acids in dogs injected with epinephrine was abolished by adrenalectoncy or by hypophyzectomy (SHAFRIR, SUSSMAN and STEINBERG 1960).

Another hormonal interrelationship exists between epinephrine and thyroid hormone. Tissues of rats treated with propylthiouracyl released very little fatty acids and did not respond to the addition of epinephrine. Conversely, in tissues of rats treated with triiodothyronine both basal release and response to epinephrine were exaggerated (DEBONS and SCHWARTZ 1961; DEYKIN and VAUGHAN 1963). Release of free fatty acids by adipose tissue from rats treated with triiodothyronine or propylthiouracyl showed that the greater accumulation of fatty acids in the medium of tissues from triiodothyronine treated rats was at the expense of preformed tissue free fatty acids. The rates of both lipolysis and esterification were greater in these tissues so that no net change in total free fatty acids took place. However, the lipolytic system in tissues treated with triiodothyronine showed greater than normal response to epinephrine.

The release of fatty acids is also under control of the nervous system. Injection of dibenzylin, a sympathetic blocking agent, inhibited the subsequent release of acid by the tissues of fasting, diabetic, cold exposed or endotoxin treated rats (WERTHEIMER, HAMOSH and SHAFRIR 1960). Hexamethonium decreased the mobilization even in adrenalectomized dogs and must have acted on the sympathetic nerve endings in adipose tissue, and not on the humoral agent secreted by the adrenal medulla (HAVEL and GOLDFIEN 1960). Sympathetic blocking agents also abolished the release from tissues following epinephrine injections (SCHOTZ and PAGE 1960).

Very little preformed free fatty acids are present in adipose tissue and most of the release is due to lipolysis of the triglycerides. This can be seen from the concommitant release of free glycerol by the tissue (LEBOEUF, FLINN and CAHILL 1959; LYNN, MACLEOD and BROWN 1960; SHAFRIR 1960; VAUGHAN 1962).

Only a part of the fatty acids formed in adipose tissue are released, since a very effective resynthesis of triglycerides from free fatty acids takes place (SHAPIRO, CHOWERS and ROSE 1957). All the enzymes required for the resynthesis could be demonstrated in adipose tissue (ROSE and SHAPIRO 1961; STEINBERG et al. 1961). The mechanism of synthesis seems to be the same as that found for liver (see chapter III) with the exception that glycerol cannot be utilized and glycerophosphate is required. This is formed from glucose and glycogen and fatty acid release will therefore decrease when glucose metabolism is enhanced and increased when it is decelerated. The very extensive literature related to this topic has been recently reviewed (STEINBERG 1963).

As glycerol is utilized by adipose tissue to only limited extent (SHAPIRO, CHOWERS and ROSE 1957), glycerol release may serve as a convenient measure of total triglyceride lipolysis (VAUGHAN 1962; VAUGHAN and STEINBERG 1963; GORIN and SHAFRIR 1963).

The enzyme responsible for lipolytic release of fatty acids from adipose tissue triglycerides is most likely not lipoprotein lipase. The activity of this enzyme increases under conditions of maximum uptake but decreases when maximum release is induced (CHERKES and GORDON 1959; SALAMAN and ROBINSON 1961). Any function of lipoprotein lipase in the transport of fat would therefore be in the uptake and not in the release.

A lipase stimulated by epinephrine has been extracted from adipose tissue (RIZACK 1961). This lipase differed from lipoprotein lipase, being sensitive to fluoride, but little affected by EDTA, protamine, phosphate and NaCl. The activity of this enzyme increased during fasting. It thus seems to be the lipase which is responsible for the release of fatty acids from the tissue. According to RUBINSTEIN et al. (1964), the epinephrine sensitive lipase is located in the mitochondria of the adipose tissue homogenates. These authors, as well as VAUGHAN et al. (1964), found that other hormones, causing increased fatty acid release, also activate the lipase. The activity of the hormone sensitive lipase decreased during incubation of the tissue. The activity could be restored by treatment for 3 minutes with epinephrine, norepinephrine, ACTH, TSH ot glucagon. All these hormones are known to increase the phosphorylase activity of the tissue. The effects on phosphorylase are presumably mediated by cyclic 3', 5' adenosine monophosphate. It has recently been demonstrated by RIZACK (1964) that this substance also activates the lipolytic activity when incubated with epididymal fat together with ATP and Mg^{++}.

In addition to this lipase, which splits triglycerides rapidly to monoglycerides, similar to the pancreatic lipase, a specific monoglyceride lipase was found in adipose tissue. This enzyme is not affected by the hormones, but its activity seems

to be high enough to hydrolyze all the products formed by the triglyceride splitting lipase (Vaughan et al. 1964; Gobin and Shafrir 1964).

Prostaglandin E_1, a vasodepressor from seminal plasma, has been found to
counteract the fat mobilizing activities of the hormones, and the epinephrine
induced activation of the lipase in adipose tissue. Concentrations of $2.8 \times 10^{-7}M$
were effective (Steinberg et al. 1964).

The transport and metabolism of triglycerides following their absorption from
the intestine can be summarized in the following scheme.

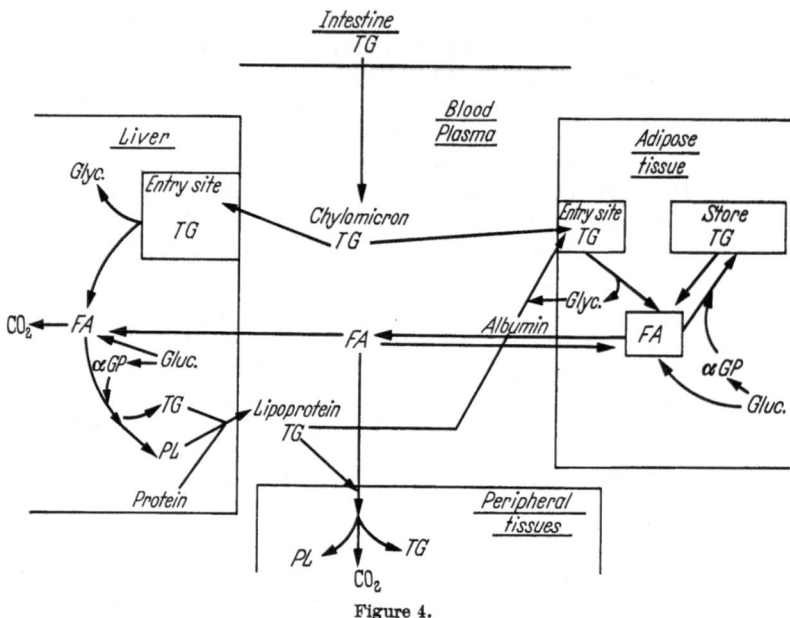

Figure 4.

References

Ailhaud, G., L. Sarda, and P. Desnuelle: Formation d'hydroxamates d'acides gras
à longues chaines par une fraction subcellulaire de muqueuse intestinale. Biochim. biophys.
Acta (Amst.) 59, 261 (1962).
Aiyar, A. S., P. Fatterpaker, and A. Sreenivasan: Lipid metabolism in liver injury caused
by carbon tetrachloride in the rat. Biochem. J. 90, 558 (1964).
Artom, C.: Role of choline in the hepatic oxidation of fat. Amer. J. clin. Nutr. 6, 221 (1958).
— G. Sarzana, C. Perrier, M. Santangelo, and E. Segré: Synthese des phospholipides o
cours de l'absorption des graisses. Arch. int. Physiol. 45, 32 (1937).
Barrett, H. M., C. H. Best, and J. H. Ridout: A study of the source of liver fat using
deuterium as an indicator. J. Physiol. (Lond.) 93, 367 (1938).
Bennet, H. S., J. H. Luft, and J. C. Hampton: Morphological classification of vertebrate
blood capillaries. Amer. J. Physiol. 196, 381 (1959).
Bennett, M. A., J. Joralemon, and P. E. Halpern: The effect of vitamin B_{12} on rat growth
and fat infiltration of the liver. J. biol. Chem. 193, 285 (1951).
Bergstöm, G., and B. Borgström: Intestinal absorption of fats. Progr. in the Chemistry of
Fats and other Lipids. 3, 352 (1955).
Bergström, S., B. Borgström, and M. Rottenberg: Intestinal Absorption and Distribution
of Fatty Acids and glycerides in the Rat. Acta phys. Sci. 25, 120 (1952).
Bernard, C.: Mémoire sur le Pancréas et la Rôle du Suc Pancréatique dans les Phénomènes
Digestifs particulièrement dans la Digestion des Matières Grasses Neutres. Paris: Bailliere
1856.
Bernhard, K., and H. Steinhauser: Fettstoffwechsel-Untersuchungen mit Deuterium als
Indikator. III. Lipid Synthese bei Inanition. Helv. chim. Acta 27, 12 (1943).

BERNHARD, K., H. WAGNER, and J. RITZEL: Versuche zur quantitativen Erfassung bei der Resorption von Neutralfett eintretenden Spaltung. Helv. chim. Acta **35**, 1404 (1952).

BEZMAN, A., I. M. FELTS, and R. S. HAVEL: Relation between incorporation of triglyceride fatty acids and heparin-released lipoprotein lipase from adipose tissue slices. J. Lipid. Res **3**, 427 (1962).

BIERMAN, E. L., and J. T. HAMLIN (1962), cited by DOLE and HAMLIN: Particulate fat in lymph and blood. Physiol. Rev. **42**, 674 (1962).

BLOOM, B., I. L. CHAIKOFF, and W. O. REINHARDT: Intestinal lymph as pathway for transport of absorbed fatty acids of different chain length. Amer. J. Physiol. **166**, 451 (1951).

BLOOMSTRAND, R., N. A. THORN, and E. H. AHRENS jr.: The absorption of fats, studied in a patient with chyluria. I. Clinical investigation. Amer. J. Med. **24**, 958 (1958).

BOLLMAN, J. L., J. C. CAIN, and J. H. GRINDLEY: Techniques for the collection of lymph from the liver, small intestine, or thoracic duct of the rat. J. Lab. clin. Med. **33**, 1349 (1948).

BORGSTRÖM, B.: On the mechanism of intestinal fat absorption. Acta physiol. scand. **25**, 140 (1952).

— On the mechanism of pancreatic lipolysis of glycerides. Biochim. biophys. Acta (Amst.) **13**, 491 (1954).

— Randomization of glyceride glycerol during absorption from the small intestine at the rat. J. biol. Chem. **214**, 671 (1955a).

— Transport of ^{14}C-decanoic acid in porta and inferior vena cava blood during absorption in the rat. Acta physiol. scand. **34**, 71 (1955b).

— In Lipide Metabolism, p. 128, Metabolism of glycerides. Ed. K. BLOCH. New York: John Wiley & Sons, Inc. 1960.

— Absorption of triglycerides. In Lipid Transport, Ed. H. C. MENG, p. 15. Springfield (Ill.:) Thomas 1964.

— A. DAHLQVIST, G. LUNDH, and J. SJÖVALL: Studies of intestinal digestion and absorption in the human. J. clin. Invest. **36**, 1521 (1957a).

— and A. F. HOFMANN: Hydrolysis of micellar solutions of long chain monoglycerides by pancreatic lipase. Biochemical Problems of Lipids, Ed. A. C. FRAZER. Amsterdam: Elsevier 1963.

— and P. JORDAN: Metabolism of chylomicron glycerides as studied by C^{14} glycerol-H^{3}palmitic acid labeled chylomicrons. Acta Soc. Med. upsalien. **64**, 185 (1959).

— C. NAITO, and T. OLIVERCRONA: Effect of ethionine on the metabolism of chylomicrons in the rat. Biochem. Pharmacol. **8**, 141 (1961).

— N. TRYDING, and G. WESTÖÖ: On the extent of hydrolysis of triglyceride ester bonds in the lumen of human small intestine during digestion. Acta physiol. scand. **40**, 241 (1957b).

BRAGDON, J. H., and R. S. GORDON: Tissue distribution of C^{14} after the intravenous injection of labeled chylomicrons and unesterified fatty acids in the rat. J. clin. Invest. **37**, 574 (1958).

— and R. J. HAVEL: In vivo effects of anti-heparin agents on serum lipids and lipoproteins. Amer. J. Physiol. **177**, 128 (1954).

BROWN, J. L., and J. M. JOHNSTON: The mechanism of intestinal utilization of monoglycerides. Biochim. biophys. Acta (Amst.) **84**, 448 (1964).

BROWN, W. D.: Reversible effects of anticoagulants and protamine in alimenraty lipemia. Quart. J. exp. Physiol. **37**, 75 (1952).

BUBLITZ, C., and E. P. KENNEDY: Synthesis of phosphatides in isolated mitochondria. J. biol. Chem. **221**, 951 (1954).

BURACK, W. R., J. PRYCE, and J. F. GOODWIN: A reversible nephrotic syndrome associated with congestive heart failure. Circulation **18**, 562 (1958).

BYERS, S. O., and M. FRIEDMAN: Site of origin of plasma triglycerides. Amer. J. Physiol. **198**, 629 (1960).

CARLSON, L. A., and L. G. EKELAND: Splanchnic production and uptake of endogenous triglycerides in the fasting state in man. J. clin. Invest. **42**, 714 (1963).

— and L. B. WADSTROEM: Studies on glycerides during the clearing reaction. Clin. chim. Acta **2**, 9 (1957).

CHERKES, A., and R. S. GORDON jr.: The liberation of lipoprotein lipase by heparin from adipose tissue incubated in vitro. J. Lipid. Res. **1**, 97 (1959).

CLARK, B., and G. HÜBSCHER: Biosynthesis of glycerides in the mucosa of the small intestine. Nature (Lond.) **185**, 35 (1960).

— — Biosynthesis of glycerides in subcellular fractions of intestinal mucosa. Biochim. biophys. Acta (Amst.) **46**, 479 (1961).

— — Glycerokinase in mucosa of the small intestine of the cat. Nature (Lond.) **195**, 599 (1962).

COLEMAN, R., and G. HÜBSCHER: Metabolism of phospholipids V. Studies of phosphatidic acid phosphatase. Biochem. biophys. Acta (Amst. **56**, 479 (1962).

CREASEY, W. A., L. HANKINS, and R. E. HANDSCHUMACHER: Fatty liver produced by orotic acid. I. Accumulation and metabolism of lipids. J. biol. Chem. **236**, 2064 (1961).

DAWSON, A. M., and K. Y. ISSELBACHER: The esterification of palmitate 1-C^{14} by homogenates of intestinal mucosa. J. clin. Invest. **39**, 150 (1960).

DEBONS, A. F., and I. L. SCHWARTZ: Dependence of the lipolytic action of epinephrine in vitro upon thyroid hormone. J. Lipid. Res. **2**, 86 (1961).

DESNUELLE, P.: Pancreatic lipase. Advanc. Enzymol. **23**, 129 (1961).

DEYKIN, D., and H. VAUGHAN: Release of free fatty acids by adipose tissue from rats treated with triiodothyronine or propylthiouracyl. J. Lipid. Res. **4**, 200 (1963).

DILUZIO, N. R.: Effect of acute ethanol intoxication on liver and plasma lipid fractions of the rat. Amer. J. Physiol. **194**, 453 (1958).

— Reticuloendothelial involvement in lipid metabolism. Ann. N. Y. Acad. Sci. **88**, 244 (1960).

DOLE, V. P.: A relation between non-esterified fatty acids in plasma and the metabolism of glucose. J. clin. Invest. **35**, 150 (1956).

— and J. T. HAMLIN: Particulate fat in lymph. and blood. Physiol. Rev. **42**, 674 (1962).

ENGELBERG, H.: Correlation of plasma heparin levels with serum lipoproteins. Acta med. scand. **151**, 161 (1955).

— Plama heparin levels in man following intravenous fat emulsions Circulation. **16**, 481 (1957).

— Human endogenous plasma lipemia clearing activity after intravenous fat emulsions. J. appl. Physiol. **12**, 292 (1958a).

— Human endogenous plasma lipemia clearing activity. J. appl. Physiol. **13**, 375 (1958b).

— Heparin lipemia clearing reaction and fat transport in man. Amer. J. clin. Nutr. 8, 21 (1960).

ENTENMAN, C., I. L. CHAIKOFF, and H. D. FRIEDLANDER: The influence of injected choline upon choline-containing and non-containing phospholipids of the liver as measured by radioactive phosphorus. J. biol. Chem. **162**, 111 (1946).

FARBER, E., M. V. SIMPSON, and H. TORVER: Studies on ethionine. II. The interference with lipid metabolism. J. biol. Chem. **182**, 91 (1950).

FAVARGER, P., R. A. COLLET, and E. CHERBULIEZ: Etude de la résorption intestinale des graisses a l'aide de deutero-glycerol et d'acides gras marqués. Helv. chim. Acta **34**, 1641 (1951).

FEIGELSON, E. B., W. W. PFAFF, A. KARMEN, and D. STEINBERG: The role of plasma free fatty acids in development of fatty liver. J. clin. Invest. **40**, 2171 (1961).

FEINBERG, H., L. RUBIN, R. HILL, C. ENTENMAN, and I. L. CHAIKOFF: Reduction of serum lipides and lipoproteins by ethionine feeding in the dog. Science **120**, 317 (1954).

FERNANDES, J., J. H. VAN DE KAMER, and H. A. WEIJERS: The absorption of fats studied in a child with chylothorax. J. clin. Invest. **34**, 1026 (1955).

— — Differences in absorption of the various fatty acids studied in children with steatorrhea. J. clin. Invest. **41**, 488 (1962).

FRAZER, A. C.: Absorption of triglyceride fat from the intestine. Physiol. Rev. **26**, 103 (1946).

FREDRICKSON, D. S., and R. S. GORDON jr.: Transport of fatty acids. Physiol. Rev. **38**, 585 (1958).

— K. ONO, and A. CHERKES: The metabolism of albumin bound C^{14}-labelled unesterified fatty acids in normal human subjects. J. clin. Invest. **37**, 1504 (1958a).

— D. L. MCCOLLESTER, and K. ONO: The role of UFA transport in chylomicron metabolism. J. clin. Invest. **37**, 1333 (1958b).

FRENCH, J. E.: The behaviour of chylomicrons in the circulation. Biochemical Problems of Lipids p. 296, Ed. A. C. FRAZER. Amsterdam: Elsevier 1963.

— and B. MORRIS: The removal of ^{14}C-labelled chylomicron fat from the circulation in rats. J. Physiol. (Lond.) **138**, 326 (1957).

— — The tissue distribution and oxidation of ^{14}C labelled chylomicron fat injected intra venously in rats. J. Physiol. (Lond.) **140**, 262 (1958).

FRIEDMAN, M. S., S. O. BYERS, and R. H. ROSENMAN: Observations concerning the production and excretion of cholesterol in mammals. Amer. J. Physiol. **177**, 77 (1954).

GAGE, S. H., and P. A. FISH: Fat digestion, absorption and assimilation in man and animals as determined by the dark-field microscope and a fat soluble dye. Amer. J. Anat. **34**, 1 (1924).

GITLIN, D., and D. CORNWELL: Plasma lipoprotein metabolism in normal individuals and nephrotic children. J. clin. Invest. **35**, 706 (1956).

GORDON jr., R. S., and A. CHERKES: Unesterified fatty acid in human plasma. J. clin. Invest. **35**, 206 (1957).

— — Production of unesterified acids from isolated adipose tissue incubated in vitro. Proc. Soc. exp. Biol. (N. Y.) **97**, 150 (1958).

GORIN, E., and E. SHAFRIR: Turnover of adipose tissue triglycerides measured by the rates of synthesis and release of triglyceride glycerol. Biochim. biophys. Acta (Amst.) **70**, 109 (1963).

— — Lipolytic activity in adipose tissue homogenates towards tri-di and monoglycerides. Biochim. biophys. Acta (Amst.) **84**, 24 (1964).

GROSSMAN, H. I., H. C. MÖLLER, and L. PALM: Effect of lipemia and heparin on free fatty acid concentration in serum in humans. Proc. Soc. exp. Biol. (N. Y.) 90, 106 (1955).

GRUNER, A., K. HILDEN, and T. HILDEN: The effect of heparin and protamine sulfate on the occurrence of chylomicrons in human blood. J. clin. Lab. Invest. 5, 241 (1953).

HÄSSLER, H. A., and K. Y. ISSELBACHER: Glycerol metabolism in the intestinal mucosa and its role in fat absorption. Amer. J. Dis. Child. 104, 543 (1962).

HAGEN, J. H.: Effect of hormones on phosphorylase activity in adipose tissue. J. biol. Chem. 236, 1023 (1961).

HAHN, P. F.: Abolishment of alimentary lipemia following injection of heparin. Science 98, 19 (1943).

HAMOSH, M., and B. SHAPIRO: Lipid release by liver slices. Amer. J. Physiol. 201, 1030 (1961).

HARRIS, P. M., and D. S. ROBINSON: Ethionine administration in the rat. 1. Effect on the liver and plasma lipids and on the disposal of dietary fat. Biochem. J. 80, 352 (1961).

HAVEL, R. J.: Evidence for the participation of lipoprotein lipase in the transport of chylomicrons. Proc. 3rd. Intern. Confer. on Biochemical Problems of Lipids, p. 265. Brussels: Erasmus, Ledeberg, Ghent 1956.

— I. M. FELTS, and C. M. VAN DUYNE: Formation and fate of endogenous triglycerides in blood plasma of the rabbit. J. Lipid Res. 3, 297 (1962).

— and D. S. FREDRICKSON: The metabolism of chylomicra. I. The removal of palmitic acid-1-14C labeled chylomicra from dog plasma. J. clin. Invest. 35, 1025 (1956).

— and A. GOLDFIEN: The role of the sympathetic nervous system in the metabolism of free fatty acids. J. Lipid. Res 1, 102 (1960).

HEIMBERG, M., H. C. MENG, and C. R. PARK: Effect of fasting and alloxan diabetes on the uptake of neutral fat by isolated perfused rat liver. Amer. J. Physiol. 195, 673 (1958a).

— — and D. BRADLEY: Effect of adrenocortical and hypophysial hormones on uptake of fat by isolated perfused liver. Amer. J. Physiol. 195, 678 (1958b).

— I. WEINSTEIN, G. DISHMON, and A. DUNKERLEY: The action of CCl₄ on the transport and metabolism of triglycerides and fatty acid by the isolated perfused rat liver and its relation to the ethiology of fatty liver. J. biol. Chem. 237, 3623 (1962a).

— — H. KLAUSNER, and M. L. WATKINS: Release and uptake of triglycerides by isolated perfused rat liver. Amer. J. Physiol. 202, 353 (1962b).

HILLYARD, L. A., C. E. CORNELIUS, and I. L. CHAIKOFF: Removal by the isolated rat liver of palmitate-1-C14 bound to albumin and of palmitate-1-C14 and cholesterol-4-C14 in chylomicrons from perfusion fluid. J. biol. Chem. 234, 2240 (1959).

HOFMANN, A. F.: The behaviour and solubility of monoglycerides in dilute micellar bile salt solution. Biochim. biophys. Acta (Amst.) 70, 306 (1963).

— and B. BORGSTRÖM: The intraluminar phase of fat digestion. J. clin. Invest. 43, 247 (1964).

HOLLENBERG, C. H.: Effect of nutrition on activity and release of lipase from rat adipose tissue. Amer. J. Physiol. 197, 667 (1959).

HÜBSCHER, G., B. CLARK, M. E. WEBB, and H. S. A. SHERRATT: Structural and enzymatic relationships in intestinal fat metabolism; In Biochemical Problems of Lipids, Ed. E. C. FRAZER, p. 209. Amsterdam-London-New York: Elsevier 1963.

ISELIN, B., and W. SCHULER: Über die Einwirkung von Heparin auf lipoprotein lipase aus Gewebe. Helv. physiol. Acta. 15, 14 (1957).

JEFFRIES, G. H.: The sites at which plasma clearing activity is produced and destroyed in the rat. Quart. J. exp. Physiol. 39, 261 (1954).

JOHNSTON, J. M.: An in vitro study of fatty acid absorption. Proc. Soc. exp. Biol. (N. Y.) 98, 836 (1958).

— The absorption of fatty acids by the isolated intestine. J. biol. Chem. 234, 1065 (1959).

— and J. H. BEARDEN: Phosphatidic acids as intermediates in fatty acid absorption. Arch. Biochem. 90, 57 (1960).

— — Intestinal phosphatidate phosphatase. Biochim. biophys. Acta (Amst.) 56, 365 (1962).

— and B. BORGSTRÖM: Intestinal uptake of micellar solutions of fatty acids and monoglycerides. Acta chem. scand. 17, 905 (1963).

— and J. L. BROWN: The intestinal utilization of doubly labelled α-monopalmitin. Biochim. biophys. Acta (Amst.) 59, 500 (1962).

JONES, H. B., J. W. GOFMAN, F. T. LINDGREN, T. P. LYON, D. M. GRAHAM, B. STRISOWER, and A. V. NICHOLS: Lipoprotein in atherosclerosis. Amer. J. Med. 11, 358 (1951).

KATES, M.: Lipolytic enzymes in lipide metabolism. Ed. K. BLOCK, p. 165. New York: Wiley 1960.

KAY, R. E., and C. ENTENMAN: The synthesis of "chylomicron like" bodies and maintenance of normal blood sugar levels by the isolated perfused rat liver. J. biol. Chem. 236, 1006 (1961).

KENNEDY, E. P., and S. B. WEISS: The function of cytidine coenzymes in the biosynthesis of phospholipides. J. biol. Chem. 222, 193 (1956).

Kinsell, L., editor: Adipose tissue an as organ. Springfield (Ill.): Thomas 1962.

Korn, E. D.: Clearing factor, a heparin-activated lipoprotein lipase. I. Isolation and characterization of the enzyme from normal rat heart. J. biol. Chem. 215, 1 (1955a).

— Clearing factor, a heparin-activated lipoprotein lipase. II. Substrate specificity and activation of coconut oil. J. biol. Chem. 215, 15 (1955b).

— and T. W. Quigley: Lipoprotein lipase of chicken adipose tissue. J. biol. Chem. 226, 833 (1957).

Kornberg, A., and W. E. Pricer, jr.: Enzymatic esterification of α-glycerophosphate by long chain fatty acids. J. biol. Chem. 204, 745 (1953).

Kyasu, J. Y., B. Bloom, and I. L. Chaikoff: The portal transport of fatty acids. J. biol. Chem. 199, 415 (1952).

Lacy, D., and A. B. Taylor: Fat absorption by epithelial cells of the small intestine of the rat. Amer. J. Anat. 110, 155 (1962).

Laurell, S.: Turnover rate of UFA in human plasma. Acta physiol. scand. 41, 158 (1957).

— Distribution of C^{14} in rats after intravenous injection of nonesterified palmitic acid 1-C^{14}. Acta physiol. scand. 46, 97 (1959a).

— Recycling of intravenously injected palmitic-1-C^{14} as esterified fatty acid in the plasma of rats and turnover rate of the plasma triglycerides. Acta physiol. scand. 47, 218 (1959b).

Leboeuf, B., and G. F. Cahill jr.: Studies on rat adipose tissue in vitro. VIII. Effect of preparations of pituitary adrenocorticotropic and growth hormone on glucose metabolism. J. biol. Chem. 236, 41 (1961).

— R. B. Flinn, and G. F. Cahill jr.: Effect of epinephrine on glucose uptake and glycerol release by adipose tissue in vitro. Proc. Soc. exp. Biol. (N. Y.) 102, 527 (1959).

Levy, S. W.: Heparin and blood lipids. Rev. canad. Biol. 17, 1 (1958).

Lynn, W. S., R. M. Macleod, and R. H. Brown: Effects of epinephrine, insulin and corticotrophin on the metabolism of rat adipose tissue. J. biol. Chem. 235, 1904 (1960).

Maling, H. M., A. Frank, and M. C. Horning: Effect of carbon tetrachloride on hepatic synthesis and release of triglycerides. Biochim. biophys. Acta (Amst.) 64, 540 (1962).

Mallov, S.: Effect of chronic ethanol intoxication on liver lipid content of rats. Proc. Soc. exp. Biol. (N. Y.) 88, 246 (1955).

— Effect of ethanol intoxication on plasma free fatty acids in the rat. Quart. J. Stud. Alcohol 22, 250 (1961).

Markscheid, L., and E. Shafrir: Assimilation of lipoprotein triglyceride in vitro: comparison of various adipose tissues and lipoproteins and effect of lipoprotein lipase inhibitors. Israel J. Chem. 1, 205 (1963).

— — Incorporation of lipoprotein borne triglycerides by adipose tissue. J. Lipid Res. 6, 247 (1965).

Marsh, J. B., and D. L. Drabkin: Experimental reconstruction of metabolic pattern of lipid nephrosis: key role of hepatic protein synthesis in hyperlipemia. Metabolism 9, 9466 (1960).

Mattson, F. H., and L. W. Beck: The specificity of pancreatic lipase for the primary hydroxyl groups of glycerides. J. biol. Chem. 219, 735 (1956).

— J. H. Benedict, J. B. Martin, and L. W. Beck: Intermediates formed during the digestion of triglycerides. J. Nutr. 48, 335 (1952).

— and R. A. Volpenhein: Rearrangement of glyceride fatty acids during digestion and absorption. J. biol. Chem. 237, 53 (1962).

McCandless, E. L., and D. B. Zilversmit: Fate of triglycerides and phospholipids of and artificial fat emulsions; disappearance from the circulation. Amer. J. Physiol. 193, 294 (1958).

Mead, J. F., and D. L. Fillerup: The transport of fatty acids in the blood. J. biol. Chem. 227, 1009 (1957).

Millington, P. F., and J. B. Finean: Electron microscopic studies of the structure of the microvilli on principal epithelial cells of rat jejunum after treatment in hypo- and hypertonic saline. J. Cell. Biol. 14, 125 (1962).

Morris, B., and J. E. French: The uptake and metabolism of ^{14}C labelled chylomicron fat by the isolated perfused liver of the rat. Quart. J. exp. Physiol. 43, 180 (1958).

Munk, I.: Zur Kenntnis der Bedeutung des Fettes und seiner Komponenten für den Stoffwechsel. Virchows Arch. Path. Anat. 80, 10 (1880).

— and A. Rosenstein: Zur Lehre von der Resorption im Darme nach Untersuchungen an einer Lymph (chylus)-fistel beim Menschen. Virchows Arch. Path. Anat. 123, 230, 484 (1891).

Nestel, P. J., R. J. Havel, and A. Bezman: Sites of initial removal of chylomicron triglyceride fatty acids from the blood. J. clin. Invest. 41, 1915 (1962).

Olivecrona, T.: Metabolism of chylomicrons labelled with C^{14}-glycerol-H^3 palmitic acid in the rat. J. Lipid Res. 3, 439 (1962a).

— The metabolism of 1-C^{14}-palmitic acid in the rat. Acta physiol. scand. 54, 295 (1962b).

OLIVECRONA, T.: The metabolism of 1-C¹⁴-palmitic acid in rats with ethionine induced fatty livers. Acta physiol. scand. **54**, 287 (1962c).
— E. P. GEORGE, and B. BORGSTRÖM: Chylomicron metabolism. Fed. Proc. **20**, 928 (1961).
PALAY, S. L., and J. P. REVEL: The morphology of fat absorption. In: Lipid transport, p. 33, Ed. H. C. MENG. Springfield (Ill.): Thomas 1964.
PFLÜGER, E.: Die Resorption der Fette vollzieht sich dadurch, daß sie in wäßrige Lösung gebracht werden. Arch. ges. Physiol. **86**, 1 (1901).
PIERCE, F. T. jr.: The interconversion of serum lipoprotein in vitro. Metabolism **3**, 142 (1954).
PLAYOUST, M. R., and K. Y. ISSELBACHER: Studies on the intestinal absorption and intramural lipolysis of a medium chain triglyceride. J. clin. Invest. **43**, 878 (1964).
RECKNAGEL, R. O., and B. LOMBARDI: Studies of biochemical changes in subcellular particles of rat liver and their relationship to a new hypothesis regarding the pathogenesis of CCl₄. J. biol. Chem. **236**, 564 (1961).
REISER, R., M. J. BRYSON, M. J. CARR, and K. A. KUIKEN: Intestinal absorption of triglycerides. J. biol. Chem. **194**, 131 (1952).
— M. C. WILLIAMS, and M. F. SORRELS: The transport and dynamic state of exogenous glycerol and palmitic acid labelled tripalmitin. J. Lipid Res. **1**, 241 (1960).
RESHEF, L., E. SHAFRIR, and B. SHAPIRO: Fat release from rat mesenteric tissue in vitro. Bull. Res. Coun. Israel E **6 A**, 306 (1957).
— — — In vitro release of unesterified fatty acids by adipose tissue. Metabolism **7**, 723 (1958).
— and B. SHAPIRO: Effect of epinephrine, cortisome and growth hormone on release of unesterified fatty acids by adipose tissue in vitro. Metabolism **9**, 551 (1960).
RIZACK, M. K.: An epinephrine sensitive lipolytic activity in adipose tissue J. biol. Chem. **236**, 657 (1961).
— Activation of adrenalin sensitive lipolytic activity from adipose tissue by adenosine 3′, 5′ phosphate. J. biol. Chem. **239**, 392 (1964).
ROBINSON, D. S.: The chemical composition of chylomicra in the rat. Quart. J. exp. Physiol. **40**, 112 (1955).
— The effect of changes in nutritional state on the lipolytic activity of rat adipose tissue. J. Lipid Res. **1**, 332 (1960).
— and J. E. FRENCH: The heparin clearing reaction and fat transport. Quart. J. exp. Physiol. **42**, 151 (1957).
— — Heparin the clearing factor lipase and fat transport. Pharmacol. Rev. **12**, 241 (1960).
— and P. M. HARRIS: The production of lipolytic activity in the circulation of the hind limb in response to heparin. Quart. J. exp. Physiol. **44**, 80 (1959).
— and A. SEAKINS: A development in the rat of fatty livers associated with reduced plasma-protein synthesis. Biochim. biophys. Acta (Amst.) **62**, 163 (1962).
RODBELL, M.: The removal and metabolism of chylomicrons by adipose tissue in vitro. J. biol. Chem. **235**, 1613 (1960).
— Location of lipoprotein lipase in fat cells of rat adipose tissue. J. biol. Chem. **239**, 753 (1964).
— R. O. SCOW, and S. CHERNICK: Removal and metabolism of triglycerides by perfused liver. J. biol. Chem. **239**, 385 (1964).
ROHDAL, K.; Editor: Fat as a tissue. New York: McGraw Hill 1963.
ROSE, G., and B. SHAPIRO: In Digestion, absorption intestinale et transport des glycérides chez les animaux supérieurs. Ed. P. DESNUELLE, Marseille, 1960. Studies in the mechanism of fat transport, by B. SHAPIRO. p. 165.
— — Enzyme systems in adipose tissue participating in fatty acid esterification. Bull. Res. Coun. Israel E **9 A**, 15 (1961).
ROSENMAN, R. H., M. FRIEDMAN, and S. O. BYERS: The causal role of plasma albumin deficiency in experimental nephrotic hyperlipemia and hypercholesterolemia. J. clin. Invest. **35**, 522 (1956).
RUBINSTEIN, D., S. CHIN, Y. NAYLOR, and J. C. BECK: Lipolytic activity of epinephrine in adipose tissue homogenates. Amer. J. Physiol. **206**, 149 (1964).
SALAMAN, M. R., and D. S. ROBINSON: The effect fasting on the clearing factor lipase activity of rat adipose tissue and plasma. In: The enzymes of lipid metabolism. p. 218. Ed. P. DESNUELLE. London: Pergamon Press 1961.
SAUNDERS, D. R., and A. M. DAWSON: Studies on the metabolism of glycerol by the small intestine in vitro and in vivo. Biochem. J. **82**, 477 (1962).
SAVARY, P., M. Y. CONSTATIN, and P. DESNUELLE: Sur la structure des triglycerides des chylomicrons lymphatiques du rat. Biochim. biophys. Acta (Amst.) **48**, 562 (1961).
— and P. DESNUELLE: Sur quelques éléments de specificité pendant l'hydrolyze enzymatique des triglycerides. Biochim. biophys. Acta (Amst.) **21**, 349 (1956).
SCHAPIRO, R. H., G. D. DRUMMEY, Y. SHIMIZU, and K. J. ISSELBACHER: Studies on the pathogenesis of ethanol induced fatty liver. J. clin. Invest. **43**, 1338 (1964).

Schmidt-Nielsen, K.: Investigations on the fat absorption in the intestine. Acta physiol. scand. 12 (Suppl. 37) (1946).

Schönheimer, R., and D. Rittenberg: Deuterium as an indicatior in the study of intermediary metabolism. J. biol. Chem. 111, 163 (1935).

Schotz, M. C., and J. H. Page: Effect of adrenergic blocking agents on the release of free fatty acid from rat adipose tissue. J. Lipid Res. 1, 466 (1960).

Seakins, A., and D. S. Robinson: The effect of administration of carbon tetrachloride on the formation of plasma lipoproteins. Biochem. J. 86, 401 (1963).

— — Changes associated with the production of fatty livers by white phosphorus and by ethanol in the rat. Biochem. J. 92, 308 (1964).

Senior, J. R., and K. Y. Isselbacher: Direct esterification of monoglycerides with palmityl coenzyme A by intestinal epithelial subcellular fractions. J. biol. Chem. 237, 1454 (1962).

— — Demonstration of an intestinal monoglyceride lipase: an enzyme with a possible role in the intracellular completion of fat digestion. J. clin. Invest. 42, 187 (1963).

Shafrir, E.: Release of glycerol during mobilization of unesterified fatty acids (UFA) from adipose tissue. Bull. Res. Coun. (Israel) E 9 A, 90 (1960).

— K. E. Sussman, and D. Steinberg: Role of the pituitary and adrenal in the mobilization of free fatty acids and lipoproteins. J. Lipid Res. 1, 459 (1960).

Shapiro, B.: Lipid dynamics in adipose tissue. Progr. Chem. Fats 4, 177 (1957).

— I. Chowers, and G. Rose: Fatty acid uptake and esterification in adipose tissue. Biochim. biophys. Acta (Amst.) 23, 115 (1957).

— D. Weissmann, V. Bentor, and E. Wertheimer: Active penetration of fat into adipose tissue. Nature (Lond.) 161, 482 (1948).

— — — Uptake of fat by adipose tissue in vitro. Metabolism 1, 396 (1952).

Sinclair, R. G.: The role of phospholipids of the intestinal mucosa in fat absorption. J. biol. Chem. 82, 117 (1929).

Singal, S. A., S. Hazan, V. P. Sydenstricker, J. M. Littlejohn: The effect of threonine deficiency on the synthesis of some phosphorus fractions in the rat. J. biol. Chem. 200, 875 (1953).

Smith, S. W., S. B. Weiss, and E. P. Kennedy: The enzymatic dephosphorylation of phosphatidic acids. J. biol. Chem. 228, 915 (1957).

Smuckler, E. A., and E. P. Benditt: CCl₄ poisoning in rats, alteration of ribosomes of the liver. Science 140, 308 (1963).

Spitzer, J. J.: Influence of protamine on alimentary lipemia. Amer. J. Physiol. 174, 43 (1953).

Standerfer, S. B., and P. Handler: Fatty liver induced by aortic acid feeding. Proc. Soc. exp. Biol. (N. Y.) 90, 270 (1955).

Stein, Y., and B. Shapiro: The synthesis of neutral glycerides by fractions of rat liver homogenates. Biochim. biophys. Acta (Amst.) 24, 197 (1957).

— — Glyceride synthesis by microsome fractions of rat liver. Biochim. biophys. Acta (Amst.) 30, 271 (1958).

— — Assimilation and dissimilation of fatty acids by the rat liver. Amer. J. Physiol. 196, 1238 (1959).

— — Uptake and metabolism of triglycerides by the rat liver. J. Lipid Res. 1, 326 (1960).

— A. Tietz, and B. Shapiro: Glyceride synthesis by rat liver mitochondria. Biochim. biophys. Acta (Amst.) 26, 286 (1957).

Steinberg, D.: Fatty acid mobilization. Mechanisms of regulation and metabolic consequences. In The Control of Lipid Metabolism, p. 111, Ed. J. K. Grant. New York: Academic Press 1963.

— M. Vaughan, and S. Margolis: Studies on triglyceride biosynthesis in homogenates of adipose tissue. J. biol. Chem. 236, 1931 (1961).

— — P. J. Nestel, D. Strand, and S. Bergström: Effects of prostaglandins on hormone induced mobilization of free fatty acids. J. clin. Invest. 43, 1533 (1964).

Stern, I., and B. Shapiro: The transport of lipids into adipose tissue. Metabolism 3, 39 (1954).

Stetten jr., D., and Y. Salcedo: The source of extra liver fat in various types of fatty liver. J. biol. Chem. 156, 27 (1944).

Swank, R. L., and S. W. Levy: Chyclomicron dissolution. Dosage and site of action of heparin. Amer. J. Physiol. 171, 208 (1952).

Tietz, A., and B. Shapiro: The synthesis of glycerides in liver homogenates. Biochim. biophys. Acta (Amst.) 19, 374 (1956).

Tzur, R., E. Tal, and B. Shapiro: Alpha-glycerophosphate as regulatory factor in fatty acid esterification. Biochim. biophys. Acta (Amst.) 84, 18 (1964).

Van de Kamer, J. H., and H. A. Weijers: Malabsorption syndrome. Fed. Proc. 20, (Suppl. 7) 335 (1961).

Van den Bosch, J., E. Evrard, A. Billiau, J. V. Jossens, and DeSomer: The role of liver and spleen in the metabolism of intravenously injected fat in rabbits. J. exp. Med. 114, 1035 (1961).

VAUGHAN, M.: Effect of hormones on phosphorylase activity in adipose tissue. J. biol. Chem. 235, 3049 (1960).
— The metabolism of adipose tissue in vitro. J. Lipid Res. 2, 293 (1961).
— The production and release of glycerol by adipose tissue incubated in vitro. J. biol. Chem. 237, 3354 (1962).
— J. E. BERGER, and D. STEINBERG: Hormone sensitive lipase and monoglyceride lipase activities in adipose tissue. J. biol. Chem. 239, 401 (1964).
— and D. STEINBERG: The effect of hormones on lipolysis and esterification of free fatty acids during incubation of adipose tissue in vitro. J. Lipid Res. 4, 193 (1963).
VENNART, G. P., V. P. PERNA, and W. B. STEWART: Fatty liver of portal type, cured by lysine plus tryptophan. J. Nutr. 61, 635 (1958).
VERZAR, F., and E. J. McDOUGALL: Absorption from the intestine. London: Longmans Green & Co. 1936.
WADDELL, M. R., R. P. GEYER, E. CLARKE, and F. J. SHARE: Function of the reticuloendothelial system in removal of emulsified fat from blood. Amer. J. Physiol. 177, 90 (1954).
WEISS, S. B., and E. P. KENNEDY: The enzymatic synthesis of triglycerides. J. Amer. chem. Soc. 78, 3550 (1956).
— — The enzymatic synthesis of triglycerides. J. biol. Chem. 235, 40 (1960).
WELLS, I. C.: Role of choline and methionine antagonists in metabolism. Amer. J. clin. Nutr. 6, 254 (1958).
WERTHEIMER, E., M. HAMOSH, and E. SHAFRIR: Factors affecting fat mobilization from adipose tissue. Amer. J. clin. Nutr. 8, 705 (1960).
— and E. SHAFRIR: Influence of hormones on adipose tissue as a center of fat metabolism. Progr. Hormone Res. 16, 467 (1960).
WHITE, Y. E., and F. L. ENGEL: A lipolytic action of epinephrine and norepinephrine on rat adipose tissue in vitro. Proc. Soc. exp. Biol. (N. Y.) 99, 375 (1958a).
— — Lipolytic action of corticotropin on rat adipose tissue in vitro. J. clin. Invest. 37, 1556 (1958b).
WINEGRAD, A. I.: Endocrine effects on adipose tissue metabolism. Vitam. and Horm. 20, 141 (1962).
YOSHIDA, A., and A. E. HARPER: Effect of threonine and choline deficiency on the metabolism of C^{14} labelled acetate and palmitate in the intact rat. J. biol. Chem. 235, 2586 (1960).
ZILVERSMIT, D. B., and N. R. DILUZIO: The role of choline in the turnover of phospholipids. Amer. J. clin. Nutr. 6, 235 (1958).

Biochemistry of Steroids

By

David Kritchevsky*

Introduction

Any discussion of the biochemistry of steroids must, of necessity, center upon the many aspects of the biochemistry of cholesterol. By nature of its prevalence in the mammalian body and its central position as a precursor of bile acids and steroid hormones, cholesterol is, biochemically, the most important steroid. Because of its wide distribution and its involvement in atherosclerotic heart disease and its *sequelae*, cholesterol has been the most widely studied of all biologically occurring steroids. The ensuing discussion will be concerned primarily with this sterol.

I. Biosynthesis

1. The Biosynthesis of Cholesterol

Historically, work on the biosynthesis of cholesterol was initiated by the studies of DEZANI (1913), who observed in balance experiments the synthesis of cholesterol in rats maintained on a cholesterolfree diet. This work was followed by similar experiments in other species (BEUMER and LEHMANN, 1923; DAM, 1930; DIRSCHERL and TRAUT, 1939). SCHOENHEIMER and BREUSCH (1933) were the first workers to attempt quantitation of cholesterol biosynthesis in intact animals, and they reported that mice maintained on bread synthesized about 1.8 mg of cholesterol daily. However, the first studies which would demonstrate the chemical nature of cholesterol biosynthesis — and which would culminate in an almost complete elucidation of the biosynthetic pathway — became possible with the availability of isotopes and of isotopically labeled compounds. RITTENBERG and SCHOENHEIMER (1937) found that cholesterol isolated from mice maintained on deuterium enriched water showed an inordinately high concentration of this isotope. Further experiments showed a direct relationship between the deuterium content of the body fluids and amount of this isotope in the isolated cholesterol. They concluded that the cholesterol is synthesized by the coupling of a number of small molecules. SONDERHOFF and THOMAS (1937) found that when yeast was grown in a medium containing trideuterioacetic acid a large excess of deuterium was present in the unsaponifiable fraction, which is primarily ergosterol. These observations led to the recognition that acetic acid is an important precursor of steroids, and the actual work on the biosynthetic pathways of steroids and polyisoprenoids had begun.

BLOCH and RITTENBERG (1942a, b) found that when deuterium-labeled acetate was fed to rats and mice the cholesterol isolated from these animals contained more deuterium than would be expected if the acetate had first been converted to water or to higher fatty acids. It was apparent that the administered deuterio-

* Supported, in part, by a Research Career Award (HE-K 6-734) and a grant (HE-03299) from the National Heart Institute, N. I. H., U. S. P. H. S.

acetate had been used directly in the biosynthetic process. The deuterium-labeled cholesterol obtained in these experiments was converted to cholesteryl chloride, and this compound was degraded by pyrolysis to yield a mixture of isooctane and isooctene (representing the side chain) and a hydrocarbon $C_{19}H_{30}$, representing the nucleus. Both pyrolytic fractions contained deuterium.

Further experiments using acetic acid labeled in the carboxyl group with ^{13}C and in the methyl group with deuterium showed conclusively that both carbon atoms of acetate participate in cholesterol biosynthesis (RITTENBERG and BLOCH, 1944, 1945). Subsequent experiments by LITTLE and BLOCH (1950) carried out with $^{14}CH_3{}^{13}COOH$ and $^{13}CH_3{}^{14}COOH$ showed that all 27 carbon atoms of cholesterol could be derived from acetate and that the ratio of incorporation of methyl/carboxyl was 15/12. Separate analysis of nucleus and side chain showed

Fig. 1

that 10 carbon atoms of the nucleus and 5 of the side chain are derived from the methyl carbon atom of acetic acid. Establishment of the origin of every carbon atom of cholesterol was achieved through a series of brilliant experiments carried out principally by BLOCH and by CORNFORTH, POPJAK and their co-workers (WÜERSCH et al., 1952; BLOCH, 1953; DAUBEN and TAKEMURA, 1953; CORN-FORTH et al., 1953, 1957). The pattern of acetate incorporation into cholesterol which emerged from this work is shown in Figure 1.

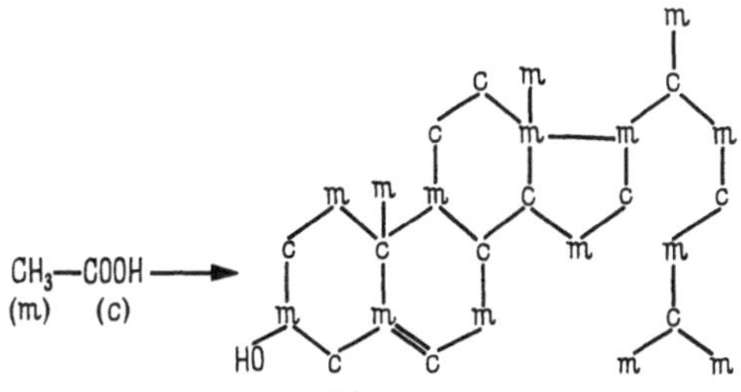

In retrospect it is convenient to relate the elucidation of the biosynthesis of cholesterol in a sequential fashion, acetate to mevalonate to sqalene to cholesterol, although this development was, in fact, not so orderly.

In the early investigations of cholesterol biosynthesis it had been shown that in addition to acetate many other low molecular weight compounds could be incorporated into cholesterol. Among these were acetoacetate and acetaldehyde (BRADY and GURIN, 1951); pyruvate (ANKER, 1948); butyrate, valerate and palmitate (BLOCH and RITTENBERG, 1944); and hexanoate and octanoate (BRADY and GURIN, 1950). The efficiency of conversion to cholesterol of many of these precursors seemed to be proportional to their ability to yield the two-carbon fragment, acetate. Observations that acetoacetate could be incorporated into cholesterol without prior breakdown to acetate (BRADY and GURIN, 1951; CUR-RAN, 1951) suggested a possible first step in the conversion of acetate and explained why compounds such as leu-

Fig. 2

cine, isovalerate and isobutyrate were also converted to cholesterol (COON and GURIN, 1949; ZABIN and BLOCH, 1950; KRITCHEVSKY and GRAY, 1951).

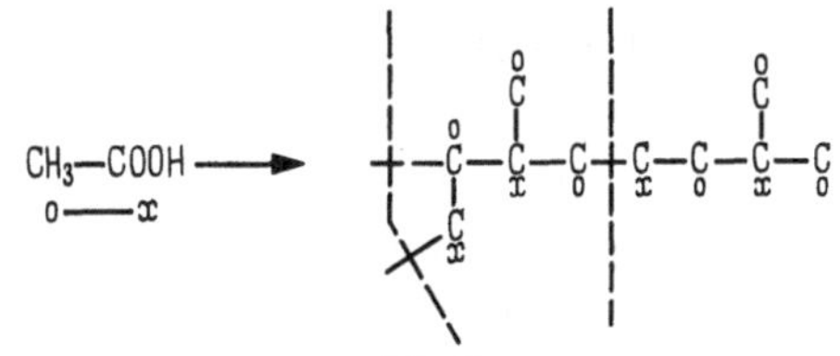

The search for precursors and pathways was brought into sharper focus through the observation by LITTLE and BLOCH (1950) that the labeling pattern of the cholesterol side chain suggested the recurrence of a five carbon atom unit (Fig. 2).

BONNER and ARREGUIN (1949) had suggested an acetate → isoprenoid inter-mediate step in the biosynthetic pathway for rubber (Fig. 3). It now became evident that the pathway of cholesterol biosynthesis must include a compound which could be derived from acetate and converted to an isoprenoid intermediate.

It was shown that hydroxymethylglutarate was synthesized in rat liver and could
be converted to cholesterol (RABINOWITZ and GURIN, 1954; RUDNEY, 1954), and

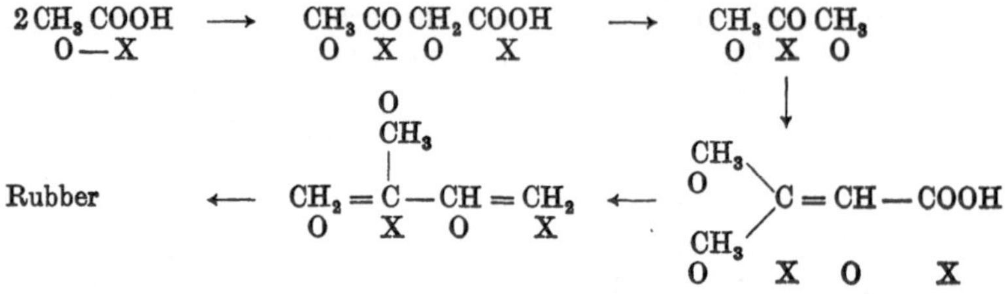

$$2\,CH_3\,COOH \longrightarrow CH_3\,CO\,CH_2\,COOH \longrightarrow CH_3\,CO\,CH_3$$
$$O-X \qquad\qquad O \quad X \quad O \quad X \qquad\qquad O \quad X \quad O$$

$$\begin{array}{c} O \\ CH_3 \\ | \end{array}$$

$$Rubber \quad\longleftarrow\quad CH_2=C-CH=CH_2 \quad\longleftarrow\quad \begin{array}{c} CH_3 \\ O \end{array}\Big\rangle C=CH-COOH$$
$$O \quad X \quad O \quad X \qquad\qquad CH_3 \Big/$$
$$O \quad X \quad O \quad X$$

Fig. 3

RUDNEY (1956) also showed that hydroxymethylglutaryl CoA is synthesized in
yeast from acetoacetyl CoA. BLOCH et al. (1954) showed that dimethylacrylate,
hydroxyisovalerate, and trans-β-methylglutaconate, all of which can arise from
acetate, may act as precursors of cholesterol. In Figure 4 the possible relationship
between these compounds is shown schematically. Speculation that hydroxymethylglutarate (HMG) might be the key intermediate in cholesterol biosynthesis
was tempered by the relatively low extent of its incorporation into this sterol.

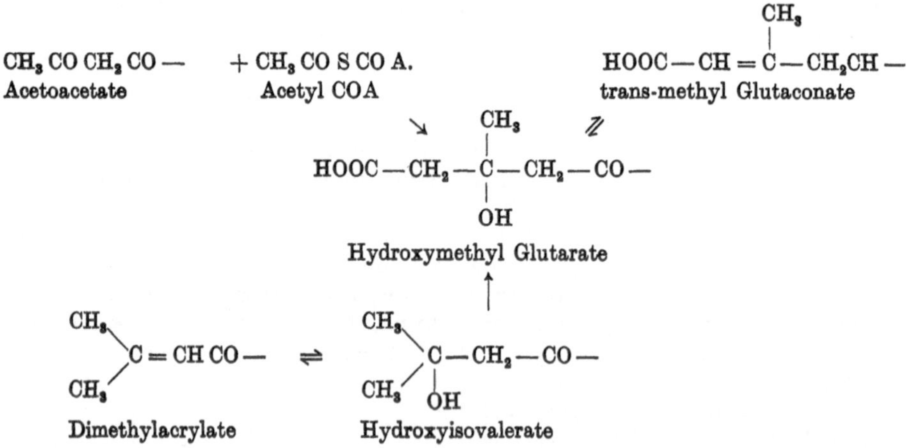

$$CH_3\,CO\,CH_2\,CO- \quad + CH_3\,CO\,S\,CO\,A. \qquad\qquad HOOC-CH=\overset{\overset{\displaystyle CH_3}{\displaystyle |}}{C}-CH_2CH-$$

Acetoacetate   Acetyl COA   trans-methyl Glutaconate

$$\searrow \qquad CH_3 \qquad \nearrow$$
$$HOOC-CH_2-\overset{\overset{\displaystyle |}{\displaystyle C}}{\underset{\underset{\displaystyle OH}{\displaystyle |}}{}}-CH_2-CO-$$

Hydroxymethyl Glutarate

$$\uparrow$$

$$\begin{array}{c} CH_3 \\ \end{array}\Big\rangle C=CH\,CO- \quad\rightleftharpoons\quad \begin{array}{c} CH_3 \\ \end{array}\Big\rangle C-CH_2-CO-$$
$$CH_3 \Big/ \qquad\qquad\qquad\qquad CH_3 \Big/ \;\; OH$$

Dimethylacrylate   Hydroxyisovalerate

Fig. 4

The breakthrough that resolved the question of the early obligatory precursor
of cholesterol came with the report of TAVORMINA, GIBBS and HUFF (1956) that
mevalonic acid (3,5-dihydroxy-3-methylvaleric acid) a factor which can replace
acetate in the culture of *Lactobacillus acidophilus* could be incorporated into
cholesterol in high yield. The similarity of mevalonic acid and hydroxymethylglutarate (HMG) is shown in Figure 5. Observations by FERGUSON et al. (1959)

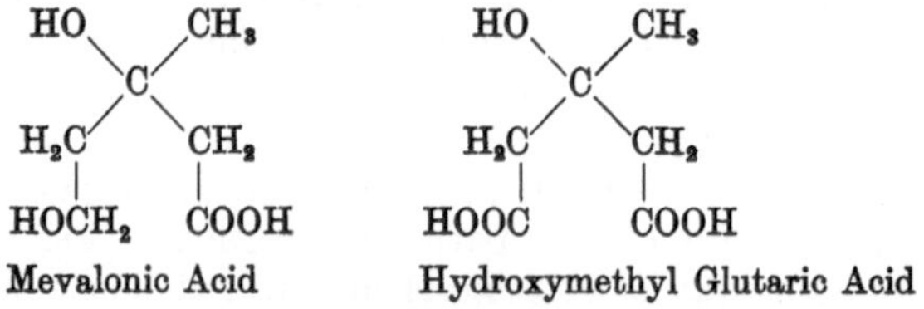

$$\begin{array}{cc} HO & CH_3 \\ & \diagdown\;C\;\diagup \\ H_2C\diagup & \diagdown CH_2 \\ | & | \\ HOCH_2 & COOH \end{array} \qquad\qquad \begin{array}{cc} HO & CH_3 \\ & \diagdown\;C\;\diagup \\ H_2C\diagup & \diagdown CH_2 \\ | & | \\ HOOC & COOH \end{array}$$

Mevalonic Acid   Hydroxymethyl Glutaric Acid

Fig. 5

that a yeast enzyme can convert HMG-CoA to mevalonate establishes its biosynthetic pathway from acetate and acetoacetate and the report of KNAUSS et al. (1959) that liver tissue can convert acetate to mevalonate strengthens the case for mevalonate as an obligatory precursor of cholesterol. LYNEN and GRASSL (1958) have established that only the (+) isomer of mevalonic acid has biological activity. TAVORMINA and GIBBS (1956) showed that about 40% of the radioactivity of DL-mevalonic acid-2-^{14}C was incorporated into cholesterol by a rat liver homogenate. Considering the facts that the carboxyl group is lost *en route* cholesterol and that only one enantiomorph of mevalonic acid is utilized, the yield of cholesterol synthesized from DL-mevalonic acid-2-^{14}C was practically 100 per cent. The conversion of HMG-CoA to mevalonic acid has been studied by DURR and RUDNEY (1960), who found that for each mole of HMG-CoA which is reduced, one mole of mevalonate is formed, two moles of NADPH are oxidized, and one mole of coenzyme A is released. The reduction is irreversible and is not stimulated by Mg^{++}, ATP or inorganic phosphorus.

The steps required to convert mevalonic acid to the "active-isoprenoid" intermediate have been worked out with some assurance. The initial step involves the phosphorylation of mevalonic acid to mevalonic acid-5-phosphate by an enzyme called mevalonic kinase. This enzyme was found in yeast by TCHEN (1958). The properties of the mevalonic kinase of liver have been described in detail by LEVY and POPJAK (1960). The kinase is inhibited by p-chloromercuribenzoate but not by iodoacetamide. The enzyme requires Mg^{++}, Mn^{++}, or Ca^{++} and ATP or inosine triphosphate. The kinase is specific for the (+) form of mevalonic acid. Mevalonic acid-5-phosphate is phosphorylated further to give mevalonic acid-5-pyrophosphate (DE WAARD and POPJAK, 1959; HENNING et al. 1959). The purified enzyme (BLOCH et al., 1959) requires a divalent metal ion for activity (Mg^{++} is preferable) and has no pronounced pH optimum. Mevalonic acid pyrophosphate then undergoes simultaneous dehydration and decarboxylation to yield isopentenylpyrophosphate (LYNEN et al., 1958; CHAYKIN et al., 1958). The enzyme concerned with the dehydration and decarboxylation has been purified (BLOCH et al., 1959) and shown to have a pH optimum between 5.5 and 7.4 and to require a divalent metal ion (Mg^{++}, Mn^{++}, Fe^{++} or Co^{++}). The series of reactions in which mevalonate is converted to isopentenylpyrophosphate is outlined in Figure 6. BRODIE et al. (1963) have established a new pathway for the biosynthesis of mevalonic acid from malonyl CoA. The importance of this particular pathway in the synthesis of sterols is still unknown.

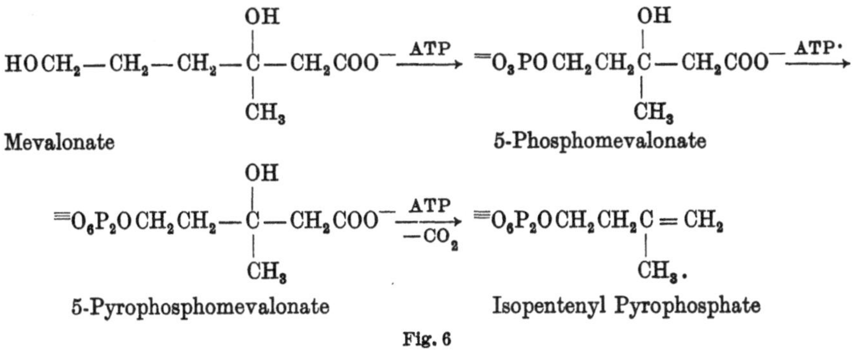

$$HOCH_2-CH_2-CH_2-\underset{\underset{CH_3}{|}}{\overset{\overset{OH}{|}}{C}}-CH_2COO^- \xrightarrow{ATP} {}^{=}O_3PO\,CH_2\,CH_2\,\underset{\underset{CH_3}{|}}{\overset{\overset{OH}{|}}{C}}-CH_2COO^- \xrightarrow{ATP\cdot}$$

Mevalonate 5-Phosphomevalonate

$$\equiv O_6P_2O\,CH_2\,CH_2-\underset{\underset{CH_3}{|}}{\overset{\overset{OH}{|}}{C}}-CH_2COO^- \xrightarrow[-CO_2]{ATP} \equiv O_6P_2O\,CH_2\,CH_2\,\underset{\underset{CH_3\cdot}{|}}{C}=CH_2$$

5-Pyrophosphomevalonate Isopentenyl Pyrophosphate

Fig. 6

Recognition of the probability that an isoprenoid precursor was involved in the biosynthesis of cholesterol led to closer examination of an old hypothesis that squalene is a precursor of cholesterol. CHANNON (1926, 1937) had investigated this possibility through feeding experiments and showed some connection between squalene feeding and cholesterol accumulation in livers of rats, but his data did not permit him to conclude that a product-precursor relationship existed. The suggestion of the role of squalene as a cholesterol precursor was initially put forth by HEILBRON et al. (1926) and by ROBINSON (1934). LANGDON and BLOCH (1953 a, b) demonstrated that squalene was indeed synthesized from acetate by rat liver and that this hydrocarbon was, in turn, converted to cholesterol. The initial product of squalene cyclization would be lanosterol, which could be converted to cholesterol after the loss of the methyl groups at positions 4,4′ and 14, hydrogenation of the side chain double bond and a shift of the nuclear double bond. WOODWARD and BLOCH (1953) proposed a mode of squalene cyclization which would yield the tetracyclic system of the steroids and in which the first product would be lanosterol. (Fig. 7). CLAYTON and BLOCH (1956 a, b) showed that lanosterol could be synthesized from acetate and converted to cholesterol *in vivo*. These findings, together with the elucidation of the pattern of incorporation of labeled acetate into squalene, left no doubt as to the major steps in the biosynthetic pathway of cholesterol. The mechanisms of formation of various intermediates were subsequently worked out.

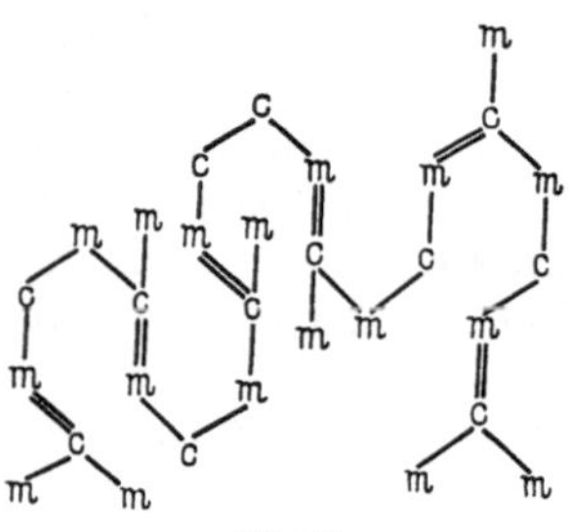

Fig. 7

The condensation of dimethyallyl pyrophosphate, an isomerization product of isopentenyl pyrophosphate, with isopentenyl pyrophosphate, has been shown to yield geranyl pyrophosphate (LYNEN et al., 1959). The enzyme, isopentenyl pyrophosphate isomerase, has been described (AGRANOFF et al., 1960). Geranyl pyrophosphate may condense with another molecule of isopentenyl pyrophosphate to yield farnesyl pyrophosphate. The enzyme farnesyl synthetase had been isolated by LYNEN et al. (1959). The reductive dimerization of two molecules of

$$CH_2 = C - CH_2CH_2OP_2O_6^{\equiv} \qquad\qquad + \quad CH_3C = CH\,CH_2\,OP_2O_6^{\equiv} \qquad\longrightarrow$$
$$\quad\quad\;\; | \qquad\qquad\qquad\qquad\qquad\qquad\qquad\qquad\;\; |$$
$$\quad\quad CH_3 \qquad\qquad\qquad\qquad\qquad\qquad\qquad\quad CH_3$$

Isopentenyl Pyrophosphate   Dimethallyl Pyrophosphate .

$$CH_3 - C = CH\,CH_2CH_2 - C = CH\,CH_2\,OP_2O_6^{\equiv} \qquad CH_2 - C - CH_2\,CH_2\,OP_2O_6^{\equiv}$$
$$\qquad\;\; | \qquad\qquad\qquad\qquad | \qquad\qquad\qquad\qquad\qquad\qquad |$$
$$\quad\;\; CH_3 \qquad\qquad\qquad CH_3 \qquad\qquad + \qquad\;\; CH_3 \qquad\qquad\qquad\longrightarrow$$

Geranyl Pyrophosphate   Isopentenyl Pyrophosphate

$$CH_3 - C = CH\,CH_2CH_2\,C = CH\,CH_2CH_2\,C = CH\,CH_2\,OP_2O_6^{\equiv} \qquad\qquad\longrightarrow$$
$$\qquad\;\; | \qquad\qquad\qquad\quad | \qquad\qquad\qquad\quad |$$
$$\quad\;\; CH_3 \qquad\qquad\qquad CH_3 \qquad\qquad\qquad CH_3 \qquad + \;\text{Farnesyl Pyrophosphate}$$

Farnesyl Pyrophosphate

$$CH_3 - C = CH\,CH_2CH_2\,C = CH\,CH_2CH_2\,C = CH\,CH_2CH_2CH = C\,CH_2CH_2CH = C\,CH_2CH_2CH = C\,CH_3$$
$$\;\; | \qquad\qquad\quad | \qquad\qquad\quad | \qquad\qquad\qquad\qquad | \qquad\qquad\qquad | \qquad\qquad\qquad |$$
$$\; CH_3 \qquad\qquad CH_3 \qquad\qquad CH_3 \qquad\qquad\qquad CH_3 \qquad\qquad\;\; CH_3 \qquad\qquad\;\; CH_3$$

Squalene

Fig. 8

farnesyl pyrophosphate, tail to tail, to yield squalene has been demonstrated by LYNEN et al. (1958, 1959). These reactions are outlined in Figure 8.

CORNFORTH and POPJAK (1959a) postulated a different mechanism for the conversion of farnesyl pyrophosphate to squalene. In their scheme, farnesyl pyrophosphate is isomerized to nerolidol pyrophosphate, and these compounds condense in a manner similar to the condensation of isopentenyl and dimethallyl pyrophosphate. The product is dehydrosqualene, which is reduced to squalene. The observation by GOODMAN and POPJAK (1960) that nerolidol is a product of hydrolysis of farnesyl pyrophosphate, and various deuterium uptake experiments by RILLING and BLOCH (1959) lend support to the Cornforth-Popjak mechanism

$$CH_3-C=CH-CH_2-CH_2-C=CH-CH_2-CH_2-C=CH\,CH_2\,OP_2O_6{}^{\equiv}$$
$$\qquad\;\; | \qquad\qquad\qquad\quad | \qquad\qquad\qquad | $$
$$\qquad\; CH_3 \qquad\qquad\qquad CH_3 \qquad\qquad\quad CH_3 \qquad\qquad\qquad\qquad +$$

Farnesyl Pyrophosphate

$$\qquad\qquad\qquad\qquad\qquad\qquad\qquad\qquad\qquad OP_2O_6{}^{\equiv}$$
$$\qquad\qquad\qquad\qquad\qquad\qquad\qquad\qquad\qquad\; |$$
$$CH_3-C=CH-CH_2-CH_2-C=CH-CH_2-CH_2-C-CH=CH_2 \qquad \longrightarrow$$
$$\qquad\;\; | \qquad\qquad\qquad\qquad | \qquad\qquad\qquad | $$
$$\qquad\; CH_3 \qquad\qquad\qquad\; CH_3 \qquad\qquad\quad CH_3$$

Nerolidol Pyrophosphate

$$R-CH_2-C=CH-CH=CH-CH=C-CH_2-R$$
$$\qquad\qquad\; | \qquad\qquad\qquad\qquad | $$
$$\qquad\qquad CH_3 \qquad\qquad\qquad\; CH_3$$

Dehydrosqualene

$$(R=CH_3-C=CH-CH_2-CH_2-C=CH-CH_2-)$$
$$\qquad\qquad\quad | \qquad\qquad\qquad\qquad | $$
$$\qquad\qquad\; CH_3 \qquad\qquad\qquad\; CH_3$$

Fig. 9

(Fig. 9). In the cyclization of squalene to lanosterol, it has been shown that no proton or hydroxyl ion from the medium is incorporated into lanosterol, but molecular oxygen is (TCHEN and BLOCH, 1957). In contrast to this finding, the formation of squalene does not require oxygen (BUCHER and McGARRAHAN, 1956).

The cyclization of squalene to lanosterol has been postulated as involving a series of 1:2 shifts, executed by two hydrogen groups and two methyl groups. Based on data from labeled acetate the 1:2 shift of the methyl groups (from carbon 8 of lanosterol to carbon 14 and the methyl group at C-14 shifting to C-13) could not be distinguished from the 1:3 shift in which the C⁸/methyl group shifts to C-13 directly. Ingenious experiments involving ¹³C-labeled precursors showed that the postulated 1:2 shift was the correct one (CORNFORTH et al., 1959 b; MAUDGAL et al., 1958) (Fig. 10).

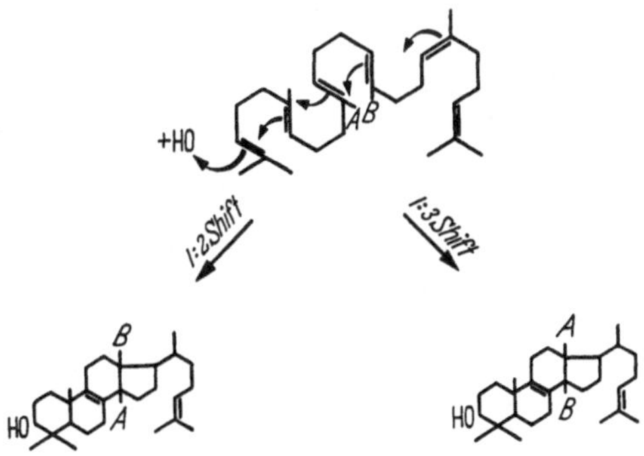

Fig. 10

The conversion of lanosterol to cholesterol involves the loss of three methyl groups (4,4′, 14), a double bond shift ($\Delta^{8,9}$ to $\Delta^{5,6}$) and a hydrogenation of the double bond at C-24. Early work by SCHWENK and WERTHESSEN (1952, 1953) had shown that in short term cholesterol biosynthesis experiments, it was possible to isolate sterols other than cholesterol of high specific activity. Among the "high counting companions" of cholesterol were lanosterol, agnosterol, and zymosterol. The conversion of zymosterol-¹⁴C to cholesterol was demonstrated by JOHNSTON

and BLOCH (1957) and by ALEXANDER and SCHWENK (1957), and the conversion
of lanosterol to cholesterol has already been noted. The three extra methyl groups
of lanosterol were shown to be lost as carbon dioxide (OLSON et al., 1957).

GAUTSCHI and BLOCH (1958) demonstrated that $\Delta^{8,24}$-4,4-dimethyl cholesta-
diene-3β-ol could be an intermediate in cholesterol biosynthesis. With the finding
that desmosterol (Δ^{24}-cholesterol) was also an intermediate in cholesterol biosynthesis (STOKES et al., 1958), it appeared that the lanosterol-cholesterol pathway

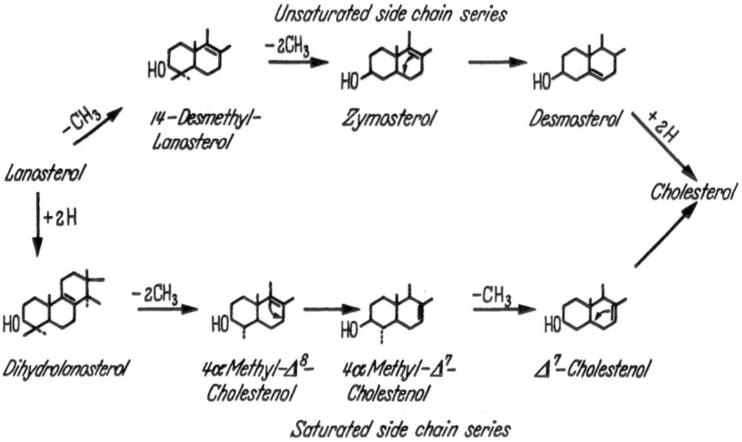

Fig. 11

was clearly marked. There is a progressive loss of methyl groups, first from C-14,
then from C-4, yielding zymosterol; a nuclear double bond shift yields desmosterol,
which is finally hydrogenated to give cholesterol. This is undoubtedly the major
pathway.

KANDUTSCH and RUSSELL (1960a—d) have reported on an alternate biosynthetic pathway which was first noted in their work with a tumor of the mouse
preputial gland. In the alternative system, the side chain of lanosterol is first
reduced to give dihydrolanosterol, which then loses two methyl groups to give
4α-methyl-Δ^8-cholestenol, which goes to the Δ^7 derivative, then loses the methyl
group at C_4 to give Δ^7-cholestenol. The latter compound is converted to cholesterol.
The alternative pathways of cholesterol biosynthesis are outlined in Figure 11.

STEINBERG and AVIGAN (1960) also recognized these two pathways in discussing the action of various drugs which influence cholesterol biosynthesis. Most
of the intermediates along the "saturated side chain" pathway from lanosterol
to cholesterol have been isolated or synthesized and shown to be convertible to
cholesterol. KANDUTSCH and RUSSELL (1960d) have shown that 24,25-dihydro-
lanosterol, 4α-methyl-Δ^8- cholestenol, Δ^7-cholestenol, and 7-dehydrocholesterol
are converted to cholesterol by cell-free homogenates of liver in yields of 18, 32.
67 and 74 per cent, respectively. AVIGAN et al. (1963) have reported the reduction
of lanosterol to 24,25-dihydrolanosterol by rat liver homogenates. WELLS and
LORAH (1960) showed that methostenol (4α-methyl-Δ^7-cholestenol) can be synthesized from acetate by rat tissue and can in turn be converted to cholesterol. The
role of 7-dehydro-cholesterol as an intermediate in the conversion of Δ^7-cholestenol
to cholesterol has also been firmly established (FRANTZ et al., 1964; DEMPSEY
et al., 1964). WILSON (1963) noted that, in skin, the "saturated side chain" pathway requires essential fatty acids and that the intermediates along this pathway
are recovered exclusively in the esterified form.

In summary, the elucidation of the pathway of cholesterol synthesis from acetate has been accomplished with only a few ancillary pieces of information still missing. The satisfactory solution of one of the most provocative problems in biochemistry has been due to the work of many investigators, but most credit must go to the contributions from the laboratories of BLOCH, LYNEN, CORNFORTH and POPJAK.

The conversion of acetate-1-^{14}C to cholesterol by a variety of rat tissues has been studied in vitro. Efficiency of conversion is greatest in newborn skin, followed by newborn brain, liver, adult skin, intestine, testes, and kidney. The liver is generally assumed to be the major source of the plasma cholesterol, and this is the target organ of most studies designed to test various aspects of cholesterol biosynthesis.

The rate of equilibration between liver and serum-free cholesterol is rapid, being attained within a few hours in dogs (ECKLES et al., 1955). In humans, the peak specific activity of the serum-free cholesterol is attained within 2—4 hours after administration of labeled acetate. Serum ester cholesterol and serum-free cholesterol equilibrate after 4—7 days (HELLMAN et al., 1954; GOULD et al., 1955). The same pattern of equilibration is observed after administration of labeled cholesterol (BIGGS et al., 1952).

Patterns of cholesterol biosynthesis and transport in the baboon parallel those observed in man (KRITCHEVSKY et al., 1965). Peak specific activity of serum-free cholesterol synthesized from mevalonic acid-2-^{14}C is reached within 4—10 hours and the free and esterified forms equilibrate by 72 hours. Peak specific activities of exogenously labeled serum-free and ester cholesterol are observed at three days. The specific activity of the total cholesterol of the serum α and β lipoproteins is equal over a 10-day period, but there is the possibility that the specific activities of the free and ester cholesterol moieties of the serum α and β lipoproteins differ. The lipoprotein cholesterol findings are similar to results reported from similar human studies (GIDEZ and EDER, 1963). The equilibration of serum and tissue cholesterol is reached at about two weeks in the dog (GOULD, 1952) and rat (CHEVALLIER, 1953) and one month in man (CHOBANIAN and HOLLANDER, 1962).

Several approaches have been made towards quantification of the cholesterol steady state in the rat. CHEVALLIER (1956) described the turnover rate of cholesterol in most tissues and calculated the amount of "replaceable cholesterol" present in each. He found (CHEVALLIER, 1960) that the cholesterol synthesized by the intestinal wall does not equilibrate with the blood cholesterol. These findings are at variance with those arising from the ingenious experiments of WILSON (1964), who attempted to quantitate cholesterol excretion and degradation in the rat and found that the major portion of fecal cholesterol of endogenous origin is derived from or is in equilibrium with the blood. Both CHEVALLIER and WILSON used isotopically labeled cholesterol administered orally, intravenously or by implantation.

Cholesterol biosynthesis is affected by dietary and hormonal factors as well as by various external influences. Cholesterogenesis is enhanced by radiation, thyroid hormones, hypophysectomy, various metal ions and surface active agents. Biosynthesis is inhibited by fasting, thyroidectomy, vanadium salts, and by feeding of cholesterol or some of its steroid precursors. These influences were reviewed by KRITCHEVSKY et al. (1960). In most cases cholesterol synthesis from acetate is more severely inhibited than is synthesis from mevalonate, suggesting that the inhibition occurs at an early step in cholesterol biosynthesis. The inhibition of cholesterol biosynthesis by cholesterol feeding was shown to possess the characteristics of a negative feedback control system (BUCHER et al., 1959).

Intensive studies by Siperstein and his co-workers (1960, 1962) showed that the primary site of depression of cholesterogenesis by exogenous cholesterol is the reduction of hydroxymethylglutaryl CoA to mevalonic acid. This type of feed-back control which had been demonstrated in a variety of animal species has also been shown to exist in man (Bhattathiry and Siperstein, 1963). In the chicken exogenous hypercholesteremia (feeding) results in suppression of cholesterogenesis, but endogenous hypercholesteremia (stilbestrol administration) does not (Saka-kida et al., 1963). The explanation for this difference may be that during stil-bestrol treatment cholesterol does not accumulate in the hepatic cell. These findings are consistent with other cases in which endogenous hypercholesteremia caused by injection of a surface active agent (Frantz and Hinkelman, 1955) or by nephrosis (Marsh and Drabkin, 1958) does not interfere with cholesterol syn-thesis.

Reasoning that a compound which might inhibit cholesterol biosynthesis could be useful for treatment of hypercholesteremia and atherosclerosis, investigators synthesized and tested a number of compounds in vitro and in vivo. With the knowledge and techniques gained from the work on cholesterogenesis, it has been possible to assign the sites at which the various compounds inhibit biosynthesis.

Redel and Cottet (1953) and Cottet et al. (1953) reported that sodium α-phenylbutyrate and related compounds lowered cholesterol levels in experi-mental animals and in man. A number of homologs and analogs of this compound have been synthesized since, and all have been found to exert an effect upon cholesterol synthesis. The site of inhibition is at the level of acetylation of co-enzyme A. Goldstein (1955) found that almost all aryl substituted short chain fatty acids interfere with acetylation of CoA and with cholesterogenesis to some extent. Blohm et al. (1959a, 1959b) reported that 1-[(4-diethylaminoethoxy) phenyl]-1-(p-tolyl)-2-(p-chlorophenyl) ethanol (MER/29) was a potent inhibitor of cholesterol biosynthesis. It was subsequently shown (Avigan et al., 1960; Frantz et al., 1960) that this compound interfered with the action of desmosterol reductase resulting in an accumulation of desmosterol in the blood and tissue of treated animals and man. Several other dialkyl aminoethanol derivatives have been tested, among them β-diethylaminoethyl-diphenylpropylacetate hydro-chloride (SKF-525A), which interferes primarily with the cyclization of squalene and 3β (β-dimethylaminoethoxy)-androst-5-en-17-one (Gordon et al., 1961), which interferes with the conversion of desmosterol to cholesterol. The diethylamino-analog behaves similarly (Phillips and Avigan, 1963).

Another compound which has a similar effect in vivo is 22,25-diazacholestanol (Dvornik and Kraml, 1963), although it has been reported to inhibit HMG-CoA reductase in vitro (Ranney and Counsell, 1962). Benzmalacene (N-(1-methyl-2,3-di-p-chlorophenylpropyl) maleamic acid (Huff and Gilfillan, 1960) is an-other potent inhibitor of cholesterol biosynthesis and appears to exert its major influence somewhere between the isopentenyl pyrophosphate and farnesyl pyro-phosphate steps. Cholestenone (Steinberg and Fredrickson, 1956) interferes with the conversion of acetate to non-saponifiable lipid but its locus of action is as yet unknown. Popjak et al. (1960) found that a number of farnesoic acid analogs also interfere with the conversion of mevalonate to cholesterol. Another compound, trans-1,4-bis(2-chlorobenzylaminomethyl dihydrochloride (AY-9944) when fed to rats, has been shown to result in an accumulation of 7-dehydro-cholesterol (Dvornik et al., 1963). The latest hypocholesteremic compound to excite the interest of workers in this field is ethyl α-p-chlorophenoxyisobutyrate (CPIB) (Thorp and Waring, 1962). From its structure, one would expect it to exert an effect on cholesterol biosynthesis at a pre-mevalonate stage. Gould et al.

(1964) have recently reported that CPIB inhibits by 70% the conversion of acetate to cholesterol but has no effect when mevalonate is the precursor. The action of drugs which affect lipid synthesis has been the subject of several excellent reviews by HOLMES (1962, 1964a, b). The formulae of some of the compounds which have been discussed are shown in Figure 12.

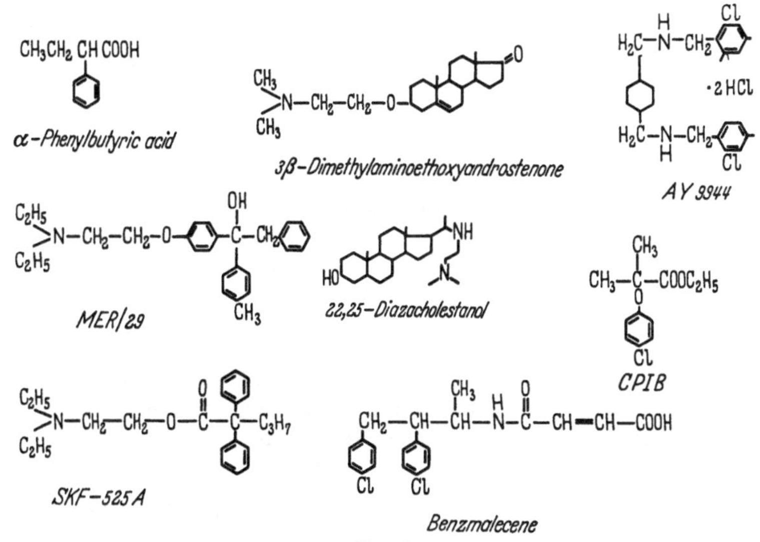

Fig. 12

2. Other Sterols

The biogenesis of a number of sterols has been investigated in the course of studies of cholesterol biogenesis and most of these have been described above. There is no question that the compounds which lie on the cholesterol biosynthetic pathway arise from the cyclization of squalene. Among these are zymosterol, which was first isolated in radioactive form after incubation of *Saccharomyces cervisiae* with acetate-1-^{14}C (SCHWENK et al., 1955), lanosterol, agnosterol and desmosterol. Desmosterol was originally isolated from chick embryo by STOKES, FISH and HICKEY (1956) and has been found to be present in developing rat brain (KRITCHEVSKY and HOLMES, 1962). Lathosterol (Δ^7-cholestenol) was shown by FIESER (1951) to be a normal companion of plasma cholesterol and its conversion to cholesterol in vivo (BIGGS et al., 1954) and in vitro (DAVIDSON et al., 1959) demonstrated (Fig. 13).

Ergosterol (Fig. 13) is a C_{28} sterol whose biosynthetic pathway, at least in the early stages, parallels that of cholesterol. The incorporation of deuterioacetate into ergosterol was shown by SONDERHOFF and THOMAS (1937). Using $^{14}CH_3{}^{13}CO_2H$ and an acetate-requiring strain of *Neurospora crassa*, OTTKE et al. (1951) showed that at least 26 of the 28 carbon atoms of ergosterol arose from acetate. Degradation experiments showed that the pattern of incorporation of the methyl and carboxyl of acetate into the side chain and carbon atoms 11 and 12 of ergosterol was similar to that seen in cholesterol (HANAHAN and WAKIL, 1953; DAUBEN and HUTTON, 1956). The extra methyl group of ergosterol (at carbon atom 24) can arise from a one carbon pool, such as formate (DANIELSSON and BLOCH, 1957; DAUBEN et al., 1957b). More extensive work on this problem showed that the extra methyl group of ergosterol is derived through a transmethylation reaction with the S-methyl group of methionine (ALEXANDER et al., 1957a,b). Finally, SCHWENK and ALEXANDER (1958) demonstrated that a cell-free yeast homogenate could convert both squalene-^{14}C and lanosterol-^{3}H to ergosterol. Whether the methylation at C-24 occurs immediately after cyclization (at a C_{30} stage) or at a C_{27} stage is not yet known.

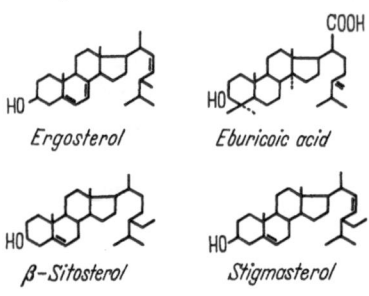

Ergosterol   Eburicoic acid

β-Sitosterol   Stigmasterol

Fig. 13

Eburicoic acid (Fig. 13), a steroid produced by certain types of fungi has been shown by DAUBEN and his co-workers (1956, 1957a, b) to possess a labeling pattern (after biosynthesis from acetate-^{14}C) that has many features in common with that of ergosterol. It is thus possible that eburicoic acid also arises from cyclization of squalene.

The biosynthesis of β-sitosterol (Fig. 13) from mevalonate has been demonstrated in several varietes of plants (BAISTED et al., 1962; NICHOLAS 1962a, b), but no further work on the pattern of labeling or on the origin of the ethyl group at C_{24} has been reported.

The incorporation of mevalonate into stigmasterol (Fig. 13) by the slime mold, *Dictyostelium discoideum* (JOHNSON et al., 1962) suggests yet another example of a sterol which may arise via squalene cyclization.

II. Conversion of Cholesterol to Other Steroids

1. Bile Acids

The first unequivocal evidence of the conversion of cholesterol to bile acids was obtained by BLOCH, BERG and RITTENBERG (1943), who isolated deuterium-labeled cholic acid following administration of cholesterol to a dog. In their study of the distribution of isotope in deuterium-labeled cholesterol (synthesized as the cholesterol-d of BLOCH, by exchange with D_2O), FUKUSHIMA and GALLAGHER (1952) found half of the isotope in the terminal isopropyl group and pointed out that about 87% of serum cholesterol had been converted to cholic acid in the BLOCH experiment. The in vivo conversion of cholesterol to cholic acid was confirmed by BYERS and BIGGS (1952), using cholesterol-^{3}H, and by BERGSTROM (1952) and SIPERSTEIN et al. (1952), using cholesterol-^{14}C. Further experiments using cholesterol-4-^{14}C and cholesterol-26-^{14}C were carried out by CHAIKOFF, SIPERSTEIN and their collaborators (SIPERSTEIN and CHAIKOFF, 1952; CHAIKOFF et al., 1952). They found that when cholesterol-4-^{14}C was administered intravenously to rats, 80—90% of the isotope was excreted in 15 days and 90% of the excreted isotope was present in the bile acids. These findings, together with their work on the excretion of $^{14}CO_2$ by rats given cholesterol-26-^{14}C, led them to conclude that between 80 and 90% of circulating cholesterol is ultimately converted to bile acid. Conversion of cholesterol to bile acid has also been observed to occur at this same high level (75—90%) in man (SIPERSTEIN and MURRAY, 1955) and in rabbits (EKDAHL and SJÖVALL, 1955). These findings establish the bile acids as the principal catabolic products of cholesterol. Isotopic data indicate that cholesterol is the obligatory precursor of bile acids (ZABIN and BARKER, 1953; STAPLE and GURIN, 1954).

The elaboration of the sequence of steps required to convert cholesterol to bile acids in vivo has been largely due to the outstanding work of BERGSTRÖM and his co-workers and has been reviewed by him (1955; 1959; 1960). The conversion of cholesterol to cholic acid requires hydrogenation of the double bond, inversion of the hydroxyl group at carbon atom 3, introduction of hydroxyl groups at carbon atoms 7 and 12 and oxidation of the side chain. BERGSTRÖM addressed himself to the problem of the order in which the various reactions took place. The technique used was to feed various suspected precursors of chloesterol to rats and then analyze the products formed in the bile. Thus, it was shown that whereas 3β-hydroxy-Δ^5-cholenic acid was not converted to cholic acid, 3α, 7α, 12α-trihydroxy-coprostanic acid was. It was thus inferred that hydroxylation was the initial step in the biosynthesis of bile acids from cholesterol. The early requirement for the intact side chain was also shown by the conversion of both 7α-hydroxycholesterol and 3α, 7α-dihydroxy-coprostane to cholic acid. On the hypothesis that the terminal isopropyl group of cholesterol was lost by methyl oxidation, to yield a 27 carbon atom trihydroxy acid, followed by β-oxidation, the conversion of 3α, 7α, 12α-trihydroxycoprostanic acid to cholic acid was indeed demonstrated. Thus they had established that the nuclear hydroxylations preceded the side chain oxidation.

Based on his examination of the bile salts of various species, HASLEWOOD (1959) had concluded that an evolutionary pattern exists which is reflected in the pathway by which the cholesterol side chain is cleaved to yield the five carbon acidic side chain of the bile acids. Thus, the older animals (shark) possess a side chain that has a 27 hydroxyl group, the reptiles mainly synthesize a 27 carboxylic acid and mammals a 25 carboxylic acid. HASLEWOOD suggested that 3α, 7α, 12α-trihydroxycoprostanic acid might be an intermediate in cholic acid formation in 1952.

Working with 3α,7α-dihydroxy-coprostane, BERGSTRÖM and LINDSTEDT (1956) found that it was readily converted to both chenodeoxycholic and cholic acids. Chenodeoxycholic acid, however, is not convertible to cholic acid. When 3α, 7α-dihydroxycoprostanic acid is administered to the rat, no cholic acid is formed. These findings suggest that the hydroxylation at C_7 may be the rate-determining step in bile acid formation. Some of the interconversions discussed above are outlined in Figure 14.

From his studies in a number of mammalian species, BERGSTRÖM (1960) concluded that the 7α hydroxyl group of the bile acids is eliminated by the action of intestinal microorganisms during the course of enterohepatic circulation. Work with the rabbit, for instance, whose major bile acid is deoxycholic acid has shown that this acid predominates because of the efficiency of the intestinal flora plus the inability of this animal to hydroxylate deoxycholic acid. The rat, on the other hand, has a potent 7α hydroxylating enzyme.

The stereospecificity of the nuclear changes has also been studied by BERGSTRÖM's group, the principal investigator in this area being SAMUELSSON. The inversion of the hydroxyl group at position 3 of cholesterol probably proceeds by way of a ketonic intermediate since it has been observed that cholesterol-3α-^{3}H loses the tritium atom in going to cholic acid. The reduction of the double bond appears to involve a stereospecific cis addition of hydrogen. Cholesterol-4-^{14}C, 6-^{3}H, when administered to bile fistula rats, gave chenodeoxycholic acid in which the ^{3}H/^{14}C ratio had not changed. Using specific enzymic 6α and 6β hydroxylations, it was shown that the tritium atom at position 6 was in the α configuration. Thus, the added hydrogens were cis and in a β orientation. In more recent work, GREEN and SAMUELSSON (1964) have studied the fate of tritium during the conversion of 3α-^{3}H-4-^{14}C and 4β-^{3}H-^{14}C-cholesterol to bile acids. They confirm the earlier suggestion that a 3-ketosteroid is involved in the epimerization at C-3; furthermore, they present evidence that the Δ^5 double bond is isomerized to the Δ^4 position prior to its reduction. A stereospecific transfer of hydrogen from the 4β to the 6β position occurs during the isomerization. The hydroxylation at C-7 does not involve a 7-keto intermediate and may proceed by direct elimination of the 7α hydrogen atom.

The in vivo work on bile acid formation has been augmented by work with liver homogenates and particulate fractions which has expanded the knowledge concerning the mechanisms involved. CHAIKOFF et al. (1952) had shown that large amounts of $^{14}CO_2$ were formed after the administration of cholesterol-26-^{14}C to

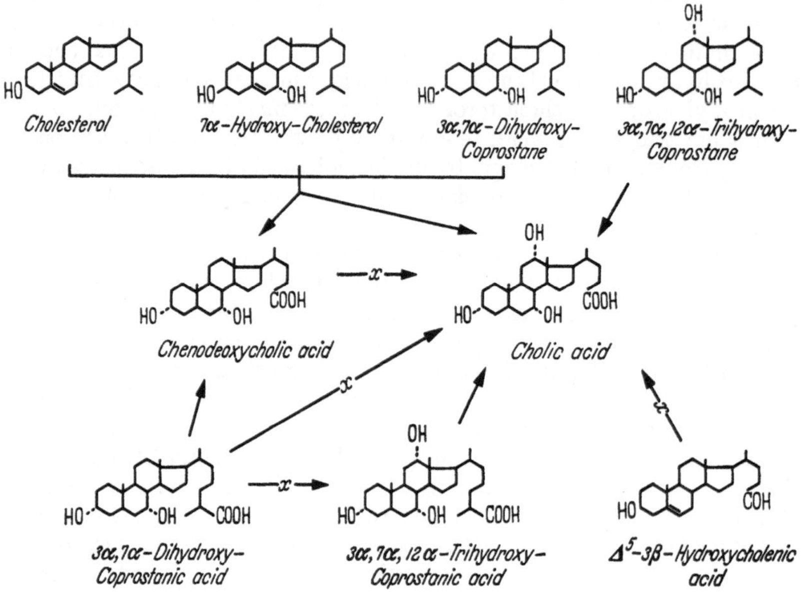

Fig. 14

intact rats. ANFINSEN and HORNING (1953) found that mouse liver homogenates were capable of oxidizing the cholesterol side chain. HORNING et al. (1957) and FREDRICKSON (1956a, b) were able to determine some of the optimal factors for this system, especially the requirement of a heat stable cofactor present in the supernatant but were not able to isolate any known normal bile acids among the reaction products, although several acids of the cholanic type were found. WHITEHOUSE, STAPLE and GURIN (1959, 1961) were able to show that rat liver mitochondrial preparations also were capable of oxidizing the cholesterol side chain to carbon dioxide. Non-hepatic mitochondrial preparations showed only a minimal oxidative capacity. BRIGGS, WHITEHOUSE and STAPLE (1959, 1961) demonstrated that cholesterol is, in fact, converted to trihydroxycoprostanic acid in the alligator and when cholesterol-26-^{14}C is used as the substrate it yields trihydroxycoprostanic-26-^{14}C acid. When this acid is incubated with rat liver mitochondrial preparations, $^{14}CO_2$ is evolved.

When trihydroxycoprostanic acid labeled in the 4 position (prepared in the same manner as the 26-labeled acid) is incubated with rat liver mitochondria, labeled cholic acid is obtained. DANIELSSON had been carrying out parallel experiments in mouse liver mitochondria, and his work yielded valuable information concerning the pattern of hydroxylation of cholesterol. Cholesterol can be converted to 26 hydroxycholesterol and also to the 3β, 7α, 26-triol. DANIELSSON also showed that liver mitochondrial preparations could convert 3α, 7α, 12α trihydroxycoprostane to 3α, 7α, 12α, 26-tetrahydroxycoprostane, 3α, 7α, 12α-trihydroxycoprostanic acid and finally to cholic acid. DANIELSON has summarized his work in a recent review (1963). SULD, STAPLE and GURIN (1962) found that trihydroxycoprostanic acid is cleaved by mitochondrial preparations to yield propionyl CoA and, presumably, cholyl CoA. The production of cholyl CoA is consistent with its known requirements for conjugation with taurine to yield taurocholic acid (SIPERSTEIN, 1955; ELLIOT, 1956). The reaction sequence is summarized in Figure 15.

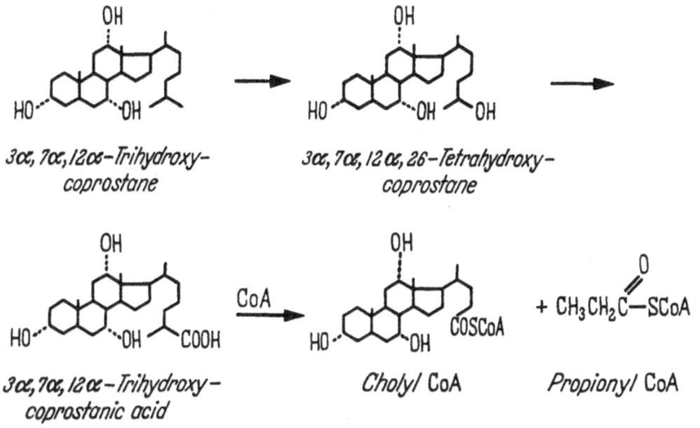

3α,7α,12α-Trihydroxy-
coprostane

3α,7α,12α,26-Tetrahydroxy-
coprostane

3α,7α,12α-Trihydroxy-
coprostanic acid

Cholyl CoA

Propionyl CoA

Fig. 15

The results obtained with the mitochondrial preparations still left the question of the mechanism of hydroxylation of cholesterol to trihydroxycoprostane incompletely answered. These preparations yield cholic acid when presented with substrates such as tri- or tetrahydroxycoprostane, but do not convert cholesterol to known bile acids. The sterol oxidase of mitochondria is apparently not highly specific and will attack the side chain of any number of cholestane or coprostane derivatives (STEVENSON and STAPLE, 1962) as well as other sterols such as ergosterol or desmosterol (KRITCHEVSKY et al., 1961, 1962). Apparently side chain oxydation will commence before the entire complement of nuclear changes required for cholic acid formation has taken place. This system is subject to a number of dietary and hormonal influences (KRITCHEVSKY, 1965). MENDELSOHN and STAPLE (1963) have recently shown that the hydroxylation of cholesterol to trihydroxycoprostane is accomplished by liver microsomal fractions which cannot, however, oxidize the side chain. Thus it appears that in vivo the nuclear changes in cholesterol are carried out by the liver microsomes and the side chain cleavage by the mitochondria.

The size of the bile acid pool in the rat is about 14—20 mg, but may vary with the diet, being lower when semi-synthetic diets are fed (ERIKSSON, 1960; PORTMAN and MURPHY, 1958). The half life of cholic and chenodeoxycholic acids is 2—3 days in normal rats (LINDSTEDT and NORMAN, 1956), but is much higher in the absence of intestinal microorganisms (LINDSTEDT and NORMAN, 1956; GUSTAFSSON et al., 1957). The intestinal flora hydrolyze the circulating bile salts and, normally, only free bile acids are found in the feces. Thyroid hormone exerts a marked effect on bile acid metabolism. In the euthyroid rat the cholic: chenodeoxycholic ratio is 4:1, but this is almost reversed in the hyperthyroid rat (ERIKSSON, 1957). The thyroid effect appears to be an inhibition of the 12α-hydroxylase, since the extent of side chain oxidation of cholesterol-26-^{14}C is the same in eu-, hyper-, or hypothyroid rats (KRITCHEVSKY et al., 1962).

In human bile, the principal bile acids are cholic, chenodeoxycholic and deoxycholic acids conjugated with taurine and glycine. The ratio of glycocholanic to taurocholanic acids is about 4:1, but is raised to 12:1 in hypothyroidism (HELL-STRÖM and SJÖVALL, 1961). The cholic acid of human bile originates from a cholesterol pool which is in equilibrium with plasma-free and bile cholesterol (ROSENFELD and HELLMAN, 1962; LINDSTEDT and AHRENS, 1961). LINDSTEDT (1957) has estimated that the cholic acid pool amounts to 1.4 gm with a half-life of 2.3 days. The chenodeoxycholic and deoxycholic acid pools are about 1.5 and 0.8 gm, respectively. It is estimated that about 0.8 gm of cholesterol is degraded to bile acids daily.

The fecal bile acids are a complex mixture due to the action of the intestinal flora. Among the fecal bile acids which have been identified are: cholic, deoxycholic, chenodeoxycholic, lithocholic, 3β-hydroxy-5β cholanic, 3 keto-5β-cholanic acid, 3α and 3β-hydroxy-12-keto-5β cholanic and 3β, 12α-dihydroxy-5β-cholanic acid.

2. Adrenocortical Steroid Hormones

The ubiquity of cholesterol in the animal body and its chemical similarity to the adrenocortical steroid hormones suggested that a product-precursor relationship might exist. This early suspicion was first confirmed by BLOCH (1945) who showed that in man, deuterium labeled cholesterol could be converted to pregnanediol, a known metabolite of progesterone. The direct conversion of cholesterol to progesterone and pregnenolone has been demonstrated (HECHTER et al., 1951; SABA et al., 1954).

The conversion of cholesterol-4-^{14}C to corticosterone and cortisol has been achieved in perfused cow adrenal (HECHTER et al., 1953) and a cell-free homogenate of cow adrenal cortex (SABA and HECHTER, 1955). In man, administration of labeled cholesterol yields the characteristic urinary metabolites of cortisol (WERBIN and LEROY, 1954, 1955). The conversion by human ovarian tissue of labeled acetate to progesterone (SWEAT et al., 1960) and other hormones (RYAN and SMITH, 1961) has also been reported. If cholesterol is indeed the precursor of the adrenocortical steroids, a predictable pattern of labeling should appear in hormones synthesized from labeled acetate. CASPI et al. (1956, 1957, 1962) have shown this to be the case.

The conversion of cholesterol to adrenocortical steroids requires the removal of six carbon atoms from the side chain plus appropriate side chain and nuclear oxidations. From the work of STAPLE et al. (1956), CONSTANTOPOULOS and TCHEN (1961), HALKERSTON et al. (1961) and SHIMIZU et al. (1962) the conversion of cholesterol to pregnenolone can now be pictured as involving two hydroxylations

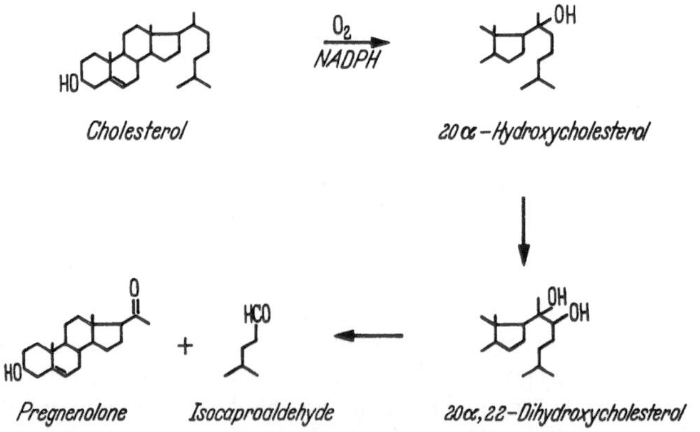

Cholesterol 20α-Hydroxycholesterol

Pregnenolone   Isocaproaldehyde 20α, 22-Dihydroxycholesterol

Fig. 16

to give first 20α-hydroxycholesterol, then 20α, 22-dihydroxycholesterol followed by scission of the side chain to yield pregnenolone and isocaproaldehyde (Fig. 16). The conversion of pregnenolone to progesterone is effected by a 3β-hydroxysteroid dehydrogenase found in the microsomal fraction of adrenal tissue (BEYER and SAMUELS, 1956). From progesterone, corticosterone arises by sequential oxidations at carbon atom 21, then at carbon 11β. In the formation of cortisol, a hydroxylation to give 17α-hydroxyprogesterone precedes the other nuclear oxidations. The enzymes involved in these reactions have been reviewed by HAYANO et al. (1956)

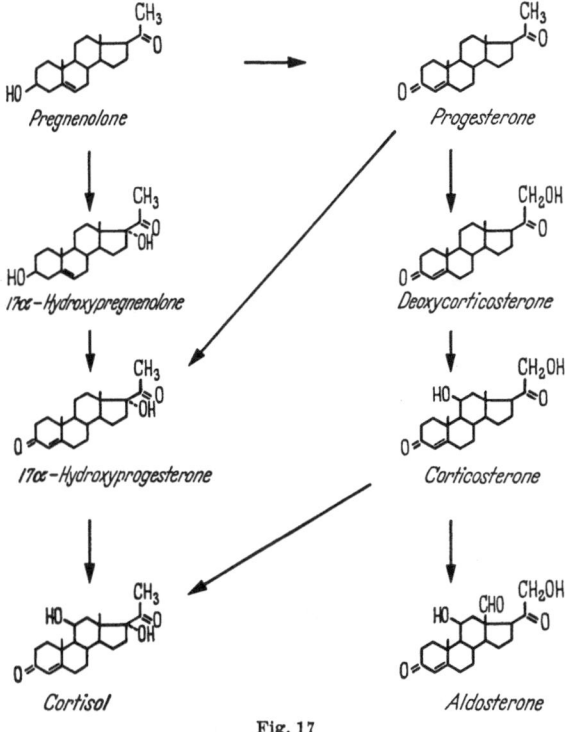

Fig. 17

(Fig. 17). An alternate route to the adrenocortical steroids which does not require the intermediary of progesterone has been discussed by HECHTER (1958). The synthesis of aldosterone requires an additional oxidation at C_{18}. It is known that progesterone, deoxycorticosterone and corticosterone can all be converted to aldosterone under certain conditions, but no definite assignment of the sequence of nuclear oxidations is possible at the present time.

3. Sex Hormones

The suggestion that cholesterol may be a precursor of all gonadal hormones was first made by BUTENANDT and KUDSZUS in 1935. Several pathways exist for the production of the androgens, all involving a 21 carbon atom intermediate. In one sequence of changes, progesterone is converted to 17α-hydroxyprogesterone which is cleaved to acetic acid and androstenedione which, in turn, is reduced to testosterone (LYNN and BROWN, 1956; SLAUNWHITE and SAMUELS, 1956). The conversion of pregnenolone to dehydroepiandrosterone has been observed (GOLDSTEIN et al., 1960) and it very probably involves 17-hydroxylation as a preliminary step (SOLOMON et al., 1960). A third pathway in which preliminary oxidation at carbon 17 is not required, but which takes progesterone directly to testosterone has been suggested by KASE et al. (1961) (Fig. 18).

The in vivo conversion of cholesterol to esterone in man has been demonstrated (WERBIN et al., 1957) and RABINOWITZ (1957) has shown that preparations of testicular tissue may convert cholesterol directly into estradiol. BAGGETT et al.

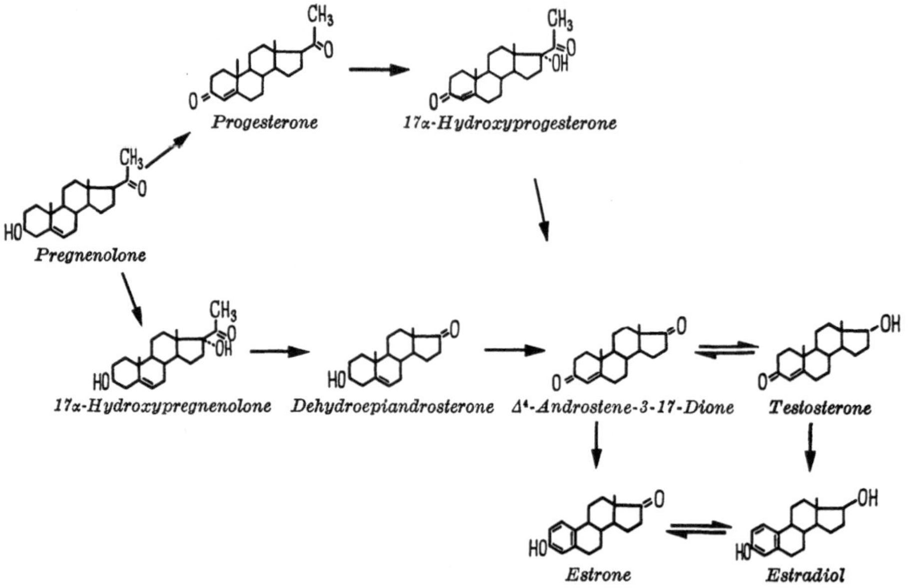

Fig. 18

(1956) have established the convertability of testosterone to estrogens. In this process the C_{19} methyl group is lost. MEYER (1955a, b) and DORFMAN (1956) have indicated that oxygenation of the angular methyl group precedes its loss and the subsequent aromatization of the A ring. The methyl group which is eliminated in the conversion of androgens to estrogens is not lost as carbon dioxide, as in conversion of lanosterol to zymosterol, but is shown to appear as formaldehyde (BREUER and GRILL, 1961). There is evidence for a NAD-linked estradiol-17β-dehydrogenase which catalyzes interconnections between estrone and 17β-estradiol (LANGER and ENGEL, 1958). Estradiol can be converted to estriol by human (ENGEL et al., 1958) and rat (HAGOPIAN and LEVY, 1958) liver.

The foregoing established a series of reactions linking cholesterol with the biogenesis of both male and female sex hormones. The alteration of cholesterol proceeds via 17α-hydroxyprogesterone which gives rise to the androgens which, in turn, are converted to estrogens. Recent work from LIEBERMAN's laboratory indicates that cholesterol sulfate may, in fact, be the immediate precursor of the gonadal steroid hormones (CALVIN et al., 1963, 1964; ROBERTS et al., 1964). Cholesterol sulfate has been established as a naturally occurring entity (DRAYER et al., 1964).

4. Neutral Sterols

A number of neutral sterols of endogenous origin have been isolated from the feces of man and of various experimental animals. Among these are cholesterol, cholestanol, coprostanol, epicoprostanol, cholestanone, coprostanone, lathosterol,

Δ^7-coprostenol, 7-dehydro-cholesterol and methostenol. The sterols of the feces are derived from bile, intestinal secretions, sloughed mucosal cells and are further altered by the action of intestinal microorganisms. Most of the sterols listed above arise in the tissues and many of them are precursors, rather than metabolites, of cholesterol. The cholesterol present in the intestine is primarily of endogenous origin. STANLEY and CHENG (1956) have calculated a daily intestinal secretion of 2 gm of endogenous cholesterol in man. This amount of cholesterol is generally greater than the daily dietary intake and even with the knowledge that less than half of the dietary cholesterol is absorbed, it must be assumed that dietary cholesterol does not contribute greatly to the amount of this sterol normally found in the intestine. This discussion will be limited to only two of the fecal sterols, coprostanol (5β-cholestan-3β-ol) and cholestanol (5α-cholestan-3β-ol) (Fig. 19).

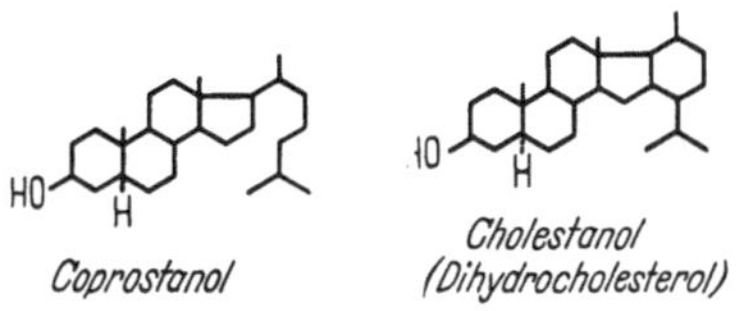

Coprostanol   Cholestanol (Dihydrocholesterol)

Fig. 19

Quantitatively, coprostanol is the most important fecal sterol. It is of interest that in dogs (SCHOENHEIMER et al., 1935) and cats (BONDZYNSKI and HUMNICKI, 1896) a meat diet is required for production of coprostanol, other diets resulting in excretion of cholesterol alone. ROSENHEIM and WEBSTER (1941, 1943) suggested that the mechanism of conversion of cholesterol to coprostanol required oxidation of cholesterol to Δ^4-cholestenone followed by stepwise reduction to coprostanone, then coprostanol. They reported spectroscopic evidence for the presence of cholestenone in feces. The formation of coprostanol from cholesterol has been accomplished in vitro using suspensions of feces (DAM, 1934; SNOG-KJAER, 1955). The hydrogenation is due to the action of microorganisms since there is no coprostanol found in the feces of rats treated with antibiotics (COLEMAN and BAUMANN, 1957) or in germ-free rats (DANIELSSON and GUSTAFSSON, 1959).

ROSENFELD and his co-workers (1954, 1956, 1964) have studied the mechanism of reduction of cholesterol to coprostanol using cholesterol labeled at the 3α position with deuterium or tritium and in the 4 position with carbon-14. Their data indicate that the coprostanol formed exhibits up to 81% retention of the isotope at the 3α position; thus, there is no oxidation at that position. However, the variable incorporation of hydrogen isotope into the B ring leaves the complete course of the conversion in doubt. The possibility exists that the products are the results of the action of more than one organism.

Cholestanol (also commonly called dihydrocholesterol) appears to accompany cholesterol in most sterol samples of mammalian origin. It is present as 1—3% of serum (SCHOENHEIMER et al., 1930) and relatively high concentrations (2—10%) are found in various tissues of the rabbit and guinea pig (WERBIN et al., 1962; MOSBACH et al., 1963).

In several insects and in certain microorganisms which require cholesterol for growth, this requirement can be met or spared by cholestanol (CLAYTON, 1964; SMITH, 1964). This sterol is generally not metabolized and is believed to replace cholesterol in structural elements of the cell (CLAYTON and BLOCH, 1963).

Recently, WERBIN et al. (1962) showed that cholesterol could be converted to coprostanol in the guinea pig, but their data did not permit them to exclude the possibility that the saturated sterol had arisen from the action of microorganisms in the intestinal tract. In a new series of experiments, WERBIN et al. (1964) demonstrated the conversion of cholesterol to cholestanol in the germ-free guinea pig, leaving little doubt that this reaction actually takes place in the tissues of the guinea pig. SHEFER, MILCH and MOSBACH (1964) have also studied the

6*

84 DAVID KRITCHEVSKY:

biosynthesis of cholestanol in the rabbit and guinea pig, using as precursors labeled acetate, mevalonate, cholestenone, desmosterol and cholesterol. In their hands, rabbit liver and intestine converted only cholestenone to cholestanol. In the rabbit adrenal both cholestenone and mevalonate were precursors of cholestanol. In the guinea pig mevalonate gave rise to cholestanol in liver, intestine and adrenal.

The discrepancies between the findings of WERBIN and of SHEFER suggest either a basic difference in biosynthesis between rabbit and guinea pig or may reflect a rate difference since the WERBIN experiment animals were maintained on a

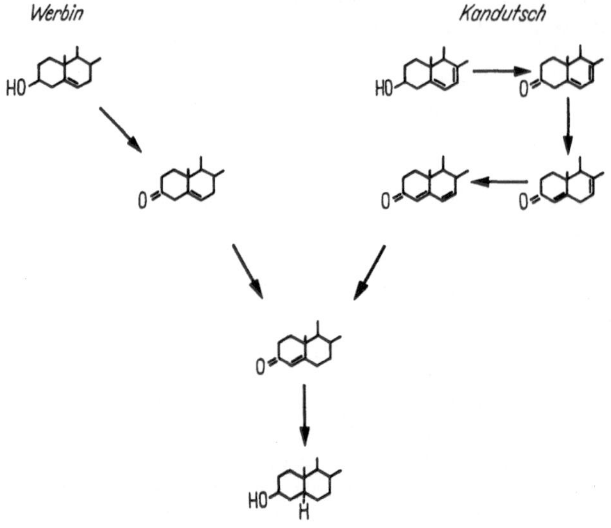

Two pathways for Cholestanol biosynthesis
Fig. 20

cholesterol diet for four days whereas SHEFER terminated the experiment within 24 hours after administration of isotope. The rapid conversion of cholestenone to cholestanol had previously been shown in rats (ANKER and BLOCH, 1949; STOKES et al., 1955) and in birds (NICHOLS et al., 1960). Two mechanisms for cholestanol biosynthesis, both involving cholestenone have been proposed. WERBIN et al. (1964) suggest a sequence from cholesterol which includes the following steps: cholesterol → Δ^5-cholestenone → Δ^4-cholestenone → cholestanone → cholestanol. KANDUTSCH (1963) proposes the conversion of a cholesterol precursor to 7-dehydrocholesterol → $\Delta^{5,7}$-cholestadiene-3-one → $\Delta^{4,7}$-cholestadien-3-one → $\Delta^{4,6}$-cholestadiene-3-one → cholestanol (Fig. 20). The complete elucidation of the pathway of cholestanol biosynthesis and the question of a possible species difference in biosynthesis of this stanol must await further work.

References

AGRANOFF, B. W., H. EGGERER, V. HENNING, and F. LYNEN: Biosynthesis of terpenes. VII. Isopentenyl pyrophosphate isomerase. J. biol. Chem. **235**, 326 (1960).
ALEXANDER, G. J., A. M. GOLD, and E. SCHWENK: The methyl group of methionine as a source of C_{28} in ergosterol. J. Amer. Chem. Soc. **79**, 2967 (1957a).
— and E. SCHWENK: Studies on biosynthesis of cholesterol. IX. Zymosterol as a precursor of cholesterol. Arch. Biochem. **66**, 381 (1957a).
— — Transfer of the methyl group of methionine to carbon-24 of ergosterol. J. Amer. Chem. Soc. **79**, 4554 (1957b).

ANFINSEN jr., C. B., and M. G. HORNING: Enzymatic degradation of the cholesterol side chain in cell-free preparations. J. Amer. Chem. Soc. 75, 1511 (1953).

ANKER, H. S.: Some aspects of the metabolism of pyruvic acid in the intact animal. J. biol. Chem. 176, 1337 (1948).

— and K. BLOCH: On the metabolism of $\Delta^{4,5}$-cholestenone. J. biol. Chem. 178, 971 (1949).

AVIGAN, J., D. S. GOODMAN, and D. STEINBERG: Studies of cholesterol biosynthesis. IV. Reduction of lanosterol to 24,25-dihydrolanosterol by rat liver homogenates. J. biol. Chem. 238, 1283 (1963).

— D. STEINBERG, H. E. VROMAN, M. J. THOMPSON, and E. MOSETTIG: Studies of cholesterol biosynthesis. I. The identification of desmosterol in serum and tissues of animals and man treated with MER-29. J. biol. Chem. 235, 3123 (1960).

BAGGETT, B., L. L. ENGEL, K. SAVARD, and R. I. DORFMAN: Conversion of testosterone-3-C^{14} to C^{14}-Estradiol by human ovarian tissue. J. biol. Chem. 221, 931 (1956).

BAISTED, D. J., E. CAPSTACK jr., and W. R. NES: The biosynthesis of β-Amyrin and β-Sitosterol in germinating seeds of Pisum sativum. Biochemistry 1, 537 (1962).

BERGSTRÖM, S.: The formation of bile acids from cholesterol in the rat. Kungl. Fysiograf. Sällskap. Lund. Forh. 22, 1 (1952).

— Formation and metabolism of bile acids. Rec. Chem. Progr. 16, 63 (1955).

— Bile acids: formation and metabolism. In: The Biosynthesis of Terpenes and Sterols, ed. G. E. W. WOLSTENHOLME and M. O'CONNOR, p. 185. London: Churchill 1959.

— H. DANIELSSON, and B. SAMUELSSON: Formation and metabolism of bile acids. In: Lipide Metabolism, ed. K. BLOCH, p. 291. New York: Wiley 1960.

— and S. LINDSTEDT: The formation of cholic acid from 3α, 7α-dihydroxycoprostane in the rat. Biochim. biophys. Acta (Amst.) 19, 556 (1956).

BEUMER, H., u. F. LEHMANN: Über die Cholesterinbildung im Tierkörper. Z. ges. exp. Med. 37, 274 (1923).

BEYER, K. F., and L. T. SAMUELS: Distribution of steroid-3β-ol-dehydrogenase in cellular structures of the adrenal gland. J. biol. Chem. 219, 69 (1956).

BHATTATHIRY, E. P. M., and M. D. SIPERSTEIN: Feedback control of cholesterol synthesis in man. J. clin. Invest. 42, 1613 (1963).

BIGGS, M. W., D. KRITCHEVSKY, D. COLMAN, J. W. GOFMAN, H. B. JONES, F. T. LINDGREN, G. HYDE, and T. P. LYON: Observations on the fate of ingested cholesterol in man. Circulation 6, 359 (1952).

— R. M. LEMMON, and F. T. PIERCE jr.: Observations on Δ^7-cholesterol metabolism in the rabbit. Arch. Biochem. 51, 155 (1954).

BLOCH, K.: The biological conversion of cholesterol to pregnanediol. J. biol. Chem. 157, 661 (1945).

— Über die Herkunft des Kohlenstoff-atoms 7 in Cholesterin. Ein Beitrag zur Kenntnis der Biosynthese der Steroide. Helv. chim. Acta. 36, 1611 (1953).

— B. N. BERG, and D. RITTENBERG: The biological conversion of cholesterol to cholic acid. J. biol. Chem. 149, 511 (1943).

— S. CHAYKIN, A. H. PHILLIPS, and A. DE WAARD: Mevalonic acid pyrophosphate and isopentenylpyrophosphate. J. biol. Chem. 234, 2595 (1959).

— L. C. CLARK, and I. HARARY: Utilization of branched chain acids in cholesterol synthesis. J. biol. Chem. 211, 687 (1954).

— and D. RITTENBERG: The biological formation of cholesterol from acetic acid. J. biol. Chem. 143, 297 (1942a).

— — On the utilization of acetic acid for cholesterol formation. J. biol. Chem. 145, 625 (1942b).

— — Sources of acetic acid in the animal body. J. biol. Chem. 155, 243 (1944).

BLOHM, T. R., T. KARIYA, and W. M. LAUGHLIN: Effects of MER-29, a cholesterol synthesis inhibitor on mammalian tissue lipids. Arch. Biochem. 85, 250 (1959b).

— and R. D. MACKENZIE: Specific inhibition of cholesterol biosynthesis by a synthetic compound (MER-29). Arch. Biochem. 85, 245 (1959a).

BONDZYNSKI, S., u. V. HUMNICKI: Über das Schicksal des Cholesterins im tierischen Organismus. Z. physiol. Chem. 22, 396 (1896).

BONNER, J., and B. ARREGUIN: The biochemistry of rubber formation in the guayule. I. Rubber formation in seedlings. Arch. Biochem. 21, 109 (1949).

BRADY, R. O., and S. GURIN: The biosynthesis of radioactive fatty acids and cholesterol. J. biol. Chem. 186, 461 (1950).

— — The synthesis of radioactive cholesterol and fatty acids in vitro. J. biol. Chem. 189, 371 (1951).

BREUER, H., u. P. GRILL: Bildung von Formaldehyd bei der Aromatisierung neutraler Steroide zu phenolischen Steroiden. Hoppe-Seylers Z. physiol. Chem. 324, 254 (1961).

BRIGGS, T., M. W. WHITEHOUSE, and E. STAPLE: Formation of bile acids from cholesterol in the alligator. Arch. Biochem. 85, 275 (1959).
— — — Metabolism of trihydroxycoprostanic acid: formation from cholesterol in the alligator and conversion to cholic acid and carbon dioxide in vitro by rat liver mitochondria. J. biol. Chem. 236, 688 (1961).
BRODIE, J. D., G. WASSON, and J. W. PORTER: The participation of malonyl coenzyme A in the biosynthesis of mevalonic acid. J. biol. Chem. 238, 1294 (1963).
BUCHER, N. L. R., and K. McGARRAHAN: The biosynthesis of cholesterol from acetate-1-C^{14} by cellular fractions of rat liver. J. biol. Chem. 222, 1 (1956).
— — E. GOULD, and A. V. LOUD: Cholesterol biosynthesis in preparations of liver from normal, fasting, x-irradiated, cholesterol-fed, triton, or Δ^4-cholesten-3-one treated rats. J. biol. Chem. 234, 262 (1959).
BUTENANDT, A., u. H. KUDSZUS: Über Androstendion, einen hochwirksam männlichen Prägungsstoff. Ein Beitrag zur Genese der Keimdrüsenhormone. Hoppe-Seylers Z. physiol. Chem. 237, 75 (1935).
BYERS, S. O., and M. W. BIGGS: Cholic acid and cholesterol: studies concerning possible intraconversion. Arch. Biochem. 39, 301 (1952).
CALVIN, H. I., and S. LIEBERMAN: Evidence that steroid sulfates serve as biosynthetic intermediates. II. In vitro conversion of pregnenolone-^{3}H-sulfate-^{35}S to 17α hydroxypregnenolone-^{3}H-sulfate-^{35}S. Biochemistry 3, 259 (1964).
— R. L. VANDEWIELE, and S. LIEBERMAN: Evidence that steroid sulfates serve as biosynthetic intermediates: in vivo conversion of pregnenolone-sulfate-S^{35} to dehydroisoandrosterone-sulfate-S^{35}. Biochemistry 2, 648 (1963).
CASPI, E., R. I. DORFMAN, B. T. KHAN, G. ROSENFELD, and W. SCHMID: Degradation of corticosteroids. VI. Origin of the carbon atoms of steroid hormones biosynthesized in vitro in the bovine adrenal from acetate-1-C^{14}. J. biol. Chem. 237, 2085 (1962).
— G. ROSENFELD, and R. I. DORFMAN: Degration of cortisol-C^{14} and corticosterone-C^{14} biosynthesized from acetate-1-C^{14}. J. org. Chem. 21, 814 (1956).
— F. UNGAR, and R. I. DORFMAN: Degradation of 3α, 17α, 21-trihydroxypregnan-20-one-C^{14} biosynthesized from acetate-1-C^{14} by a Cushing's patient. J. org. Chem. 22, 326 (1957).
CHAIKOFF, I. L., M. D. SIPERSTEIN, W. G. DAUBEN, H. L. BRADLOW, J. F. EASTHAM, G. M. TOMKINS, J. R. MEIER, R. W. CHEN, S. HOTTA, and P. A. SRERE: C^{14}-Cholesterol. II. Oxidation of carbons 4 and 26 to carbon dioxide by the intact rat. J. biol. Chem. 194, 413 (1952).
CHANNON, H. J.: The biological significance of the unsaponifiable matter of oils. I. Experiments with the unsaturated hydrocarbon squalene. Biochem. J. 20, 400 (1926).
— and G. R. TRISTRAM: The effect of the administration of squalene and other hydrocarbons on cholesterol metabolism in the rat. Biochem. J. 31, 738 (1937).
CHAYKIN, S., J. LAW, A. H. PHILLIPS, T. T. TCHEN, and K. BLOCH: Phosphorylated intermediates in the synthesis of squalene. Proc. Nat. Acad. Sci. (Wash.) 44, 998 (1958).
CHEVALLIER, F.: Application des méthodes isotopiques . l'étude de l'état dynamique des constituants organiques. Ann. Nutr. (Paris) 7, 225 (1953).
— L'espace cholestérol du rat. Arch. Sci. physiol. 10, 249 (1956).
— Détermination des quantités de stérols excrétés et sécrétes, et de la fraction du cholestérol des parois digestives renouvelé par transfert. Bull. Soc. Chim. biol. (Paris) 42, 1633 (1960).
CHOBANIAN, A. V., and W. HOLLANDER: Body cholesterol metabolism in man. I. The equilibration of serum and tissue cholesterol. J. clin. Invest. 41, 1732 (1962).
CLAYTON, R. B.: The utilization of sterols by insects. J. Lipid Res. 5, 3 (1964).
— and K. BLOCH: Biological synthesis of lanosterol and agnosterol. J. biol. Chem. 218, 305 (1956a).
— — The biological conversion of lanosterol to cholesterol. J. biol. Chem. 218, 319 (1956b).
— — Sterol utilization by the hide beetle, Dermestes vulpinus. J. biol. Chem. 238, 586 (1963).
COLEMAN, D. L., and C. A. BAUMANN: Intestinal sterols. III. Effects of age, sex and diet. Arch. Biochem. 66, 226 (1957).
CONSTANTOPOULOS, G., and T. T. TCHEN: Cleavage of cholesterol side chain by adrenal cortex. I. Cofactor requirement and product of cleavage. J. biol. Chem. 236, 65 (1961).
COON, M. J., and S. GURIN: Studies on the conversion of radioactive leucine to acetoacetate. J. biol. Chem. 180, 1159 (1949).
CORNFORTH, J. W., R. H. CORNFORTH, A. PELTER, M. G. HORNING, and G. POPJAK: Studies on the biosynthesis of cholesterol. 7. Rearrangements of methyl groups during enzymic cyclisation of squalene. Tetrahedron 5, 311 (1959b).
— I. Y. GORE, and G. POPJAK: Studies on the biosynthesis of cholesterol. 4. Degradation of rings C and D. Biochem. J. 65, 94 (1957).
— G. D. HUNTER, and G. POPJAK: Studies of cholesterol biosynthesis. I. A new chemical degradation of cholesterol. Biochem J. 54, 590 (1953).
— and G. POPJAK: Mechanism of biosynthesis of squalene from sesquiterpenoids. Tetrahedron Letters 19, 29 (1959a).

COTTET, J., J. VIGNALOU, J. REDEL et COLAS-BELCOUR: Propriétés hypocholésterolémiantes de acides phényl-éthyl-acétique (22TH) et phényl-méthyl-acétique (4082TH). Bull. mem. Soc. méd. Hôp. (Paris) **69**, 903 (1953).

CURRAN, G. L.: Utilization of acetoacetic acid in cholesterol synthesis by surviving rat liver. J. biol. Chem. **191**, 775 (1951).

DAM, H.: Über die Cholesterinsynthese im Tierkörper. Biochem. Z. **220**, 158 (1930).

— The formation of coprosterol in the intestine. II. The action of intestinal bacteria on cholesterol. Biochem. J. **28**, 820 (1934).

DANIELSSON, H.: Present status of research on catabolism and excretion of cholesterol. In: Advanc. Lipid Res. Vol. I, ed. R. PAOLETTI and D. KRITCHEVSKY, p. 335. New York: Academic Press 1963.

— and K. BLOCH: On the origin of C_{28} in ergosterol. J. Amer. chem. Soc. **79**, 500 (1957).

— and B. GUSTAFSSON: On serum cholesterol levels and neutral fecal sterols in germ free rats. Arch. Biochem. **83**, 482 (1959).

DAUBEN, W. G., G. J. FONKEN, and G. A. BOSWELL: The biosynthetic precursor of the extra carbon atom in the side-chain of steroids. J. Amer. chem. Soc. **79**, 1000 (1957b).

— and T. W. HUTTON: The biosynthesis of steroids and triterpenes. The origin of carbons 11 and 12 of ergosterol. J. Amer. chem. Soc. **78**, 2647 (1956).

— and K. H. TAKEMURA: A study of conversion of acetate to cholesterol via squalene. J. Amer. chem. Soc. **75**, 6302 (1953).

DAVIDSON, A. G., E. G. DULIT, and I. D. FRANTZ jr.: Conversion of tritiated lathosterol to cholesterol by cell-free preparations of rat liver. Fed. Proc. **16**, 169 (1957).

DEMPSEY, M. E., J. D. SEATON, G. J. SCHROEPFER jr., and R. W. TROCKMAN: The intermediary role of $\Delta^{5,7}$-cholestadien-3β-ol in cholesterol biosynthesis. J. biol. Chem. **239**, 1381 (1964).

DE WAARD, A., and G. POPJAK: Studies on the biosynthesis of cholesterol. 9. Formation of phosphorylated derivatives of mevalonic acid in liver-enzyme preparations. Biochem. J. **73**, 410 (1959).

DEZANI, S.: Richerche sulla genesi della colesterina. G. Accad. Med. Torino. **19**, 149 (1913).

DIRSCHERL, W., u. H. TRAUT: Zur Frage der Cholesterinbildung im Tierkörper. Hoppe-Seylers Z. physiol. Chem. **262**, 61 (1939).

DORFMAN, R.I.: Metabolism of androgens, estrogens and corticoids. Amer. J. Med. **21**, 679 (1956).

DRAYER, N. M., K. D. ROBERTS, L. BANDI, and S. LIEBERMAN: The isolation of cholesterol sulfate from bovine adrenals. J. biol. Chem. **239**, PC 3112 (1964).

DURR, I. F., and H. RUDNEY: The reduction of β-hydroxy-β-methyl-glutaryl coenzyme A to mevalonic acid. J. biol. Chem. **235**, 2572 (1960).

DVORNIK, D., and M. KRAML: Accumulation of 24-dehydrocholesterol in rats treated with 22,25-diazacholestanol. Proc. Soc. exp. Biol. (N. Y.) **112**, 1012 (1963).

— — J. DUBUC, M. GIVNER, and R. GAUDRY: A novel mode of inhibition of cholesterol biosynthesis. J. Amer. chem. Soc. **85**, 3309 (1963).

ECKLES, N. E., C. B. TAYLOR, D. J. CAMPBELL, and R. G. GOULD: The origin of plasma cholesterol and the rates of equilibration of liver, plasma and erythrocyte cholesterol. J. Lab. clin. Med. **46**, 359 (1955).

EKDAHL, P. H., and J. SJÖVALL: Formation of bile acids from cholesterol in the rabbit. Acta physiol. scand. **34**, 329 (1955).

ELLIOTT, W. H.: The enzymic synthesis of taurocholic acid: a qualitative study. Biochem. J. **62**, 433 (1956).

ENGEL, L. L., B. BAGGETT, and M. HALLA: The formation of ^{14}C-labelled estriol from 16-^{14}C-estradiol-17β by human fetal liver slices. Biochim. biophys. Acta (Amst.) **30**, 435 (1958).

ERIKSSON, S.: Influence of thyroid on excretion of bile acids and cholesterol in the rat. Proc. Soc. exp. Biol. (N. Y.) **94**, 582 (1957).

— Bile acid pool in the rat. Acta physiol. scand. **48**, 439 (1960).

FERGUSON, J. J., I. F. DURR, and H. RUDNEY: The biosynthesis of mevalonic acid. Proc. Nat. Acad. Sci. (Wash.) **45**, 499 (1959).

FIESER, L. F.: A companion of cholesterol. J. Amer. chem. Soc. **73**, 5007 (1951).

FRANTZ jr., I. D., and B. T. HINKELMAN. Acceleration of hepatic cholesterol synthesis by Triton WR-1339, J exp. Med. **101**, 225 (1955).

— M. L. MOBBERLEY, and G. SCHROEPFER jr.: Effects of MER-29 on the intermediary metabolism of cholesterol. Progr. cardiovasc. Dis. **2**, 511 (1960).

— A. T. SANGHVI, and G. J. SCHROEPFER jr.: Irreversibility of the biogenetic sequence from Δ^7-cholesten-3β-ol through $\Delta^{5,7}$-cholestadien-3β-ol to cholesterol. J. biol. Chem. **239**, 1007 (1964).

FREDRICKSON, D. S.: The conversion of cholesterol-4-C^{14} to acids and other products by liver mitochondria. J. biol. Chem. **222**, 109 (1956a).

— and K. ONO: The in vitro production of 25- and 26-hydroxycholesterol and their in vivo metabolism. Biochim. biophys. Acta (Amst.) **22**, 183 (1956b).

FUKUSHIMA, D. K., and T. F. GALLAGHER: Isotopic distribution in cholesterol after platinum-catalyzed hydrogen-deuterium exchange. J. biol. Chem. **198**, 861 (1952).

GAUTSCHI, F., and K. BLOCH: Synthesis of isomeric 4,4-dimethyl-cholestenols and identification of a lanosterol metabolite. J. biol. Chem. **233**, 1343 (1958).

GIDEZ, L. I., and H. A. EDER: Cholesterol turnover in man. In: Proc. First Int. Pharmacol. Meeting, Vol. 2, Effects of Drugs on Synthesis and Mobilization of Lipids. eds. E. C. HORNING, and P. LINDGREN, p. 67. Oxford: Pergamon-Press 1963.

GOLDSTEIN, F. B.: Studies on aromatic acids in relation to phenylpyruvic oligophrenia. Thesis, McGill University, Montreal (1955).

GOLDSTEIN, M., M. GUT, and R. I. DORFMAN: Conversion of pregnenolone to dehydroepiandrosterone. Biochim. biophys. Acta (Amst.) **38**, 190 (1960).

GOODMAN, D. S., and G. POPJAK: Studies on the biosynthesis of cholesterol. XII. Synthesis of allyl pyrophosphates from mevalonate and their conversion into squalene with liver enzymes. J. Lipid Res. **1**, 286 (1960).

GORDON, S., E. W. CANTRALL, W. P. CEKLENIAK, H. J. ALBERS, R. LITTELL, and S. BERNSTEIN: The hypocholesteremic effect of 3β-(β-dimethyl-aminoethoxy)-androst-5-en-17-one and its mechanism of action. Biochem. biophys. Res. Commun. **6**, 359 (1961).

GOULD, R. G.: Lipid metabolism in arteriosclerosis. Amer. J. Med. **11**, 209 (1951).

— D. R. AVOY, and E. A. SWYRYD: Effect of α-p-chlorophenoxyisobutyrate (CPIB) on cholesterol (Abstract). Circulation **30**. (Suppl. III) 11 (1964).

— G. V. LEROY, G. T. OKITA, J. J. KABARA, P. KEEGAN, and D. M. BERGENSTAL: The use of C^{14}-labeled acetate to study cholesterol metabolism in man. J. Lab. clin. Med. **40**, 374 (1955).

GREEN, K., and B. SAMUELSSON: Mechanisms of bile acid biosynthesis studied with 3α-^{3}H and 4β-^{3}H-cholesterol. J. biol. Chem. **239**, 2804 (1964).

GUSTAFSSON, B., S. BERGSTRÖM, S. LINDSTEDT, and A. NORMAN: Turnover and nature of fecal bile acids in germfree and infected rats fed cholic acid-24-C^{14}. Proc. Soc. exp. Biol. (N. Y.) **94**, 467 (1957).

HAGOPIAN, M., and L. K. LEVY: The conversion of 16-^{14}C-17β-estradiol to estriol by isolated rat livers. Biochim. biophys. Acta (Amst.) **30**, 641 (1958).

HALKERSTON, I. D. K., J. EICHHORN, and O. HECHTER: A requirement for reduced triphosphopyridine nucleotide for cholesterol side chain cleavage by mitochondrial fractions of bovine adrenal cortex. J. biol. Chem. **236**, 374 (1961).

HANAHAN, D. J., and S. J. WAKIL: The origin of some of the carbon atoms of the side chain of C^{14}-ergosterol. J. Amer. chem. Soc. **75**, 273 (1953).

HASLEWOOD, G. A. D.: Comparative studies of "bile salts." 5. Bile salts of Crocodylidae. Biochem. J. **52**, 583 (1952).

— Specific comparison as an aid in the study of the process sterols → bile salts. In: The Biosynthesis of Terpenes and Sterols, ed. G. E. W. WOLSTENHOLME, and M. O'CONNOR, p. 206. London: Churchill 1959.

HAYANO, M., N. SABA, R. I. DORFMAN, and O. HECHTER: Some aspects of the biogenesis of adrenal steroid hormones. Recent Progr. Hormone Res. **12**, 79 (1956).

HECHTER, O.: Conversion of cholesterol to steroid hormones. In: Cholesterol, ed. R. P. COOK, p. 309. New York: Academic-Press 1958.

— M. M. SOLOMON, A. ZAFFARONI, and G. PINCUS: Transformation of cholesterol and acetate to adrenal cortical hormones. Arch. Biochem. **46**, 201 (1953).

— A. ZAFFARONI, R. P. JACOBSEN, H. LEVY, R. W. JEANLOZ, V. SCHENKER, and G. PINCUS: The nature and the biogenesis of the adrenal secretory product. Recent Progr. Hormone Res. **6**, 215 (1951).

HEILBRON, I. M., E. D. KAMM, and W. M. OWENS: Unsaponifiable matter from the oils of elasmobranch fish. I. Contribution to the study of the constitution of squalene (spinacene). J. chem. Soc. **1926**, 1630.

HELLMAN, L., R. S. ROSENFELD, and T. F. GALLAGHER: Cholesterol synthesis from C^{14}-acetate in man. J. clin. Invest. **33**, 142 (1954).

HELLSTRÖM, K., and J. SJÖVALL: Conjugation of bile acids in patients with hypothyroidism. J. Atheroscler. Res. **1**, 205 (1961).

HENNING, V., E. M. MÖSLEIN, and F. LYNEN: Biosynthesis of terpenes V. Formation of 5-pyrophosphomevalonic acid by phosphomevalonic kinase. Arch. Biochem. **83**, 259(1959).

HOLMES, W. L.: Drugs affecting lipid synthesis. In: Lipid Pharmacology, ed. R. PAOLETTI, p. 131. New York: Academic-Press 1964.

— Drugs affecting lipid synthesis. J. Amer. Oil Chem. Soc. **41**, 702 (1964b).

— and N. W. DI TULLIO: Inhibitors of cholesterol biosynthesis which act at or beyond the mevalonic acid stage. Amer. J. clin. Nutr. **10**, 310 (1962).

HORNING, M. G., D. S. FREDRICKSON, and C. B. ANFINSEN: Studies on the enzymatic degradation of the cholesterol side chain. II. Requirements of the mitochondrial system. Arch. Biochem. **71**, 266 (1957).

HUFF, J. W., and J. L. GILFILLAN: Benzmalacene: inhibition of cholesterol biosynthesis and hypocholesteremic effects in rats. Proc. Soc. exp. Biol. (N. Y.) 103, 41 (1960).

JOHNSON, D. F., B. E. WRIGHT, and E. HEFTMANN: Biogenesis of Δ^{22}-Stigmasten-3β-ol in Dictyostelium discoideum. Arch. Biochem. 97, 232 (1962).

JOHNSTON, J. D., and K. BLOCH: In vitro conversion of zymosterol and dihydrozymosterol to cholesterol. J. Amer. chem. Soc. 79, 1145 (1957).

KANDUTSCH, A. A.: Metabolism of cholesta-4,7-diene-3-one and cholesta-4,6-dien-3-one by mouse liver microsomes. J. Lipid Res. 4, 179 (1963).

— and A. E. RUSSELL: Preputial gland tumor sterols. I. The occurrence of 24,25-dihydro-lanosterol and a comparison with liver and normal gland. J. biol. Chem. 234, 2037 (1960a).

— — Preputial gland tumor sterols. II. The identification of 4-α-methyl-Δ^8-cholesten-3β-ol. J. biol. Chem. 235, 2253 (1960b).

— — Preputial gland tumor sterols. III. A metabolic pathway from lanosterol to cholesterol. J. biol. Chem. 235, 2256 (1960c).

— — Intermediates in a pathway from lanosterol to cholesterol. Fed. Proc. 19, 237 (1960d).

KASE, N., E. FORCHIELLI, and R. I. DORFMAN: In vitro production of testosterone and androst-4-ene-3, 17-dione in a human ovarian homogenate. Acta endocr. (Kbh.) 37, 19 (1961).

KNAUSS, H. J., J. W. PORTER, and G. WASSON: The biosynthesis of mevalonic acid from 1-C^{14} acetate by a rat liver enzyme system. J. biol. Chem. 234, 2835 (1959).

KRITCHEVSKY, D.: Factors influencing the oxidation of cholesterol by rat liver mitochondria. In: Metabolism of Lipids as Related to Atherosclerosis, ed. F. KUMMEROW, p. 106. Springfield (Ill.): Thomas 1965.

— M. C. COTTRELL, and S. A. TEPPER: Oxidation of cholesterol by rat liver mitochondria: effect of thyroactive compounds. J. Cell. comp. Physiol. 60, 105 (1962).

— and I. GRAY: Biosynthesis of cholesterol from isobutyrate. Experientia (Basel) 7, 183 (1951).

— and W. L. HOLMES: Occurence of desmosterol in developing rat brain. Biochem. biophys. Res. Commun. 7, 128 (1962).

— and E. STAPLE: Oxidation of desmosterol by rat liver mitochondria. Naturwissenschaften 49, 109 (1962).

— — and M. W. WHITEHOUSE: Regulation of cholesterol biosynthesis and catabolism. Amer. J. clin. Nutr. 8, 411 (1960).

— — Oxidation of ergosterol by rat and mouse liver mitochondria. Proc. Soc. exp. Biol. (N. Y.) 106, 704 (1961).

— N. T. WERTHESSEN, and I. SHAPIRO: Studies on the biosynthesis of lipids in the baboon. Biosynthesis and transport of cholesterol. Clin. chim. Acta 11, 44 (1965).

LANGDON, R. G., and K. BLOCH: The biosynthesis af squalene. J. biol. Chem. 200, 129 (1953a).

— — The utilization of squalene in the biosynthesis of cholesterol. J. biol. Chem. 200, 135 (1953b).

LANGER, L. J., and L. L. ENGEL: Human placental estradiol-17β dehydrogenase. I. Concentration, characterization and assay. J. biol. Chem. 233, 583 (1958).

LEVY, H. R., and G. POPJAK: Studies on the biosynthesis of cholesterol. 10. Mevalonic kinase and phosphomevalonic kinase from liver. Biochem. J. 75, 417 (1960).

LINDSTEDT, S.: Turnover of cholic acid in man. Acta physiol. scand. 40, 1 (1957).

— and E. H. AHRENS jr.: Conversion of cholesterol to bile acids in man. Proc. Soc. exp. Biol. (N. Y.) 108, 286 (1961).

— and A. NORMAN: Turnover of bile acids in the rat. Acta physiol. scand. 38, 121 (1956).

LITTLE, H. N., and K. BLOCH: Studies on the utilization of acetic acid for the biological synthesis of cholesterol. J. biol. Chem. 183, 33 (1950).

LYNEN, F., B. W. AGRANOFF, H. EGGERER, V. HENNING u. E. M. MÖSLEIN: γ,γ-Dimethyl-allyl-pyrophosphat und Geranyl-pyrophosphat, biologische Vorstufen des Squalens. Angew. Chem. 71, 657 (1959).

— H. EGGERER, V. HENNING u. I. KESSELL: Farnesyl-pyrophosphat und 3-Methyl-Δ^3-butenyl-1-pyrophosphat, die biologischen Vorstufen des Squalens. Angew. Chem. 70, 738 (1958).

— u. M. GRASSL: Zur Biosynthese der Terpene. II. Darstellung von (—) Mevalonsäure durch bakterielle Racematspaltung. Hoppe-Seylers Z. physiol. Chem. 313, 291 (1958).

LYNN jr., W. S., and R. BROWN: Mechanism of in vitro steroid oxidation. Biochim. biophys. Acta (Amst.) 21, 403 (1956).

MARSH, J. B., and D. L. DRABKIN: Metabolic channeling in experimental nephrosis. V. Lipide metabolism in the early stages of the disease. J. biol. Chem. 230, 1083 (1958).

MAUDGAL, R. K., T. T. TCHEN, and K. BLOCH: 1,2-methyl shifts in the cyclization of squalene to lanosterol. J. Amer. chem. Soc. 80, 2589 (1958).

MENDELSOHN, D., and E. STAPLE: The in vitro catabolism of cholesterol: formation of 3α, 7α, 12α-trihydroxycoprostane from cholesterol in rat liver. Biochemistry 2, 577 (1963).] ! ..

Meyer, A. S.: 19-hydroxylation of 4-androstene-3, 17-dione and dehydroepiandrosterone by bovine adrenal glands. Experientia (Basel) 11, 99 (1955a).
— Conversion of 19-hydroxy-Δ^4-androstene-3,17-dione to estrone by endocrine tissue. Biochim. biophys. Acta (Amst.) 17, 441 (1955b).
Mosbach, E. H., J. Blum, E. Arroyo, and S. Milch: A new method for the determination of dihydrocholesterol in tissues. An. Biochem. 5, 158 (1963).
Nicholas, H. J.: Biosynthesis of β-sitosterol and pentacyclic triterpenes of salvia officinalis. J. biol. Chem. 237, 1476 (1962a).
— Biosynthesis of sclareol, β-sitosterol and oleanolic acid from mevalonic acid-2-C^{14}. J. biol. Chem. 237, 1481 (1962b).
Nichols jr., C. W., S. Lindsay, D. D. Chapman, and I. L. Chaikoff: Prolonged Δ^4-cholestenone feeding in birds. Circulation Res. 8, 16 (1960).
Olson, J. A., M. Lindberg, and K. Bloch: On the demethylation of lanosterol to cholesterol. J. biol. Chem. 226, 941 (1957).
Ottke, R. C., E. L. Tatum, I. Zabin, and K. Bloch: Isotopic acetate and isovalerate in the synthesis of ergosterol by neurospora. J. biol. Chem. 189, 429 (1951).
Phillips, W. A., and J. Avigan: Inhibition of cholesterol biosynthesis in the rat by 3β-(-2 diethylaminoethoxy) androst-5-en-17-one hydrochloride. Proc. Soc. exp. Biol. (N. Y.) 112, 233 (1963).
Popjak, G., R. H. Cornforth, and K. Clifford: Inhibition of cholesterol biosynthesis by farnesoic acid and its analogues. Lancet 1960/I, 1270.
Portman, O. W., and P. Murphy: Excretion of bile acids and β-hydroxysterols by rats. Arch. Biochem. 76, 367 (1958).
Rabinowitz, J. L.: Biosynthesis of radioactive 17β-estradiol. IV. Substrate utilization by testicular homogenates. Atompraxis 5, 1 (1959).
— and S. Gurin: Biosynthesis of cholesterol and β-hydroxy-β-methylglutaric acid by extracts of liver. J. biol. Chem. 208, 307 (1954).
Ranney, R. W., and R. E. Counsell: An azasterol that inhibits cholesterol synthesis in vitro. Proc. Soc. exp. Biol. (N. Y.) 109, 820 (1962).
Redel, J., et J. Cottet: Action hypocholéstérolémiante de quelques acides acétiques disubstitués. C.R. Acad. Sci. (Paris) 236, 2553 (1953).
Rilling, H. C., and K. Bloch: On the mechanism of squalene biogenesis from mevalonic acid. J. biol. Chem. 234, 1424 (1959).
Rittenberg, D., and K. Bloch: The utilization of acetic acid for fatty acid synthesis. J. biol. Chem. 154, 311 (1944).
— — The utilization of acetic acid for the synthesis of fatty acids. J. biol. Chem. 160, 417 (1945).
— and R. Schoenheimer: Deuterium as an indicator in the study of intermediary metabolism XI. Further studies on the biological uptake of deuterium into organic substances with special reference to fat and cholesterol formation. J. biol. Chem. 121, 235 (1937).
Roberts, K. D., L. Bandi, H. I. Calvin, W. D. Drucker, and S. Lieberman: Evidence that cholesterol sulfate is a precursor of steroid hormones. J. Amer. chem. Soc. 86, 958 (1964).
Robinson, R.: Structure of cholesterol. J. Soc. chem. Ind. 53, 1062 (1934).
Rosenfeld, R. S., and T. F. Gallagher: Further studies of the biotransformation of cholesterol to coprostanol. Steroids 4, 515 (1964).
— D. K. Fukushima, L. Hellman, and T. F. Gallagher: The transformation of cholesterol to coprostanol. J. biol. Chem. 211, 301 (1954).
— and L. Hellman: Excretion of steroid acids in man. Arch. Biochem. 97, 406 (1962).
— — and T. F. Gallagher: The transformation of cholesterol-3d to coprostanol-d. Location of deuterium in coprostanol. J. biol. Chem. 222, 321 (1956).
Rosenheim, O., and T. A. Webster: A dietary factor concerned in coprosterol formation. Biochem. J. 35, 920 (1941).
— — The mechanism of coprosterol formation in vivo. 1. Cholestenone as an intermediate. Biochem. J. 37, 513 (1943).
Rudney, H.: The synthesis of β-hydroxy-β-methylglutaric acid in rat liver homogenates. J. Amer. chem. Soc. 76, 2595 (1954).
— Biosynthesis of β-hydroxy-β-methyl-glutaric acid (HMG). Fed. Proc. 15, 342 (1956).
Ryan, K. J., and O. W. Smith: Biogenesis of estrogens by the human ovary. IV. Formation of neutral steroid intermediates. J. biol. Chem. 236, 2207 (1961).
Saba, N., and O. Hechter: Cholesterol-4-C^{14} metabolism in adrenal homogenates. Fed. Proc. 14, 775 (1955).
— — and D. Stone: Conversion of cholesterol to pregnenolone in bovine adrenal homogenates. J. Amer. chem. Soc. 76, 3862 (1954).
Sakakida, H., C. C. Shediac, and M. D. Siperstein: Effect of endogenous and exogenous cholesterol on the feedback control of cholesterol synthesis. J. clin. Invest. 42, 1521 (1963).

SCHOENHEIMER, R., H. v. BEHRING u. R. HUMMEL: Untersuchung der Sterine aus verschiedenen Organen auf ihren Gehalt an gesättigten Sterinen. Hoppe-Seylers Z. physiol. Chem. 192, 93 (1930).
— and F. BREUSCH: Synthesis and destruction of cholesterol in the organism. J. biol. Chem. 103, 439 (1933).
— D. RITTENBERG, and M. GRAFF: Deuterium as an indicator in the study of intermediary metabolism. IV. The mechanism of coprosterol formation. J. biol. Chem. 111, 183 (1935).
SCHWENK, E., and G. J. ALEXANDER: Biogenesis of yeast sterols. II. Formation of ergosterol in yeast homogenates. Arch. Biochem. 76, 65 (1958).
— — T. H. STOUDT, and C. A. FISH: Studies on the biosynthesis of cholesterol. VII. Formation of cholesterol precursors by yeast. Arch. Biochem. 55, 274 (1955).
— and N. T. WERTHESSEN: Studies on the biosynthesis of cholesterol. III. Purification of C^{14}-cholesterol from perfusions of livers and other organs. Arch. Biochem. 40, 334 (1952).
— — Studies on the biosynthesis of cholesterol. IV. Higher counting substances accompnying C^{14}-cholesterol in the intact rat. Arch. Biochem. 42, 91 (1953).
SHEFER, S., S. MILCH, and E. H. MOSBACH: Biosynthesis of 5α-cholestan-3β-ol in the rabbit and guinea pig. J. biol. Chem. 239, 1731 (1964).
SHIMIZU, K., M. GUT, and R. I. DORFMAN: 20α, 22ξ-dihydroxycholesterol, an intermediate in the biosynthesis of pregnenolone (3β-hydroxypregn-5-en-20-one) from cholesterol. J. biol. Chem. 237, 699 (1962).
SIPERSTEIN, M. D.: Enzymatic synthesis of bile salts. Fed. Proc. 14, 282 (1955).
— and I. L. CHAIKOFF: C^{14}-cholesterol. III. Excretion of carbons 4 and 26 in feces, urine and bile. J. biol. Chem. 198, 93 (1952).
— and V. M. FAGAN: Inhibition of mevalonate synthesis by dietary cholesterol. Fed. Proc. 21, 300 (1962).
— and M. J. GUEST: Studies on the site of feedback control of cholesterol biosynthesis. J. clin. Invest. 39, 642 (1960).
— M. E. JAYKO, I. L. CHAIKOFF, and W. G. DAUBEN: Nature of the metabolic products of C^{14}-cholesterol excreted in bile and feces. Proc. Soc. exp. Biol. (N. Y.) 81, 720 (1952).
— and A. W. MURRAY: Cholesterol metabolism in man. J. clin. Invest. 34, 1449 (1955).
SLAUNWHITE jr., W. R., and L. T. SAMUELS: Progesterone as a precursor of testicular androgens. J. biol. Chem. 220, 341 (1956).
SMITH, P. F.: Relation of sterol structure to utilization in pleuro-pneumonia-like organisms. J. Lipid Res. 5, 121 (1964).
SNOG-KJAER, A., I. PRANGE, and H. DAM: On the formation of coprosterol in the intestine. Experientia (Basel) 11, 316 (1955).
— — — Conversion of cholesterol into coprosterol by bacteria in vitro. J. gen. Microbiol. 14, 256 (1956).
SOLOMON, S., A. C. CARTER, and S. LIEBERMAN: The conversion in vivo of 17α-hydroxypregnenolone to dehydroisoandrosterone and other 17-ketosteroids. J. biol. Chem. 235, 351 (1960).
SONDERHOFF, R., u. H. THOMAS: Die enzymatische Dehydrierung der Trideutero-Essigsäure. Ann. 530, 195 (1937).
STANLEY, M. M., and S. H. CHENG: Cholesterol exchange in the gastrointestinal tract in normal and abnormal subjects. Gastroenterology 30, 62 (1956).
STAPLE, E., and S. GURIN: The incorporation of radioactive acetate into biliary cholesterol and cholic acid. Biochim. biophys. Acta (Amst.) 15, 372 (1954).
— W. S. LYNN jr., and S. GURIN: An enzymatic cleavage of the cholesterol side chain. J. biol. Chem. 219, 845 (1956).
STEINBERG, D., and J. AVIGAN: Studies of cholesterol biosynthesis. II. The role of desmosterol in the biosynthesis of cholesterol. J. biol. Chem. 235, 3127 (1960).
— and D. S. FREDRICKSON: Inhibitors of cholesterol biosynthesis and the problem of hypercholesterolemia. Ann. N. Y. Acad. Sci. 64, 579 (1956).
STEVENSON, E., and E. STAPLE: Oxidation of various simple steroids by the cholesterol oxidase system. Arch. Biochem. 97, 485 (1962).
STOKES, W. M., W. A. FISH, and F. C. HICKEY: The fate of injected cholestenone in the intact rat. J. biol. Chem. 213, 325 (1955).
— — — Metabolism of cholesterol in the chick embryo. II. Isolation and chemical nature of two companion sterols. J. biol. Chem. 220, 415 (1956).
— F. C. HICKEY, and W. A. FISH: Sterol metabolism. 1. The occurrence of desmosterol (24-dehydrocholesterol) in rat skin and its conversion in vivo to cholesterol. J. biol. Chem. 232, 347 (1958).
SULD, H. M., E. STAPLE, and S. GURIN: Mechanism of formation of bile acids from cholesterol: Oxidation of 3β-cholestane-3α, 7α, 12α-triol and formation of propionic acid from the side chain by rat liver mitochondria. J. biol. Chem. 237, 338 (1962).

SWEAT, M. L., D. L. BERLINER, M. J. BRYSON, C. NABORS jr., J. HASKELL, and E. G. HOLM-
  STRÖM: The synthesis and metabolism of progesterone in the human and bovine ovary.
  Biochim. biophys. Acta (Amst.) 40, 289 (1960).
TAVORMINA, P. A., and M. H. GIBBS: The metabolism of β, γ-dihydroxy-β-methylvaleric acid
  by liver homogenates. J. Amer. chem. Soc. 78, 6210 (1956).
— M. H. GIBBS, and J. W. HUFF: The utilization of β-hydroxy-β-methyl-γ,δ-valerolactone in
  cholesterol biosynthesis. J. Amer. chem. Soc. 78, 4498 (1956).
TCHEN, T. T.: Mevalonic kinase: purification and properties. J. biol. Chem. 233, 1100 (1958).
— and K. BLOCH: On the mechanism of enzymatic cyclization of squalene. J. biol. Chem. 226,
  931 (1957).
THORP, J. M., and W. S. WARING: Modification of metabolism and distribution of lipids by
  ethyl chlorophenoxyisobutyrate. Nature (Lond.) 194, 948 (1962).
WELLS, W. W., and C. L. LORAH: The incorporation of acetate-1-C^{14} into methostenol of rat
  tissue and the conversion of synthetic methostenol-4-C^{14} to cholesterol in vivo. J. biol.
  Chem. 235, 978 (1960).
WERBIN, H., I. L. CHAIKOFF, and M. R. IMADA: 5α-cholestan-3β-ol: Its distribution in
  tissues and its synthesis from cholesterol in the guinea pig. J. biol. Chem. 237, 2072 (1962).
— — and B. P. PHILLIPS: Conversion of cholesterol to 5α-cholestan-3β-ol in germfree guinea
  pigs. Biochemistry 3, 1558 (1964).
— and G. V. LEROY: Cholesterol — A precursor of tetrahydrocortisone in man. J. Amer.
  chem. Soc. 76, 5260 (1954).
— — Cholesterol — A precursor of tetrahydrocortisone (THF) and 11-ketoetiocholanolone in
  man. Fed. Proc. 14, 303 (1955).
— J. PLOTZ, G. V. LEROY, and E. M. DAVIS: Cholesterol — A precursor of estrone in vivo.
  J. Amer. chem. Soc. 79, 1012 (1957).
WHITEHOUSE, M. W., E. STAPLE, and S. GURIN: Catabolism in vitro of cholesterol. I. Oxidation
  of the terminal methyl groups of cholesterol to carbon dioxide by rat liver preparations.
  J. biol. Chem. 234, 276 (1959).
— — — Catabolism in vitro of cholesterol. II. Further studies on the oxidation of cholesterol
  by rat liver mitochondria. J. biol. Chem. 236, 68 (1961a).
WILSON, J. D.: Studies on the regulation of cholesterol synthesis in the skin and preputial
  gland of the rat. Adv. in Biology of Skin, IV, eds. W. MONTAGNA, R. A. ELLIS, and A. F.
  SILVER, p. 148. London: Pergamon 1963.
— The quantification of cholesterol excretion and degradation in the isotopic steady state in
  the rat: the influence of dietary cholesterol. J. Lipid Res. 5, 409 (1964).
WOODWARD, R. B., and K. BLOCH: The cyclization of squalene in cholesterol biosynthesis.
  J. Amer. chem. Soc. 75, 2023 (1953).
WÜERSCH, J. R., R. L. HUANG, and K. BLOCH: The origin of the isooctyl side chain of chole-
  sterol. J. biol. Chem. 195, 439 (1952).
ZABIN, I., and W. F. BARKER: The conversion of cholesterol and acetate to cholic acid. J. biol.
  Chem. 205, 633 (1953).
— and K. BLOCH: The formation of ketone from isovaleric acid. J. biol. Chem. 185, 117 (1950).

Biochemistry of Phosphatides

By

R. J. Rossiter

Introduction

This discussion will be confined to a general description of the biosynthesis and degradation of the glycerophosphatides commonly found in animal tissues. Reference will be made to the glycerophosphatides of plants and bacteria for comparative purposes only. Even with these severe restrictions, it will be possible to refer to no more than a small selection of the many important papers that have appeared on the subject during the past few years.

I. Biosynthesis of glycerophosphatides

When a suitably labelled precursor is administered to an animal, the label appears in the glycerophosphatides of most tissues. This is true for a wide variety of precursors, including orthophosphate labelled with P^{32}; fatty acid labelled with H^3, C^{14}, I^{131}, or elaidic acid; acetate labelled with H^3 or C^{14}; glycerol labelled with C^{14}; choline, ethanolamine, or serine, labelled with C^{14}, N^{15}, or H^3; inositol labelled with C^{14} or H^3, etc.

Similar labelling experiments carried out *in vitro* with slice or cell-free preparations suggest that in most animal tissues the glycerophosphatides are formed *in situ* from appropriate precursors of low molecular weight. Such isotope experiments, although they demonstrate that the synthesis of a particular glycerophosphatide can occur in a given tissue, provide little information concerning the metabolic pathways involved. Of recent years, largely as the result of the notable contributions of KENNEDY (1961), much has been learned concerning the biosynthesis of the glycerophosphatides. Recent reviews are those of KENNEDY (1961, 1962), ROSSITER and STRICKLAND (1960), ROSSITER (1960, 1964) and ANSELL and HAWTHORNE (1964).

1. Phosphatidic Acid

The parent compound of the glycerophosphatides is L-α-phosphatidic acid (I), a substance now known to be an important intermediate in the biosynthesis of most of these lipids.

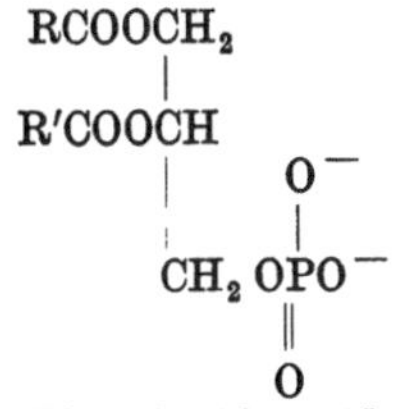

$$
\begin{array}{l}
\text{RCOOCH}_2 \\
\text{R'COOCH} \\
\qquad\quad\; \text{O}^- \\
\qquad\quad\; | \\
\text{CH}_2\,\text{OPO}^- \\
\qquad\quad\; \| \\
\qquad\quad\; \text{O}
\end{array}
$$

L-α-Phosphatidic acid   (I)

When cell-free tissue preparations are incubated in the presence of inorganic P^{32}, much of the radioactivity may be recovered from phosphatidic acid, whereas very little radioactivity is present in the other glycerophosphatides. Also in similar cell-free preparations of liver (KORNBERG and PRICER 1952a, KENNEDY 1953) or brain (McMURRAY et al. 1957) the radioactivity of P^{32}-labelled α-glycerophosphate appears chiefly in the phosphatidic acid.

KORNBERG and PRICER (1953a) showed that guinea pig liver contains an acyl CoA* synthetase system (Acid: CoA ligase (AMP) EC 6.2.1.3) capable of catalysing the activation of long-chain fatty acids with the formation of thioesters of CoA according to the overall equation:

$$\text{Fatty acid} + \text{ATP} + \text{CoA} \rightleftharpoons \text{acyl CoA} + \text{AMP} + \text{PP}_1 \tag{1}$$

Subsequently, a similar reaction was observed in brain (VIGNAIS, GALLAGHER and ZABIN 1958) and other tissues (SENIOR and ISSELBACHER 1960).

VIGNAIS and ZABIN (1958) provided evidence that the reaction, like the activation of acetate, occurs in the following two steps:

$$\text{Fatty acid} + \text{ATP} \rightleftharpoons \text{acyl adenylate} + \text{PP}_1 \tag{2}$$

$$\text{Acyl adenylate} + \text{CoA} \rightleftharpoons \text{acyl CoA} + \text{AMP} \tag{3}$$

KORNBERG and PRICER (1953b) further showed that liver contains enzymes (acyltransferases) capable of catalysing the esterification of L-α-glycerophosphate by acyl CoA to yield phosphatidic acid. Presumably the esterification takes place in two stages:

$$\text{L-}\alpha\text{-glycerophosphate} + \underset{\text{CoA}}{\text{acyl}} \rightarrow \text{L-}\alpha\text{-lysophosphatidic} + \text{CoA} \tag{4}$$
$$\text{acid}$$

$$\underset{\text{acid}}{\text{L-}\alpha\text{-lysophosphatidic}} + \underset{\text{CoA}}{\text{acyl}} \rightarrow \underset{\text{acid}}{\text{L-}\alpha\text{-phosphatidic}} + \text{CoA} \tag{5}$$

Similar enzymes occur in many tissues (PIERINGER and HOKIN 1962b, BRANDES, OLLEY and SHAPIRO 1963).

Glycerol is not esterified by the enzymes catalysing Reactions 4 and 5, nor is glycerol-C^{14} readily incorporated into the phosphatidic acid of cell-free tissue preparations. These findings suggest that glycerophosphate is the more immediate precursor of phosphatidic acid. Such a possibility was suggested by the earlier experiments of ZILVERSMIT, ENTENMAN and CHAIKOFF (1948) and POPJÁK and MUIR (1950), who investigated the specific radioactivity of the α-glycerophosphate in the tissues of animals after the administration of inorganic P^{32}. The glycerophosphate may be formed by the action of L-α-glycerolphosphate dehydrogenase (L-glycerol-3-phosphate: NAD-oxidoreductase EC 1.1.1.8) on the glycolysis intermediate dihydroxyacetone phosphate, or by the direct transfer of a phosphoryl group to glycerol from ATP. The enzyme catalysing the latter reaction, glycerokinase (ATP: glycerol phosphotransferase EC 2.7.1.30), was partially purified by BUBLITZ and KENNEDY (1954) and was obtained in crystalline form by WIELAND and SUYTER (1957).

There is now good evidence that the reaction sequence described above is not the only pathway leading to the formation of phosphatidic acid. PIERINGER and HOKIN (1962a) showed that lysophosphatidic acid may be formed by the phos-

---

* The following abbreviations are used: CoA, coenzyme A; AMP, adenosine 5'-monophosphate; ADP, adenosine 5'-diphosphate; ATP, adenosine 5'-triphosphate; CMP, cytidine 5'-monophosphate; CDP, cytidine 5'-diphosphate; CTP, cytidine 5'-triphosphate; P_1, inorganic orthophosphate; PP_1, inorganic pyrophosphate; NAD, nicotinamide adenine dinucleotide; GPC, glycerolphosphorylcholine; GPE, glycerolphosphorylethanolamine; GPI, glycerolphosphorylinositol.

phorylation of monoglyceride by ATP, a reaction catalysed by a soluble brain enzyme, monoglyceride kinase:

$$\text{Monoglyceride} + \text{ATP} \rightarrow \text{L-}\alpha\text{-lysophosphatidic acid} + \text{ADP} \qquad (6)$$

It is also known from the work of HOKIN and HOKIN (1959) and STRICKLAND (1962) that phosphatidic acid may be formed by the phosphorylation of D-α, β-diglyceride from ATP, a reaction catalysed by the enzyme diglyceride kinase:

$$\text{D-}\alpha,\beta\text{-diglyceride} + \text{ATP} \rightarrow \text{L-}\alpha\text{-phosphatidic acid} + \text{ADP} \qquad (7)$$

In addition, CLARK and HÜBSCHER (1963) and SENIOR and ISSELBACHER (1962) have shown that a tissue such as intestinal mucosa contains an enzyme, monoglyceride acyltransferase, that catalyses the acylation of monoglyceride from acyl CoA:

$$\text{Monoglyceride} + \text{acyl CoA} \rightarrow \text{diglyceride} + \text{CoA} \qquad (8)$$

The reactions leading to the biosynthesis of phosphatidic acid are summarized in Figure 1.

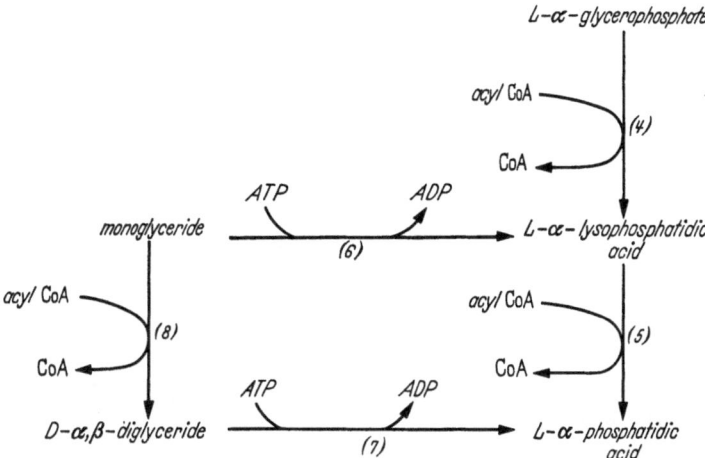

Figure 1. Biosynthesis of phosphatidic acid. Figures in parentheses refer to equations in text.

In the biosynthesis of many of the glycerophosphatides, phosphatidic acid is first dephosphorylated. SMITH, WEISS and KENNEDY (1957) showed that liver contains an enzyme, phosphatidic acid phosphatase (L-α-phosphatidate phosphohydrolase EC 3.1.3.4), which removes phosphate from phosphatidic acid with the formation of D-α,β-diglyceride (II):

$$\text{L-}\alpha\text{-phosphatidic acid} \rightarrow \text{D-}\alpha,\beta\text{-diglyceride} + \text{P}_i \qquad (9)$$

Similar enzymes occur in many tissues. D-α,β-diglyceride so formed may be converted into many of the glycerophosphatides (see below) or, as demonstrated by WEISS, KENNEDY and KIYASU (1960), it may be esterified by a diglyceride acyltransferase (Acyl-CoA: 1,2-diglyceride O-acyltransferase EC 2.3.1.d) to give triglyceride:

$$\text{D-}\alpha,\beta\text{-diglyceride} + \text{acyl CoA} \rightarrow \text{triglyceride} + \text{CoA} \qquad (10)$$

The occurrence of Reaction 9 provides an explanation of the frequently reported finding that radioactivity from P^{32}-labelled L-α-glycerophosphate is not incorporated into the major glycerophosphatides in cell-free tissue preparations, whereas radioactivity from C^{14}-labelled glycerophosphate is readily incorporated (STRICKLAND et al. 1963).

2. Phosphatidyl choline (Lecithin)

The early experiments of RILEY (1944), in which labelled phosphorylcholine was administered to rats *in vivo*, suggested that this substance is not an immediate precursor of lecithin (III). Subsequently, however, KORNBERG and PRICER (1952b) showed that phosphorylcholine, doubly labelled with C^{14} and P^{32}, is incorporated as a unit into the lecithin of a rat liver preparation. Radioactivity from both C^{14}-labelled (KENNEDY 1954, STRICKLAND et al. 1963) and P^{32}-labelled (RODBELL and HANAHAN 1955, McMURRAY et al. 1957) phosphorylcholine is incorporated into the lecithin of a wide variety of tissue preparations. The phosphorylcholine may be formed by the phosphorylation of choline by ATP, a reaction catalysed by the enzyme, choline kinase (ATP: choline phosphotransferase EC 2.7.1.32), partially purified from yeast by WITTENBERG and KORNBERG (1953), and now known to occur in a variety of tissues.

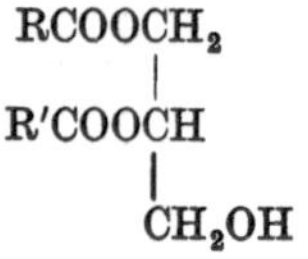

$$RCOOCH_2$$
$$|$$
$$R'COOCH \qquad\qquad\qquad\qquad\qquad\qquad (II)$$
$$|$$
$$CH_2OH$$

D-α,β-Diglyceride

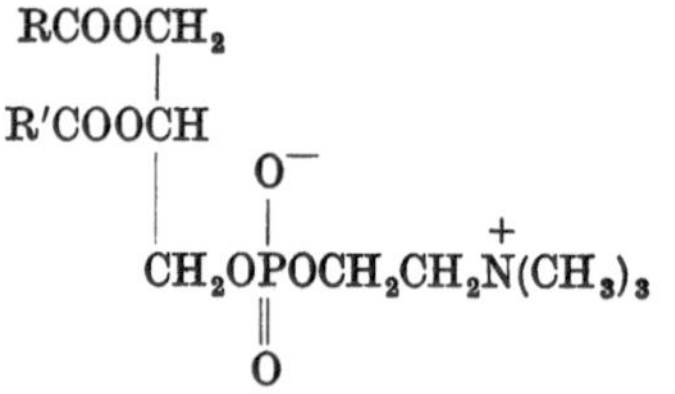

$$RCOOCH_2$$
$$|$$
$$R'COOCH$$
$$| \qquad\quad O^- \qquad\qquad\qquad\qquad\qquad (III)$$
$$| \qquad\quad | \qquad\qquad\qquad +$$
$$CH_2OPOCH_2CH_2\overset{+}{N}(CH_3)_3$$
$$\qquad\quad ||$$
$$\qquad\quad O$$

L-α-Lecithin
(L-α-Phosphatidyl choline)

A major advance in the understanding of the biosynthesis of the glycerophosphatides was the discovery by KENNEDY and WEISS (1956) of the role of nucleotides of cytosine in the biosynthesis of the glycerophosphatides. Cytidine 5'-triphosphate (CTP) was shown to be necessary for the incorporation of phosphorylcholine into lecithin by liver preparations. Similar observations have been reported for brain (McMURRAY et al. 1957, STRICKLAND et al. 1963) and other tissues. The nucleotide requirement is specific for CTP, none of the other nucleoside 5'-triphosphates being active. KENNEDY and WEISS (1956) showed that CTP combines with phosphorylcholine to form the intermediate CDP-choline (IV) according to the equation:

$$Phosphorylcholine + CTP \rightleftharpoons CDP\text{-}choline + PP_i \qquad\qquad (11)$$

CDP-choline has been characterized and synthesized (KENNEDY 1956). It occurs in a number of tissues (KENNEDY and WEISS 1956) including brain (ANSELL and BAYLISS 1961) and yeast (BERGER and GIMENEZ 1956). The properties of the enzyme phosphorylcholine-cytidyl transferase (CTP: cholinephosphate cytidylyltransferase EC 2.7.7.15) catalysing Reaction 11 have been studied by BORKENHAGEN and KENNEDY (1957), who showed that the enzyme readily catalyses the reverse reaction, i.e. the pyrophosphorolysis of CDP-choline, with the formation of phosphorylcholine and CTP.

KENNEDY and WEISS (1956) further showed that chicken liver contains a second enzyme capable of forming lecithin (III) by the transfer of phosphorylcholine from CDP-choline (IV) to D-α,β-diglyceride (II) according to the equation:

$$CDP\text{-}choline + D\text{-}\alpha,\beta\text{-}diglyceride \rightleftharpoons L\text{-}\alpha\text{-}lecithin + CMP \qquad\qquad (12)$$

The enzyme catalysing this reaction, phosphorylcholine-glyceride transferase (CDP-choline: 1,2-diglyceride cholinephosphotransferase EC 2.7.8.2), was partially purified from liver by WEISS, SMITH and KENNEDY (1958), who showed that it catalyses the reverse reaction, i.e. the "cytidylolysis" of lecithin with the formation of CDP-choline and D-α,β-diglyceride.

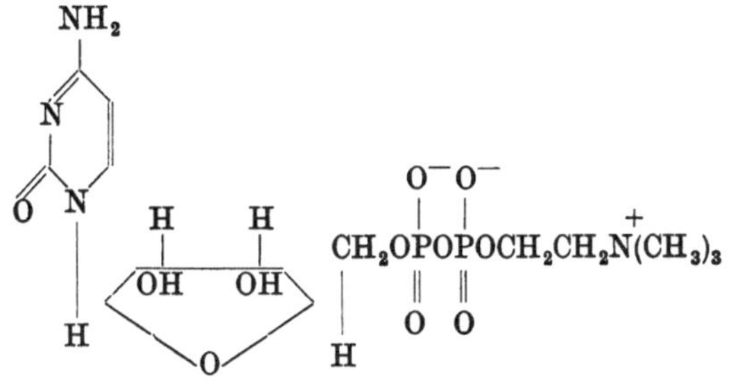

(IV)

CDP-choline

The enzymes leading to the biosynthesis of lecithin by the pathways outlined above (Reactions 11 and 12) are not restricted to liver. They have been demonstrated in brain (STRICKLAND et al. 1963) seminal vesicle (WILLIAMS-ASHMAN and BANKS 1956) and intestinal mucosa (GURR and HÜBSCHER 1964). Experiments such as those of MIANI and BUCCIANTE (1958), in which inorganic P^{32} was administered to rats, and those of GØRANSSON (1964), in which labelled fatty acids were given, provided evidence that this pathway for the biosynthesis of lecithin is operative *in vivo*.

Although it is well established that lecithin may be formed by the above sequence of reactions, it should not be concluded that this is the only pathway, nor indeed the major pathway, for the biosynthesis of lecithin in all tissues. Of great interest is the finding of BREMER and GREENBERG (1961) that lecithin may be formed by the transfer of methyl groups from S-adenosyl methionine to phosphatidyl ethanolamine (V). Presumably the methylation takes place in three stages according to the following sequence of reactions:

Phosphatidyl + S-adenosyl → phosphatidyl + S-adenosyl
ethanolamine   methionine   monomethyl-   homocysteine   (13)
                              ethanolamine

Phosphatidyl + S-adenosyl → phosphatidyl + S-adenosyl
monomethyl-   methionine   dimethyl-   homocysteine   (14)
ethanolamine   ethanolamine

Phosphatidyl + S-adenosyl → L-α-lecithin + S-adenosyl
dimethyl-   methionine   homocysteine   (15)
ethanolamine

Although these reactions take place in a number of tissues (GIBSON, WILSON and UDENFRIEND 1961, LAW, ZALKIN and KANESHIRO 1963, ROSSITER and DONISCH 1964), experiments by ANSELL and his associates carried out both *in vitro* (CHOJNACKI et al. 1964) and *in vivo* (ANSELL and SPANNER 1962) suggest that they are not very active in brain tissue. On the other hand, it is known that 2-dimethylaminoethanol occurs in a tissue such as brain (HONEGGER and HONEGGER 1960) and that 2-dimethylaminoethanol labelled with C^{14} is incorporated into the lipids of brain and liver *in vivo* (GROTH, BAIN and PFEIFFER 1958). It is now clear that glycerophosphatides containing mono- and di-methylaminoethanol may be formed from the appropriate bases by pathways involving CDP-intermediates. The reactions are analogous to Reactions 11 and 12 for the synthesis of lecithin (Ansell and Chojnacki 1962 a, b).

$$RCOOCH_2$$
$$|$$
$$R'COOCH$$
$$|\quad O^-$$
$$|\quad |\quad +$$
$$CH_2OPOCH_2CH_2NH_3 \qquad\qquad (V)$$
$$\|$$
$$O$$

L-α-Phosphatidyl ethanolamine

The work of Nyc and associates on the lipids of *Neurospora crassa* is of particular interest in relation to the biosynthesis of lecithin. The phospholipid of a choline-requiring mutant contains the phosphatidyl esters of both mono- and dimethylaminoethanol (Hall and Nyc 1961). Nutritional studies with appropriate mutants of this organism have shown that lecithin may be formed (a) from choline by the cytosine nucleotide pathway (Reactions 11 and 12), (b) from phosphatidyl ethanolamine by the methylation pathway (Reactions 13, 14 and 15) and (c) from mono- and di-methylaminoethanol by the incorporation of the base into lipid, presumably by way of CDP-intermediates, followed by methylation. The relative contributions of these pathways can be influenced by mutations and by nutritional supplementation of the culture medium (Crocken and Nyc 1964).

Many of the reactions leading to the biosynthesis of lecithin are summarized in Figure 2. The sequences shown in the figure do not represent all of the possibilities however. For example, Lands and Merkl (1963) have shown that in liver preparations lecithin may be formed as the result of the acylation of lysolecithin (VI) by acyl CoA:

$$\text{L-α-lysolecithin} + \text{acyl CoA} \rightarrow \text{L-α-lecithin} + \text{CoA} \qquad (16)$$

A similar reaction takes place in brain (Webster and Alpern 1964). The acyltransferase enzyme of liver shows a preferential esterification of unsaturated fatty acids with the β-hydroxyl group of α'-acylglycerolphosphorylcholine and of saturated fatty acids with the α'-hydroxyl group of β-acylglycerolphosphorylcholine (Lands and Merkl 1963).

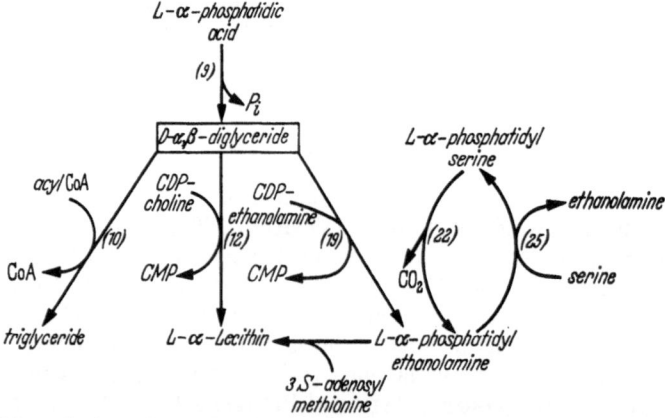

Figure 2. Biosynthesis of glycerophosphatides. Figures in parentheses refer to equations in text.

3. Choline Plasmalogen

It is now generally agreed that choline plasmalogen (VII) may be represented by the unsaturated ether structure of RAPPORT and co-workers (RAPPORT et al. 1957, RAPPORT and FRANZL 1957a), who suggest that the compound be referred to as phosphatidal choline.

Information concerning the biosynthesis of choline plasmalogen is somewhat limited. Most of the work on the biological formation of plasmalogens has been done on ethanolamine plasmalogen (see below) rather than choline plasmalogen. An exception is the report of KEENAN, BROWN and MARKS (1961), who showed that C^{14}-labelled fatty acids are incorporated in both the acyl ester group and the

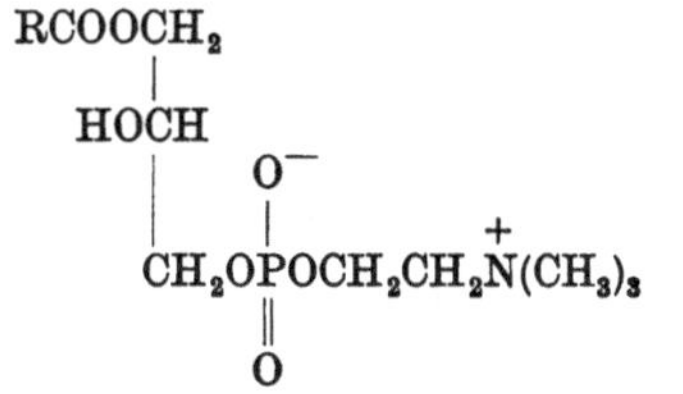

$$RCOOCH_2$$
$$|$$
$$HOCH \qquad O^-$$
$$| \qquad |$$
$$CH_2OPOCH_2CH_2\overset{+}{N}(CH_3)_3 \qquad (VI)$$
$$\|$$
$$O$$

L-α-Lysolecithin
(α′-Acyl L-α-glycerolphosphorylcholine)

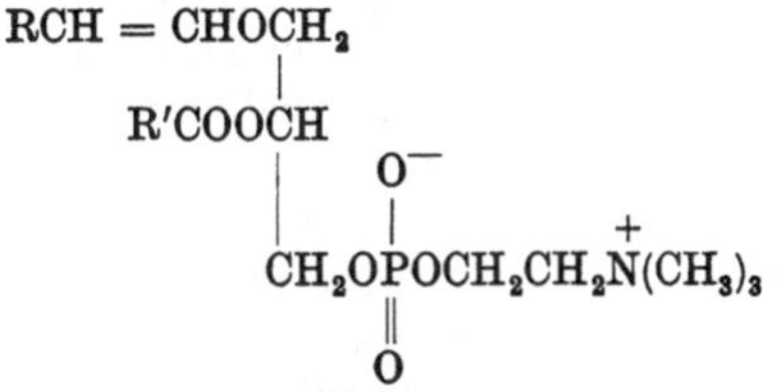

$$RCH = CHOCH_2$$
$$|$$
$$R'COOCH \qquad O^-$$
$$| \qquad |$$
$$CH_2OPOCH_2CH_2\overset{+}{N}(CH_3)_3 \qquad (VII)$$
$$\|$$
$$O$$

Choline plasmalogen
(L-α-Phosphatidal choline)

unsaturated ether group of the choline plasmalogen of perfused dog heart. In these experiments the ester group was preferentially labelled.

An important step was the finding of KIYASU and KENNEDY (1960) that rat liver contains an enzyme that is able to catalyse the formation of choline plasmalogen from CDP-choline and plasmalogenic diglyceride:

$$\begin{matrix} \text{CDP-} + \text{plasmalogenic} \rightleftharpoons \text{choline} + \text{CMP} \\ \text{choline} \quad \text{diglyceride} \quad \text{plasmalogen} \end{matrix} \qquad (17)$$

The plasmalogenic diglyceride, prepared enzymically by the action of phospholipase C on the choline-containing phospholipid of beef heart, is defined as a D-α,β-diglyceride in which the ester at the α′-position is replaced by an unsaturated ether. The reaction is catalysed by a choline-phosphotransferase enzyme similar to the phosphorylcholine-glyceride transferase shown to participate in the biosynthesis of lecithin (Reaction 12). A similar reaction occurs in brain (McMURRAY 1964b).

It is also known from the work of SRIBNEY and KENNEDY (1958) that many tissues contain an enzyme (CDP-choline: ceramide cholinephosphotransferase EC 2.7.8.a) capable of transfering phosphorylcholine from CDP-choline to ceramide with the formation of sphingomyelin:

$$\text{CDP-choline} + \text{ceramide} \rightleftharpoons \text{sphingomyelin} + \text{CMP} \qquad (18)$$

Thus CDP-choline is the precursor of three phosphatides (Figure 3). It may donate phosphorylcholine to D-α,β-diglyceride with the formation of lecithin

7*

(Reaction 12), to plasmalogenic diglyceride with the formation of choline plasmalogen (Reaction 17), or to ceramide with the formation of sphingomyelin (Reaction 18).

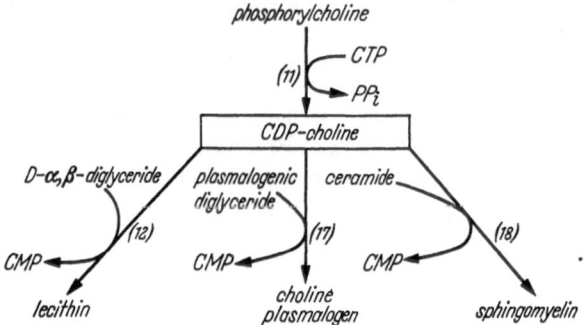

Figure 3. Biosynthesis of choline-containing phosphatides. Figures in parentheses refer to equations in
text.

4. Phosphatidyl Ethanolamine

Early work on the formation of phosphatidyl ethanolamine (V) gave little
information concerning the intermediates involved. For example, the experiments
of Chargaff and Keston (1940), in which labelled phosphorylethanolamine was
administered to rats *in vivo*, suggested that this substance was not a direct precursor. The demonstration that phosphorylcholine was an immediate precursor
of lecithin and the discovery of the cytosine nucleotide pathway (Reactions 11
and 12) led to a reinvestigation of the matter. Kennedy and Weiss (1956) demonstrated the presence of an enzyme, phosphorylethanolamine-cytidyl transferase (CTP: ethanolaminephosphate cytidylyltransferase EC 2.7.7.14), catalysing
the formation of the intermediate CDP-ethanolamine (cf Reaction 11) in many
tissues. Phosphatidyl ethanolamine is formed as the result of the transfer of
phosphorylethanolamine from CDP-ethanolamine to D-α,β-diglyceride:

$$\text{CDP-ethanolamine} + \text{D-}\alpha, \beta\text{-diglyceride} \rightleftharpoons \text{L-}\alpha\text{-phosphatidyl ethanolamine} + \text{CMP} \tag{19}$$

The above reaction is catalysed by the enzyme phosphorylethanolamine-
glyceride transferase (CDP-ethanolamine: 1,2-diglyceride ethanolaminephosphotransferase EC 2.7.8.1). Similar enzymes are present in brain tissue (McMurray
1964b).

As stressed for the biosynthesis of lecithin, the possibility of alternative pathways should be borne in mind. An example is the demonstration by Merkl and
Lands (1963) of the enzymic acylation of lysophosphatidyl ethanolamine to form
phosphatidyl ethanolamine by a reaction similar to that described for the acylation
of lysolecithin to form lecithin (Reaction 16).

In *Escherichia coli* phosphatidyl ethanolamine is one of the principal glycerophosphatides (Kanfer and Kennedy 1963). Recently, Kanfer and Kennedy
(1964) showed that in this organism the glycerophosphatides are formed by a
second quite distinct pathway involving the liponucleotide CDP-diglyceride (VIII).
This unusual substance, first described by Agranoff, Bradley and Brady (1958),
is now known to be an intermediate in the formation of a number of the glycerophosphatides. It is formed in both liver (Paulus and Kennedy 1960) and brain
(Thompson, Strickland and Rossiter 1963) by a cytidylyltransferase reaction.

A cytidylyl group is transferred from CTP to L-α-phosphatidic acid (I), with the formation of CDP-diglyceride and pyrophosphate:

$$\underset{\text{acid}}{\text{L-α-phosphatidic}} + \text{CTP} \rightleftharpoons \underset{\text{diglyceride}}{\text{CDP-}} + \text{PP}_i \qquad (20)$$

In a cell-free preparation from *E. coli* KANFER and KENNEDY (1964) demonstrated the presence of a phosphatidyltransferase that catalyses the transfer of a phosphatidyl group from CDP-diglyceride to L-serine with the formation of phosphatidyl serine (IX):

$$\underset{\text{diglyceride}}{\text{CDP-}} + \text{L-serine} \rightleftharpoons \underset{\text{L-serine}}{\text{L-α-phosphatidyl}} + \text{CMP} \qquad (21)$$

The phosphatidyl serine so formed is then decarboxylated to yield phosphatidyl ethanolamine (V):

$$\underset{\text{L-serine}}{\text{L-α-phosphatidyl}} \rightarrow \underset{\text{ethanolamine}}{\text{L-α-phosphatidyl}} + CO_2 \qquad (22)$$

Thus, whereas in mammalian tissue phosphatidyl ethanolamine is formed by way of CDP-ethanolamine (Reaction 19), and incidentally may be methylated to form lecithin (Figure 2), in *E. coli* phosphatidyl ethanolamine is derived from phosphatidyl serine (Reaction 22), which is formed by way of CDP-diglyceride (Reaction 21, Figure 4).

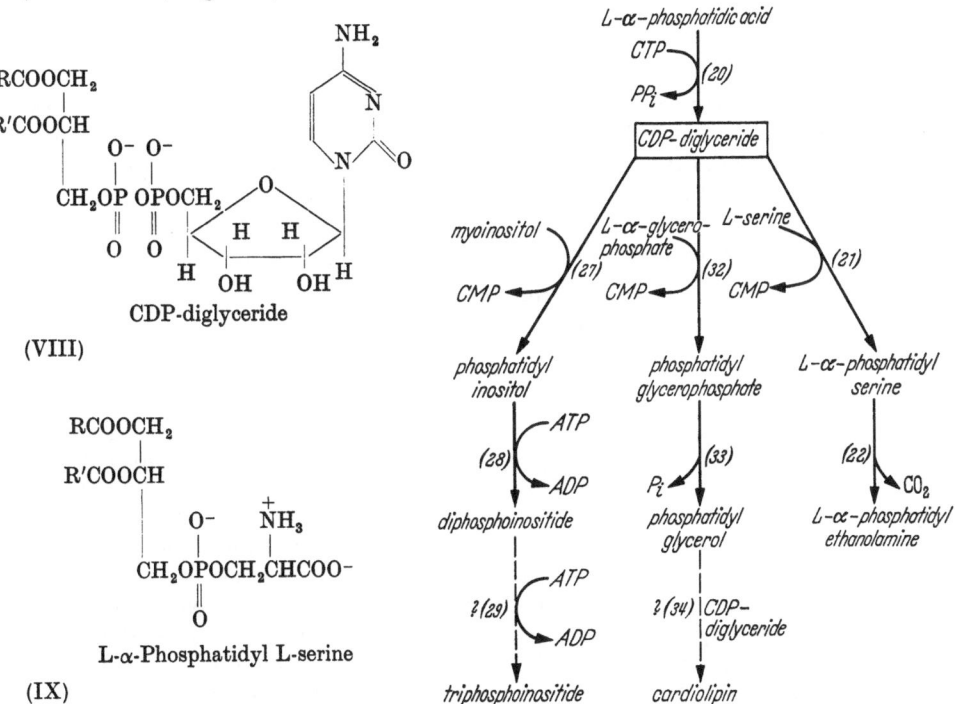

Figure 4. CDP-diglyceride reactions. Figures in parentheses refer to equations in text.

5. Ethanolamine Plasmalogen

The principal plasmalogen of brain contains ethanolamine rather than choline. The work of RAPPORT and associates (RAPPORT et al. 1957, RAPPORT and FRANZL 1957b) indicates that the structure of this compound is analogous to that previously described for choline plasmalogen, i.e. phosphatidal ethanolamine (X).

KOREY and ORCHEN (1959) showed that if acetate-1-C^{14} or palmitate-1-C^{14} is administered to rats, radioactivity may be recovered from both the acyl ester and the unsaturated ether side-chains of brain plasmalogens. With acetate-C^{14} more radioactivity was incorporated into the unsaturated ether, whereas with palmitate-C^{14} more radioactivity was incorporated into the ester. CARR, HAERLE and EILER (1963) reported that in rat brain homogenates palmitate-1-C^{14}, but not palmitaldehyde-C^{14}, may serve as a precursor of the unsaturated ether side-chain, but that much less radioactivity may be recovered from the unsaturated ether side-chain than from the acyl ester group. GAMBAL and MONTY (1959) claimed that the incorporation of radioactivity from palmitate-1-C^{14} into the unsaturated ether side-chain was stimulated by the addition of CTP and ethanolamine, a finding that suggests a cytosine nucleotide might be an intermediate in

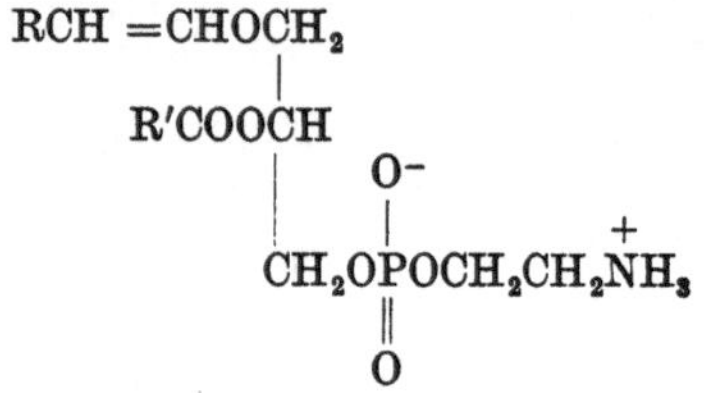

$$
\begin{array}{l}
\text{RCH} =\text{CHOCH}_2 \\
\qquad | \\
\text{R'COOCH} \\
\qquad | \qquad\quad \text{O}^- \\
\qquad | \qquad\quad | \qquad\qquad + \\
\text{CH}_2\text{OPOCH}_2\text{CH}_2\text{NH}_3 \\
\qquad\qquad || \\
\qquad\qquad \text{O}
\end{array}
\qquad (X)
$$

Ethanolamine plasmalogen
(L-α-Phosphatidal ethanolamine)

the formation of ethanolamine plasmalogen. It was not surprising, therefore, when KIYASU and KENNEDY (1960) described an ethanolaminephosphotransferase enzyme in rat liver that catalyses the transfer of phosphorylethanolamine from CDP-ethanolamine to plasmalogenic diglyceride:

$$
\begin{array}{ll}
\text{CDP-} \quad + \quad \text{plasmalogenic} \rightleftharpoons \text{ethanolamine} + \text{CMP} \\
\text{ethanolamine} \quad \text{diglyceride} \qquad\quad \text{plasmalogen}
\end{array}
\qquad (23)
$$

This reaction is analogous to that previously described for the biosynthesis of choline plasmalogen (Reaction 17). It also occurs in brain tissue (McMURRAY 1964 b).

6. Glycerol Ether Phosphatides

As early as 1949 BRANTE (1949) reported that brain contains a phospholipid other than sphingomyelin, the phosphorus of which is not rendered water-soluble by mild alkaline and acid hydrolysis. Subsequently CARTER, SMITH and JONES (1958) showed that egg yolk contains a phosphorylethanolamine derivative of batyl alcohol, a lipid that on mild alkaline and acid hydrolysis behaves as the phospholipid originally described by BRANTE. Similar phospholipids have been described in a variety of tissues (EDGAR and SMITS 1959, HANAHAN and WATTS 1961, CRONE and BRIDGES 1962, THOMPSON and HANAHAN 1963a, RENKONEN and HIRVISALO 1963). SVENNERHOLM and THORIN (1960) described the separation of such a lipid from ox and human brain. They provided evidence that the naturally occurring compound is esterified in the β-position, so that it may be represented as α'-alkoxy-β-acyl-α-glycerolphosphorylethanolamine (XI). The occurrence of such a glycerol ether phosphatide in brain also has been reported by ANSELL and SPANNER (1963), who distinguished it from the cyclic acetal of glycerolphosphorylethanolamine (XII) that may arise as an artifact from ethanolamine plasmalogen under certain conditions of hydrolysis (DAVENPORT and DAWSON 1962, PIETRUSZKO and GRAY 1962).

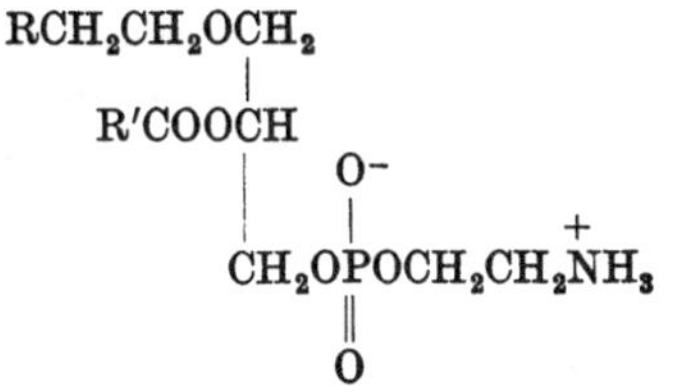

$$RCH_2CH_2OCH_2$$
$$R'COOCH$$
$$CH_2OPOCH_2CH_2NH_3^+ \quad O^-$$
$$O$$

(XI)

Glycerol ether phosphatide
(α'-Alkoxy-β-acyl L-α-glycerol-phosphorylethanolamine)

$$O—CH_2$$
$$R—CH_2—CH$$
$$O—CH$$
$$CH_2OPOCH_2CH_2NH_3^+ \quad O^-$$
$$O$$

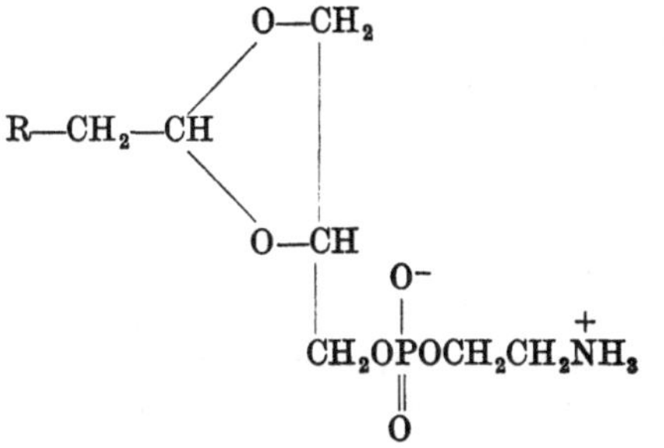

(XII)

Cyclic acetal of glycerol-phosphorylethanolamine

McMurray (1964b) reported that when homogenates of young rat brain are incubated in the presence of CDP-ethanolamine-C^{14}, the specific radioactivity of the glycerol ether phosphatide greatly exceeds that of either phosphatidyl ethanolamine or ethanolamine plasmalogen, a finding that suggests that the glycerol ether phosphatide of brain may be formed as the result of the enzymic transfer of phosphorylethanolamine from CDP-ethanolamine to some as yet unknown acceptor by an ethanolamine phosphotransferase:

$$\text{CDP-ethanolamine} + \text{unknown acceptor} \rightleftharpoons \text{glycerol ether phosphatide} + \text{CMP} \tag{24}$$

The work of Thompson and Hanahan (1963b), who studied the incorporation of radioactivity from glucose-6-C^{14} into the phospholipids of bone marrow cells *in vitro*, suggests that plasmalogen may be the precursor of glycerol ether phosphatide. On the other hand, the experiments of Magee (1965) on the incorporation of inorganic P^{32} into the lipids of cat brain slices, like those of McMurray (1964b) referred to above, show that the specific radioactivity of the glycerol ether phosphatide greatly exceeds that of ethanolamine plasmalogen.

7. Phosphatidyl Serine

The work of Hübscher (1962) and Borkenhagen, Kennedy and Fielding (1961) indicates that in mammalian tissues phosphatidyl serine (IX) is not formed by the transfer of O-phosphoserine from CDP-serine to D-α,β-diglyceride by a reaction analogous to those already described for the formation of lecithin and phosphatidyl ethanolamine (Reactions 12 and 19). Apparently free serine and not O-phosphoserine is the immediate precursor of phosphatidyl serine. Serine displaces ethanolamine from phosphatidyl ethanolamine in an enzymic reaction activated by Ca^{2+} and not requiring ATP:

$$\text{L-}\alpha\text{-phosphatidyl ethanolamine} + \text{L-serine} \rightleftharpoons \text{L-}\alpha\text{-phosphatidyl L-serine} + \text{ethanolamine} \tag{25}$$

There is evidence that in certain enzyme preparations the addition of CMP and ATP may be necessary for the formation of serine-containing phospholipids, suggesting that phosphatidyl serine also may be formed by a second pathway as yet not defined (ARTOM and WAINER 1963, MIRAS, MANTZOS and LEVIS 1964).

In addition, BORKENHAGEN et al. (1961) showed that in mammalian tissues phosphatidyl serine formed as described above may be decarboxylated to give phosphatidyl ethanolamine (V), a reaction already described as the principal pathway leading to the formation of phosphatidyl ethanolamine in *E. coli* (Reaction 22). The decarboxylation takes place in many tissues (ANSELL and SPANNER 1962, McMURRAY 1964a, ROSSITER and DONISCH 1964). Reactions 25 and 22 together lead to a glycerophosphatide cycle (see Figure 2), the overall effect of which is the decarboxylation of free serine to give ethanolamine (sum of Reactions 25 and 22):

$$\text{L-serine} \rightarrow \text{ethanolamine} + CO_2 \tag{26}$$

The conversion of serine to ethanolamine by brain and liver preparations has been known for a long time (see WILSON, GIBSON and UDENFRIEND 1960).

Reference has been made already to the recent findings of KANFER and KENNEDY (1964), who showed that in cell-free extracts of *E. coli* phosphatidyl serine is formed by a different pathway. A phosphatidyl group is transferred from CDP-diglyceride to L-serine by a highly specific enzyme L-serine-CMP phosphatidyltransferase (Reaction 21). In this organism most of the phosphatidyl serine so formed is decarboxylated to yield phosphatidyl ethanolamine (Reaction 22).

8. Phosphatidyl Inositol

Phosphatidyl inositol (XIII) occurs in a wide variety of tissues, but the concentration in brain is particularly high (see HAWTHORNE and KEMP 1964, for a review of brain phosphoinositides). Polymannosides of phosphatidyl inositol occur in *Mycobacterium tuberculosis* (BALLOU, VILKAS and LEDERER 1963) and phosphatidyl inositol derivatives of various types probably have quite a wide distribution in nature (CARTER et al. 1958, KLENK and HENDRICKS 1961).

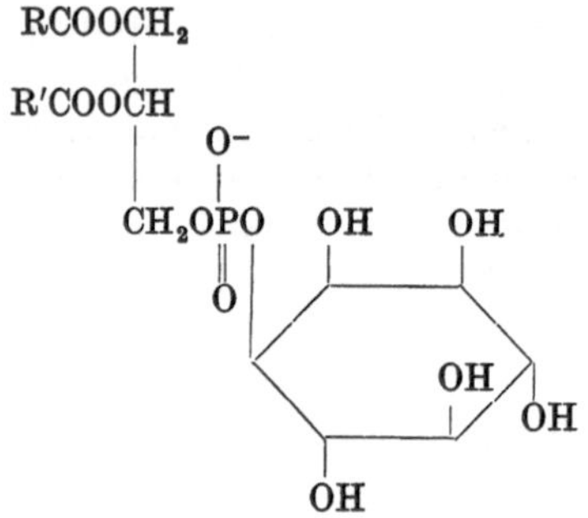

$$
\begin{array}{l}
RCOOCH_2 \\
\quad | \\
R'COOCH \\
\quad | \quad\quad O^- \\
\quad | \quad\quad | \\
CH_2OPO \quad OH \quad\quad OH \\
\quad\quad \| \\
\quad\quad O
\end{array}
\tag{XIII}
$$

Monophosphoinositide (Phosphatidyl-L-myoinositol)

The finding of McMURRAY et al. (1957) that the addition of CTP increases the incorporation of inorganic P^{32} into the phosphatidyl inositol of brain preparations implicated a cytosine nucleotide in the biosynthesis of this lipid. It is now believed that phosphatidyl inositol is formed by a phosphatidyltransferase reaction in which a phosphatidyl group is transferred to free myoinositol from CDP-diglyceride:

$$
\begin{array}{ll}
\text{CDP-} & + \text{ myoinositol} \rightleftharpoons \text{l-phosphatidyl} + \text{CMP} \\
\text{diglyceride} & \quad\quad\quad\quad\quad\quad\quad \text{L-myoinositol}
\end{array}
\tag{27}
$$

This reaction occurs in kidney (AGRANOFF et al. 1958), liver (PAULUS and KENNEDY 1960) and brain (THOMPSON et al. 1963).

KEENAN and HOKIN (1964) showed that lysophosphatidyl inositol occurs in pigeon pancreas and that this compound may be esterified by an acyltransferase reaction analogous to the enzymic acylation of lysolecithin (Reaction 16).

9. Polyphosphoinositides

The early investigations of FOLCH (1949) indicated that brain tissue contains a diphosphoinositide, a lipid which yields inositol diphosphate as a major hydrolysis product. More recent work has shown, however, that the polyphosphoinositides of brain are more complex than was hitherto suspected (HÖRHAMMER, WAGNER and RICHTER 1958, HÖRHAMMER, WAGNER and HÖLZL 1960, BROCKERHOFF and BALLOU 1961, DITTMER and DAWSON 1961, ELLIS, GALLIARD and HAWTHORNE 1963). In addition to a diphosphoinositide, brain contains a monophosphoinositide and a triphosphoinositide. The important investigations of BROCKERHOFF and BALLOU (1961) and DAWSON and DITTMER (1961) have established the structures of brain monophosphoinositide, diphosphoinositide and triphosphoinositide as 1-phosphatidyl-L-myoinositol (XIII), 1-phosphatidyl-L-myoinositol-4-phosphate (XIV) and 1-phosphatidyl-L-myoinositol-4,5-diphosphate (XV), respectively. The recent publications of WAGNER et al. (1963), OLIVER, GARDINER and ROSSITER (1964), SANTIAGO-CALVO et al. (1964) and EICHBERG and DAWSON (1964) show that the polyphosphoinositides are not confined to brain. They occur in all mammalian tissues examined.

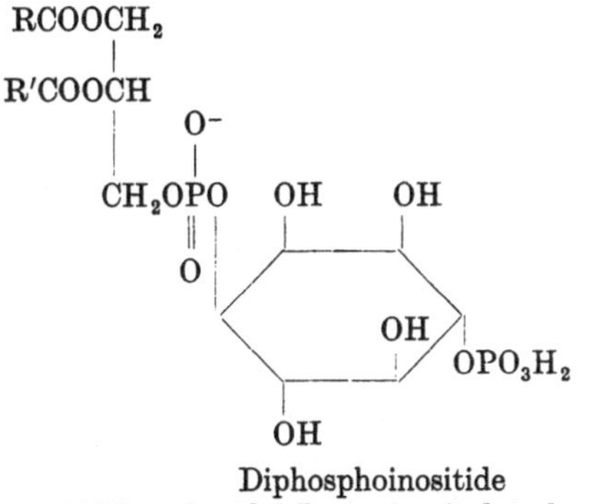

(XIV)

Diphosphoinositide
(1-Phosphatidyl-L-myoinositol 4-phosphate)

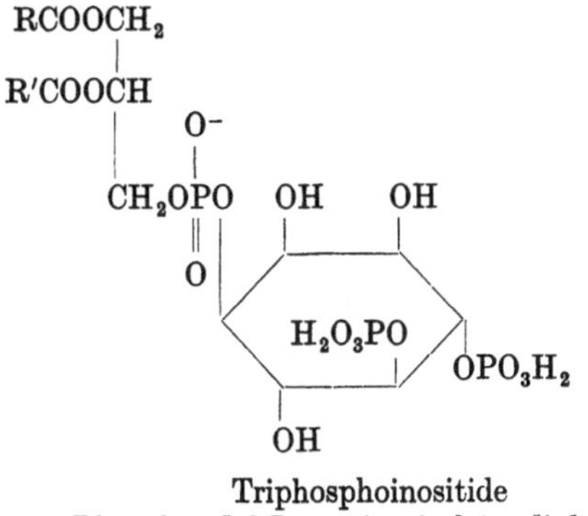

(XV)

Triphosphoinositide
(1-Phosphatidyl-L-myoinositol 4,5-diphosphate)

Brockerhoff and Ballou (1962a) showed that when slices of rabbit brain are incubated with inorganic P^{32} most of the radioactivity in the polyphosphoinositides may be recovered from the monoesterified phosphate groups, the specific radioactivity of which greatly exceeds that of the diester phosphate. Similar results were obtained by Palmer and Rossiter (1965). In experiments in which inorganic P^{32} was administered to rats *in vivo*, Wagner et al. (1962) also found the specific radioactivity of the polyphosphoinositides to be very high. Brockerhoff and Ballou (1962a) reported that for the diester phosphate the molar radioactivities of the phosphoinositides are in the order monophosphoinositide > diphosphoinositide > triphosphoinositide. With both inositol-H^3 and glycerol-C^{14} as precursors the molar radioactivities of the phosphoinositides were reported to be in the same order (Brockerhoff and Ballou 1962b).

Brockerhoff and Ballou (1962a, b) suggested that diphosphoinositide and triphosphoinositide are formed by the successive phosphorylation of the monophosphoinositide by ATP:

$$\begin{array}{ll} \text{1-phosphatidyl-} + \text{ATP} \rightarrow \text{1-phosphatidyl-} + \text{ADP} \\ \text{L-myoinositol} \qquad\qquad \text{L-myoinositol-} \\ \qquad\qquad\qquad\qquad \text{4-monophosphate} \end{array} \qquad (28)$$

$$\begin{array}{ll} \text{1-phosphatidyl-} + \text{ATP} \rightarrow \text{1-phosphatidyl-} + \text{ADP} \\ \text{L-myoinositol-} \qquad\quad\; \text{L-myoinositol-} \\ \text{4-monophosphate} \qquad\;\; \text{4,5-diphosphate} \end{array} \qquad (29)$$

Recently Colodzin and Kennedy (1964) have provided evidence for the occurrence of Reaction 28 in a cell-free preparation of rat brain.

An alternative possibility for the biosynthesis of diphosphoinositide is that myoinositol is first phosphorylated by ATP:

$$\text{Myoinositol} + \text{ATP} \rightarrow \text{inositol monophosphate} + \text{ADP} \qquad (30)$$

The inositol monophosphate could then receive a phosphatidyl group from CDP-diglyceride to form phosphatidyl inositol monophosphate by a reaction analogous to Reaction 27 leading to the formation of phosphatidyl inositol:

$$\begin{array}{ll} \text{CDP-} \qquad + \text{ myoinositol} \quad \rightleftharpoons \text{phosphatidyl} + \text{CMP} \\ \text{diglyceride} \quad \text{ monophosphate} \quad\; \text{inositol} \\ \qquad\qquad\qquad\qquad\qquad\qquad\; \text{monophosphate} \end{array} \qquad (31)$$

It is known that inositol monophosphate occurs in mammalian tissues (Hübscher and Hawthorne 1957) and in fish liver (Tsuyuki and Idler 1961). After the administration of myoinositol-C^{14}, the specific radioactivity of inositol monophosphate is such that it cannot be derived from the hydrolysis of phosphatidyl inositol (Tsuyuki and Idler 1961, Galliard and Hawthorne 1963). Although

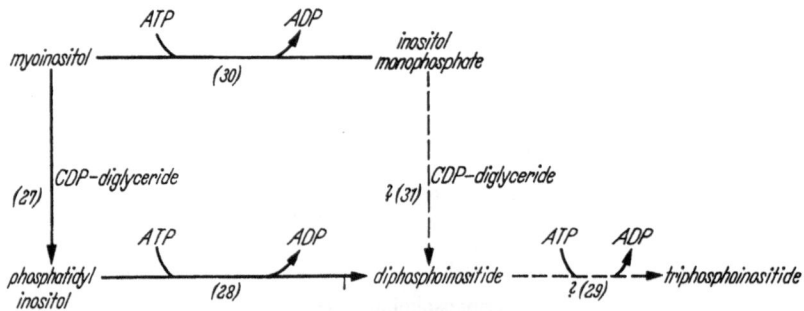

Figure 5. Biosynthesis of phosphoinositides. Figures in parentheses refer to equations in text.

a myoinositol kinase was not demonstrated in mammalian tissue by PAULUS and KENNEDY (1960), HOFFMAN-OSTENHOF, JUNGWIRTH and DAWID (1958) described the occurence of an enzyme catalysing Reaction 30 in yeast. As far as we are aware there is at the present time no direct evidence for the occurence of either Reaction 31 or Reaction 29.

Possible pathways leading to the formation of the polyphosphoinositides are shown in Figure 5.

10. Phosphatidyl Glycerol

Phosphatidyl glycerol (XVI) is a prominent glycerophosphatide of plants (BENSON and MARUO 1958) and micro-organisms (reviewed by MACFARLANE 1964a) and its occurence has been reported in mammalian mitochondria (STRICK-LAND and BENSON 1960). MACFARLANE (1962) showed that phosphatidyl glycerol is the lipid component of the lipoamino acids of *Clostridium perfringens* and other Gram-positive bacteria (HOUTSMULLER and VAN DEENEN 1963). These compounds are O-amino acid esters of phosphatidyl glycerol, in which the amino acid is esterified to the α'-carbon of the non-acylated glycerol moiety. Usually only one amino acid (lysine, ornithine, or alanine) is present in each bacterial species. Apparently similar compounds have not been detected either in Gram-negative bacteria or in animal tissues (MACFARLANE 1964b).

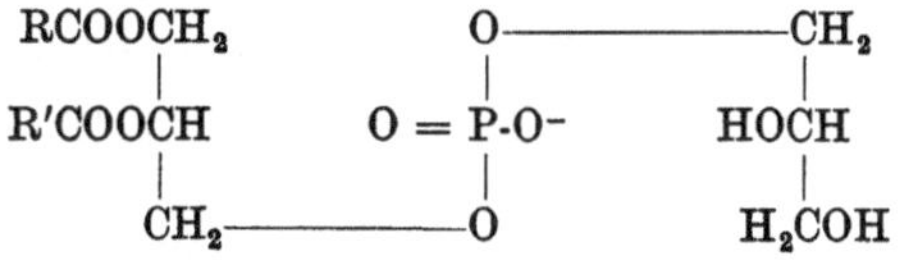

$$
\begin{array}{ccc}
\text{RCOOCH}_2 & \text{O} \longrightarrow \text{CH}_2 & \\
| & | & \\
\text{R'COOCH} \quad \text{O} = \text{P-O}^- & \text{HOCH} & \text{(XVI)} \\
| & | & \\
\text{CH}_2 \longrightarrow \text{O} & \text{H}_2\text{COH} &
\end{array}
$$

L-α-phosphatidyl glycerol

KIYASU, PIERINGER, PAULUS and KENNEDY (1963) showed that in liver and other animal tissues phosphatidyl glycerol is formed by the transfer of a phosphatidyl group from CDP-diglyceride (VIII) to L-α-glycerophosphate, with the formation of phosphatidyl glycerophosphate:

$$
\begin{array}{ll}
\text{CDP-} & + \text{L-}\alpha\text{-glycero-} \rightarrow \text{L-}\alpha\text{-phosphatidyl} + \text{CMP} \qquad (32) \\
\text{diglyceride} & \text{phosphate} \qquad \text{glycerophosphate}
\end{array}
$$

The L-α-phosphatidyl glycerophosphate so formed is dephosphorylated to yield L-α-phosphatidyl glycerol:

$$
\begin{array}{ll}
\text{L-}\alpha\text{-phosphatidyl} \rightarrow \text{L-}\alpha\text{-phosphatidyl} + \text{P}_i \qquad (33) \\
\text{glycerophosphate} \qquad \text{glycerol}
\end{array}
$$

Phosphatidyl glycerophosphate does not occur in high concentrations, but KATES, SASTRY and YENGOYAN (1963) reported the presence of a diether analogue of phosphatidyl glycerophosphate in *Halobacterium cutirubrum*, an extreme halophilic bacterium.

It is of interest that the phosphatidyl glycerol produced by these reactions has the same configuration (L-α-phosphatidyl-D-glycerol or 1,2-diacylglycerol-3-phosphoryl-1'-glycerol, according to HIRSCHMANN 1960) as the naturally occurring phosphatidyl glycerol of plants (BENSON and MIYANO 1961, HAVERKATE and VAN DEENEN 1964). Reactions 32 and 33 take place in cell-free extracts of *E. coli* (KANFER and KENNEDY 1964) and in brain (POSSMAYER and STRICK-LAND 1964).

11. Cardiolipin

Polyglycerophosphatides are known to have a wide distribution in nature. A major polyglycerophosphatide is cardiolipin, which occurs in animals (PANGBORN 1942), plants (BENSON and STRICKLAND 1960) and bacteria (MACFARLANE 1964a). In animals cardiolipin is a prominent lipid of mitochondria (STRICKLAND and BENSON 1960, FLEISCHER et al. 1962, MACFARLANE 1964a, EICHBERG, WHITTAKER and DAWSON 1964). MACFARLANE (1958) proposed the structure of bis-(diacyl-glycerophosphoryl)-glycerol or diphosphatidyl glycerol (XVII). As pointed out by MACFARLANE (1964c) there is reason to believe that cardiolipin is not triphosphatidyl glycerol as proposed by ROSE (1964). Recently the structure of cardiolipin (XVII) and also its absolute configuration has been confirmed by LE COCQ and BALLOU (1964) (see chapter I).

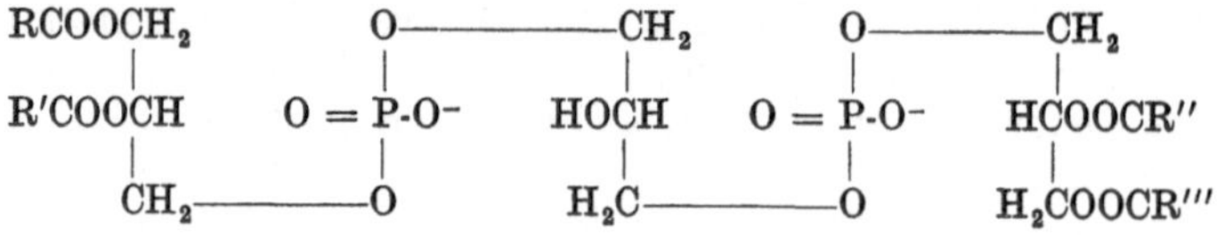

$$
\begin{array}{ccccc}
\text{RCOOCH}_2 & \text{O}\!-\!\!-\!\!-\!\text{CH}_2 & \text{O}\!-\!\!-\!\!-\!\text{CH}_2 \\
| & | & | & | & | \\
\text{R'COOCH} & \text{O}=\text{P-O}^- & \text{HOCH} & \text{O}=\text{P-O}^- & \text{HCOOCR}'' \quad\text{(XVII)} \\
| & | & | & | & | \\
\text{CH}_2\!-\!\!-\!\!-\!\text{O} & & \text{H}_2\text{C}\!-\!\!-\!\!-\!\text{O} & & \text{H}_2\text{COOCR}''' \\
\end{array}
$$

Cardiolipin

KIYASU et al. (1963) suggested that in the synthesis of cardiolipin the function of CDP-diglyceride as a donor of phosphatidyl groups might be extended to include the transfer of a phosphatidyl group to phosphatidyl glycerol:

$$
\underset{\text{diglyceride}}{\text{CDP-}} + \underset{\text{glycerol}}{\text{phosphatidyl}} \rightarrow \text{cardiolipin} + \text{CMP} \tag{34}
$$

This is an attractive hypothesis, but at the present time there is no experimental evidence in favour of such a reaction. Reactions involving CDP-diglyceride are summarized in Figure 4.

II. Degradation of Glycerophosphatides

Enzymes capable of degrading glycerophosphatides are found in snake venoms, plants and bacteria. It is only recently, however, that the presence of many of these enzymes has been established beyond question in animal tissues, for in much of the earlier work bacterial contamination was not adequately controlled.

The enzymes that hydrolyse the glycerophosphatides have been referred to variously as lecithinases, lecithases, lecitholipases, phosphatidolipases, phosphatidases, or phospholipases. Following the Enzyme Commission these enzymes will be referred to as *phospholipases*.

Four major phospholipases are known. Unfortunately, much confusion still exists concerning terminology. Phospholipase A (phosphatide acyl-hydrolase EC 3.1.1.4) liberates a fatty acid from the β-position of the glycerophosphatide molecule, with the formation of the corresponding lysoglycerophosphatide. Phospholipase B or lysophospholipase (lysolecithin acyl-hydrolase EC 3.1.1.5) preferentially removes the remaining fatty acid from the α'-position of the lysoglycerophosphatide, with the formation of a phosphodiester of glycerol and the corresponding base. Under certain circumstances (see below) this enzyme also may remove the fatty acid esterified in the β-position of an intact glycerophosphatide. For this reason phospholipase B is preferred to lysophospholipase as a trivial name. Phospholipase C (phosphatidyl choline cholinephosphohydrolase EC 3.1.4.3) hydrolyses the ester linkage between glycerol and phosphate, with the formation of the appropriate phosphorylated base and α, β-diglyceride. Phospholipase D (phosphatidyl choline phosphatidohydrolase EC 3.1.4.4) liberates the base with the formation of phosphatidic acid. The sites of action of the phospholipases are represented in XVIII.

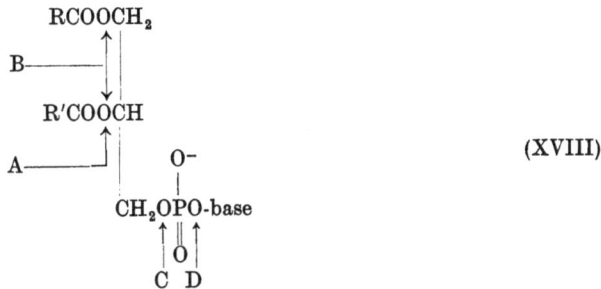

(XVIII)

Sites of action of phospholipases

A review summarizing the classical work on phospholipases is that of ERCOLI (1940). More recent reviews have been prepared by ROSSITER (1960), KATES (1960) and ANSELL and HAWTHORNE (1964).

1. Phosphatidyl Choline (Lecithin)

a) **Phospholipase A.** Phospholipase A forms L-α-lysolecithin (VI) from L-α-lecithin (III) by the removal of the fatty acid esterified in the β-position:

$$\text{L-}\alpha\text{-lecithin} + H_2O \rightarrow \text{L-}\alpha\text{-lysolecithin} + \text{fatty acid} \tag{35}$$

The enzyme has a very wide distribution, being present in snake venoms, animal tissues, plants, bacteria and fungi. Venom phospholipase A was crystallized by DE (1944).

A finding of interest is the discovery of HANAHAN (1952) that the activity of phospholipase A is increased by the addition of diethyl ether, a property the enzyme shares with other phospholipases. DAWSON (1963) concluded that the stimulatory effect of ether on the hydrolysis of lecithin by phospholipase A is the result of penetration of ether molecules into the lipid micelle. Such a penetration causes a wider spacing of the molecules of lecithin orientated in the lipid-water interface, allowing more ready access of the enzyme to the susceptible acyl ester bond. Also the fatty acids liberated in the enzymic reaction will be more readily removed from the surface of the lecithin micelles. Such fatty acids will be replaced by fresh substrate molecules and so will not impede the action of the enzyme. It should also be pointed out that phospholipids oriented in a lipoprotein complex are more readily hydrolysed by phospholipase A than is a suspension of purified lecithin (CONDREA et al. 1963).

Phospholipase A, which is inactive towards lysolecithin (FAIRBAIRN 1945), is capable of removing both saturated and unsaturated fatty acids from lecithins, but at different rates (HANAHAN, RODBELL and TURNER 1954, LONG and PENNY 1957). LONG and PENNY (1957) showed that the enzyme can remove fatty acid from both natural and synthetic L-α-lecithins, but not from D-α-lecithins. The effect of the enzyme on a series of synthetic substrates was investigated by VAN DEENEN and DE HAAS (1963).

There is now considerable evidence that it is the fatty acid esterified in the β-position that is selectively detached with the production of α'-acyl-α-glycerolphosphorylcholine (VI) (TATTRIE 1959, HANAHAN, BROCKERHOFF and BARRON

1960, DE HAAS, DAEMEN and VAN DEENEN 1962). DE HAAS and VAN DEENEN (1963) showed that the enzyme also catalyses the release of one fatty acid from synthetic β-lecithins with the formation of an optically active α-acyl-β-glycerol-phosphorylcholine. They conclude that in general terms phospholipase A catalyses the hydrolysis of the acyl ester linkage adjacent to the glycerophosphoric acid ester bond, but only if the fatty acid to be released occupies the appropriate steric configuration.

b) Phospholipase B (lysophospholipase). Phospholipase B removes the remaining fatty acid esterified in the α'-position from lysolecithin with the formation of glycerolphosphorylcholine (GPC):

$$\text{L-}\alpha\text{-lysolecithin} + H_2O \rightarrow \text{L-}\alpha\text{-GPC} + \text{fatty acid} \tag{36}$$

The enzyme occurs in animal tissues, wasp venom, plants and moulds. SHAPIRO (1953) obtained a crystalline preparation from pancreas. The phospholipase B of *Penicillium notatum* attacks lysolecithin, but is inactive towards lecithin (FAIRBAIRN 1948, UZIEL and HANAHAN 1956). More recently DAWSON (1958a, b) made the significant finding that lecithin micelles may be attacked by phospholipase B of *P. notatum* if the system is activated by the addition of certain acidic lipids such as phosphatidyl inositol or cardiolipin. BANGHAM and DAWSON (1959, 1960) showed that before the enzyme can hydrolyse lecithin micelles the *zeta*-potential must be negative (see also, DAWSON and BANGHAM 1959). This can be provided by introducing long-chain anions, such as phosphatidyl inositol or cardiolipin, into the micelle, or by adding a polyvalent anion such as $Fe(CN)_6{}^{3-}$ to the bulk buffer phase. The introduction of amphipathic cations, such as stearylamine, or addition to the buffer of polyvalent cations, such as Ca^{2+} or $UO_2{}^{2+}$ inhibits the activity of the enzyme.

c) Phospholipase C. In 1941 MACFARLANE and KNIGHT (1941) showed that the toxin of *Clostridium perfringens* contains an enzyme that liberates phosphoryl-choline from lecithin with the formation of diglyceride (II):

$$\text{L-}\alpha\text{-lecithin} + H_2O \rightarrow \text{D-}\alpha,\beta\text{-diglyceride} + \text{phosphorylcholine} \tag{37}$$

Phospholipase C occurs principally in bacterial toxins and snake venoms, but it has been reported in animal tissue (DRUZHININA and KRITZMAN 1952). The enzyme is able to liberate phosphorylcholine from sphingomyelin (MACFARLANE 1948) but not from lysolecithin or GPC (ZAMECNIK, BREWSTER and LIPMANN 1947).

BANGHAM and DAWSON (1962) showed that, in contrast to phospholipase B, a positive *zeta*-potential is necessary for phospholipase C activity. This can be obtained either by introducing long-chain cations into the lecithin micelle or by adding polyvalent cations to the buffer. In this instance long-chain anions and polyvalent anions are inhibitory. These experiments again indicate the importance of electrokinetic potentials in influencing the activity of enzymes capable of degrading the glycerophosphatides.

d) Phospholipase D. Although an enzyme with phospholipase D activity had been postulated for many years, it was not until 1947 that HANAHAN and CHAIKOFF (1947) demonstrated the presence in plant tissue of an enzyme capable of releasing choline from lecithin with the formation of phosphatidic acid (I):

$$\text{L-}\alpha\text{-lecithin} + H_2O \rightarrow \text{L-}\alpha\text{-phosphatidic acid} + \text{choline} \tag{38}$$

Phospholipase D occurs widely in the plant kingdom, but the enzyme has not been reported in animal tissues. Although it shows greater activity towards glycerophosphatides with the L-α structure, apparently the enzyme is able to release choline from β-lecithin, but less rapidly (DAVIDSON and LONG 1958). The enzyme does not liberate choline from lysolecithin, GPC or phosphorylcholine (KATES 1956).

Phospholipase D resembles phospholipase A in that it is stimulated by diethyl ether and other organic solvents (KATES 1957) and it resembles phospholipase B in that it is activited by phosphatidyl inositol (WEISS, SPIEGEL and TITUS 1959) and anionic detergents, whereas cationic detergents are inhibitory (KATES 1957). Presumably these amphipathic substances modify the activity of the enzyme by affecting the *zeta*-potential as described above.

e) GPC Diesterase. Many early studies indicated that choline may be formed enzymically from lecithin in the absence of phospholipase D. HAYAISHI and KORNBERG (1954) demonstrated the presence in *Serratia plymuthica* of a GPC diesterase (L-3-glycerylphosphorylcholine glycerophosphohydrolase EC 3.1.4.2) capable of liberating choline from GPC:

$$\text{L-}\alpha\text{-GPC} + \text{H}_2\text{O} \rightarrow \text{L-}\alpha\text{-glycerophosphate} + \text{choline} \qquad (39)$$

The enzyme is now known to occur widely in animal tissues and bacteria. It is unable to form free choline from lecithin, lysolecithin or phosphorylcholine (DAWSON 1956a).

f) Phosphomonoesterases. It is well known that both acid and alkaline phosphomonoesterases (orthophosphoric monoester phosphohydrolase EC 3.1.3.1 and EC 3.1.3.2) are widely distributed in nature. These enzymes are able to split glycerophosphate formed by the action of GPC diesterase (Reaction 39) into glycerol and orthophosphate:

$$\text{L-}\alpha\text{-glycerophosphate} + \text{H}_2\text{O} \rightarrow \text{glycerol} + \text{P}_\text{I} \qquad (40)$$

Phosphomonoesterases also are capable of hydrolysing the ester bond of phosphorylcholine:

$$\text{Phosphorylcholine} + \text{H}_2\text{O} \rightarrow \text{choline} + \text{P}_\text{I} \qquad (41)$$

In the degradation of lecithin there is little evidence that phosphorylcholine may arise from GPC by the action of GPC diesterase, but phosphorylcholine is known to be produced by the action of bacterial phospholipase C on lecithin.

Pathways leading to the degradation of lecithin are summarized in Figure 6. It will be noted that lecithin may be broken down by three different pathways, initiated by phospholipase A, phospholipase C, or phospholipase D. In animal tissues lecithin is converted into lysolecithin, GPC, glycerophosphate and glycerol by the successive actions of phospholipase A (Reaction 35), phospholipase B (Reaction 36), GPC diesterase (Reaction 39) and phosphomonoesterase (Reaction 40). In bacteria phospholipase C converts lecithin into diglyceride and phosphorylcholine (Reaction 37), which is further hydrolysed by phosphomonoesterase (Reaction 41).

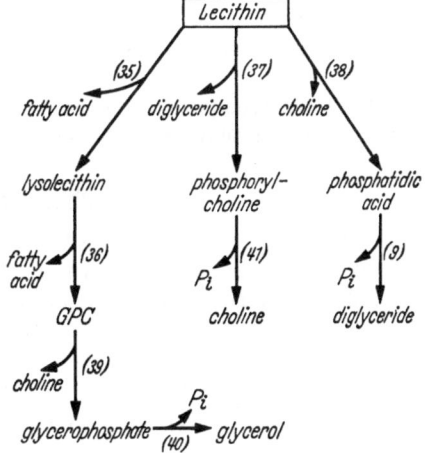

Figure 6. Degradation of lecithin. Figures in parentheses refer to equations in text.

In plants phospholipase D converts lecithin into choline and phosphatidic acid (Reaction 38), which is further broken down by phosphatidic acid phosphatase (Reaction 9).

2. Phosphatidyl Ethanolamine

In animal tissues phosphatidyl ethanolamine (V) is degraded by a series of reactions similar to those described for lecithin. Phospholipase A removes one molecule of fatty acid from phosphatidyl ethanolamine (Fairbairn 1948, Long and Penny 1957) and phospholipase B removes a second molecule from the lysophosphatidyl ethanolamine so formed (Fairbairn 1948, Dawson 1956b). The reactions are in every way similar to Reactions 35 and 36. The glycerolphosphorylethanolamine (GPE) formed by these reactions is further broken down into glycerophosphate and ethanolamine by a diesterase similar to that catalysing Reaction 39 (Dawson 1956a).

It was previously thought that bacterial phospholipase C does not act upon phosphatidyl ethanolamine (MacFarlane 1948, Zamecnik et al. 1947). Recently, however, de Gier, de Haas and van Deenen (1961) showed that the phospholipase C of *Clostridium perfringens* is able to release phosphorylethanolamine from phosphatidyl ethanolamine by a reaction similar to Reaction 37, provided that lecithin is added to the reaction mixture. Bangham and Dawson (1962) reported comparable findings and suggested that the addition of lecithin reduces the net negative charge on the phosphatidyl ethanolamine micelles, thus permitting the formation of an enzyme-substrate complex. In addition, it is now known that phospholipase C obtained from *Bacillus cereus* acts upon phosphatidyl ethanolamine in the absence of added lecithin (Chu 1949, de Gier et al. 1961).

Plant phospholipase D removes ethanolamine from phosphatidyl ethanolamine, with the formation of phosphatidic acid by a reaction similar to Reaction 38 (Kates 1956, Davidson and Long 1958). There is no evidence that either phospholipase C or phospholipase D plays a role in the breakdown of phosphatidyl ethanolamine in animal tissue.

3. Phosphatidyl Serine

It is highly likely that phosphatidyl serine is broken down in animal tissues by a series of reactions similar to those already described for lecithin and phosphatidyl ethanolamine. Both phosphalipase A (Long and Penny 1957) and phospholipase B (Fairbairn 1948) remove fatty acids from serine glycerophosphatides. Also phospholipase C is reported to be inactive (MacFarlane 1948, Zamecnik et al. 1947), whereas phospholipase D degrades phosphatidyl serine into free serine and phosphatidic acid (Kates 1956).

4. Phosphatidyl Glycerol

The experiments of Haverkate and van Deenen (1964) indicate that phosphatidyl glycerol is broken down by the same enzymes that degrade lecithin. Phospholipases A, B, C (from *Bacillus cereus*, but not from *Clostridium perfringens*) and D all act upon phosphatidyl glycerol with the formation of the expected hydrolysis products.

Houtsmuller and van Deenen (1963) reported that both phospholipase A and phospholipase C show activity towards the O-ornithine ester of phosphatidyl glycerol.

5. Cardiolipin

van Deenen and de Haas (1963) demonstrated that cardiolipin is hydrolysed by phospholipase A, the product of the reaction being lysocardiolipin (Marinetti 1964).

6. Phosphatidic Acid

It seems probable that the fatty acids of phosphatidic acid also are removed by phospholipases A and B (RIMON and SHAPIRO 1959). The phosphate group is detached by a specific enzyme, phosphatidic acid phosphatase (L-α-phosphatidate phosphohydrolase EC 3.1.3.4), first discovered by SMITH et al. (1957) (Reaction 9). As noted previously, this enzyme plays an important role in the synthesis of glycerophosphatides. The enzyme, which has a wide distribution in animal tissue, was studied in some detail by COLEMAN and HÜBSCHER (1962).

7. Plasmalogens

The acyl ester group is removed from plasmalogens by the same enzyme (phospholipase A) that releases the fatty acid esterified in the β-position of the diacylglycerophosphatides. Thus RAPPORT and FRANZL (1957a) reported that the acyl ester linkage of choline plasmalogen is hydrolysed by phospholipase A to yield a lysoplasmalogen (now known to be α'-alkenyl-α-glycerolphosphorylcholine) by a reaction analogous to Reaction 35. LONG and PENNY (1957) reported similar findings for ethanolamine plasmalogen. The acyl ester linkage of choline plasmalogen is attacked less readily than the acyl ester linkage of the corresponding diacyl compound (GOTTFRIED and RAPPORT 1962).

Apparently the unsaturated ether group is removed by specific enzymes. WARNER and LANDS (1961) reported the presence in the microsomal fraction of rat liver of an enzyme that hydrolyses the vinyl ether linkage of choline lysoplasmalogen (α'-alkenyl-α-glycerolphosphorylcholine) to yield GPC. The enzyme does not act upon the corresponding ethanolamine compound or upon choline plasmalogen itself. On the other hand, ANSELL and SPANNER (1964) described an enzyme in brain preparations that hydrolyses the vinyl ether linkage of both ethanolamine lysoplasmalogen, to yield GPE, and ethanolamine plasmalogen itself to yield β-acyl-α-glycerolphosphorylethanolamine. The two enzymes thus differ considerably in their substrate specificities.

The experiments of KIYASU and KENNEDY (1960) and McMURRAY (1964b) indicate that phospholipase C is active in removing phosphorylcholine from choline plasmalogen. HACK and FERRANS (1959) also report that choline plasmalogen is hydrolysed by both phospholipase C and phospholipase D.

8. Phosphatidyl Inositol

Phosphatidyl inositol may be degraded by one of two pathways. DAWSON (1959) showed that an enzyme preparation from *P. notatum* breaks down phosphatidyl inositol by a series of reactions analogous to those catalysed by phospholipase A (Reaction 35) phospholipase B or lysophospholipase (Reaction 36) GPC-diesterase (Reaction 39) and phosphomonoesterase (Reaction 40). KEMP, HÜBSCHER and HAWTHORNE (1961) reported a similar degradation of phosphatidyl inositol by a rat liver enzyme preparation. The liver enzyme does not attack lecithin or any of the other glycerophosphatides, whereas the *P. notatum* enzyme of DAWSON (1959) hydrolyses lysolecithin.

A second enzyme active towards phosphatidyl inositol is present in ox pancreas (DAWSON 1959) and rat liver (KEMP et al. 1961). With this enzyme the lipid is broken down into diglyceride and inositol monophosphate by a reaction analogous to the hydrolysis of lecithin by phospholipase C (Reaction 37). The enzyme does not hydrolyse lecithin.

Thus phosphatidyl inositol may be broken down by enzymes similar to the phospholipases A, B and C that attack other glycerophosphatides, but apparently quite distinct from these enzymes. Kemp et al. (1961) suggested that the enzymes responsible for the degradation of phosphatidyl inositol be referred to as phosphoinositidases. Until these enzymes have been purified further and the possible effects of cationic and anionic amphipathic substances have been fully explored, such a suggestion would appear to be premature.

9. Polyphosphoinositides

Polyphosphoinositides are readily broken down in tissue preparations. Thompson and Dawson (1964a) showed that in extracts of brain tissue polyphosphoinositides may be degraded by one of two pathways. For example, triphosphoinositide may be hydrolysed by a specific triphosphoinositide phosphodiesterase to yield diglyceride and inositol triphosphate:

$$\begin{array}{l} \text{phosphatidyl} + H_2O \rightarrow \text{diglyceride} + \text{inositol} \\ \text{inositol} \qquad\qquad\qquad\qquad\qquad \text{triphosphate} \\ \text{triphosphate} \end{array} \qquad (42)$$

Alternatively, triphosphoinositide may be hydrolysed by a specific triphosphoinositide phosphomonoesterase to give diphosphoinositide and inorganic orthophosphate:

$$\begin{array}{l} \text{Phosphatidyl} + H_2O \rightarrow \text{phosphatidyl} + Pi \\ \text{inositol} \qquad\qquad\qquad\quad \text{inositol} \\ \text{triphosphate} \qquad\qquad\quad\ \text{diphosphate} \end{array} \qquad (43)$$

A preparation of triphosphoinositide phosphodiesterase free from the monoesterase was obtained from ox brain (Thompson and Dawson 1964b). It catalyses the removal of diglyceride from both triphosphoinositide and diphosphoinositide. The enzyme is different from the phospholipase C that catalyses the formation of diglyceride from lecithin (Reaction 37). It is also different from the enzyme that catalyses the formation of diglyceride from phosphatidyl inositol described above. The activity of triphosphoinositide phosphodiesterase is increased by substances that combine with the substrate to decrease the negative charges of the phosphate groups. Thus the enzyme is activated by the addition of Mg^{2+} or Ca^{2+} ions, amphipathic cations, such as cetyltrimethylammonium bromide, or by the addition of basic proteins, such as protamine or histone. Anionic amphipathic substances, such as sodium hexadecyl sulphate or ganglioside, are inhibitory.

A preparation of triphosphoinositide phosphomonoesterase also was obtained from ox brain (Dawson and Thompson 1964). The enzyme is specific for triphosphoinositide and presumably diphosphoinositide also. It displays some activity towards inositol triphosphate, but most phosphomonoesters are not hydrolysed. Triphosphoinositide phosphomonoesterase, like the corresponding phosphodiesterase, is activated by the addition of divalent cations, long-chain bases and basic proteins. This activation is abolished by anionic amphipathic substances.

Pathways leading to the degradation of the phosphoinositides are summarized in Figure 7. The polyphosphoinositides may be broken down into the corresponding inositol polyphosphate and diglyceride by the specific phosphodiesterase (Reaction 42), or they may be dephosphorylated by the specific phosphomonoesterase to yield phosphatidyl inositol (Reaction 43). The phosphatidyl inositol may then be degraded through lysophosphatidyl inositol, GPI and glycerophosphate, by reactions analogous to those catalysed by phospholipase A, phospholipase B, phosphodiesterase and phosphomonoesterase, i. e. by reactions similar to Reaction 35, 36, 39 and 40, already described for the degradation of lecithin. Alternatively, the

phosphatidyl inositol may be hydrolysed to give diglyceride and inositol monophosphate by a reaction similar to that catalysed by phospholipase C in the
degradation of lecithin (cf. Reaction 37). Inositol monophosphate, formed either
as the result of this reaction or by the dephosphorylation of the inositol polyphosphates formed by Reaction 42, may then be split into inositol and inorganic
orthophosphate by a non-specific phosphomonoesterase (cf. Reaction 41).

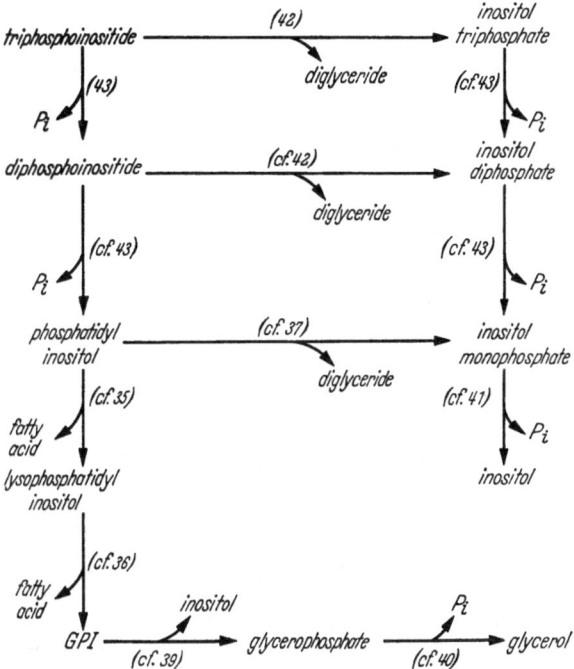

Figure 7. Degradation of phosphoinositides. Figures in parentheses refer to equations in Text.

III. Conclusion

In most tissues the glycerophosphatides are synthesized *in situ* from appropriate precursors of low molecular weight. The phosphodiester group characteristic
of the glycerophosphatides is formed by way of one of a number of CDP-intermediates. These cytosine nucleotides (e. g. CDP-choline and CDP-diglyceride) are
then able to serve as donors of essential groups (e.g. phosphorylcholine, phosphatidyl
group), which are passed on to appropriate acceptors with the formation of the
lipid. It is seen that the metabolic pathways are by no means the same for each
of the glycerophosphatides. In some instances a glycerophosphatide may be derived from another glycerophosphatide, i.e. the biosynthesis involves a lipid-to-lipid
transformation, a reaction that probably takes place while the lipid is oriented in
membranous structures.

The degradation of the glycerophosphatides may be brought about by a variety
of enzymes with a wide distribution in nature. The activity of many of these
enzymes is altered considerably (1) by the addition of substances, such as ethyl
ether, that can penetrate into the lipid micelle and alter the spacing of the molecules oriented at the lipid-water interface and (2) by the presence in the water
phase of polyvalent cations or anions that can modify the surface charge in the

more polar regions of the lipid molecules. For these reasons, the activity of many
of the phospholipases may be modified greatly by the addition of cationic and
anionic amphipathic substances, molecules that are able to penetrate the lipid
micelle and at the same time are able to alter the charge at the lipid-water interface.

References

AGRANOFF, B. W., R. M. BRADLEY, and R. O. BRADY: The enzymatic synthesis of inositol
   phosphatide. J. biol. Chem. **233**, 1077—83 (1958).
ANSELL, G. B., and B. J. BAYLISS: The cytidine diphosphate choline content of rat brain.
   Biochem. J. 78, 209—13 (1961).
— and T. CHOJNACKI: Incorporation of 1-0-Phosphoryl-2-dimethylaminoethanol and phosphorylcholine into the phospholipids of brain and liver dispersions. Nature (Lond.) **196**,
   545—47 (1962a).
— — The incorporation of the 0-phosphate esters of N-methylaminoethanols into the phospholipids of brain and liver dispersions. Biochem. J. 85, 21p—32p (1962b).
— and J. N. HAWTHORNE: Phospholipids. Amsterdam: Elsevier 1964.
— and S. SPANNER: The incorporation of the radioactivity of (3-¹⁴C) serine into brain glycerophospholipids. Biochem. J. 84, 12p—13p (1962).
— — The occurrence of a long-chain ether analogue of phosphatidyl ethanolamine in brain
   tissue. Biochem. J. 88, 56—64 (1963).
— — The enzymic cleavage of the vinyl ether linkage in brain ethanolamine plasmalogen.
   Biochem. J. 90, 19p—20p (1964).
ARTOM, C., and A. WAINER: Incorporation of serine into the lipids of liver fractions. Fed. Proc.
   22, 415 (1963).
BALLOU, C. E., E. VILKAS, and E. LEDERER: Structural studies on the myo-inositol phos-
   pholipids of *Mycobacterium tuberculosis* (var. *bovis*, strain BCG). J. biol. Chem. **238**,
   69—76 (1963).
BANGHAM, A. D., and R. M. C. DAWSON: The relation between the activity of a lecithinase
   and the electrophoretic charge of the substrate. Biochem. J. 72, 486—92 (1959).
— — The physicochemical requirements for the action of *Penicillium notatum* phospholipase
   B on unimolecular films of lecithin. Biochem. J. 75, 133—38 (1960).
— — Electrokinetic requirements for the reaction between *Cl. Perfringens* α-toxin (phospholipase C) and phospholipid substrates. Biochim. biophys. Acta (Amst.) 59, 103—15 (1962).
BENSON, A. A., and B. MARUO: Plant phospholipids. I. Identification of the phosphatidyl
   glycerols. Biochim. biophys. Acta (Amst.) 27, 189—95 (1958).
— and M. MIYANO: The phosphatidylglycerol and sulpholipid of plants. Asymmetry of the
   glycerol moiety. Biochem. J. 81, 31p (1961).
— and E. H. STRICKLAND: Plant Phospholipids. III. Identification of diphosphatidyl glycerol.
   Biochim. biophys. Acta (Amst.) 41, 328—33 (1960).
BERGER, L., and W. T. GIMENEZ: Crystallization of cytidine diphosphate choline from yeast.
   Science 124, 81 (1956).
BORKENHAGEN, L. F., and E. P. KENNEDY: The enzymatic synthesis of cytidine diphosphate
   choline. J. biol. Chem. 227, 951—62 (1957).
— — and L. FIELDING: Enzymatic formation and decarboxylation of phosphatidylserine.
   J. biol. Chem. 236, PC28—PC29 (1961).
BRANDES, R., J. OLLEY, and B. SHAPIRO: Assay of glycerol phosphate acyltransferase in liver
   particles. Biochem. J. 86, 244—47 (1963).
BRANTE, G.: Studies on lipids in the nervous system. With special reference to quantitative
   chemical determination and topical distribution. Acta physiol.. scand. 18, Suppl. 63, 1—189
   (1949).
BREMER, J., and D. M. GREENBERG: Methyl transfering enzyme system of microsomes in the
   biosynthesis of lecithin (phosphatidylcholine). Biochim. biophys. Acta (Amst.) 46, 205—16
   (1961).
BROCKERHOFF, H., and C. E. BALLOU: The structure of the phosphoinositide complex of beef
   brain. J. biol. Chem. 236, 1907—11 (1961).
— — Phosphate incorporation in brain phosphoinositides. J. biol. Chem. 237, 49—52 (1962a).
— — On the metabolism of the brain phosphoinositide complex. J. biol. Chem. 237, 1764—66
   (1962b).
BUBLITZ, C., and E. P. KENNEDY: Synthesis of phosphatides in isolated mitochondria. III.
   The enzymatic phosphorylation of glycerol. J. biol. Chem. 211, 951—61 (1954).
CARR, H. G., H. HAERLE, and J. J. EILER: Phospholipid and plasmalogen synthesis in rat-
   brain homogenates. Biochim. biophys. Acta (Amst.) 70, 205—7 (1963).

CARTER, H. E., R. H. GIGG, J. H. LAW, T. NAKAYAMA, and E. WEBER: Biochemistry of sphingolipids. XI. Structure of phytoglycolipide. J. biol. Chem. 233, 1309—14 (1958).
— D. B. SMITH, and D. N. JONES: A new ethanolamine-containing lipid from egg yolk. J. biol. Chem. 232, 681—94 (1958).
CHARGAFF, E., and A. S. KESTON: The metabolism of aminoethylphosphoric acid, followed by means of the radioactive phosphorus isotope. J. biol. Chem. 134, 515—22 (1940).
CHOJNACKI, T., T. KORZYBSKI, and G. B. ANSELL: The methylation of natural and unnatural analogues of ^{32}P-labelled phosphatidylethanolamine by brain and liver tissue. Biochem. J. 90, 18P—19P (1964).
CHU, H. P.: The lecithinase of Bacillus cereus and its comparison with Clostridium welchii α-toxin. J. gen. Microbiol. 3, 255—73 (1949).
CLARK, B., and G. HÜBSCHER: Monoglyceride transacylase of rat-intestinal mucosa. Biochim. biophys. Acta (Amst.) 70, 43—52 (1963).
COLEMAN, R., and G. HÜBSCHER: Metabolism of phospholipids. V. Studies of phosphatidic acid phosphatase. Biochim. biophys. Acta (Amst.) 56, 479—90 (1962).
COLODZIN, M., and E. P. KENNEDY: Biosynthesis of diphosphoinositide in brain. Fed. Proc. 23, 229 (1964).
CONDREA, E., C. KLIBANSKY, R. KERET, and A. DE VRIES: Action of bovine and human pancreatic phospholipase A on lipoprotein-bound phospholipids. Nature (Lond.) 200, 1096—97 (1963).
CROCKEN, B. J., and J. F. NYC: Phospholipid variations in mutant strains of Neurospora crassa. J. biol. Chem. 239, 1727—30 (1964).
CRONE, H. D., and R. G. BRIDGES: Phospholipids of the house fly Musca domestica stable to hydrolysis by mild alkali and acid. Biochem. J. 84, 101P (1962).
DAVENPORT, J. B., and R. M. C. DAWSON: The formation of cyclic acetals during the acid hydrolysis of lysoplasmalogens. Biochem. J. 84, 490—96 (1962).
DAVIDSON, F. M., and C. LONG: The structure of the naturally occurring phosphoglycerides. 4. Action of cabbage-leaf phospholipase D on ovolecithin and related substances. Biochem. J. 69, 458—66 (1958).
DAWSON, R. M. C.: Liver glycerylphosphorylcholine diesterase. Biochem. J. 62, 689—93 (1956a).
— The phospholipase B of liver. Biochem. J. 64, 192—96 (1956b).
— The identification of two lipid components in liver which enable Penicillium notatum extract to hydrolyse lecithin. Biochem. J. 68, 352—60 (1958a).
— Studies on the hydrolysis of lecithin by a Penicillium notatum phospholipase B preparation. Biochem. J. 70, 559—70 (1958b).
— Studies on the enzymic hydrolysis of monophosphoinositide by phospholipase preparations from P. Notatum and ox pancreas. Biochem. biophys. Acta (Amst.) 33, 68—77 (1959).
— On the mechanism of action of phospholipase A. Biochem J. 88, 414—23 (1963).
— and A. D. BANGHAM: The activation of surface films of lecithin by amphipathic molecules. Biochem. J. 72, 493—96 (1959).
— and J. C. DITTMER: Evidence for the structure of brain triphosphoinositide from hydrolytic degradation studies. Biochem. J. 81, 540—45 (1961).
— and W. THOMPSON: The triphosphoinositide phosphomonoesterase of brain tissue. Biochem. J. 91, 244—50 (1964).
DE, S. S.: Physico-chemical studies on haemolysin. Part I. Crystalline haemolysin (lecithinase). Ann. Biochem. exp. Med. (Calcutta) 4, 45—56 (1944).
DEENEN, L. L. M. VAN, and G. H. DE HAAS: The substrate specificity of phospholipase A. Biochim. biophys. Acta (Amst.) 70, 538—53 (1963).
DITTMER, J. C., and R. M. C. DAWSON: The isolation of a new lipid, triphosphoinositide, and monophosphoinositide from ox brain. Biochem. J. 81, 535—40 (1961).
DRUZHININA, K. V., and M. G. KRITZMAN: Biokhimiya 17, 77 (1952).
EDGAR, G. W. F., and G. SMITS: Alkali-stable phospholipids during the development of the rabbit brain. J. Neurochem. 3, 316—21 (1959).
EICHBERG, J., and R. M. C. DAWSON: Distribution of polyphosphoinositides in tissues and cell fractions. Biochem. J. 93, 23P (1964).
— V. P. WHITTAKER, and R. M. C. DAWSON: Distribution of lipids in subcellular particles of guinea-pig brain. Biochem. J. 92, 91—100 (1964).
ELLIS, R. B., T. GALLIARD, and J. N. HAWTHORNE: Phosphoinositides. 5. The inositol lipids of ox brain. Biochem. J. 88, 125—31 (1963).
ERCOLI, A.: in F. F. NORD, and R. WEIDENHAGEN: Handbuch der Enzymologie, Vol. 1, p.480. Leipzig: Akademische Verlagsgesellschaft 1940.
FAIRBAIRN, D.: The phospholipase of the venom of the cottonmouth mocassin (Agkistrodon piscivorus L.) J. biol. Chem. 157, 633—44 (1945).
— The preparation and properties of a lysophospholipase from Penicillium notatum. J. biol. Chem. 173, 705—14 (1948).

FLEISCHER, S., G. BRIERLEY, H. KLOUWEN, and D. B. SLAUTTERBACK: The role of phospholipids in electron transfer. J. biol. Chem. **237**, 3264—72 (1962).

FOLCH, J.: Brain diphosphoinositide, a new phosphatide having inositol metadiphosphate as
a constituent. J. biol. Chem. **177**, 505—19 (1949).

GALLIARD, T., and J. N. HAWTHORNE: Metabolism of *myo*-inositol in mammalian liver. Biochem. J. **88**, 38P (1963).

GAMBAL, D., and K. J. MONTY: The biosynthesis of plasmalogens. Fed. Proc. **18**, 232 (1959).

GIBSON, K. D., J. D. WILSON, and S. UDENFRIEND: The enzymatic conversion of phospholipid ethanolamine to phospholipid choline in rat liver. J. biol. Chem. **236**, 673—79 (1961).

GIER, J. DE, G. H. DE HAAS, and L. L. M. VAN DEENEN: Action of phospholipase from
Clostridium welchii and *Bacillus cereus* on red-cell membranes. Biochem. J. **81**, 33P—34P
(1961).

GØRANSSON, G.: The incorporation of palmitic acid and oleic acid into liver lipids by the rat.
Biochem. J. **92**, 41P—42P (1964).

GOTTFRIED, E. L., and M. M. RAPPORT: I. Isolation and characterization of phosphatidyl
choline, a pure native plasmalogen. J. biol. Chem. **237**, 329—33 (1962).

GROTH, D. P., J. A. BAIN, and C. C. PFEIFFER: The comparative distribution of C^{14}-labelled
2-dimethylaminoethanol and choline in the mouse. J. Pharmacol. exp. Ther. **124**, 290—95
(1958).

GURR, M. I., and G. HÜBSCHER: Cytidine diphosphate choline: 1,2-diglyceride choline-
phosphotransferase in intestinal mucosa. Biochem. J. **92**, 10P (1964).

DE HAAS, G. H., F. J. M. DAEMEN, and L. L. M. VAN DEENEN: The site of action of phosphatide acyl-hydrolase (phospholipase A) on mixed-acid phosphatides containing a polyunsaturated fatty acid. Biochim. biophys. Acta (Amst.) **65**, 260—70 (1962).

— and L. L. M. VAN DEENEN: The sterospecific action of phospholipase A on β-lecithins.
Biochim. biophys. Acta (Amst.) **70**, 469—71 (1963).

HACK, M. H., and V. J. FERRANS: Papierchromatographische analyse von plasmalogenen.
Hoppe-Seylers Z. physiol. Chem. **315**, 157—62 (1959).

HALL, M. O., and J. F. NYC: The isolation and characterization of phospholipids containing
mono- and dimethylethanolamine from *Neurospora crassa*. J. Lipid Res. **2**, 321—27 (1961).

HANAHAN, D. J.: The enzymatic degradation of phosphatidyl choline in diethyl ether. J. biol.
Chem. **195**, 199—206 (1952).

— H. BROCKERHOFF, and E. J. BARRON: The site of attack of phospholipase (lecithinase) A.
J. biol. Chem. **235**, 1917—23 (1960).

— and I. L. CHAIKOFF: The phosphorus-containing lipides of the carrot. J. biol. Chem. **168**,
233—40 (1947).

— M. RODBELL, and L. D. TURNER: Enzymatic formation of monopalmitoleyl- and mono-
palmitoyllecithin (lysolecithins). J. biol. Chem. **206**, 431—41 (1954).

— and R. WATTS: The isolation of an α'-alkoxy-β-acyl-α-glycerophosphorylethanolamine
from bovine erythrocytes. J. biol. Chem. **236**, PC59—PC60 (1961).

HAVERKATE, F., and L. L. M. VAN DEENEN: The stereochemical configuration of phosphatidyl
glycerol. Biochim. biophys. Acta (Amst.) **84**, 106—8 (1964).

HAWTHORNE, J. N., and P. KEMP: The brain phosphoinositides. Adv. Lipid Res. **2**, 127—66
(1964).

HAYAISHI, O., and A. KORNBERG: Metabolism of phospholipides by bacterial enzymes. J. biol.
Chem. **206**, 647—63 (1954).

HIRSCHMANN, H.: The nature of substrate asymmetry in stereoselective reactions. J. biol.
Chem. **235**, 2762—67 (1960).

HOFFMANN-OSTENHOF, O., C. JUNGWIRTH, and I. B. DAWID: Enzymic phosphorylation of
myo-inositol by enzyme from yeast. Naturwissenschaften **45**, 265 (1958).

HOKIN, M. R., and L. E. HOKIN: The synthesis of phosphatidic acid from diglyceride and
adenosine triphosphate in extracts of brain microsomes. J. biol. Chem. **234**, 1381—86 (1959).

HONEGGER, C. G., and R. HONEGGER: Volatile amines in brain. Nature (Lond.) **185**, 530—32
(1960).

HÖRHAMMER, L., H. WAGNER, and J. HÖLZL: Über die Inositphosphatide des Rinderhirns.
Biochem. Z. **332**, 269—76 (1960).

— H. WAGNER, and G. RICHTER: Über die Inositphosphatide des Rinderhirns und der Soja-
bohne. Biochem. Z. **330**, 591—94 (1958).

HOUTSMULLER, U. M. T., and L. L. M. VAN DEENEN: Identification of a bacterial phospholipid
as an *O*-ornithine ester of phosphatidyl glycerol. Biochim. biophys. Acta (Amst.) **70**,
211—13 (1963).

HÜBSCHER, G.: Metabolism of phospholipids. VI. The effect of metal ions on the incorporation
of L-serine into phosphatidyl serine. Biochim. biophys. Acta (Amst.) **57**, 555—61 (1962).

— and J. N. HAWTHORNE: The isolation of inositol monophosphate from liver. Biochem.
J. **67**, 523—27 (1957).

KANFER, J., and E. P. KENNEDY: Metabolism and function of bacterial lipids. I. Metabolism of phospholipids in *Escherichia coli* B. J. biol. Chem. 238, 2919—22 (1963).
— — Metabolism and function of bacterial lipids. II. Biosynthesis of phospholipids in *Escherichia coli*. J. biol. Chem. 239, 1720—26 (1964).
KATES, M.: Hydrolysis of glycerolphosphatides by plastid phosphatidase C. Canad. J. Biochem. 34, 967—80 (1956).
— Effects of solvents and surface-active agents on plastid phosphatidase C activity. Canad. J. Biochem. 35, 127—42 (1957).
— in K. BLOCH: Lipolytic Enzymes. Lipide Metabolism, p. 165. New York: John Wiley 1960.
— P. S. SASTRY, and L. S. YENGOYAN: Isolation and characterization of a diether analog of phosphatidyl glycerophosphate from *Halobacterium cutirubrum*. Biochim. biophys. Acta (Amst.) 70, 705—7 (1963).
KEENAN, R. W., J. B. BROWN, and B. H. MARKS: Plasmalogen and ester phospholipid biosynthesis in dog-heart-lung preparations. Biochim. biophys. Acta (Amst.) 51, 226—29 (1961).
— and L. E. HOKIN: The enzymatic acylation of lysophosphatidylinositol. J. biol. Chem. 239, 2123—29 (1964).
KEMP, P., G. HÜBSCHER, and J. N. HAWTHORNE: Phosphoinositides. 3. Enzymic hydrolysis of inositol-containing phospholipids. Biochem. J. 79, 193—208 (1961).
KENNEDY, E. P.: Synthesis of phosphatides in isolated mitochondria. J. biol. Chem. 201, 399—412 (1953).
— Synthesis of phosphatides in isolated mitochondria. II. Incorporation of choline into lecithin. J. biol. Chem. 209, 525—35 (1954).
— The synthesis of cytidine diphosphate choline, cytidine diphosphate ethanolamine, and related compounds. J. biol. Chem. 222, 185—91 (1956).
— Biosynthesis of complex lipids. Fed. Proc. 20, 934 (1961).
— The metabolism and function of complex lipids. Harvey Lect. 57, 143—71 (1962).
— and S. B. WEISS: The function of cytidine co-enzymes in the biosynthesis of phospholipids. J. biol. Chem. 222, 193—214 (1956).
KIYASU, J. Y., and E. P. KENNEDY: The enzymatic synthesis of plasmalogens. J. biol. Chem. 235, 2590—94 (1960).
— R. A. PIERINGER, H. PAULUS, and E. P. KENNEDY: The biosynthesis of phosphatidylglycerol. J. biol. Chem. 238, 2293—98 (1963).
KLENK, E., and U. W. HENDRICKS: An inositol phosphatide containing carbohydrate isolated from human brain. Biochim. biophys. Acta (Amst.) 50, 602—3 (1961).
KOREY, S. R., and M. ORCHEN: Plasmalogens of the nervous system. I. Deposition in developing rat brain and incorporation of C^{14} isotope from acetate and palmitate into the α,β-unsaturated ether chain. Arch. Biochem. 83, 381—89 (1959).
KORNBERG, A., and W. E. PRICER: Enzymatic synthesis of phosphorus-containing lipides. J. Amer. chem. Soc. 74, 1617 (1952a).
— — Studies on the enzymatic synthesis of phospholipids. Fed. Proc. 11, 242 (1952b).
— — Enzymatic synthesis of the coenzyme A derivatives of long-chain fatty acids. J. biol. Chem. 204, 329—43 (1953a).
— — Enzymatic esterification of α-glycerophosphate by long chain fatty acids. J. biol. Chem. 204, 345—57 (1953b).
LANDS, W. E. M., and I. MERKL: Metabolism of glycerolipids. III. Reactivity of various acyl esters of co-enzyme A with α'-acylglycerophosphorylcholine, and positional specificities in lecithin synthesis. J. biol. Chem. 238, 898—904 (1963).
LAW, J. H., H. ZALKIN, and T. KANESHIRO: Transmethylation reactions in bacterial lipids. Biochim. biophys. Acta (Amst.) 70, 143—51 (1963).
Le COCQ, J., and C. E. BALLOU: On the structure of cardiolipin. Biochem. 3, 976 (1964).
LONG, C., and I. F. PENNY: The structure of the naturally occurring phosphoglycerides. 3. Action of moccasin-venom phospholipase A on ovolecithin and related substances. Biochem. J. 65, 382—89 (1957).
MacFARLANE, M. G.: The biochemistry of bacterial toxins. 2. The enzymic specificity of *Clostridium welchii* lecithinase. Biochem .J. 42, 587—90 (1948).
— Structure of cardiolipin. Nature (Lond.) 182, 946 (1958).
— Characterizations of lipoamino-acids as O-aminoacid esters of phosphatidyl-glycerol. Nature (Lond.) 196, 136—38 (1962).
— Phosphatidylglycerols and lipoamino acids. Advanc. Lipid Res. 2, 91—125 (1964a).
— in R. M. C. DAWSON, and D. N. RHODES: Lipids of bacterial membranes. Metabolism and Physiological Significance of Lipids, p. 399. London: John Wiley 1964b.
— The structure of cardiolipin. Biochem. J. 92, 12C—14C (1964c).
— and B. C. J. G. KNIGHT: The biochemistry of bacterial toxins. 1. The lecithinase activity of *Cl. welchii* toxins. Biochem. J. 35, 884—902 (1941).
MAGEE, W. L.: To be published.

Marinetti, G. V.: Hydrolysis of cardiolipin by snake venom phospholipase A. Biochim. biophys. Acta (Amst.) **84**, 55—59 (1964).

McMurray, W. C.: Metabolism of phosphatides in developing rat brain. — I. Incorporation of radioactive precursors. J. Neurochem. **11**, 287—99 (1964a).

— Metabolism of phosphatides in developing rat brain. — II. Labelling of plasmalogens and other alkali-stable lipids from radioactive cytosine nucleotides. J. Neurochem. **11**, 315—26 (1964b).

— K. P. Strickland, J. F. Berry, and R. J. Rossiter: Incorporation of ^{32}P-labelled intermediates into the phospholipids of cell-free preparations of rat brain. Biochem. J. **66**, 634 (1957).

Merkl, I., and W. E. M. Lands: Metabolism of glycerolipids. IV. Synthesis of phosphatidylethanolamine. J. biol. Chem. **238**, 905—6 (1963).

Miani, N., and G. Bucciante: La posizione occupata dalla fosforilcolina, citidindifosfatocolina, α-glicerilfosforilcolina e da altri corpi analoghi nel ciclo metabolico di alcuni fosfatidi encefalici. Experientia (Basel) **14**, 10 (1958).

Miras, C. J., J. Mantzos, and G. Levis: Incorporation of L-[3-^{14}C] serine into microsomal phospholipids of human leucocytes. Biochim. biophys. Acta (Amst.) **84**, 101—3 (1964).

Oliver, G. L., R. J. Gardiner, and R. J. Rossiter: Distribution of free inositol, phosphatidyl inositol and polyphosphoinositides in tissues. Proc. Canad. Fed. biol. Soc. **7**, 27 (1964).

Palmer, F. B., and R. J. Rossiter: A simple procedure for the study of inositol phosphatides in cat brain slices. Canad. J. Biochem. **43**, 671—83 (1965).

Pangborn, M. C.: Isolation and purification of a serologically active phospholipid from beef heart. J. biol. Chem. **143**, 247—56 (1942).

Paulus, H., and E. P. Kennedy: The enzymatic synthesis of inositol monophosphatide. J. biol. Chem. **235**, 1303—11 (1960).

Pieringer, R. A., and L. E. Hokin: Biosynthesis of lysophosphatidic acid from monoglyceride and adenosine triphosphate. J. biol. Chem. **237**, 653—58 (1962a).

— — Biosynthesis of phosphatidic acid from lysophosphatidic acid and palmityl coenzyme A. J. biol. Chem. **237**, 659—63 (1962b).

Pietruszko, R., and G. M. Gray: The products of mild alkaline and mild acid hydrolysis of plasmalogens. Biochim. biophys. Acta (Amst.) **56**, 232—39 (1962).

Popják, G., and H. Muir: In search of a phospholipin precursor. Biochem. J. **46**, 103—13 (1950).

Possmayer, F., and K. P. Strickland: The role of CMP-containing compounds in the biosynthesis of brain phospholipids. Proc. Canad. Fed. biol. Soc. **7**, 33 (1964).

Rapport, M. M., and R. E. Franzl: The structure of plasmalogens. I. Hydrolysis of phosphatidal choline by lecithinase A. J. biol. Chem. **225**, 851—57 (1957a).

— — The structure of plasmalogens. III. The nature and significance of the aldehydogenic linkage. J. Neurochem. **1**, 303—10 (1957b).

— B. Lerner, N. Alonzo, and R. Franzl: The structure of plasmalogens. II. Crystalline lysophosphatidal ethanolamine (acetal phospholipide). J. biol. Chem. **225**, 859—867 (1957).

Renkonen, O., and E. L. Hirvisalo: The alkoxy lecithins of ox-heart. Biochem. J. **89**, 29 P (1963).

Riley, R. F.: Metabolism of phosphorylcholine. II. Partition of phosphorylcholine phosphorus between blood phosphate fractions. III. Partition of phosphorylcholine phosphorus between tissues. IV. Distribution of phosphorylcholine phosphorus in tissue lipids. J. biol. Chem. **153**, 535—49 (1944).

Rimon, A., and B. Shapiro: Properties and specificity of pancreatic phospholipase A. Biochem. J. **71**, 620—23 (1959).

Rodbell, M., and D. J. Hanahan: Lecithin synthesis in liver. J. biol. Chem. **214**, 607—18 (1955).

Rose, H. G.: Studies on the molecular structure in rat liver cardiolipin. Biochim. biophys. Acta (Amst.) **84**, 109 (1964).

Rossiter, R. J.: in D. M. Greenberg: Metabolism of phosphatides. Metabolic Pathways: 2nd Edit., Vol. 1, p. 357. New York: Academic Press 1960.

— in R. M. C. Dawson, and D. N. Rhodes: Biosynthesis of lipids in the nervous system. Metabolism and Physiological Significance of Lipids, p. 511. London: John Wiley 1964.

— and V. Donisch: Formation of phospholipids in Ehrlich ascites tumor. Canad. Fed. biol. Soc. **7**, 6 (1964).

— and K. P. Strickland: in K. Bloch: The metabolism and function of phosphatides, p. 69. Lipide Metabolism: New York: John Wiley 1960.

Santiago-Calvo, E., S. Mule, C. M. Redman, M. R. Hokin, and L. E. Hokin: The chromatographic separation of polyphosphoinositides and studies of their turnover in various tissues. Biochim. biophys. Acta (Amst.) **84**, 550—62 (1964).

Senior, J. R., and K. J. Isselbacher: Activation of long-chain fatty acids by rat-gut mucosa. Biochim. biophys. Acta (Amst.) **44**, 399—400 (1960).

— — Glyceride synthesis by membranous structures derived from rat-gut epithelial cells. Fed. Proc. **21**, 288 (1962).

SHAPIRO, B.: Purification and properties of a lysolecithinase from pancreas. Biochem. J. **53**, 663—66 (1953).

SMITH, S. W., S. B. WEISS, and E. P. KENNEDY: The enzymatic dephosphorylation of phosphatidic acids. J. biol. Chem. 228, 915—22 (1957).

SRIBNEY, M., and E. P. KENNEDY: The enzymatic synthesis of sphingomyelin. J. biol. Chem. 233, 1315—22 (1958).

STRICKLAND, E. H., and A. A. BENSON: Neutron activation paper chromatographic analysis of phosphatides in mammalian cell fractions. Arch. Biochem. 88, 344—48 (1960).

STRICKLAND, K. P.: Phosphorylation of diglycerides by rat brain. Canad. J. Biochem. **40**, 247—59 (1962).

— D. SUBRAHMANYAM, E. T. PRITCHARD, W. THOMPSON, and R. J. ROSSITER: Biosynthesis of lecithin in brain. Participation of cytidine diphosphate choline and phosphatidic acid. Biochem. J. 87, 128—36 (1963).

SVENNERHOLM, L., and H. THORIN: Isolation of "kephalin B" from cerebral lipids. Biochim. biophys. Acta (Amst.) 41, 371—72 (1960).

TATTRIE, N. H.: Positional distribution of saturated and unsaturated fatty acids on egg lecithin. J. Lipid Res. 1, 60—5 (1959).

THOMPSON, G. A., and D. J. HANAHAN: Identification of α-glyceryl ether phospholipids as major lipid constituents in two species of terrestrial slug. J. biol. Chem. **238**, 2628—31 (1963a).

— — Studies on the nature and formation of α-glyceryl ether lipids in bovine bone marrow. Biochemistry 2, 641—46 (1963b).

THOMPSON, W., and R. M. C. DAWSON: The hydrolysis of triphosphoinositide by extracts of ox brain. Biochem. J. **91**, 233—36 (1964a).

— — The triphosphoinositide phosphodiesterase of brain tissue. Biochem. J. **91**, 237—43 (1964b).

— K. P. STRICKLAND, and R. J. ROSSITER: Biosynthesis of phosphatidyl inositol in rat brain. Biochem. J. 87, 136—42 (1963).

TSUYUKI, H., and D. R. IDLER: The metabolism of inositol in salmon. III. The biochemical reactions of 2-C^{14}-myoinositol in coho liver. Canad. J. Biochem. **39**, 1037—42 (1961).

UZIEL, M., and D. J. HANAHAN: An enzymatic route to L-α-glyceryl-phosphorylcholine. J. biol. Chem. 220, 1—7 (1956).

VIGNAIS, P. M., C. H. GALLAGHER, and I. ZABIN: Activation and oxidation of long-chain fatty acids by rat brain. J. Neurochem. 2, 283—87 (1958).

VIGNAIS, P. V., and I. ZABIN: Synthesis and properties of palmityl adenylate palmityl coenzyme A, and palmityl glutathione. Biochim. biophys. Acta (Amst.) **29**, 263—69 (1958).

WAGNER, H., J. HÖLZL, A. LISSAU, and L. HÖRHAMMER: Papierchromatographie von Phosphatiden. III. Mitteilung. Quantitative papierchromatographische Bestimmung von Phosphatiden und Phosphatidsäuren in Rattenorganen. Biochem. Z. **339**, 34—45 (1963).

— A. LISSAU, J. HÖLZL, and L. HÖRHAMMER: The incorporation of P^{32} into the inositol phosphatides of rat brain. J. Lipid Res. **3**, 177—80 (1962).

WARNER, H. R., and W. E. M. LANDS: The metabolism of plasmalogen: Enzymatic hydrolysis of the vinyl ether. J. biol. Chem. 236, 2404—9 (1961).

WEBSTER, C. R., and R. J. ALPERN: Studies on the acylation of lysolecithin by rat brain. Biochem. J. 90, 35—42 (1964).

WEISS, H., H. E. SPIEGEL, and E. TITUS: Isolation of an activator for phospholipase D. Nature (Lond.) 183, 1393—94 (1959).

WEISS, S. B., E. P. KENNEDY, and J. Y. KIYASU: The enzymatic synthesis of triglycerides. J. biol. Chem. 235, 40—44 (1960).

— S. W. SMITH, and E. P. KENNEDY: The enzymatic formation of lecithin from cytidine diphosphate choline and D-1,2-diglyceride. J. biol. Chem. 231, 53—64 (1958).

WIELAND, O., and M. SUYTER: Glycerokinase: Isolierung und Eigenschaften des Enzyms. Biochem. Z. 329, 320—31 (1957).

WILLIAMS-ASHMAN, H. G., and J. BANKS: Participation of cytidine coenzymes in the metabolism of choline by seminal vesicle. J. Biol. Chem. 223, 509—21 (1956).

WILSON, J. D., K. D. GIBSON, and S. UDENFRIEND: Studies on the conversion *in vitro* of serine to ethanolamine by rat liver and brain. J. biol. Chem. 235, 3539—43 (1960).

WITTENBERG, J., and A. KORNBERG: Choline phosphokinase. J. biol. Chem. 202, 431—44 (1953).

ZAMECNIK, P. C., L. E. BREWSTER, and F. LIPMANN: A manometric method for measuring the activity of *Cl. welchii* lecithinase and a description of certain properties of this enzyme. J. exp. Med. 85, 381—94 (1947).

ZILVERSMIT, D. B., C. ENTENMAN, and I. L. CHAIKOFF: The measurement of turnover of the various phospholipids in liver and plasma of the dog and its application to the mechanism of action of choline. J. biol. Chem. 176, 193 (1948).

Biochemistry
of Sphingosine Containing Lipids

By

Robert M. Burton

Introduction

The sphingolipids are a class of compounds quite analogous to the lipid series derived from glycerol. Just as glycerol can form a series of phosphorous containing complex lipids, i. e., lecithin, cephalin, etc. (cf. chap. by ROSSITER, p. 93), sphingosine can combine with fatty acids, phosphorous, and bases to give rise to the sphingomyelins. The glycerides can form complex lipids with sugars (PUTNAM and HASSID 1954, CARTER et al. 1956) — and, in a similar manner, sphingosine can form a series of complex sugar-containing lipids, i.e., psychosine, cerebrosides, cerebroside sulfate and gangliosides (DEUEL 1951, CELMER and CARTER 1952). The chemistry of the glycerol and sphingosine containing lipids has been reviewed in other chapters in this volume. The similarity of structure between phosphatidylcholine and sphingomyelin is apparent. Thus the 1 carbon is substituted with phosphoryl choline and carbons 2 and 3 contain long chain fatty acid and/or hydrocarbon residues. In the case of glycerol carbon 3 is substituted with a fatty acid, whereas sphingomyelin contains a hydrocarbon residue joined by carbon-carbon covalent bonding to carbon 3 as an integral part of the sphingosine molecule. If indeed the properties of the glycerol and sphingosine containing lipids are similar, as illustrated by the phosphoryl choline containing derivatives, then one can ask what are the roles of these classes of lipids and why are both classes important to the physiological functioning of animals ? The clue to the answer to these questions may be derived from the cellular and subcellular distribution of these lipids. Because the glycerol containing lipids are rapidly metabolized and their component parts readily utilized either anabolically or catabolically, whereas the sphingosine-containing lipids appear to be metabolized slowly yielding sphingosine which itself resides not in the major metabolic pathways and is metabolized slowly, it may be suggested that the sphingolipids participate as structural components in those parts of the cells which demand stability, for example the myelin sheath of axones, and the glycerides participate in storage as the triglycerides (such as adipose tissue) or in structures where the turnover of components may be more rapid (such as the plasma membranes of cells).

It is the purpose of this chapter to review the pathways of synthesis and degradation of the sphingolipids and to describe the enzymatic steps insofar as they are known. The results of *in vivo* studies on incorporation of precursor materials into the sphingolipids and the resultant turnover data thus derived will be presented. Selected studies of the lipidosis involving the sphingolipids will be presented and discussed in terms of tissue composition and *in vivo* and *in vitro* studies. The possible relevance of the antigenic properties of the sphingolipids will be discussed in relationship to these diseases.

Nomenclature*

Sphingosine, the parent base of the sphingolipids, has been identified both by degradation and synthesis to be D-erythro-1,3-dihydroxy-2-amino-4-trans-octadecene (cf. chap. by STOFFEL, p. 1. Also LEVENE and WEST 1914; KLENK 1929; CARTER 1947; CARTER and HUMISTON 1951; CARTER et al. 1953, JENNY and GROB 1953, MISLOW 1953, KISS et al. 1954, MARINETTI and STOTZ 1954, KLENK and FAILLARD 1955, CARTER et al. 1956). The recent discovery of a 20-carbon sphingosine indicates that sphingosine itself is only one of a homologous series of compounds. (PROSTENIK and MAJHOFER-ORESCANIN 1960, KLENK and GIELEN 1961, STANACEV and CHARGAFF 1962, SAMBASIVARAO and McCLUER 1964, KARLSSON 1964). In this chapter sphingosine will refer to the 18-carbon compound defined above. Members of the series will be referred to collectively as sphingosines and individually will be represented as follows:

sphingosine or 18:sphingosine = parent compound
20:sphingosine = D-*erythro*-1,3-dihydroxy-2-amino-4-*trans*-eicosene
Dihydrosphingosine or 18:dihydrosphingosine = D-*erythro*-1,3-dihydroxy-2-amino-octadecane
20:dihydrosphingosine = D-*erythro*-1,3-dihydroxy-2-amino-eicosane
phytosphingosine or 18:phytosphingosine = D-*erythro*-1,3,4-trihydroxy-2-amino-octadecane
20:phytosphingosine = D-*erythro*-1,3,4-trihydroxy-2-amino-eicosane

In this system the use of the numbers is equivalent to that employed currently with the shorthand representation of fatty acids (cf KISHIMOTO and RADIN 1964). Thus, the number of carbon atoms in the molecule is indicated by the 18 or 20.

Ceramide, the fatty acid amide of the sphingosines:
N-stearyl sphingosine or N-n-tetracosanoyl 18:sphingosine
Psychosine, the O^1-glycosides of the sphingosines:
O^1-glucosyl sphingosine or 1-O-glucosyl 18:sphingosine

Cerebroside, is the name given to the glycosyl derivative of ceramide or alternately to the fatty acyl derivative of psychosine. In general the cerebrosides will be considered to be derivatives of a ceramide family of compounds. Thus, specific cerebrosides will be designated as follows:

glucosyl ceramide = O^1-glucosyl ceramide
galactosyl ceramide = O^1-galactosyl ceramide

An example of the complete definition of a cerebroside would be, N-2-hydroxy-tetracosanoyl-O^1-galactosyl 18:sphingosine. Such compounds as cytolipin-H (cytoside) will be designated as lactosyl ceramide or galactosyl $(1 \rightarrow 4)$ glucosyl ceramide. The oligosaccharide moieties of the glycosphingolipids will be in general denoted by standard abbreviation, i.e. gal $(1 \rightarrow 4)$ glc-ceramide. Frequently the numbers

---

* Abbreviations to be employed are presented in the text (this section, nomenclature) or are as follows: glucose, glc; galactose, gal; galactosamine, galN; N-acetyl-galactosamine, galNAc; N-acetylneuraminic acid (a sialic acid), neuNAc; sphingosine, sph; ceramide or N-acyl sphingosine, cer; psychosine or O^1-galactosyl sphingosine, psy; specific acyls by first three letters, e.g. palmityl, pal and stearyl, ste; phosphoryl choline, PCh or P-choline; coenzyme A, CoA or CoASH; coenzyme A esters of fatty acids, acyl-SCoA; diphosphopyridine nucleotide, DPN; triphosphopyridine nucleotide, TPN; DPNH and TPNH, the reduced forms; adenosine triphosphate, ATP; adenosine diphosphate, ADP; adenosine-5'-phosphosulfate, APS; 3'-phospho-adenosine-5'-phosphosulfate, PAPS; pyrophosphate, PP; uridine diphosphogalactose, UDP gal; uridine diphosphoglucose, UDP glc; uridine diphospho (N-acetyl) galactosamine, UDP gal NAc; cytidine monophosphate (N-acetyl) neuraminic acid, CMP neuNAc; cytidine diphosphocholine, CDP-choline.

indicating the glycosidic linkages will be omitted. Thus the abbreviated notation would be gal-glc-ceramide or lac-ceramide for cytolipin-H.

Sphingoplasmalogens, a new class of glycolipids recently described by Kochetkov et al. (1963, 1964), contains a vinyl ether (at carbon 3 of the sphingosine) in a cerebroside structure:

O^3-alkenylcerebroside or
O^1-galactosyl, O^3-alkenyl N-cerebronyl 18:sphingosine

Cerebroside sulfate, a sulfuric acid ester of cerebroside: 3′-sulfogalactosyl ceramide (Yamakawa et al. 1962, Stoffyn and Stoffyn 1963, Taketomi and Yamakawa 1964).

Gangliosides are oligosaccharide derivatives of ceramide which contain N-acetyl-neuraminic acid. Gangliosides exist as a family whose chemistry is reviewed in an earlier chapter (Stoffel page 1—39). In general the various gangliosides will be identified according to the numbering system presented in tables on page 22 and 214. When appropriate, ganglioside structure will be designated chemically as illustrated in the example which follows:

For ganglioside B4, N-acetylneuraminyl-(2 → 3)-galactosyl-(1 → 3)-N-acetyl-galactosaminyl-(1 → 4)[N-acetylneuraminyl-(2 → 3)]galactosyl-(1 → 4)-glu-cosyl ceramide or abbreviated NeuNAc-Gal-GalNAc (NeuNAc) Gal-Glc-ceramide.

Sphingomyelin, the diester of phosphoric acid with choline and ceramide: O^1-phosphorylcholine ceramide.

I. Studies on the Synthesis of Sphingolipids
Sphingosine and Dihydrosphingosine

With the elucidation of the structure of 18:sphingosine, Zabin and Mead (1953) suggested that the hydrocarbon portion of the sphingosine might arise from acetate in the same manner that fatty acids arise from acetate and that the polar end of the molecule might be derived from ethanolamine. Sprinson and Coulon (1954) investigated the synthesis of the polar end of sphingosine by the use of isotopic ethanolamine and precursors of ethanolamine such as glycine and serine. In general both groups of workers approach the problem methodologically from the same point of view. In both cases the appropriate isotopically labeled compounds were administered intraperitoneally to rats. Zabin and Mead used rats 20 days of age and administered the isotope daily for five days whereas Sprinson and Coulon used animals 25 to 27 days old, administering the isotopic material for 19 days. When the animals were killed Zabin and Mead isolated the sphingosine from the total sphingosine-contained lipids whereas Sprinson and Coulon isolated cerebrosides from which they subsequently isolated the sphingosine. Zabin and Mead catalytically hydrogenated their isolated sphingosine to form dihydro-sphingosine prior to degradation by periodic acid oxidation. The sphingosine fraction isolated by Sprinson and Coulon was directly oxidized with periodate. Formaldehyde formed from carbon 1 was distilled and isolated as a dimedon derivative. The formic acid derived from carbon 2 was converted to carbon dioxide and collected. A long chain aldehyde was recovered as the 2,4-dinitrophenol-hydrazine derivative (Sprinson and Coulon, 1954) or as a semicarbazide (Zabin and Mead, 1954). Zabin and Mead converted the semicarbazide to palmitic acid by alkaline permanganate. Bromine oxidation of the silver salt of palmitic acid yielded, in a step-wise manner, carbon 3, carbon 4, and carbon 5 of the sphingosine.

The results of these experiments have been recalculated from the data of ZABIN and MEAD (1953, 1954) and SPRINSON and COULON (1954) and are presented in Table 1. It is immediately apparent from this data that acetate labelled in either the one or two positions gives rise exclusively to the hydrocarbon portion of the sphingosine. Degradation of the palmitic acid derived from the sphingosine labelled with acetate-2-^{14}C shows that carbon 4 is 3 to 5 times richer in ^{14}C than carbons 3 or 5. This is consistent with the pattern observed during fatty acid synthesis

Table 1. *Distribution of isotope in rat brain Sphingosine*

Isotope donor (*designates isotope)	CH$_2$-CH-CH-CH$_2$-CH$_2$-(CH$_2$)$_{12}$-CH$_3$ OH NH$_2$ OH					
	1 %	2 %	3 %	4 %	5 %	18 %
	C1	C2	C3	C4	C5	C3-18
CH$_3$————C*OOH	0	0				99
C*H$_3$————COOH	3	2	2	10	3	
H————C*OOH	64	10				16
C*H$_2$—C*H$_2$ / OH NH$_2$	7	12				57
C*H$_2$—CH$_2$ / OH NH$_2$	2½	2½				95
CH$_2$————C*OOH / NH$_2$	7	8				92
C*H$_2$————COOH / NH$_2$	27	50				23
C*H$_2$—CH————COOH / OH NH$_2$	65	2				33

Determined after reduction to dihydrosphingosine (see text). Adopted from the data of ZABIN and MEAD (1953, 1954) and SPRINSON and COULON (1954).

from acetate. Of considerable interest is the observation that ethanolamine is a poor precursor of the polar end of the sphingosine; up to 95% of the radioactivity derived from ethanolamine-2-^{14}C is in carbon atoms 3 to 18. While glycine-1-^{14}C induced radioactivity primarily in the hydrocarbon portion, formate-^{14}C labelled carbon one to the extent of 64%. These observations therefore suggested that the prime precursor of the polar-end of sphingosine is serine. Glycine-2-^{14}C may be converted *in vivo* by "active" formate to serine-2-^{14}C. If this were the donor, it would be expected that radioactivity would appear in carbon 2 of the sphingosine. The data in Table 1 shows 50% of the radioactivity from glycine-2-^{14}C resides in carbon 2. Similarly the administration of serine-3-^{14}C, which should give rise to carbon 1 of the sphingosine, does induce 65% of the ^{14}C into this position. On this basis it was proposed that the sphingosines are synthesized by the condensation of palmitic acid or a palmitic acid derivative and serine, concurrent with the decarboxylation of the serine.

In vivo studies indicate the formation of sphingosine as formulated in the following reaction:

$$COOH$$
$$[CH_3—(CH_2)_{14}—COOH] + H—\overset{|}{\underset{|}{C}}—CH_2OH \qquad (1)$$
$$NH_2$$

$$\downarrow$$

$$CH_3—(CH_2)_{12}—CH = CH—\overset{H}{\underset{|}{C}}—\overset{H}{\underset{|}{C}}—CH_2OH + CO_2 + [H_2O] + [H]$$
$$\underset{OH}{\,}\quad\underset{NH_2}{\,}$$

With this reaction in mind, Brady and Koval (1957, 1958) demonstrated that incubating DL-serine-3-^{14}C in the presence of pyridoxal phosphate, magnesium chloride, TPN, DPN, and an unidentified substance present in a kochsaft prepared from rat liver would yield sphingosine containing radioactivity in the presence of a dialyzed brain supernatant preparation. Subsequent studies by Brady and Koval (1957, 1958) and Brady et al. (1958) have delineated an enzyme system capable of the step-wise synthesis of 18:sphingosine.

Cell-free particles obtained from the brains of rats 12 to 18 days old were used as the enzyme-system source. These particles sediment at $3 \times 10^6 \times$ g-min but not at $6 \times 10^5 \times$ g-min. In some experiments these particles were washed and resuspended in potassium phosphate buffer (pH 7.4), sonic irradiated at 9 KC for 10 min. at -2°C, and following centrifuging at $6 \times 10^6 \times$ g-min yielded a soluble enzyme-system preparation. When L-serine-U-^{14}C was incubated with this enzyme preparation and cofactors (CoASH, ATP, pyridoxal phosphate, and a TPNH generating system composed of glucose-6-phosphate, magnesium chloride and glucose-6-phosphate dehydrogenase) labelled sphingosine was formed which contained 88% of the carbon-14 in carbons 1 and 2. Palmitic acid-1-^{14}C yielded labelled sphingosine when incubated under similar conditions. The presence of CoA and ATP facilitated the incorporation of the palmitic acid. The substitution of palmityl-SCoA was effective in replacing the palmitic acid, CoA and ATP requirements. A consideration of the reaction formulated above would suggest that the principle donor of the hydrocarbon portion must be at the oxidation level of palmitaldehyde. Possible reactants such as beef heart plasmalogens were ineffective in the synthesis of sphingosine. In the early studies palmitaldehyde was not effective. However, subsequent studies showed this to be a solubility problem and that a balance could be obtained between the Tween 20 concentration necessary to solubilize palmitaldehyde and the inhibitory effect of Tween 20 on the enzyme system. Under this condition palmitaldehyde was as effective an acceptor for DL-serine-3-^{14}C radioactivity as was palmityl CoA plus TPNH. Thus 0.12 μmoles pal-SCoA plus TPNH (generating system) gave 293 cpm/μmoles sphingosine and 0.12 μmoles palmitaldehyde plus 1.2 mg Tween 20 gave 296 cpm/μmoles sphingosine. Control, no long chain compound additions, gave 37 cpm/μmoles sphingosine (All three reaction mixtures contained DL-serine-3-^{14}C, enzyme preparation, and cofactors as appropriate). Since the reaction yielding sphingosine is the condensation of palmitaldehyde with serine, the formation of palmitaldehyde from palmityl-SCoA must occur in the enzyme preparations. Spectrophotometric evidence for the oxidation of TPNH by palmityl-SCoA and for the reduction of both TPN and DPN by palmitaldehyde, in the presence of CoA, has been obtained by Brady et al. (1958). This reaction, as formulated below, is similar to the aldehyde dehydrogenase reported by Burton and Stadtman (1953).

$$CH_3(CH_2)_{14}CO \overset{O}{\underset{SCoA}{\diagup\diagdown}} + TPNH + H^+ \rightleftharpoons CH_3(CH_2)_{14}C \overset{O}{\underset{H}{\diagup\diagdown}} + TPN^+ + CoASH \qquad (2)$$

The reaction of L-serine-U-^{14}C with pal-SCoA plus TPNH and the brain enzyme system to yield sphingosine has been shown to proceed readily. The question of the incorporation of ethanolamine was investigated by BRADY et al. (1958). Using the system under the conditions appropriate for the incorporation of serine, no formation of sphingosine was seen when serine was replaced by ethanolamine.

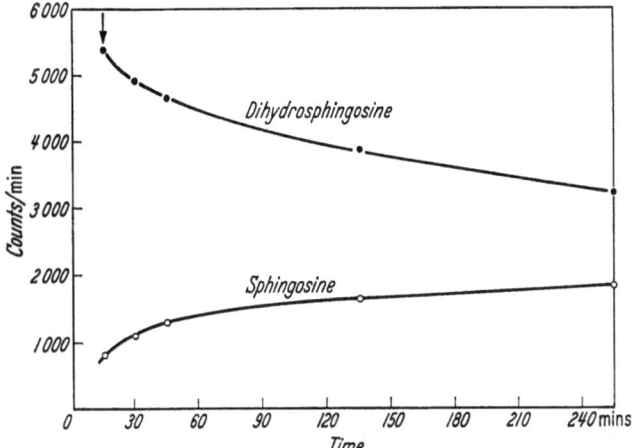

Fig. 1. Kinetic study of the conversion of L-serine-U-C^{14} to dihydrosphingosine (●) and sphingosine (○). The experimental details are described in the text. From BRADY and KOVAL (1958)

In addition, it was shown that serine could form a complex with pyridoxal phosphate in the presence of nickel nitrate. This complex, with an absorption maximum at 940 mμ, was taken as evidence for formation of a schiff-base. Again, under conditions in which serine formed this complex, ethanolamine failed to form a schiff-base. BRADY et al. (1958) have suggested that the inactivity of ethanolamine may be due to its failure to form a pyridoxal phosphate intermediate.

Two final questions remained, first, is the product of the reaction of serine with palmitaldehyde dihydrosphingosine or sphingosine and second, does an enzyme exist in this brain enzyme system which will convert dihydrosphingosine to sphingosine?

BRADY and his colleagues (1958) studied the incorporation of serine-^{14}C into sphingosine and dihydrosphingosine by withdrawing aliquots from the reaction mixture and separating the saturated from the unsaturated sphingosines on silicic acid columns. Figure 1 pictures the time course of incorporation of serine radioactivity into the sphingosines. It may be seen that dihydrosphingosine is highly radioactive at the early time periods and decreases in radioactivity with increasing time, whereas sphingosine has little radioactivity at the beginning but shows a concomitant increase in radioactivity with the fall in the dihydrosphingosine radioactivity. This of course indicates that the product of the condensation of serine with palmitaldehyde is the saturated base. Figure 2 illustrates the oxidation of the dihydrosphingosine by this rat brain enzyme system under conditions in which sphingosine is not oxidized. Safranin-T served as the electron acceptor. The oxidation of dihydrosphingosine is indicated by the reduction of optical density at 520 mμ due to the safranin-T. Final proof of the oxidation of dihydrosphingosine was an experiment in which 1.5 mμ moles was incubated with the brain enzyme preparation at pH 7.8 for six hours under oxygen (37°C) in the presence of Tween 20, magnesium chloride, nicotinamide, DPN, TPN, and 5 mg phenazine methosulfate. At the end of this time the sphingosine content was measured and indicated a conversion of 5.8% of the saturated to the unsaturated form.

The configuration of the sphingosine formed during incubations of serine-C[14] and palmityl-SCoA with rat brain homogenates was determined by Fujino and Zabin (1962a, b). In these experiments, carrier *erythro*-sphingosine and carrier *threo*-sphingosine were added to the homogenates to trap the newly synthesized radioactive sphingosines. The *erythro*- and *threo*-forms were separated by crystallization as the tri-benzoyl derivatives of the dihydrosphingosine (following reduction) and by thin-layer chromatography of the free bases. In all experiments, only the *erythro*-form contained radioactivity (sufficient to account for the total amount incorporated in the homogenate) and the *threo*-forms were essentially non-radioactive.

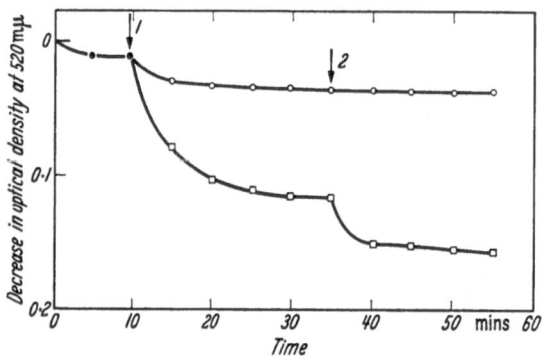

Fig. 2. Spectrophotometric measurement of the reduction of Safranin T by dihydrosphingosine (□) and sphingosine (○). At Arrow 1, 0.4 μmole of sphingosine and dihydrosphingosine hydrochlorides suspended in 10 mg. of bovine serum albumin were added to the respective cuvettes: At Arrow 2, 0.2 μmole of additional substrate was added. From Brady and Koval (1958)

Reactions summarizing the formation of the sphingosines are illustrated in the following 3 equations:

$$CH_3(CH_2)_{12}CH_2CH_2C\overset{O}{\underset{SCoA}{\diagdown}} + TPNH + H^+ \rightleftharpoons CH_3(CH_2)_{12}CH_2CH_2C\overset{O}{\underset{H}{\diagdown}} + TPN^+ + CoASH \quad (3)$$

$$CH_3(CH_2)_{12}CH_2CH_2C\overset{O}{\underset{O}{\diagdown}} + HC\overset{COOH}{\underset{NH_2}{\diagup}}\overset{Pyridoxal}{\underset{OH}{\xrightarrow{Phosphate}}} CH_3(CH_2)_{12}CH_2CH_2-CH-CH-CH_2 + CO_2 \quad (4)$$
$$\underset{OH}{\quad}\underset{NH_2}{\quad}\underset{OH}{\quad}$$

$$CH_3(CH_2)_{12}CH_2CH_2-CHCHCH_2 + (Flavin?) \rightleftharpoons \quad (5)$$
$$\underset{OH}{\quad}\underset{NH_2}{\quad}\underset{OH}{\quad}$$

$$\rightleftharpoons (Flavin-H_2?) + CH_3(CH_2)_{12}CH=CH-CHCHCH_2$$
$$\underset{OH}{\quad}\underset{NH_2}{\quad}\underset{OH}{\quad}$$

It is of interest to mention that sphingosines occur in organisms, such as fungi (Oda, 1952), corn (Carter et al., 1954) and yeast (Stodola and Wickerham, 1960) in addition to animal tissues. The predominate form present in non-animal cells is phytosphingosine. In addition, 18:sphingosine has been found in both plants (Carter et al., 1961) and yeast (Stodola et al., 1962), as well as the 20:phyto-sphingosine (in yeast, Prostenik and Stanacev, 1958) and 18:dehydrophyto-sphingosine (D-*erythro*-1,3,4-trihydroxy-2-amino-trans-octa-decene; in soybean, Mueller, 1953). In addition to their existence intracellularly as complex sphingo-lipids, the yeast, *Hansenula ciferri*, excretes both the tetracetyl-18:phytosphingo-sine and triacetyl-18:dihydrosphingosine. (Wickerham and Stodola, 1960; Sto-dola et al., 1962). The yield of the extracellular sphingosines is about 100—200 mg per liter of yeast culture fluid. This suggests that additional enzymatic studies on the biosynthesis of the sphingosines and sphingolipids could be carried out fruitfully using *Hansenula ciferri*, and other microorganisms.

Ceramides have been isolated from a number of tissues. It is not known if the tissue ceramides arrive by synthesis, as intermediates in the formation of other sphingosine containing lipids, or whether they represent degradative products of the more complex lipids. Evidence for the synthesis of ceramide by rat brain homogenates was obtained by ZABIN (1957). ZABIN employed a reaction mixture similar to that of BRADY and coworkers (1957, 1958) which actively synthesized sphingosine from serine-3-[14]C. The radioactive sphingosine in the ceramides isolated was used as the index of ceramide synthesis. Under these conditions ceramide labelled with carbon-14 could be isolated from the reaction mixture in the presence of palmityl-SCoA. The addition of nonisotopic sphingosine reduced the extent of radioactivity incorporated from serine-3-^{14}C into the ceramides.

Recently GATT has obtained an enzyme preparation from rat brain which catalyzes the hydrolytic cleavage of the amide linkage of ceramide. This enzyme has been purified 110-fold. Both liver and kidney have been found to possess ceramide hydrolase activity. The soluble enzyme was completely dependent upon sodium cholate or related detergents, no metal requirements were noted, and an enzyme pH optimum of near 5 was seen. Substrates such as N-oleyl-18:sphingosine, N-palmitoyl-18:sphingosine, N-palmitoyl-18:dihydrosphingosine and N-stearoyl-18:sphingosine were readily hydrolyzed. Neither N-lignoceryl-18:dihydrosphingosine nor N-acetyl-18:sphingosine were hydrolyzed by this enzyme preparation. It was noted that the hydrolytic products of the reaction inhibited the hydrolysis. In fact, this enzyme preparation showed the ability to form ceramide from the products, i.e. 18:sphingosine and fatty acid. The synthetic reaction showed a pH optimum of near 5, a requirement for the cholate salt, and the absence of a requirement for ATP or CoA. The substitution of palmityl-SCoA for the free fatty acid resulted in a reduction of the synthesis of the ceramide. It would appear that the synthesis of the ceramide by the Gatt enzyme represents a different activity than the palmityl-SCoA enzyme described by ZABIN. It is of interest to note that the enzyme prepared by GATT, while synthesizing ceramide, failed to form cerebroside from O^1-galactosyl-18:sphingosine and palmitic acid.

Psychosine, galactosyl sphingosine, may be synthesized from UDP-galactose and sphingosine in the presence of a UDP-galactose:sphingosine transferase present in guinea pig brain and spinal cord homogenates. This is formulated in the following reactions:

$$UDPgal + CH_3(CH_2)_{12}CH = CH - \underset{\underset{OH}{|}}{CH} - \underset{\underset{NH_2}{|}}{CH} - CH_2OH \rightarrow \qquad (6)$$

$$CH_3(CH_2)_{12}CH = CH - \underset{\underset{OH}{|}}{CH} - \underset{\underset{NH_2}{|}}{CH} - \underset{\underset{O-gal}{|}}{CH_2} + UDP$$

Experiments reported by CLELAND and KENNEDY (1960) showed that the enzyme activity was present to the greatest extent in the microsomal fraction prepared by centrifugation at 2.52×10^6 g-min. This enzyme preparation possessed the ability to incorporate the galactose moiety from UDP-galactose into psychosine. The substitution of galactose-1-phosphate and UDP-glucose for the UDP-galactose provided the effective synthesis of psychosine demonstrating the presence in these preparations of UDP-glucose:galactose-1-phosphate transferase activity. Neither galactose-1-phosphate nor free galactose would catalyze the formation of psychosine. It is shown in Table 2 that the galactose acceptor is rather non-specific. The better acceptors are DL-*erythro*-18:dihydrosphingosine and the

Table 2. *UDP-galactose: sphingosine transferase Specificity*

Sphingosine	Relative Activity[*] Guinea Pig Brain %	Young Rat Brain %
Configuration		
D-*erythro* ——————18:dihydrosph.	92	81
DL-*erythro-trans* ————18:sph.	100*	100*
DL-*erythro-cis* ————18:sph.	43	50
DL-*erythro*——————17:sph. (cyne)**	80	
DL-1-hydroxy-2-amino-octadecane	52	65
DL-*threo*——————18:dihydrosph.	18	
DL-*threo-trans* ————18:sph.	25	
DL-*threo-cis* ————18:sph.	47	
DL-*threo*——————18:sph. (cyne)***	34	40

Recalculated from Data of Cleland and Kennedy (1960).

* Reference sphingosine; activity arbitrarily set equal to 100%. All activities corrected for endogenous reaction (9% in guinea pig and 20% in rat).

** DL-*erythro*-1,3-dihydroxy-2-amino-heptadecyne.

*** DL-*threo*-1,3-dihydroxy-2-amino-octadecyne.

DL-*erythro*-18:sphingosine. Both the guinea pig and young rat enzyme activity with dihydrosphingosine was 80 and 90% of sphingosine. A change in configuration of the double bond from *trans* to *cis* results in a reduction in activity. Restoration of the linear structure by the introduction of an acetylenic bond at carbon 4 yields a compound with a reaction rate of 78% of sphingosine. The 3-hydroxy functional group was shown to be required for maximal activity. That the *erythro* configuration is the preferred form is demonstrated by the low reaction rate with the *threo*-sphingosines, where reaction rates vary from 17 to 48% of the maximal rate (with the *erythro* sphingosine). Phytosphingosine showed only 38% of the maximal activity with the guinea pig brain enzyme.

It is interesting to note that crude homogenates of guinea pig brain incubated with UDP-galactose-1-^{14}C and acceptors showed the ability to galactosylate DL-*erythro-trans*-18:sphingosine and, in addition, the N-acetyl *erythro-trans*-18:-sphingosine to the extent of 16% of the maximal rate (Cleland and Kennedy, 1960). On the other hand, DL-*threo-trans*-18:sphingosine was galactosylated only to the extent of 28% whereas N-acetyl-*threo-trans*-18:sphingosine accepted the galactose at 72% of the rate with *erythro*-trans-18:sphingosine. The ability to transfer galactose from UDP-galactose to the ceramide was lost during the enzyme purification which selected for the UDPgal:sphingosine transferase activity.

Cerebrosides synthesis can occur potentially by two routes: 1) the acylation of psychosine to yield cerebroside, and 2) the galactosylation of ceramide. The acylation of psychosine can occur *in vitro* as demonstrated by Brady (1962) and suggested by the work of Cleland and Kennedy (1960). Brady prepared microsomes from the brains of young rats (14 day old; sedimented at 3×10^6 g-min.). When these microsomal preparations were incubated in phosphate buffer (pH 7.8) with stearyl-1-^{14}C-SCoA, Tween-20, magnesium chloride and ATP, incorporation into cerebrosides of the radioactivity in the stearic acid occurred in the presence of psychosine but not in the presence of sphingosine (unless UDP-glucose was present also).

Burton, Sodd and Brady (1958) employed a crude system from rat brain for the investigation of the biosynthesis of cerebroside. The assay employed was the incorporation of radioactivity from galactose-1-^{14}C into cerebroside. The cerebrosides were isolated on a mixed-bed resin column (see RADIN et al., 1955) which removes psychosine from the cerebroside isolated. The enzyme source was the microsomal fraction prepared from rat brain (14 to 18 day old) which also provided the acceptor for the galactosyl moiety. The best galactosyl donors were UDP-galactose and those systems which give rise to UDP-galactose, i.e., galactose-1-phosphate in the presence of UDP-galactose or galactose + ATP in the presence of UDP-glucose. Galactose, galactose + ATP, galactose + UDP-glucose or galactose-1-phosphate alone showed only negligible synthesis of cerebrosides. While the total incorporation of radioactivity into the cerebrosides was small, it should be born in mind that dependence upon an endogenous acceptor was involved and no detergents were employed (as has been demonstrated subsequently to be necessary in these synthetic systems). The cerebroside isolated from the neutral glycolipid fraction was identified by chromatography on silicic acid and compared with the point of elution of known cerebroside, by its solubility characteristics, by its infrared spectrum, and by the fact that it contained the proportionate amount of galactose. Methanolysis of the cerebroside yielded methyl galactoside which contained the radioactivity. The best interpretation of these data suggests that the endogenous acceptor was ceramide and the reaction may be formulated as in the following equation:

$$\text{UDPgal} + \begin{array}{c} \text{R}-\text{CH}-\text{CH}-\text{CH}_2 \\ \quad\ \ |\quad\ \ |\quad\ \ | \\ \quad\ \ \text{OH}\ \ \text{NH}\ \ \text{OH} \\ \qquad\quad | \\ \qquad\quad \text{C}=\text{O} \\ \qquad\quad | \\ \qquad\quad \text{R}_1 \end{array} \longrightarrow \begin{array}{c} \text{R}-\text{CH}-\text{CH}-\text{CH}_2 \\ \quad\ \ |\quad\ \ |\quad\ \ | \\ \quad\ \ \text{OH}\ \ \text{NH}\ \ \text{O-gal} \\ \qquad\quad | \\ \qquad\quad \text{C}=\text{O} \\ \qquad\quad | \\ \qquad\quad \text{R}_1 \end{array} + \text{UDP} \qquad (7)$$

Had synthesis occurred via psychosine, the presence of α-hydroxy-lignoceryl-SCoA or α-hydroxy-lignoceric acid, ATP, and the fatty acid activating system would have been required to convert the psychosine to the cerebroside. In addition more recent experiments have shown a stimulation of the incorporation of radioactivity from UDP-galactose-1-^{14}C into cerebroside by the addition of exogenous ceramide (isolated from cerebroside) in a reaction mixture containing brain microsomes and 2% n-butanol (BURTON, unpublished data).

Cerebroside sulfate has not been synthesized *in vitro*, as yet[*]. However, HEALD and ROBINSON (1961) have shown that a sulfatide contains radioactivity after the aerobic incubation of slices of guinea pig brain tissue with $^{35}SO_4^{2-}$ and glucose. The sulfatide isolated was soluble in chloroform-methanol (2—1) and failed to partition into an aqueous phase. Further identification of the sulfolipid was not made. GOLDBERG (1961) has postulated several pathways which may be involved in cerebroside sulfate synthesis. The initial steps are the activations of sulfate to 3′-phosphoadenosine-5′-phosphosulfate, i.e., PAPS, as described by BANDURSKI et al. (1956, 1958), WILSON and BANDURSKI (1956), and ROBBINS and LIPMANN (1956, 1958a, b).

$$\text{ATP} + \text{SO}_4^{2-} \rightleftharpoons \text{APS} + \text{PP} \qquad (8)$$

$$\text{ATP} + \text{APS} \rightarrow \text{PAPS} + \text{ADP} \qquad (9)$$

---

[*] A recent abstract and verbal report by McKHANN, LEVY, and Ho (1965) reports the *in vitro* synthesis of cerebroside sulfate by a microsomal enzyme system from young rat brain (18—22 days old). Sonic irradiation of the microsomal fractions resulted in the solublization of a sulfokinase system. The complete synthesis required the microsomal fraction of brain, $^{35}SO_4^{2-}$, ATP, cerebrosides, and a non-ionic detergent (BRIJ 96). The reaction reported would be consistant with equations 8, 9, and 10. No incorporation of ^{35}S-sulfate into a cholesterol ester nor an exchange with unlabelled cerebroside sulfate was observed.

The sulfate from PAPS would then be transferred to a lipid acceptor such as cerebroside or psychosine,

$$\left.\begin{array}{c}\text{cerebroside}\\\text{psychosine}\end{array}\right\} + \text{PAPS} \to \left.\begin{array}{c}\text{cerebroside sulfate}\\\text{psychosine sulfate}\end{array}\right\} + \text{PAP} \qquad (10)$$

or a nucleotide intermediate,

$$\text{UDP-galactose} + \text{PAPS} \to \text{UDP-galactose-sulfate} + \text{PAP} \qquad (11)$$

In Goldberg's experiments (1960a, b), PAP ^{35}S incubated with extracts prepared from rat kidney, liver and brain yielded a radioactive lipid which was not identified. The addition of cerebrosides and psychosine failed to increase the incorporation of $^{35}SO_4^{2-}$ from PAPS. However, N-acetyl sphingosine did increase the yield of a $^{35}SO_4^{2-}$ labeled lipid identified tentatively as O-sulfo-N-acetyl sphingosine. No formations of UDP-galactose-$^{35}SO_4$ was observed in this system (Goldberg, 1960a). It should be noted that Strominger (1955) has found UDP-(N-acetyl)galactosamine-4-sulfate in hen oviduct. Investigation of the dynamic aspect of cerebroside sulfate in brain (*in vivo*) will be discussed in a later section.

Gangliosides. Considerable information on the incorporation *in vivo* of various carbohydrate precursors into gangliosides has recently become available (Radin et al., 1957, Moser and Karnovsky, 1959, Burton et al., 1963, and Suzuki and Korey, 1963). These studies have not produced evidence for a specific type of pathway. Burton et al. (1959) and Burton (1960) have discussed possible routes of biosynthesis. The possible routes are diagrammatically presented as follows:

$$\text{UDPglc} + \left\{\begin{array}{c}\text{sphingosine}\\\text{ceramide}\end{array}\right\} \to \left\{\begin{array}{c}\text{psychosine}\\\text{cerebroside}\end{array}\right\} + \text{UDPgal} \qquad (12)$$

$$\searrow \text{UDPgalNAc}$$

$$\searrow \text{CMPneuNAc}$$

$$\searrow \boxed{\text{gangliosides}}$$

$$\text{UDPglc} \overset{\text{UDPgal}}{\underset{\text{UDPgalNAc}}{- \to - \to}} \overset{\text{CMPneuNAc}}{\longrightarrow} \text{UDPglc}-\text{gal}-\text{galNAc}-\text{gal}-\text{NeuNAc} + \left\{\begin{array}{c}\text{sphingosine}\\\text{ceramide}\end{array}\right.$$

$$\underset{\text{neuNAc}}{|} \qquad (13)$$

In essence the question may be formulated, are gangliosides synthesized step-wise, i.e., by the addition of monosaccharide units, to give the final product, the ganglioside family, or, by analogy to bacterial cell wall synthesis (Strominger, 1963), is the oligosaccharide moiety synthesized as a nucleotide and then transferred, intact, to the acceptor which gives rise to the ganglioside family. Of course one may visualize a scheme in which part of the oligosaccharide moiety is built on a nucleotide and part added as monosaccharide units to form the finished product. During experiments conducted to study the *in vivo* incorporation of glucose-1-^{14}C radioactivity into cerebrosides and gangliosides of young rat brain, the nucleotide fraction of these rat brains was extracted by cold perchloric acid according to the procedure of Schmitz et al. (1954). Chromatography of these fractions on paper yielded a series of nucleotide spots (detected by ultraviolet absorption) and radioactive areas (detected by radioautography). It may be seen from Figure 3 that the UDP-glucose and UDP-galactose spots were radioactive. In addition, ultraviolet absorbing and radioactive areas were detected closer to the origin in the solvent system. These would be the region in which nucleotide oligosaccharide would be expected to appear. As yet, these materials have not been identified and the results are therefore, at best, only mildly suggestive.

It has been shown by Roseman's laboratory that the incorporation of neuraminic acid into neuraminic acid containing materials both in mammalian tissue and in bacterial systems requires the intermediate compound CMP-neuNAc (JOURDIAN et al. 1963 and AMINOFF et al. 1963). KANFER and associates studied the incorporation of neuraminic acid from CMP-neuNAc into gangliosides employing preparations of kidney from rats (12 to 14 days of age). Incubation of CMP-neuNAc-^{14}C with the glycolipid acceptor, rat kidney homogenate, and

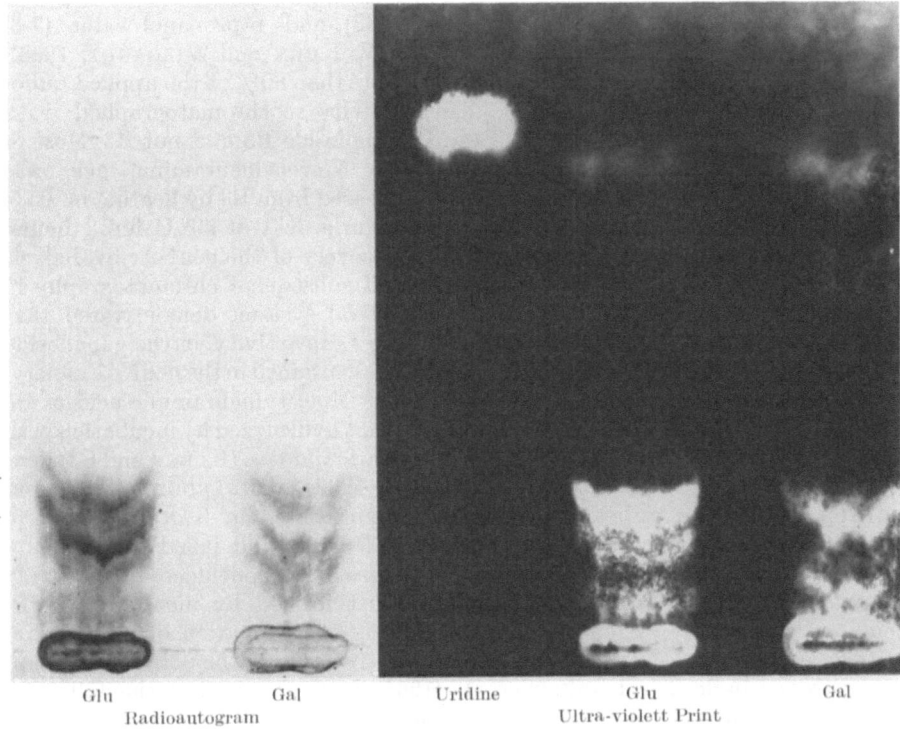

UDP gal →

UDP glc →

Glu   Gal   Uridine   Glu   Gal

Radioautogram   Ultra-violett Print

Fig. 3. Chromatogram of nucleotides isolated from young rat brain after the injection of glucose-^{14}C (Glu) and galactose-^{14}C (Gal). The nucleotides were dedected by absorbtion of ultra-violet light. Radioactivity was dedected by radioautography. From BURTON (unpublished data)

various supplements consisting of magnesium ions, glutathione, UTP, UDP-glc, UDP-gal, UDP-gluNAc and a detergent (Cutscum) resulted in incorporation of radioactivity into the ganglioside fraction. Table 3 presents results which illustrate the incorporation. Incorporation of radioactivity occurred in the absence of added acceptor to the extent of 12 or 13 fold over either the zerotime or boiled tissue control. The use of the glycolipid, gal-galNAc-gal-glc-Cer, resulted in little increase of incorporation of radioactivity over the endogenous control. However, the addition of galNAc-gal-glc-Cer as the acceptor markedly (3 fold) stimulated the incorporation of radioactive neuraminic acid when compared to the endogenous control. The addition of nonradioactive N-acetylneuraminic acid to the complete system containing CMP-neuNAc-^{14}C did not alter the incorporation of radioactivity into the ganglioside, indicating that the nucleotide bound neuraminic acid is the donor and not free neuraminic acid. It was interesting to note that in this system, as well as in other lipid synthetic systems discussed, the omission of the detergent reduced the incorporation of the radioactivity to the endogenous level.

Radioactive product formed as in Table 3 was mixed with nonradioactive carrier ganglioside, a mixture of beef brain gangliosides B4 and B3 and the ganglioside B2 from a Tay Sachs' patient. This solution was mixed thoroughly in chloroform-methanol and the gangliosides extracted by partition, extensively dialyzed, and recrystallized to constant specific activity. The radioactive product was chromatogramed on silica gel-G using thin layer techniques employing solvent systems of chloroform-methanol-formic acid (TRAMS and LAUTER, 1962) and n-propanol-water (7-3, V/V; KUHN and WIEGANDT, 1963). More than 80% of the applied radioactivity cochromatographed with ganglioside B3 and not B2. Most of the N-acetylneuraminic acid was released from B3 by heating in .05 N sulfuric acid at 80° C for 2 hours. Recovery of the neuNAc by dialysis and subsequent chromatography in several systems demonstrated that the radioactivity in the ganglioside was contained in the neuNAc moiety. The N-acetylneuraminic acid of B3 is not hydrolyzed by incubation with neuraminidase (KLENK and GIELEN,

Table 3. *Incorporation of N-acetylneuraminic acid from CMP-neuNAc-^{14}C into gangliosides*

Lipid Acceptor Added	Ganglioside Radioactivity Total CPM
1. galNAc-gal-glc-cer	2300
2. gal-galNAc-gal-glc-cer	903
3. CONTROLS	
Acceptor omitted	703
Tissue boiled	60
Zero time aliquot	54
4. galNAc-gal-glc-cer (plus non-radioactive neuNAc)	2300
5. galNAc-gal-glc-cer (detergent omitted)	703

See text for details
Data from KANFER et al. (1964).

1960, KUHN et al. 1960, TRAMS and LAUTER, 1962, SVENNERHOLM, 1962, and BURTON, 1963). The radioactive ganglioside synthesized in KANFER's *in vitro* system was incubated with neuraminidase for 5 hours and failed to show any release of radioactivity. For these reasons it has been concluded by KANFER, BRADY et al. (1964) that the metabolic product formed by incubating CMP-neuNAc-^{14}C with the system described results in the formation of gal-galNAc-gal(neuNAc-^{14}C)-glc-Cer, i.e. B3. In view of the structure of the obligatory acceptor, galNAc-gal-glc-Cer, KANFER et al. (1964) have formulated the following series of reactions to explain the synthesis of ganglioside B3.

$$galNAc\text{-}gal\text{-}glc\text{-}cer + CMP\text{-}neuNAc \rightarrow galNAc\text{-}gal\text{-}glc\text{-}cer + CMP \qquad (14)$$
$$|$$
$$neuNAc$$
$$(ganglioside\ B2)$$

$$galNAc\text{-}gal\text{-}glc\text{-}cer + [UDP\text{-}gal] \rightarrow gal\text{-}galNAc\text{-}gal\text{-}glc\text{-}cer + UDP \qquad (15)$$
$$| \qquad\qquad\qquad\qquad |$$
$$neuNAc \qquad\qquad\qquad neuNAc$$
$$(ganglioside\ B2) \qquad\qquad (ganglioside\ B3)$$

This involves the intermediate formation of Tay Sach's ganglioside (B2) and its subsequent galactosylation (by UDP-gal?). In these experiments the requirement for the nucleotide sugar is uncertain and inconsistent. No evidence was presented that ganglioside B2 was formed as the intermediate. Since the enzyme system as formulated requires two steps, it should be possible to acquire evidence for the intermediate by the use of cold ganglioside B2 in the complete system to trap any radioactive ganglioside B2 formed before its conversion to B3. Then, it should be possible to incubate ganglioside B2 with UDP-gal-^{14}C to demonstrate the synthesis of B3 with radioactivity in the terminal galactose.

An oral report from ROSEMAN's laboratory (BASU and KAUFMAN, 1965) described the incorporation *in vitro* of neuNAc from CMPneuNAc into gangliosides. The enzyme source was brain tissue particles from chick embryos

(9—11 days old embryos). A mixture of detergents was necessary for activity, e.g. Triton-CF54 plus Tween 80. While both gal-glu-cer and gal-galNAc-gal-glu-cer served as acceptors for the neuNAc, different enzymes appear to be involved based on differential heat inactivation studies. In general, only one neuNAc was added to each acceptor yielding gangliosides with neuraminidase sensitivity. A minor product formed from gal-galNAc-gal-glu-cer contained two neuNAc per mole. The identification of these products is being investigated. While lactose can accept neuNAc from CMPneuNAc in this system, it appears to do so less readily than the glycosphingolipid acceptor. In contrast to KANFER's systems (equation 14), the embryo chick brain particles did not appear to significantly catalyze the transfer of neu-NAc from the nucleotide to galNAc-gal-glu-cer. Both gal-cer and glu-cer were without acceptor activity.

KOREY, GONATAS, and STEIN reported in 1963 that glucose-^{14}C could be incorporated into gangliosides by preparations of brain tissue incubated *in vitro*.

Table 4. *Incorporation of radioactivity from D-glucose-U-^{14}C into rat brain gangliosides in vitro*

Ganglioside Components	Radioactivity (total cpm/molar ratio of component)
N-Acetylneuraminic acid (total)	215
Hexoses	184
N-acetylgalactosamine	55
Ceramide	340

Data adapted from SUZUKI (1964)

An extension of this work by SUZUKI (1964) led to the description of a cell free, rat brain microsomal system which appears to incorporate D-glucose-U-^{14}C into gangliosides. The reaction mixture employed contained both microsomes and the soluble supernatant fraction (prepared from 12—13 days old rat brain), 1 μc D-glucose-U-^{14}C, ribonuclease, creatine phosphate, creatine phosphokinase, ATP, sodium chloride, potassium chloride, magnesium chloride, and Tris buffer pH 7.8. When the reaction mixture was incubated at 37° in air measurable incorporation of radioactivity into all of the individual gangliosides isolated occurred in 5 minutes with maximal incorporation occurring within 15 minutes. Table 4 shows the distribution of radioactivity among the various components of the gangliosides. These results are reported as the total counts per minute in each component divided by the molar ratio of that component in the ganglioside. It may be noticed that all components of the ganglioside contain radioactivity i.e. the N-acetylneuraminic acid, glucose, galactose, N-acetyl-galactosamine, and the ceramide. Because experiments of this type are highly important in our understanding of ganglioside biosynthesis, several specific criticisms must be considered and documented in a subsequent report by SUZUKI. First, the observation that *all* components of the ganglioside contain radioactivity is disturbing. This indicates that the glucose must be converted to the other saccharides necessary. In addition, the glucose-U-^{14}C must be converted to acetate which in turn participates in the synthesis of palmitic acid, palmitaldehyde and stearic acid for the formation of radioactive ceramide. The time course of the reaction is extremely rapid in the experiment reported to be consistent with such a complex series of reactions to be *totally* finished within thirty minutes. In addition, *in vivo* experiments (BURTON et al. 1963) indicate a rapid and selective incorporation of sugars into the hexoses and N-acetylneuraminic acid but not into the ceramide moiety in the initial 24 hour period. Second, the extent of incorporation is very small, being less than 0.1%. And third, at variance with other *in vitro* ceramide and glycolipid systems reported, no detergent was required for this complex system of synthetic reactions. This latter point may of course account for the low extent of incorporation of radioactivity.

Sphingomyelin. WEISS and KENNEDY (1956) have described the synthesis of lecithin from CDP-choline and a diglyceride. An analogous reaction was reported by SRIBNEY and KENNEDY (1958) to be involved in the biosynthesis of sphingomyelin. This reaction is formulated below:

$$\text{CDP-choline} + \text{ceramide} \rightarrow \text{sphingomyelin} + \text{CMP} \tag{16}$$

The initial investigation showed that both the mitochondrial fraction and the microsomal fraction prepared from fresh frozen chicken livers contained approximately equivalent amounts of CDP-choline:ceramide transferase activity. In

Table 5. *Synthesis of sphingomyelin by chicken liver particles*

Lipid Acceptor Added	Sphingomyelin formed* mμmoles
Experiment A:	
1. None — endogenous control	2
2. 18:sphingosine	1
3. Ceramide	
a) phospholipase D hydrolysis of sphingomyelin	1
b) acid hydrolysis of cerebroside	66
c) sphingosine refluxed with acetic acid in sulfuric acid	120
d) sphingosine refluxed with propionic acid in sulfuric acid	540
Experiment B:	
1. N-acetyl-DL-*erythro-trans*-18:sphingosine	4
2. N-acetyl-DL-*threo-trans*-18:sphingosine	105
Experiment C:	
1. N-acetyl-DL-*erythro-trans*-18:sphingosine	5
2. N-acetyl-DL-*threo-trans*-18:sphingosine	83
3. N-acetyl-DL-*erythro-cis*-18:sphingosine	1
4. N-acetyl-DL-*threo-cis*-18:sphingosine	1

* Calculated from radioactivity incorporated from CDP-choline-[14]C.
See text for other details of the experiment.
Data from SRIBNEY and KENNEDY (1958)

general, a particulate preparation from liver was used in a reaction mixture containing cysteine, Tris buffer at pH 7.4, Tween 20, magnesium chloride, CDP-choline 1,2-^{14}C, and the lipid acceptor. Incubation was at 37° C for 2 hours. Under these conditions neither sphingosine nor ceramide prepared from sphingomyelin by the hydrolytic action of phospholipase D (from *Clostridium perfringens* type A toxin) would serve as an acceptor for the radioactive choline from the CDP-choline (see Table 5, A). On the other hand, ceramide isolated after acid hydrolysis of cerebroside readily formed sphingomyelin in the presence of CDP-choline and the enzyme preparation. When sphingosine was refluxed with acetic acid in sulfuric acid solution or with propionic acid in sulfuric acid solution an acceptor was obtained which was highly effective in the formation of sphingomyelin.

The question, "why was ceramide prepared by acid hydrolysis effective as an acceptor for choline and the more native ceramide produced enzymatically by the action of the enzyme phospholipase D not effective?" was resolved by the data reported in Table 5, B and C. It may be seen that N-acetyl-DL-*erythro-trans*-18:sphingosine is a poor acceptor (this appears to be the natural configuration of sphingosine see CARTER et al. 1956 and CLELAND and KENNEDY, 1958) whereas the N-acetyl-DL-*threo-trans*-18:sphingosine was highly effective as an acceptor. It may be recalled from the studies of CARTER and FUJINO (1956) that acid hydrolysis of the sphingolipids occurs in part by migration of the acyl group on the nitrogen to the oxygen on carbon-3 accompanied by an inversion of the carbon-

3 hydroxyl group configuration i.e. from *erythro* to *threo*. The acyl group on the oxygen is then hydrolyzed. It would seem that the *threo* configuration of the ceramide is necessary in order for it to accept choline, *in vitro*, and that this configuration may be produced by the acid hydrolysis of sphingolipid or by the acetylation or propionylation of sphingosine in the presence of an acid catalyst. The formation of ceramide by the enzymatic technique does not lead to inversion of configuration of carbon-3 and therefore yields an inactive ceramide. The data in Table 5, C indicates that the *trans* configuration of the double bond is essential for activity whereas the *cis* configuration is incompatible with acceptor ability. Other experiments indicated that the N-acetyl-DL-*threo*-18:dihydrosphingosine and the N-acetyl-18:phytosphingosine were ineffective as choline acceptors. Both

Table 6. *Determinations of the configuration (threo or erythro) of sphingosine in sphingomyelin from chicken liver and beef heart*

Sphingosine source	Ceramide used as acceptor	Sphingomyelin synthesized* mμmoles	Conclusion: sphingosine configuration
Chicken liver	N-acetyl sphingosine (natural configuration)	20	*erythro*
	N-acetyl sphingosine (refluxed with acetic acid in sulfuric acid)	150	*threo*
Beef heart	N-acetyl sphingosine (natural configuration)	20	*erythro*
	N-acetyl sphingosine (refluxed with acetic acid in sulfuric acid)	175	*threo*

* From CDP-choline-C[14] using CDP-choline:ceramide Transferase.
Details are given in the text.
Data from SRIBNEY and KENNNEDY (1958).

N-acetyl-DL-*threo*-1,3-dihydroxy-2-amino-octadecyne and the N-octanyl-derivative were quite effective in the formation of sphingomyelin. The acetylenic derivatives of the D-*erythro* configuration were not active.

Since the natural configuration of the sphingosines is *erythro* in all the lipids studied, the question arose could the conversion of the *threo* to the *erythro* form occur during synthesis of sphingomyelin? This was answered by a study of the product formed during *in vitro* synthesis. The product was identified as sphingomyelin based on a number of criteria, (1) position of elution from a silicic acid-celite column, (2) the recrystallization of the product to a specific activity equivalent to that of 96% of the specific activity of the CDP-choline-^{14}C employed in the synthesis, (3) stability to alkali, (4) the ratio of nitrogen to phosphorus was equal to 2.08, (5) insolubility in ether and acetone, (6) infrared spectrum and (7) the ability of phospholipase D to hydrolyze the product to yield a ceramide. Because of its stereo specificity, the CDP-choline: ceramide transferase was employed to confirm the configuration of the sphingosine in sphingomyelin isolated from chicken liver and beef heart. In these experiments the sphingomyelin was hydrolyzed with barium hydroxide (a procedure which retains the configuration of the sphingosine, CARTER et al., 1956) and the sphingosine was converted to the N-acetyl sphingosine by acetylation with acetic anhydride in ether (CARTER et al., 1947). The ceramide thus formed retained its natural configuration and was employed as an acceptor in the CDP-choline:ceramide transferase reaction. The results are presented in Table 6. It may be seen that the ceramides formed from the sphingosine which retained their native configuration were inactive as acceptors of choline, whereas refluxing these ceramides with acetic acid in sulfuric acid solution yielded ceramides which were active as acceptors. It may be concluded that the configuration of the sphingosines occurring in tissue sphingomyelin are of *erythro* form. The radioactive product of the CDP-choline: ceramide transferase, identified as a sphingomyelin (see above), was hydrolyzed by phospholipase D and the resultant ceramide was isolated and studied as an acceptor in the transferase reaction. It served as an effective acceptor of choline from the CDP-choline in the presence of the enzyme. This indicates that the enzyme preparation studied (CDP-choline: ceramide transferase) does not convert the *threo*-sphingomyelin to the *erythro*-sphingomyelin form as a step in the synthesis itself or as a separate enzyme activity.

A study of the effect of the fatty acid carbon number on the ability of the ceramide to participate in the transferase reaction showed that in the absence of Tween 20 the most effective choline acceptor was the N-acetyl (*threo*) sphingosine. Other ceramides were relatively ineffective. In the presence of Tween 20 an increase in the carbon number of the fatty acid moiety was accompanied by an increased ability to form sphingomyelin until n-octanoic acid, thereafter a rapid fall off of activity occurred. Of the longer chain ceramides, N-palmityl-DL-*threo-trans*-18:sphingosine was completely inactive in the enzymatic system even in the presence of Tween 20, however both N-oleyl and N-linoleyl derivatives of the *threo-trans*-18:sphingosine formed sphingomyelin readily. Both of the unsaturated ceramides were more easily emulsified in water with Tween 20 than the saturated palmitic acid derivative.

The pH optimum of the CDP-choline: ceramide transferase occurred between 7.5 and 8.0. Manganese was necessary for the reaction, magnesium being less effective and calcium inhibitory. The enzyme is completely specific for CDP-choline; UDP-choline, ADP-choline, GDP-choline had no activity. The CDP-choline: ceramide transferase occurs in guinea pig and hog liver as well as in the liver, kidney, spleen, and brain of the young rat (10—20 days old).

Enzymes which degrade sphingolipids: All of the enzyme systems described which degrade the sphingolipids appear to be hydrolytic in nature. Thus the complex sphingolipids are hydrolyzed to yield ceramide which in turn is hydrolyzed to sphingosine and a free fatty acid. An enzymatic system which hydrolyzes ceramide has been described by Gatt (1963) and was reviewed in the section on the synthesis of ceramide (p. 129). The subsequent metabolism of free fatty acids must occur and these systems are reviewed in chapter 2. The metabolism of sphingosine has not been described as yet, but undoubtedly will occur by oxidation of carbon 1,2 and 3 to yield a fatty acid which will then be metabolized by the conventional fatty acid metabolizing system.

Cerebrosides: In 1936, Thannhauser and Reichel (1936) reported the presence of enzymes in both spleen and brain which will catalyze the hydrolysis of the carbohydrate moiety (galactose) from cerebroside. These systems were essentially whole tissue preparations and involved long incubation periods under toluene to achieve significant hydrolysis. Recently, Morozova and Promyslov (1960) have attempted to repeat the experiment of Thannhauser and Reichel and failed to demonstrate the hydrolysis of cerebroside by brain tissue preparations. A new sensitive approach to the study of the metabolism of glucosyl ceramide has been undertaken by Brady, Kanfer and Shapiro (1964). These workers synthesized O^1-glucosyl(1-^{14}C)-N-stearyl 18:sphingosine and O^1-glucosyl N-stearyl (1-^{14}C) 18:sphingosine and employed these isotopic substrates in their investigation of the enzyme system. In an initial experiment Brady et al. (1964) incubated

0.5 μmoles of (glucose-1-^{14}C) cerebroside (243,000 cpm) in the presence of a detergent (Cutscum; isooctyl phenoxypolyoxyethanol), phosphate buffer (pH 7), and 70 milligrams of spleen supernatant protein from which cellular debris and whole cells had been removed. This reaction mixture was incubated at 37° for 15 hours and the liberated carbon dioxide was trapped by Hyamine in a center well. The radioactivity of the liberated carbon dioxide was measured and is reported in Table 7.

Table 7. *Metabolism of (glucose-1-^{14}C) cerebroside by rat spleen and human spleen enzyme preparations*

Gas phase	Incubation Mixture*	Radioactivity in Carbon Dioxide	
		Rat spleen cpm	Human spleen cpm
98% O_2— 2% CO_2	Complete system	36,250	6,960
	Complete system (Boiled enzymes)	53	66
	Complete system (Non-incubated control)	25	34
98% N_2— 2% CO_2	Complete system	3,415	—

* Complete system contained (glucose-1-^{14}C) cerebroside (243,000 cpm; 0,5 μmole), Cutscum, potassium phosphate buffer (pH 7.0) and supernatant liquid from either rat spleen or human spleen (70 mg protein).

The reaction may be schematically written as follows:

$$glu\text{-}cer + H_2O \rightarrow glu + cer \\ + O_2 \xrightarrow{\quad} CO_2 \tag{17}$$

It may be seen that under aerobic conditions about 15% of the cerebroside radioactivity was recovered as carbon dioxide from the rat spleen preparation, whereas incubation under nitrogen resulted in a marked reduction in the conversion of the radioactivity to CO_2. Human spleen oxidized the cerebroside to carbon dioxide but to a much less extent than the rat spleen preparation. Further studies indicated that this enzyme system resided almost exclusively in the soluble portion of spleen tissue (100,000 × g supernatant) and could be purified by employing ammonium sulfate, alcohol, acetone and pH precipitation techniques. The final enzyme preparation was 82 × more active in removing glucose from the cerebroside than the initial spleen supernatant which served as source material. The purified protein fraction catalyzed hydrolysis of 12 mμmoles of glucose containing cerebroside per milligram of protein in 1 hour of incubation. The pH optimum for hydrolysis was 6.0. This preparation did not hydrolyze galactosyl ceramide or chloronitrophenol-D-galactopyranoside. Because of variation in the ratios of enzyme activities on different substrates, it appears that the glucosyl ceramide hydrolase is an enzyme different from those which hydrolyzed p-nitrophenol-β-D-glucopyranoside and p-nitrophenol-β-D-acetamido-2-deoxyglucopyranoside. K_m of the glucosyl ceramide hydrolase was estimated at 3.2×10^{-6} M. The products of the enzymatic hydrolysis of cerebroside were isolated and determined to be glucose and N-stearyl-18:sphingosine. This corresponds to the reaction as formulated:

$$O^1\text{-glucosyl-N-stearyl-sphingosine} + H_2O \rightarrow glucose + N\text{-stearyl-sphingosine} \tag{18}$$
$$[\text{cerebroside}] \qquad\qquad\qquad\qquad [\text{ceramide}]$$

HAJRA and RADIN (1965) have described a similar type of enzyme activity in pig brain preparations. The 100,000 × g supernatant fraction catalyzes the hydrolysis of galactose containing cerebrosides.

$$O^1\text{-galactosyl-N-stearyl sphingosine} + H_2O \quad \rightarrow \quad (18\text{a})$$
$$[\text{cerebroside}]$$
$$\text{galactose} + \text{N-stearyl sphingosine}$$
$$[\text{ceramide}]$$

The index of hydrolysis was the formation of ste ($-1-^{14}C$)-sph from cerebrosides containing stearic-$1-^{14}C$ acid. The use of a detergent mixture containing sodium cholate was required for hydrolysis. The enzyme showed maximum activity at pH 4.5, at which point both the enzyme and cholate precipitated. Other substrates included naturally occurring cerebrosides (galactose containing) and showed the formation of ceramides containing normal and α-hydroxy fatty acid. Enzyme activity was seen also in rat brain, spleen, and kidney.

Cerebroside sulfate: FUJINO and NEGISHI (1957) have surveyed a number of mammalian tissues and microorganisms searching for enzymes which will hydrolyze cerebroside sulfate according to the following reaction:

$$SO^-_4\text{-gal-cer} + H_2O \quad \rightarrow \text{gal-cer} + SO^{2-}_4 \quad (19)$$
$$(\text{cerebroside sulfate}) \qquad (\text{cerebroside})$$

Cerebroside sulfatase activity was observed only in shell fish preparations. The sulfatase preparation from Abalone liver* was incubated with cerebroside sulfate (about 80 μgrams sulfate), acetate buffer at pH 5.2, and toluene. After 3 hours at 25^0, inorganic sulfate was determined. No inorganic sulfate was detected in the absence of the abalone enzyme preparation. In the presence of the enzyme about 12 μgrams of inorganic sulfate were observed corresponding to 14% hydrolysis of the cerebroside sulfate. No additional hydrolysis occurred during the next 21 hours. Of the other shell fish examined, neither the scallop nor the round clam would hydrolyze cerebroside sulfate and the oyster appeared to only have limited activity. The abalone liver sulfatase would not hydrolyze phenolsulfate or glucosulfate whereas chondroitin sulfate was readily hydrolyzed. In addition, no galactosidase activity was observed at pH 3.6 nor was amidase activity observed at pH 7.

Because turnover studies indicate that cerebroside sulfate can be degraded (see below, *in vivo* studies) MEHL and JATZKEWITZ (1963) recently investigated swine kidney for cerebroside sulfatase activity. These workers employed a particulate preparation from kidney which had been exposed to butyl alcohol and then to calcium chloride. After centrifugation the protein fraction was concentrated on Sephadex G-25 and collected by the use of sodium acetate buffer (pH 4.5) with sodium chloride. Cerebroside sulfate ($-^{35}S$) was employed in the assay for sulfatase activity. Following incubation, cold carrier sulfate was added to the reaction vessel and inorganic sulfate precipated with benzidine, filtered, and the radioactivity of the precipitate determined. In one experiment reported the reaction mixture was chromatographed on thin layer before and after incubation. The sulfatase showed a pH optimum at 4.5 and a linearity of sulfate liberated V^s time during 4 hours of incubation at 37^0. The sulfatase specific activity of the best preparation liberated 33 μmoles of inorganic sulfate from cerebroside sulfate per gram protein in 1 hour at 37^0. Similar to the abalone liver sulfatase preparation, the swine kidney sulfatase preparation also was able to hydrolyze chondroitin

---

* The enzyme was prepared from shell fish liver by the procedure of SODA (1956). Abalone livers were crushed in acetone and transferred to a small wire basket in a beaker containing acetone. With agitation of the basket, the crushed liver separated into a fine powder which passed through the wire mesh and a fibrous material which remained in the basket. Acetone was removed by decantation and the fine powder residue was mixed with fresh acetone. This was repeated to completely dehydrate and defat the protein. The material was air dried yielding a brownish green powder in a yield of 8 to 10% of the abalone liver. A 20% suspension of the acetone powder in water was allowed to autolyze at 25^0 for 2 days. The suspension was centrifuged and the supernatant employed as a sulfatase preparation.

sulfate. It would be interesting to compare the ratios of the cerebroside sulfatase activity with the chondroitin sulfatase activity during the various stages involved in the purification of both the abalone liver and the swine kidney sulfatase preparation. This would suggest whether or not these sulfatase activities were separate or identical.

Ganglioside: A gangliosidase system has been described by KOREY and STEIN (1962, 1963a, b) as being present in the brains of both young rats (11 to 16 days) and humans (normal and Tay-Sachs brain tissue). In their experiments, tissue from the young rats was homogenized briefly in Tris buffer (pH 7.0) containing calcium, magnesium, potassium, sodium, and phosphate. This homogenate was incubated with gangliosides under nitrogen at 37⁰ for various lengths of time between 15 minutes and 3 hours. After incubation, the reaction mixture was extracted with chloroform-methanol and partitioned with water according to FOLCH et al. (1951). The aqueous phase was concentrated under nitrogen and dialyzed overnight at 4⁰. The contents of the dialysis tubing were analyzed for the components of gangliosides. Using the loss of the ganglioside components, (after dialysis) as an index of activity e.g. N-acetylneuraminic acid, hexoses, and N-acetylgalactosamine, it was observed that hydrolytic activity occurred only in anaerobic systems. Oxygen appeared to inhibit the reaction. On the other hand, preincubation of the enzyme preparation under nitrogen for one hour followed by 2 hours of incubation in air after the addition of ganglioside substrate, showed satisfactory hydrolysis of the

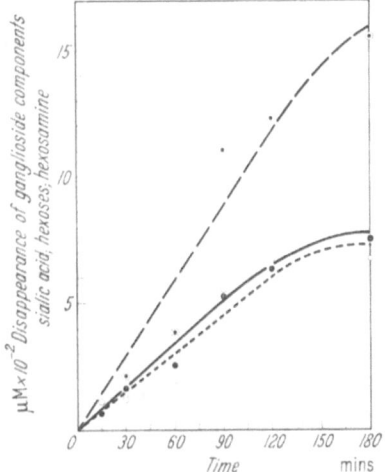

Fig. 4. Rate of degradation of added gangliosides plus gangliosides of enzymatic component as measured by sialic acid, hexoses, hexosamine. Enzyme, weanling rat brain. Added ganglioside, beef brain. ○ – – ○ Hexoses; ●———● Sialic acid; ○ · · · · · ○ Hexosamine. From KOREY and STEIN (1963)

ganglioside. Figure 4 indicates the time course of hydrolysis of the gangliosides (endogenous rat and beef brain gangliosides) as measured by the liberation of N-acetylneuraminic acid, hexoses, and hexosamine. Analysis of the beef brain ganglioside used as substrate in this experiment indicated a ratio of N-acetylneuraminic acid:hexose:N-acetylgalactosamine:sphingosine of 1.00:1.78:0.75: 0.96*. It is interesting to note from the figure that the loss of the ganglioside components occur in this same ratio. Specifically the ratios were, in the same order, 1.00:1.58:0.58:0.61. The loss of the components of ganglioside in proportion to the ratios in the ganglioside molecule suggest that the gangliosidase system hydrolyzes each ganglioside molecule completely, at least the oligosaccharide unit (no effort was made to determine the ceramide content after hydrolysis). Evidence on this point exists in the inability of these workers to demonstrate the presence of glucosyl ceramide or galNAc-gal-glc-ceramide in either the aqueous or organic phases following incubation. It was observed with interest that gangliosides prepared from the brain of a Tay-Sachs patient appeared to stimulate the hydrolysis of normal human or beef brain ganglioside by the rat brain gangliosidase system.

* The ratios of the components of the ganglioside added and determined during the course of hydrolysis must be reconciled with the current structures of gangliosides as demonstrated by KLENK et al. (1962, 1963) and KUHN and WEIGANDT (1963a, b, 1964). cf Chapter by STOFFEL.

Continuing their studies, it was observed by Korey and Stein that human tissue obtained by biopsy required incubation under nitrogen to demonstrate gangliosidase activity. However, tissue obtained post-mortem did not require preincubation under nitrogen. This has suggested to these workers that the gangliosidase enzyme system exists particulately bound and may be released from the particles only after death. With this interpretation, metabolic control of ganglioside levels could reside in the binding of, or liberation of, the gangliosidase system by subcellular particles thus permitting accumulation or degradation of gangliosides as required. This may be, or be related to, the lysozyme subcellular fraction of brain tissue. This type of control could exist in addition to, or in lieu of, feed back regulation of the biosynthetic pathway for ganglioside formation.

The cerebral cortex adjacent to a subfrontal meningioma (adult male) was used to prepare a gangliosidase system (Korey and Stein, 1963b). The cortical tissue was homogenized in Tris buffer (pH 7.3) containing cysteine. Normal butanol was added to the homogenate to give a final concentration of 10% V/V. This was stirred for 50 minutes, centrifuged, and the supernatant obtained lyophilized. The lyophilized brain was suspended in buffer and centrifuged. The clear supernatant was incubated for 3 hours at 37° under nitrogen with gangliosides prepared from normal human brain and/or from Tay-Sachs brain tissue. Analysis of the non-dialyzable gangliosides remaining showed a net loss of N-acetylneuraminic acid, hexoses, and N-acetylgalactosamine when compared to values for suitable controls. These results therefore are analogous to the experiments with rat brain homogenates. Similar experiments conducted with an enzyme preparation (butanol procedure described) from the biopsy specimen of a patient with Tay-Sachs disease indicated the presence of an active neuraminidase and a less active N-acetylgalactosaminidase. The ability of this enzyme preparation to hydrolytically remove the hexose components was markedly reduced.

Carubelli, Trucco and Caputto (1962) surveyed neuraminidase activity in various mammalian organs. They used as their indicator substrate N-acetylneuraminyl lactose and measured the liberation of N-acetylneuraminic acid. The highest content of neuraminidase activity in the rat was found to occur in lactating mammary glands which was 20 fold higher than non-lactating glands. Liver was next highest being only 30% higher than brain. Lower activities were observed in the small intestines, kidney, spleen, and testes.

An interpretation of these experiments would suggest that the gangliosidase system consists of a series of individual hydrolases, the limiting rate of the total hydrolysis being the first hydrolase, i.e. the neuraminidase activity. This would be illustrated by the following sequence of reactions:

$$\text{neuNAc-gal-galNAc-gal-glc-cer} \xrightarrow[\text{hydrolase 1}]{H_2O} \text{gal-galNAc-gal-glc-cer} + \text{neuNAc} \qquad (20)$$
$$|\qquad\qquad\qquad\qquad\qquad\qquad\qquad\qquad |$$
$$\text{neuNAc}\qquad\qquad\qquad\qquad\qquad\qquad\text{neuNAc}$$

$$\text{gal-galNAc-gal-glc-cer} \xrightarrow[\text{hydrolase 2}]{H_2O} \text{galNAc-gal-glc-cer} + \text{gal} \qquad (21)$$
$$|\qquad\qquad\qquad\qquad\qquad\qquad\qquad |$$
$$\text{neuNAc}\qquad\qquad\qquad\qquad\text{neuNAc}$$

$$\text{galNAc-gal-glc-cer} \xrightarrow[\text{hydrolase 3}]{H_2O} \text{neuNAc-gal-glc-cer} + \text{galNAc} \qquad (22)$$
$$|$$
$$\text{neuNAc}$$

$$\text{neuNAc-gal-glc-cer} \xrightarrow[\text{hydrolase 4}]{H_2O} \text{gal-glc-cer} + \text{neuNAc} \qquad (23)$$

$$\text{gal-glc-cer} \xrightarrow[\text{hydrolase 5}]{H_2O} \text{glc-cer} + \text{gal} \qquad (24)$$

$$\text{glc-cer} \xrightarrow[\text{hydrolase 6}]{H_2O} \text{cer} + \text{glc} \qquad (25)$$

The individual reactions are placed in the above sequence primarily to account for the neuraminidase lability of only one of the two N-acetylneuraminic acid of ganglioside B 4 even though the N-acetylneuraminic acid of ganglioside B1 is labile. It would appear that either the N-acetylgalactosamine or galactose moiety, or both, inhibit hydrolysis of the proximal N-acetylneuraminic acid. Thus, hydrolase 1 and 4 (reactions 20 and 23) may be identical. An alternate suggestion, that the gangliosidase initially cleaves the entire oligosaccharide unit from the ceramide and that this unit is the dialyzable carbohydrate portion lost during the assay procedure was not compatible with the enzyme experiment utilizing pathological tissue or with the failure to find such an oligosaccharide unit in the recovered dialyzable fraction.

Sphingomyelin: The degradation of sphingomyelin most likely occurs in a manner similar to that of the other sphingolipids, i.e. the removal of the groupings attached to carbon 1 to liberate a ceramide, the ceramide being subsequently metabolized as discussed earlier. Phospholipase D from sources such as *Clostridium perfringens* type A toxin will hydrolyze the phosphocholine moiety from sphingomyelin, in a manner analogous to the hydrolysis of lecithin (See its use in the biosynthesis of sphingomyelin as described earlier). Recent studies by HELLER and SHAPIRO (1963) describe the hydrolysis of sphingomyelin by a phospholipase D type of reaction. The hydrolase involved was purified from an acetone powder preparation of rat liver and is contained in the sedimented particles. The reaction yields ceramide and phosphocholine as formulated below:

$$\text{choline}-\overset{O}{\overset{\|}{P}}-O-\text{cer} + H_2O \rightarrow \text{cer} + \text{choline}-\overset{O}{\overset{\|}{P}}-OH \qquad (26)$$
$$\qquad\quad |\qquad\qquad\qquad\qquad\qquad\qquad\quad |$$
$$\qquad\quad -O\qquad\qquad\qquad\qquad\qquad\qquad\quad O-$$

The enzyme is stabile for months at $-18°$, shows a pH optimum between 5 and 5.5, and is activated by pyridine, acetyl trimethylammonium bromide, Triton X-100, and cholate. The activity of the particles was greater with sphingomyelin than with lecithin, however after sonification and centrifugation the supernatant contained more activity toward lecithin than sphingomyelin. The addition of cholate to the supernatant preparation produced a 14 fold increase in the rate of hydrolysis of sphingomyelin and a reduction in the rate of hydrolysis of lecithin. In addition, dialysis of the supernatant preparation caused a loss of sphingomyelin hydrolase activity. These experiments therefore indicate the presence of two enzyme activities, one enzyme is specific for lecithin and the other enzyme has greater activity with sphingomyelin than lecithin.

In view of the similar nature of sphingomyelin and lecithin, it should be noted that the esterase, phospholipase A, is without activity upon the amide bond in sphingomyelin (FAIRBAIRN, 1945).

II. Studies on the Intact Animal

1. Developmental Studies

Sphingosine containing lipids are widely distributed throughout all tissues of the animal species studied. The quantitative estimation of cerebrosides and sphingomyelin in various animal tissues are illustrated in Table 8. Most of the tissues which have been studied show little change in the concentration of these sphingolipids with age. On the other hand, brain tissue show a characteristic

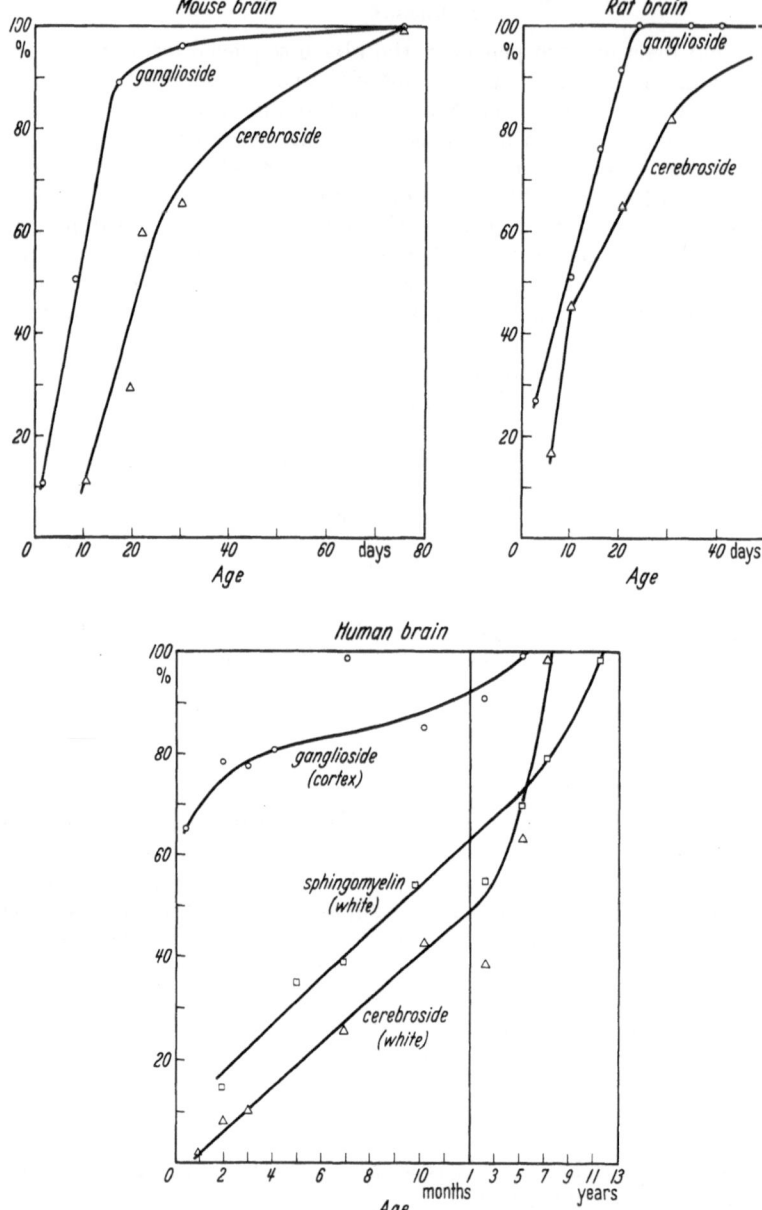

Fig. 5. The accumulation of sphingosine containing lipids in brain tissue. Mouse brain, data estimated from graph presented by FOLCH (1955) for whole tissue (points are calculated); Rat brain, whole tissue (BURTON, unpublished); Human brain, cortex or white as noted (CUMINGS et al. 1958)

increase in sphingolipids, as well as other lipids, during early *postpartum* development. This accumulation coincides with the myelination process. The accumulation of these lipids in brain tissue from mice, rats, and humans illustrated in Figure 5 are derived from the data of FOLCH et al. (1955), BURTON (unpublished) and CUM-MINGS et al. (1958). In all cases a rapid accumulation of these lipids occurs in the first few weeks of life, approaching a plateau at near adult level of the lipids.* Thereafter little change in the lipid composition occurs in the normal animal.

Table 8. *Cerebroside and sphingomyelin content of rat tissues*

	cerebroside (% dry weight)		sphingomyelin (% dry weight)	
	15 days old	70 days old	15 days old	70 days old
Brain	3.8	8.4	3.9	4.3
Liver	0.1	0.1	0.4	0.4
Spleen	0.6	0.8	0.5	1.1
Lung	0.9	0.9	2.0	2.6
Kidney	1.2	1.3	1.0	1.8
Heart	2.3	1.4	1.0	0.5
Skeletal muscle	1.5	3.6	0.5	0.2
Testes	1.9	4.0	1.1	1.0
Thymus	1.3	1.1	0.9	0.7

Data from WILLIAMS et al. (1945) and DEUEL (1951).

In certain disease processes i.e. the lipidosis, additional accumulation of some of these lipids occurs to an abnormal extent. Then too, there are disease processes in which the level of the lipids decrease and a resultant demyelination of axones occurs. These diseases will be discussed in a later section.

2. Studies Conducted in Vivo with Isotopes

Efforts to elucidate the biological pathways involved in the synthesis and degradation of the sphingolipids have been carried out in living animals by administering the appropriate precursor compounds labelled with radioactive iso-topes. In addition, these studies were aimed at answering the question "is the myelin sheath of nerve cells a stable structural component or do the lipids of the myelin sheath, in fact, turn-over and exist in a dynamic state ?" From the data previously presented it is apparent that the biosynthesis of sphingosine containing lipids occurs most rapidly in the brain of young animals. Therefore, most of the experiments to be reported below were carried out using animals at the peak period of the rate of myelination and refer to brain tissue. Little data is available on the incorporation of sphingolipid precursors into lipids of other tissues. First, the incorporation of radioactive isotopes from precursors to sphingosine will be discussed. Next, the incorporation of labeled precursors into the carbohydrate moieties of sphingolipids will be described. Finally, the incorporation of precursors into the fatty acids moieties of the sphingolipids will be presented. A brief ac-counting of several studies involving the metabolism of radioactive sphingolipids administered to intact animals will be given. A discussion of possible interpretation of all of these data will then follow.

a) Sphingosine

An account of the early work of ZABIN and MEAD (1953, 1954) and SPRINSON and COULON (1954) on the incorporation of carbon-14 labeled acetate and serine

---

* An interesting recent observation by ROSENBERG and STERN (1965) indicates that the sphingosine in gangliosides occurs primarily as 18:sphingosine in the newborn rat. At 2 to 5 weeks of age 20:sphingosine begins to accummulate in the gangliosides until approximately equal amounts of the homologues are present. Only 18:sphingosine was found in cerebrosides and sphingomyelin.

into sphingosine was described on page 124. Mature rats were employed in these experiments and injected repeatedly with large doses of the isotopic compound. BURTON and his co-workers (1963) injected DL-serine-3-^{14}C intraperitoneally into young rats of various ages from 1 to 30 days old. Twenty-four hours later the animals were killed, the brains removed, and the cerebrosides and gangliosides isolated and their radioactivity determined. Maximum incorporation of radioactivity occurred in animals between eleven and sixteen or seventeen days of age. The younger animals and older animals showed reduced rates of incorporation. A study of the time-course of incorporation of DL-serine-3-^{14}C into rats fourteen days of age showed peak incorporation to occur twenty-four hours following administration of the isotope. Thereafter, a decline in the total amount of radioactivity in the lipid fraction occurred. In these experiments, considerable incorporation of the serine radioactivity occurred in a non-specific manner; the radioactivity of the serine entered general metabolic pathways and appeared in the gangliosides, for example, as carbohydrate as well as being specifically incorporated into the sphingosine. Previously, DAVISON and his colleagues (1959) had injected DL-serine-3-^{14}C into eleven day old rabbits. The rabbits were killed at various time intervals after injection, from one day to 192 days. The cholesterol, cerebrosides and sphingomyelin were isolated and radioactivities determined. The radioactivity was found to persist in these lipids for a considerable period of time, being present in appreciable amounts even six months post injection. This suggested to DAVISON et al. (1959) that myelin, which contains these lipids, is a stable component and turns-over very slowly. This appeared to be true for brain tissue as well as sciatic nerve.

b) Carbohydrates

The first experiments on the incorporation of galactose-1-^{14}C into the carbohydrate moieties of cerebrosides, cerebroside sulphate, and gangliosides were conducted by RADIN et al. in 1957. These findings indicated a rapid incorporation of the sugar into the cerebroside and ganglioside fractions (reaching a maximum at near twenty-four hours following the injection) and a slower incorporation into the cerebroside sulphate fraction (reaching a maximum somewhat after forty-eight hours). Thereafter a rather slow loss of radioactivity occurred in both the cerebroside and ganglioside fractions. Similar data by BURTON and co-workers in 1958 and 1963 confirmed these results and showed, in addition, that the incorporation of radioactivity was greatest during the period at which the rats were undergoing rapid myelination, i.e. ten to sixteen or seventeen days of age. Somewhat different results were obtained by MOSER and KARNOVSKY (1959) who studied the incorporation of radioactive glucose and galactose into the brain lipids of young mice. In these experiments, maximum incorporation of radioactivity into cerebrosides occured one hour after the administration of the isotopic sugars. Thereafter, a plateau existed for a few hours followed by a subsequent decrease in radioactivity. Studying the incorporation of radioactivity of glucose-^{14}C one hour after administering the sugar (maximum incorporation) as a function of age showed relatively little change in the specific activity of the total brain lipids from 2 to 23 days old, whereas older animals (30—180 days old) were somewhat less successful in incorporating the sugar. Incorporation of radioactivity into a specific lipid, the cerebrosides, showed a very sharp maximum for total incorporations at twenty-two days of age. The total incorporation of radioactivity into the ganglioside fraction showed a less pronounced peak with incorporation occurring maximally in animals between the ages of about eight to thirty days. In these experiments MOSER and KARNOVSKY (1959) injected glucose-6-^{14}C and recovered the hexose unit from cerebrosides as well as the galactose, glucose and galactosamine from the gangliosides. The distribution of the radioactivity in these sugars was determined and compared with the distribution of the radioactivity in blood hexose and in the glucose derived from glycogen. It was found that the galactose derived from the cerebroside contained 94% of the radioactivity in Carbon 6, whereas the galactose derived from the ganglioside contained 82% in Carbon 6 and the glucose from the ganglioside possessed 102% in Carbon 6. The radioactivity in galactosamine appeared to be considerably more random with only 62% residing in Carbon 6. For comparison, blood glucose contained 80% in Carbon 6 and 14% in Carbons 1, 2 and 3 and glucose derived from glycogen contained only 57% in Carbon 6 and 42% in Carbons 1, 2 and 3. This, of course, indicates a very direct incorporation of the glucose into the sphingosine glycolipids.

The incorporation of carbon-14 labeled D-galactose and D-glucose radioactivity into gangliosides has been studied most extensively by BURTON et al. (1963), and recently by SUZUKI and KOREY (1963). In addition, the incorporation of D-glucosamine-1-^{14}C has been studied by BURTON et al. (1963). Several fundamental differences in the data reported from these two laboratories should be noted. Whereas SUZUKI and KOREY (1963) used rats seven days of age and killed them at intervals to a maximum time lapse of five hours, BURTON and co-workers (1963) used rats thirteen to fourteen days old and killed them at intervals up to seventy-two hours. Most of the data reported by BURTON et al. (1963) were derived from animals killed at twelve and twenty-four hours after the injection. BURTON et al. (1963) observed the incorporation of radioactivity primarily into the two gangliosides containing two moles of neuNAc per mole ganglioside. They failed to observe any mono-neuNAc containing gangliosides upon chromatography either visually after staining or by radioactivity measurements, prior to the exposure of the ganglioside fraction to neuraminidase or to mild acid hydrolysis. On the other hand, SUZUKI and KOREY (1963) isolated four ganglioside fractions including a mono-neuNAc containing ganglioside. In both of these studies the specific activities of the different gangliosides were similar. The specific activities of the individual components of the gangliosides were shown by SUZUKI and KOREY to be higher for the glucose, galactose and "stable" neuNAc than for the enzymatically labile neuNAc and galactosamine. This suggested to these workers that the two N-acetylneuraminic acids on the ganglioside molecule were derived from different pools. This is in contrast to the work of BURTON et al. (1963) who showed that the glucose, galactose, and galactosamine moieties had approximately the same specific activities and that of the N-acetylneuraminic acids was lower. In addition, both molecules of neuNAc possess the same specific activity. This is consistent with the pattern observed in experiments involving the incorporation of glucosamine radioactivity. In these experiments none of the hexoses were labelled, whereas the amino sugars, i.e. the N-acetyl galactosamine and N-acetylneuraminic acids, were labeled with approximately the same specific activities. Both the stable and the enzymatically labile neuNAc had the same specific activities. The same labeling patterns were shown by both B4 and C3 gangliosides. Turn-over studies conducted over a six month interval indicated that the half-times for B4 and C3 are the same (BURTON, unpublished data).

c) Sulfate

While the first mention of a sulfolipid in brain tissue was in 1884 (THUDICHUM), definitive studies on the structure of cerebroside sulfates are still in progress (YAMAKAWA et al. 1962; STOFFYN and STOFFYN 1963; TAKETOMI and YAMAKAWA 1964). Similarly, the metabolism of cerebroside sulfates is largely unknown. Brain tissue contains large amounts of cerebroside sulfate. However, other tissues do contain sulfolipids, e.g. kidney (Landsteiner and Levene, 1925), lung (Sammartino, 1921), liver (Koch, 1907 and Goldberg, 1960a), muscle, testis, submaxillary gland (Koch, 1907) and spleen, adrenals (Blix, 1933). Green and Robinson (1960) administered ^{35}S-sulfate to adult rats (150 g body weight) and isolated the cerebroside sulfates and determined their radioactivity as a function of time after the injection. Results of this study are illustrated in Fig. 6. It may be seen that rapid incorporation of sulfate into the lipid fraction occurred in all tissues studied, i.e. brain, kidney, liver, spleen, and a mastocytoma. The incorporation into heart tissue was very low. No sulfate-containing lipid was extracted from blood cells or plasma. Whereas the turn-over of the sulfate in liver, spleen, and the mastocytoma was rapid, radioactivity persisted in brain and kidney tissues for many days. In the study conducted by Radin et al. (1957) on galactolipid metabolism in the brain, it was observed that the injection of galactose-^{14}C or sulfate-^{35}S resulted in the labeling of cerebroside sulfate. Fig.7, adapted from Radin et al. (1957), illustrates the persistence of radioactivity in the cerebroside sulfate fraction from brain tissue when sodium sulfate-^{35}S is administered.

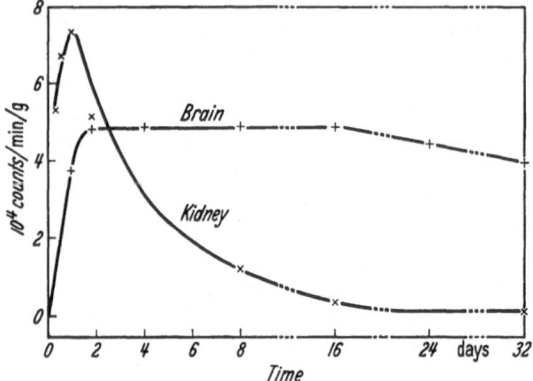

Fig. 6a. ^{35}S-content of cerebroside sulfate as a function of time

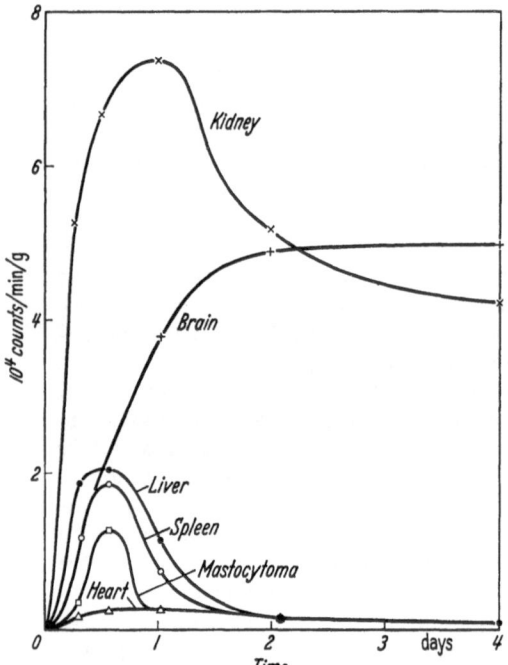

Fig. 6b. ^{35}S-content of cerebroside sulfate as a function of time. From Green and Robinson (1960)

Other authors have confirmed the radioactive sulfate incorporation data (Green and Robinson, 1960; Bakke and Cornatzer, 1961; Davison and Gregson, 1962; Kataoka, 1962; and Burton, unpublished data). While Burton (unpublished data) has obtained results consistent with those of Radin's for the persistence of radioactive sulfate in the cerebroside sulfate fraction, Burton's experiments indicate the same rate of loss of radioactivity due to ^{14}C in the carbohydrate moieties of cerebroside and cerebroside sulfate whereas Radin et al. found a retension of ^{14}C as well as ^{35}S. Hauser (1964) and others (Bakke and Cornatzer, 1961, Davison and Gregson, 1962) have observed that the cerebroside:cerebroside sulfate ratio in brain tissue appears to remain constant even though these lipids accumulate with age. Thus Hauser (1964) found ratios of 3 in 20 day-old rats and 4 in adult animals. Further experiments need to be carried out to determine if the 30% difference in ratios between young and adult rats is significant and to examine in more detail the turn-over rates of the individual components of the cerebrosides and cerebroside sulfates in the various subcellular fractions of brain tissue.

d) Fatty acids: The incorporation *in vivo* of radioactive acetate into the sphingosine moiety of the sphingolipids was discussed in an earlier section. The use of radioactive acetate to study the *in vivo* synthesis of the fatty acid moieties of cerebrosides (HAJRA and RADIN, 1962, 1963a, b) and gangliosides (BARTSCH, 1963) has yielded much interesting data. HAJRA and RADIN (1963a, b) injected weanling rats with tritium-labeled acetate, the animals were killed and the cerebrosides were isolated from the brain tissue. The fatty acids of the cerebrosides

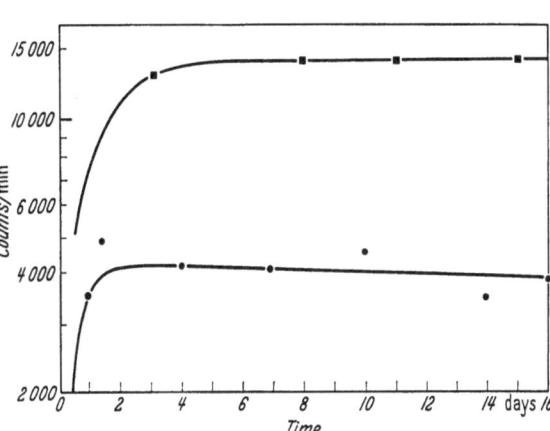

Fig. 7. ³⁵S-content of rat brain lipids as a function of time. ■ values obtained with 83 μc. of Na₂S³⁵O₄ in rats weighing 78 gm.; ● values obtained with 88 μc. in rats weighing 245 gm. From RADIN et al. (1957)

were obtained by hydrolysis followed by a combination of column chromatography and gas-liquid chromatography. Fig. 8 presents the time course of the incorporation of radioactivity into individual fatty acids when acetate-³H is the precursor. It may be seen that at the first time period studied, i.e. 4 hours post-injection, a high level of radioactivity was present in the long chain-length normal saturated fatty acids of the cerebrosides. A rapid loss of radioactivity occurred during the next eight hours reaching a minimum at 12 hours post-injection. Thereafter, a slow increase in total radioactivity of the 20:0, 22:0, and especially the 24:0 acids occurred. After a short burst of increased radioactivity at 24 hours, the total radioactivity of 18:0 acids from the cerebrosides decreased with time. The clever use of acetate-³H for studying fatty acid turn-over minimized the recycling of the radioactive label. Parenterally administered acetate is rapidly metabolized (GOULD et al., 1949; and HUTCHENS et al., 1954), thus the incorporation of

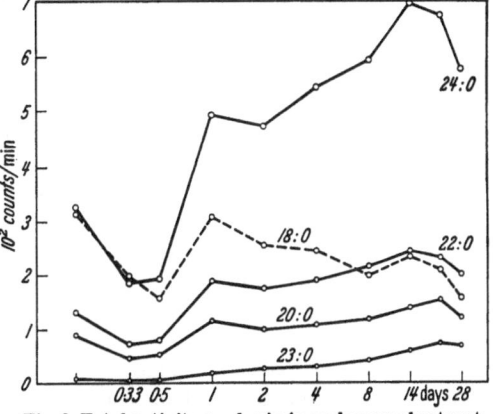

Fig. 8. Total activity per brain in each normal saturated cerebroside acid. From HAJRA and RADIN (1963)

radioactivity from acetate-³H must occur within the first few hours post-injection. The recycling of radioactivity from ³H-labeled fatty acids is prevented by the loss of the isotope (as tritiumwater) during the catabolism of the fatty acids. The dilution of the isotope in body water largely eliminates the incorporation of ³H from water as a factor in labeling the longer chain fatty acids. On the other hand, chain elongation would permit the continued increase in *total* radioactivity of each fatty acid from radioactive fatty acids of shorter chain length. An interpretation of the data of Hajra and Radin, Fig. 8, indicates the presences of two "pools" of cerebroside. One "pool" which can turn-over rapidly, hence the rapid labeling and subsequent loss of label (the first 12 hours) and a stable "pool" which is labeled slowly and turns-over slowly. It could be suggested that the stable "pool" contains long chain fatty acids, e.g. 24:0, and the more labile "pool" has a high percentage of stearic acid.* This data indicates also that a chain-elongation mechanism must be operating for the formation of the 20:0, 22:0, and 24:0 fatty acids

Table 9. *Incorporation of radioactivity into brain lipids**

Lipid isolated	Fatty acid administered:		
	$1-^{14}C$ Lignoceric Acid	$1-^{14}C$ Palmitic Acid	$1-^{14}C$ Acetic Acid
	Incorporation of Radioactivity as m μmoles precursor/μmole lipid		
Ceramide	4.0	1.0	0.8
Ceramide-sphingosine moiety	0.2	0.7	0.5
Ceramide-fatty acids moiety	3.2	0.2	0.4
Cerebrosides	0.8	1.4	2.6
Cerebrosides-sphingosine moiety	0.2	0.7	0.8
Cerebrosides-fatty acids moiety	0.6	0.6	0.9
Sphingomyelin	2.1	2.0	0.8
Sphingomyelin-sphingosine moiety	0.1	1.0	0.3
Sphingomyelin-fatty acids moiety	2.0	0.8	0.5

* Adapted from Gatt (1963).

(see Fig. 4 in Hajra and Radin, 1963b). The ratios of radioactivity from acetate-1-^{14}C incorporated into the cerebroside fatty acids (carboxyl carbon:α-carbon i.e. C1:C2) was 6.5 and 10.5 for 22h:0 and 24h:0, but was only 0.35 for 23h:0. Hajra and Radin (1962, 1963a,b) suggest that in brain the fatty acids with an odd-number of carbons are derived from those with an even-number of carbons by decarboxylation.

Gatt and his co-workers (Fields and Gatt, 1963, Gatt and Shapiro, 1960, and Gatt, 1963) have synthesized 1-^{14}C-lignoceric acid and showed that it was readily absorbed from the intestinal tract. It was incorporated into various lipids after parenteral administration. Intravenous 1-^{14}C-lignoceric acid was taken-up primarily by the liver, where 18—50% of the radioactivity injected could be found. The lipid classes containing phosphatic acid or sphingosine were highly labeled with the 24:0 fatty acid. Neutral fats contained less radioactivity, but had incorporated some 24:0. Under normal conditions the neutral fats and phosphatic acid lipids do not contain lignoceric acid. When given by an intracerebral injection, the 1-^{14}C-lignoceric acid was incorporated into sphingomyelin, cerebrosides, and neutral lipids. Table 9, adapted from Gatt (1963) illustrates the incorporation of radioactivity from 1-^{14}C-acetate, 1-^{14}C-palmitate, and 1-^{14}C-lignocerate into the components of ceramide, cerebrosides, and sphingomyelins of brain tissue. When acetate-1-^{14}C and palmitate-1-^{14}C are the radioactive precursors administered, the sphingolipids contain approximately an equal distribution of radioactivity between the sphingosine moiety and the fatty acid moiety. A tendency for palmitate to preferentially label the sphingosine may be noted in the ceramide data. Palmitate is a precursor of sphingosine (see Brady et al.

---

* A similar relationship appears to be true of the sphingomyelins. Pilz and Jatzkewitz (1964) have reported that sphingomyelins in white matter of brain tissue contain primarily 24:0 and 24:1 acids, whereas grey matter sphingomyelin was found to have stearic acid as the primary fatty acid. This suggests that the structural units, as in myelin, are of the very long chain length fatty acids types.

1957, 1958a,b). On the other hand, when lignoceric-1-^{14}C acid was administered the radioactivity resided primarily in the fatty acid moiety whether the lipid isolated was the ceramide, the cerebroside, or the sphingomyelin.

HAJRA and RADIN (1963c) injected emulsions* of 1-^{14}C-palmitate, 1-^{14}C-stearate, 1-^{14}C-lignocerate, and 1-^{14}C-cerebronate into the brain tissue of young rats. They observed that all of these fatty acids were incorporated into the sphingolipids. Consistent with the chain elongation mechanism, the 1-^{14}C-palmitate and 1-^{14}C-stearate gave rise to radioactive lignocerate and cerebronate in which the carboxyl groups were *not* radioactive. While the 1-^{14}C-lignocerate radioactivity appeared as 1-^{14}C-cerebronate in the sphingolipids, the 1-^{14}C-cerebronate administered did not give rise to radioactive lignoceric or other non-hydroxylated fatty acids.

The results of GATT can be compared to related experiments conducted by BARTSCH (1964) who injected acetate-1-^{14}C intracerebrally into rats fourteen days of age. Litter mates were killed at intervals from one day to twelve weeks after administration of the isotope. All of the sphingosine-containing lipids became radioactive, reaching a maximum at one day; thereafter showing a slow decrease in radioactivity. In these experiments almost 80% of the total radioactivity of the sphingolipids could be accounted for as fatty acids. Some incorporation of the acetate radioactivity into the sphingosine moiety did occur and was proportional to the amount of acetate carbon-14 incorporated into the fatty acids of the cerebrosides, sphingomyelins, and gangliosides. These experiments are especially interesting because of the disproportionate distribution of the radioactivity incorporated from the acetate between the sphingosine and the fatty acids. This suggests that a difference in pool-sizes exists between the various precursors leading to the sphingolipids. Or possibly, that the pathway for the biosynthesis of sphingosine may not, in fact, involve palmityl-SCoA, the expected intermediate common both to higher fatty acid synthesis and to sphingosine synthesis.

3. Cerebroside and Ceramide Metabolism

Gaucher's disease is characterized chemically by the accumulation of cerebroside (most probably glucosyl-ceramide, see SUOMI and AGRANOFF, 1964; BRANDE, 1963; and KLENK, 1955) in the reticulo endothelial system. In an effort to produce this disease in an experimental situation, CHRISTIANSON (1941) conducted experiments upon the rabbit in which he administered (orally and intraperitoneally) large amounts of cerebrosides (galactosyl ceramides). After a prolonged period of continuous administration of cerebrosides, the rabbit tissues were shown to accumulate cerebrosides and lesions were observed histologically similar to those seen in Gaucher's disease. Similar experiments were conducted in 1955 by BURTON in which cerebroside (galactosyl ceramide) suspensions in water were administered intraperitoneally daily to rats. No tissue accumulation of cerebrosides was noted after a three months interval indicating a mechanism for the elimination of galactosyl ceramide by metabolism and/or excretion. To study this aspect in greater detail tritium random-labelled cerebroside (galactosyl-ceramide) was prepared and administered in small amounts to rhesus monkeys. Samples of the blood, total urine and total feces, collected daily, as well as tissues obtained at autopsy were examined for radioactivity and cerebrosides. Fig. 9 presents data from BURTON et al. (unpublished) which indicates the level of radioactivity derived from the tritiated cerebroside present in blood plasma over the thirty-seven days duration of the

---

* Sodium palmitate and stearate were suspended in water with bovine serum albumin by heat and ultrasonic irradiation. Potassium lignocerate and cerebronate were emulsified with polyoxyethylene stearate G-2159.

experiment. It also illustrates the urinary excretion of tritium throughout this period of time. 60% of the intravenously administered radioisotope was excreted in the urine in the thirty-seven day interval. The excretory product was determined to be primarily water. The shape of the curve indicating radioactivity in the blood plasma (little radioactivity was found associated with the red blood cell) indicates a rapid uptake of the tritiated galactosyl ceramide by tissues with a subsequent re-distribution, at least of the radioactivity, being reflected by a secondary peak level of radioactivity of the blood plasma. The radioactivity present in the tissues of monkeys killed one hour and eight hours after the administration of the radioactive cerebroside was present almost exclusively as cerebroside. On the other hand, the monkey killed thirty-seven days following the injection showed that the radioactivity resided primarily in non-cerebroside components. It was noted that throughout these experiments the radioactivity present in liver was relatively constant, whereas the radioactivity in spleen and in abdominal fat showed a progressive increase with time. It should be remarked that the physical properties of the tritiated cerebroside, while closely resembling non-radioactive cerebroside, were different in respect to crystallinity and reduced ability to hydrate. Due to the reduced ability of the tritiated cerebroside to hydrate, the material injected was particulate rather than a smooth colloidal suspension. The data reported suggest that the larger particles were filtered from the blood by lung tissue. Nevertheless, these studies do indicate that *in vivo* the rhesus monkey can totally metabolize galactosyl ceramide as indicated by the large outpouring of radioactive water in the urine. They further show that tritiated cerebroside has little access to central nervous system tissue.

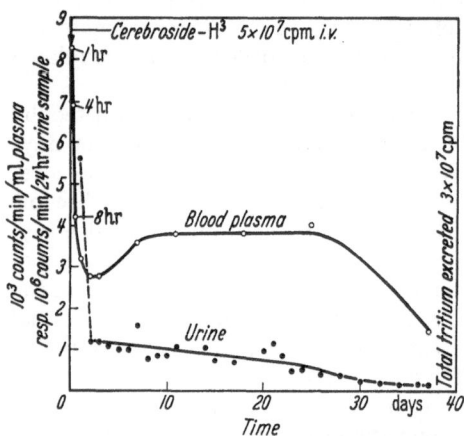

Fig. 9. Excretion of tritium after the intravenous infusion of cerebroside-³H to the monkey. From BURTON, SODD and LEWIS (unpublished data)

KOPACZYK and RADIN (1964, 1965) prepared cerebroside (galactosyl ceramide) labeled with lignoceryl-1-^{14}C acid and ceramide labeled with stearyl-1-^{14}C acid. These lipids were administered as emulsions intracerebrally to rats fifteen days of age. The data derived from animals killed two days following the injection are presented in Table 10. These data show small, but significant, metabolism of the intracerebrally injected cerebroside and ceramide. This metabolism is reflected by the appearance of radioactive fatty acids in other sphingolipids than those injected. For example, radioactivity from the stearyl(-1-^{14}C)-sphingosine was found in cerebrosides, cerebroside sulfate, gangliosides, and sphingomyelin. Radioactivity from O^1-galactosyl-N-lignoceryl(-1-^{14}C)-sphingosine appeared in ceramides, the hydroxy fatty acids of cerebrosides, cerebroside sulfate and sphingomyelin. This accounts for 1.7% and 3.2% of the injected ceramide and cerebroside radioactivity respectively. Total radioactivity recovered after 2 days, was 38% from cerebroside and 13% from ceramide.

It was shown that considerably more radioactivity was present as the fatty acids than as sphingosine. A small fraction of the radioactivity appeared in cholesterol, reflecting metabolism of the lipid to radioactive acetate and subsequent synthesis of cholesterol. This suggests that part of the radioactivity recovered in the sphingolipids could have been derived from a similar pool of radioactive acetate. The radioactive ceramide administered gave rise to an appreciable quantity of sphingomyelin. The radioactive cerebroside yielded ceramide in which all of the radioactivity was present in the carboxyl carbon of the fatty acid and whose specific activity was 5700 cpm/μmole. The cerebroside radioactivity also appeared in the sphingomyelin fraction whose specific activity was 3600 cpm/μmole.

Table 10. *Radioactivity in cerebral lipids after intracerebral injection of cerebroside-*^{14}C *and ceramide-*^{14}C

	Compound Administered	
Cerebral Lipid isolated	Cerebroside (gal-lignoceryl-(1—^{14}C)-sph) % total radioactivity	Ceramide (stearyl-(1—^{14}C)-sph) % total radioactivity
Ceramides	0.45* (5700 cpm/μmole)	—
Cerebrosides	—	0.26 (equal specific activities in normal and hydroxy fatty acids)
Cerebroside — hydroxy fatty acids	1.07 (8.4% in carboxyl group)	—
Cerebroside sulfate	0.09	0.05
Sphingomyelin	1.63** (3600 cpm/μmole)	1.3
Gangliosides	—	0.13***

Data from Kopaczyk and Radin (1964, 1965).

* All radioactivity in carboxyl carbon.
** 95.2% ^{14}C as lignoceric acid (90.3% ^{14}C in carboxyl carbon).
*** 16:0—15.4% ^{14}C, 18:0—62.4% ^{14}C, 20:0—22.2% ^{14}C.

Both of these data are consistent with the precursor-product relationship expected if ceramide, rather than sphingosine and fatty acid, was the precursor of the sphingomyelin. This is, of course, consistent with the *in vitro* data discussed earlier. It would have been interesting to know the amount of sphingomyelin and ceramide present in these brain tissues and, if possible, to know the quantity of "newly-synthesized" sphingomyelin formed. This would permit a better evaluation of the specific activities and their consistency with the precursor-product relationship. Some of the radioactivity derived from the cerebroside appeared in cerebroside hydroxy-fatty acids. However, only 8.4% of the radioactivity resided in the carboxyl carbon. This indicates that the fatty acids in cerebrosides cannot be directly hydroxylated and, in this case, undoubtedly arose from metabolic products of the lignoceryl-1-^{14}C derived from the cerebroside injected. While radioactivity from the stearyl(-1-^{14}C) sphingosine appeared in the isolated cerebroside, it was present in equivalent amounts in both the normal saturated and hydroxy-saturated fatty acids. These observations suggest that ceramide is not an intermediate in the synthesis of cerebroside, because if ceramide were an intermediate then the radioactive cerebroside synthesized should have contained more radioactivity in the saturated fatty acid moiety than in the hydroxy-fatty acid. It was noted that a little radioactivity appeared in the cerebroside sulfate fraction from both the cerebroside-^{14}C and ceramide-^{14}C injected animals. Unfortunately, the data does not permit answering the question of direct sulfation of cerebrosides.

a) **Turnover Studies:** In a steady state condition, the turnover of a lipid is a measure of the rate of destruction of the lipid and its replacement by synthesis.

In general the turnover is presented numerically as the time required to change or alter one-half of the molecules present, i.e. the half-time ($t^1/_2$). The turnover of lipids *in vivo* must be approached by the use of isotopes. The general technique is to administer isotopically labeled precursor material to the animal, to allow sufficient time for the precursor to be incorporated into the lipid under study, and then to measure the rate of loss of the isotope from the lipid. A plot of the log of the per cent isotope remaining in the lipid vs time normally gives a linear plot from which the half-time can be estimated. Such a plot is presented in Fig. 10 for the depletion of carbon-14 from gangliosides (BURTON et al., 1964). The label was introduced by administering glucose-1-^{14}C and glucosamine-1-^{14}C. It may be seen that the half-time of gangliosides is approximately 24 days when the isotopic precursor was glucosamine, whereas the time for half turnover was approximately 10 days when the precursor was glucose-1-^{14}C. It is apparent that one must ask the question in these experiments: "What does the half-time we have measured represent? Does it adequately reflect the turnover of the lipids or does it reflect only the turnover of *a component* of the lipids?" In the ganglioside example, we know from previous work that glucosamine-1-^{14}C labels only the aminosugars in the ganglioside molecule and that the glucose-1-^{14}C labels all of the carbohydrate components of gangliosides (BURTON et al., 1963). It may be seen that in the one case (glucose) the turnover time is much more rapid than in the other case (galactosamine). A reasonable interpretation of these data is to consider that the turnover

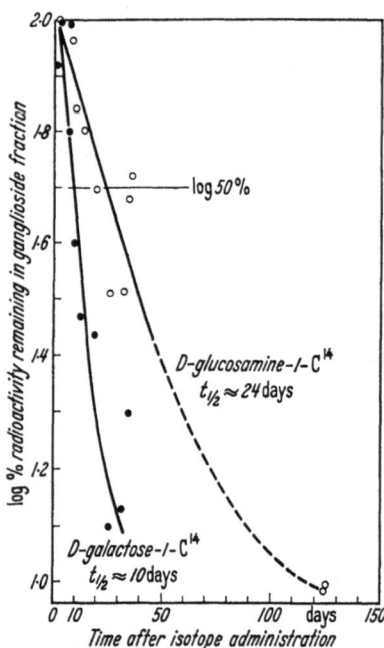

Fig. 10. Gangliosides turnover in rat brain. From BURTON (unpublished data)

time of the ganglioside carbohydrate moiety is less than 10 days. As the carbohydrate units are liberated from the oligosaccharide they enter pools of different sizes, thus, the galactose and glucose enter large pools, which are interconvertible. The isotope is diluted by the nonlabeled sugars in these pools. In addition, the metabolic demand upon the glucose pool is large, since the primary source of energy for brain tissue is, of course, glucose. The net result is a reduction in the specific activity of the glucose and galactose present in brain by dilution and metabolism. As the gangliosides which have been degraded are replaced by synthesis the radioactivity reincorporated from glucose and galactose pools would be very small. On the other hand, the N-acetyl neuraminic acid and N-acetyl galactosamine pools are small (BURTON et al., 1963). There is little metabolic demand for these aminosugars in brain tissue. The net result is only a slight decrease in the specific radioactivity of the aminosugars being enzymatically removed from the gangliosides. The aminosugars used in the *re*synthesis of gangliosides will be of a relatively high specific activity and the gangliosides thus formed will contain considerable radioactivity. This data (Fig. 10) therefore indicates that gangliosides undergo turnover with a half-time considerably less than 10 days as measured by radioactivity in the oligosaccharide moiety. It gives no indication of the turnover of either the fatty acids or sphingosine moieties.

Similar studies designed to measure the turnover of cerebrosides of brain tissue have been carried out by a number of investigators. DAVISON et al. (1959) employed serine-3-^{14}C to label brain cerebrosides and computed the turnover rate to be near 200 days. On the other hand HAJRA and RADIN (1964) administered acetate-^{14}C and measured the rate of loss of radioactivity from the fatty acid moieties of the cerebrosides. In the latter experiments the half-time was near 42 days. When the hexose of the cerebrosides is labeled by means of glucose-1-^{14}C or galactose-1-^{14}C, the rate of depletion of the isotope indicated a half-time of near 40 days (BURTON, et al, 1964). These data indicate that cerebrosides turn over slowly in brain, at a rate near 40 days, as measured by the hexose and fatty acid moieties. The data derived from the serine experiment undoubtedly indicates that the sphingosine pool in brain is small and that this compound is reused in the synthesis of the sphingolipids.

Recent data obtained by BURTON (unpublished) on the turnover of cerebrosides sulfates showing the persistence of radioactivity in the brain tissue cerebroside sulfate, when sulfate-^{35}S is the label, indicates that the sulfate pool is small and that considerable reuse of the isotopic sulfate occurs. In these same experiments, a more rapid turnover of the hexose moiety of the cerebroside sulfate occurred than of the sulfate moiety. In fact, the half-time for the rate of loss of radioactivity from the hexose unit of cerebroside sulfate was identical with the rate of loss of the carbohydrate unit from cerebroside.

The net result of these turnover studies is to show that lipids in brain are a part of the dynamic biochemistry of the body — even though they may function primarily as structural components. These data strongly suggest that considerable caution must be exerted in the interpretation of isotopic experiments conducted *in vivo*, especially when complex compounds are being studied. It emphasizes the need to know more than the radioactivity in the lipid. Other perimeters, such as pool sizes, turnover rates of the pools themselves, permeability, cellular barriers (such as the blood-brain barrier) and other related factors must be determined before a full explanation of the isotope data can be made.

b) Metabolic Pathways: The results of all of the studies carried out both *in vitro* and *in vivo* on the metabolism of the sphingosine containing lipids may be summarized diagrammatically to illustrate the relationships between the various lipids. Such a scheme is presented in Metabolic Pathways 1, below. It is readily seen that the incorporation of serine into the sphingosine lipids occurs primarily into the sphingosine moiety. With time some incorporation occurs via the conversion of serine to acetate and, hence, incorporation both into the sphingosine moiety as well as into the fatty acid unit. The 18:dihydrosphingosine is readily converted to the 18:sphingosine which may be acylated to give rise to N-acyl sphingosine hence to sphingomyelin. In addition, carbohydrate may be added to 18:sphingosine to give rise to psychosine, which then may give rise to cerebroside by acylation. Since the routes of formation of the sphingosine containing sulfatides are unknown, only possible pathways of formation are indicated. Again, speculative pathways are indicated for the synthesis of the gangliosides from the sphingosine and sphingosine derivatives. No indication is shown for the two possible major routes of ganglioside formation i.e. "step-wise" synthesis, via a sequence of nucleotide hexose donors and "one-step" synthesis via a nucleotide oligosaccharide donor. In addition, no indication of the different fatty acid profiles for the various sphingolipids is made.

A large part of the sphingolipids are present as glycolipids. Metabolic Pathway 2, shown below, indicates the known routes of formation of the major nucleotide monosaccharide intermediates i.e. UDPgal, UDPglc, UDPgalNAc and CMPneu-

NAc. It is immediately apparent that these pathways are interrelated, thus glucose and galactose are interconvertible and can give rise to aminosugars. It is, however, more difficult for the aminosugars to give rise to glucose and galactose derivatives.

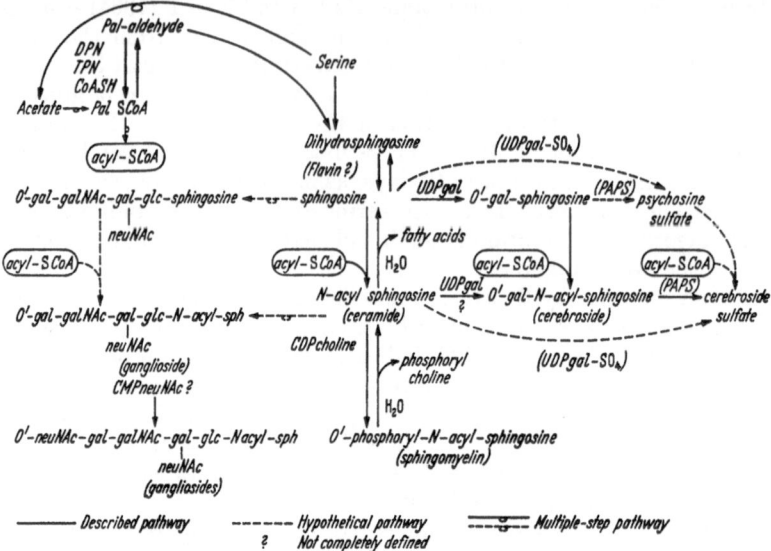

Pathway 1. Summary diagram showing reactions involved in metabolism of the sphingolipids. The individual reactions are described in the text. No indication has been made of the specific fatty acids involved — in some cases they are long chain (24:) and in some cases medium chain (18:).

While several other enzymatic routes have been observed to occur in micro-organisms, these routes have not been depicted in the above scheme.

The pathways of synthesis and degradation of sphingomyelin have not been illustrated here because they are similar to those described in another chapter (Rossiter).

Pathway 2. Reactions involved in synthesis of the nucleotide sugar intermediates. These reactions are documented in the following references: Kalckar and Maxwell (1958), Pogell and Gryder (1957), Chou and Soodak (1952), Davidson et al. (1957), Leloir and Cardini (1956), Maley et al. (1956), Cardini and Leloir (1957), Comb and Roseman (1958), Ghosh and Roseman (1961, 1962), Warren and Felsenfeld (1961, 1962), Roseman (1962) and Glaser (1963).

c) **Immunology of the Sphingolipids:** Rapport et al. (1958) and Graf and Rapport (1960) injected rabbit with human reticulum cell sarcoma cytoplasm; antisera was prepared from blood serum of these rabbits and measured using the complement fixation assay. A lipid material was isolated from human epidermoid carcinoma and its structure appeared to be a sphingosine derivative and named Cytolipin-H. Cytolipin-H reacts poorly in the complement fixation assay with antisera prepared as above, but when Cytolipin-H is mixed with auxiliary lipids (lecithin-cholesterol, 1-1) as little as 1 mμg of Cytolipin-H can be determined. This is demonstrated in Fig. 11. Cytolipin-H has been found to contain sphingosine fatty acid, glucose, and galactose in equal proportions. A comparison of Cytolipin-H with a similar material prepared from beef spleen by KLENK and RENNKAMP (1942) indicate a similar composition of these two lipids as well as identical behavior in the complement fixation assay (RAPPORT, et al., 1960). The configuration of the disaccharide residue in Cytolipin-H was determined by RAPPORT et al.

(1961) who showed that the reaction between the human tumor antisera prepared from rabbit and Cytolipin-H was specifically inhibited by lactose. The percentage inhibition was linearly related to the concentration of lactose. Control experiments indicated that cellobiose, fructose, fucose, galactose, glucose, maltose, melizitose, melibiose, raffinose, and sucrose were totally without effect even at high concentration. 25% inhibition of the complement fixation test was produced with 6×10^{-4} M lactose and 50% inhibition with 5.6×10^{-3} M lactose. This clearly indicates the structure of Cytolipin-H and the beef spleen lipid to be β-D-galactosyl (1→4) glucosyl ceramide. The acyl residue appears to be largely lignoceric acid (RAPPORT et al., 1961). Additional studies

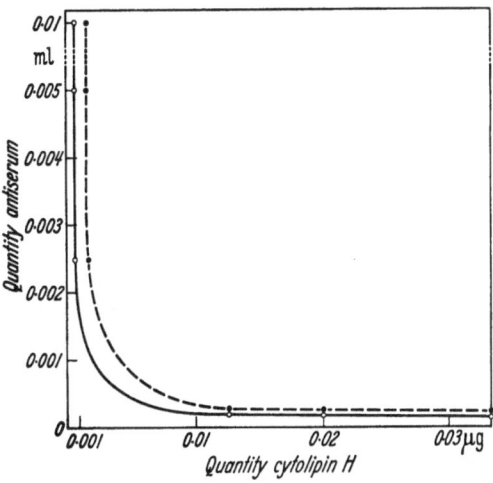

Fig. 11. Isofixation curves of cytolipin H with two antisera to human tumors determined at a sensitivity level of 3 units of complement. O · · · · · O anticarcinoma cervix serum; O————O anti-reticulum cell sarcoma serum. From RAPPORT et al. (1958)

by JOFFE and RAPPORT (1963) and RAPPORT et al. (1964) have shown the haptenic property of cerebrosides.

SOMERS, KANFER and BRADY (1964) prepared rabbit antiserum to ganglioside (prepared by the method of TRAMS and LAUTER, 1962; a mixture of B4 and C3) and "asialoganglioside" (B4 and C3 in which the neuNAc has been removed, i.e. gal(1→3)galNAc(1→4)gal(1→4)glc-cer) by the injection of red blood cells coated with the appropriate glycolipid (YOKAYAMA et al., 1963). The antiganglioside-antibodies were specific for gangliosides and showed no cross reaction with either "asialo-B4" or "asialo-B2" (i.e. aminoglycolipid of BOGOCH, 1961) in the hemagglutination assay. While the anti-"asialo-B4" antibody did not cross react with ganglioside it showed cross reactivity with "asialo-B2". These workers studied a series of lipids and carbohydrates as inhibitors of the hemagglutination test system. Of the forty-one potential inhibitors studied, only two compounds were inhibitory to the reaction of ganglioside with antiganglioside antibody. These compounds were colominic acid (a polymer [neuNAc(2→8)neuNAc]n) and N-acetylneuraminic acid itself. While ganglioside (B4 and C3) inhibited the reaction in the test system, ganglioside B2 (Tay-Sachs ganglioside) failed to inhibit. This would indicate that the terminal galactose unit was necessary for inhibition. When the anti-"asialo-B4" antibody reaction with "asialo-B4" was studied, inhibition was shown by "asialo-B2", "asialo-B4", galactosylarabinose, 6-O-β-D-galactopyranosyl-D-galactose, D-galactopyranosyl-β-1, 3-D-glucose, 4-O-β-D-galactosyl-N-acetylglucosamine, lactobionic acid, lactose, methyl 2-acetamido-2-deoxy-β-D-galactopyranoside and methyl β-D-galactopyranoside.

All of these inhibitors were β-galactosides with lactose being the most potent inhibitor. When the anti-"asialo-B4" antibody reaction with "asialo-B2" was studied, several differences in the pattern of inhibition were noted. While lactose was an inhibitor it inhibited only at a much higher concentration than with "asialo-B4". Greatest inhibition of the asialo-B2 assay system was with methyl 2-acetamido-2-deoxy-β-D-galactopyranoside. The α-anomer did not inhibit. In addition, high concentrations of monosaccharides such as D-galactose and N-acetyl-D-galactosamine were inhibitory. While these results are difficult to interpret they do indicate that the terminal sugar in "asialo-B4" is galactose and is in β (probably 1→4) linkage. It is interesting to note that Cytolipin-H was not an inhibitor in any of the system studied. Unfortunately the interpretation of this negative data is difficult since this lipid is extremely insoluble in water. It is therefore not known whether the lack of inhibition is due to the fact that the lactose portion of the ganglioside is not involved in the antibody-antigen reaction or whether the negative results are simply a question of solubility and hence concentration. It is also worthy of note that N-acetyl neuraminyl lactose did not inhibit any of the three assay systems employed in this study. Does this mean that the N-acetyl neuraminyl lactose unit does not occur in ganglioside, i.e. that the neuNAc linkage may be at a different position (see Kanfer and Brady, 1963, and the enzymatic studies of Burton 1963)? It is, of course, possible that the N-acetyl neuraminyl lactose unit, which is an interior portion of the ganglioside molecule, may not be involved in bonding the antigen-antibody together.

Taketomi and Yamakawa (1963) have approached the immunochemical study of glycolipids by use of a method involving the formation of diazo-coupled glycolipid-protein compounds. N-p-aminobenzoyl dihydropsychosine was diazotized and reacted with either egg albumin or bovine serum albumin. About 30 moles of the glycolipid combined with one mole of albumin. The product was extensively dialyzed and used to prepare anti-serum (rabbit). The antibody-antigen reaction was studied by the precipitin reaction. It was observed that anti-serum prepared by injecting psychosine-serum albumin contained antibodies to bovine serum albumin as well as to psychosine-serum albumin. No precipitin reaction was observed with egg albumin. However, psychosine-egg albumin did react with the anti-psychosine-serum albumin. This indicates that at least part of the specificity of the antigen-antibody reaction is due to the diazotized psychosine moiety. A number of sugars were examined as inhibitors of the precipitin reaction, e.g. galactose, lactose, glucose, α-methyl galactoside, and β-methyl galactoside. Both lactose and β-methyl galactoside inhibited the reaction more strongly than either the free galactose or the α-methyl galactoside. Glucose was not an inhibitor. It appears that the carbohydrate moiety is probably the antigenic determinate of the protein-coupled psychosine.

While these studies clearly indicate the ability of glycolipids to participate in antibody-antigen reactions, it would appear that the carbohydrate units are the portion of the molecule responsible for their antigenicity. A recent abstract indicates that sphingosine-protein complex can yield antibodies which are specific for sphingosine (Taketomi and Yamakawa, 1965). These immunological techniques may prove to be powerful tools for elucidating the structure of these complex glycolipids and the fact that they are antigenic would suggest that their role in disease process should be investigated.

d) **Diseases involving sphingolipids.** A consideration of the list of sphingosine containing lipids indicates a potentiality for a series of lipidoses in which each sphingolipid, in turn, might be involved. With four exceptions, such diseases have been described. To date, no lipidoses have been identified in which sphingosine (as the free base), psychosine, ceramide, or the newly reported sphingoplasmalogen, are present in excessive amounts. Deficiency diseases (e.g. the demyelinating diseases) are known in which the total sphingosine content, as well as other cellular components, is lower than in normal tissues.

The nature of the specific defect(s) is unknown for each of these diseases. The sphingolipidoses, in general, appear to be of genetic origin (STANBURY et al., 1960 and ARONSON and VOLK, 1962). It is known that the sphingosine-containing lipids turnover and exist in a steady state condition, even those lipids which are components of the more stable cellular structures (e.g. myelin sheaths). Since synthesis and destruction of the sphingolipids occur constantly throughout life, it is easy to visualize disease conditions in which the synthesis: destruction balance is altered resulting in a lipid storage condition. An *overproduction* of sphingolipids by the presence of an excessive quantity of an anabolic enzyme system seems unlikly. Examples are known of diseases in which enzymes are missing or are present in quantitatively low amounts (e.g. galactosemia, cf. KALCKAR and MAXWELL, 1958), support the concept of *under-destruction* of sphingolipids as pathogenesis of lipid storage diseases. An alternate possibility would be a defective control mechanism for regulating the rates of formation and destruction of the lipids. That such control mechanisms exist for the sphingolipids can be inferred from the isotope incorporation data of BURTON et al. (1958, 1963), MOSER and KARNOVSKY (1959), and others. In these experiments it was observed that synthesis of gangliosides and cerebrosides in brain tissue began shortly after birth, proceeded rapidly for one to two weeks, and then markedly slowed. A near steady-state condition of these lipids has been demonstrated, with a very slow rate of accumulation throughout the animal's life. The question "what initiates the rapid synthesis of cerebrosides and gangliosides and what slows or terminates this rapid process after adult levels of these brain lipids are reached?" has not been answered as yet. A consideration of metabolic pathways 1 and 2 suggest a number of possible feedback control points which could be investigated. Knowledge of these control mechanisms may enable the development of drugs capable of preventing lipid storage, e.g. sugar or nucleotide analogues, sphingosine derivatives, etc.

With the observations by several laboratories that the sphingolipids can participate in antibody production (RAPPORT et al., 1964, JOFFE and RAPPORT, 1963, SOMERS et al., 1963, and TAKETOMI and YAMAKAWA, 1963, 1965), the question truly can be raised as to the role of autoimmune responses in the etiology of the demyelinating diseases. To this end, the extensive studies of allergic encephalitis will certainly be most valuable (cf. SCHEINBERG, KIES, and ALVORD, 1965). In turn, the study of sphingolipids, both their synthesis and destruction, in these allergic demyelinating diseases may aid in unraveling the control mechanisms discussed above.

There are a number of recent reviews of the sphingolipidoses such as those of van BOGAERT et al., 1957; VOLK and SPERRY, 1959; STANBURY et al., 1960; FOLCH-PI, 1961; ARONSON and VOLK, 1962; and FOLCH-PI and BAUER, 1963. The following *selectively* document the known sphingolipid storage diseases with newer references and mention briefly several recent observations.

Cerebrosidosis (Gaucher's disease): SUOMI and AGRANOFF (1964) examined the spleens of eight patients and showed an average of a 130 fold increase over normal in the cerebroside level. The hexose component of the splenic cerebroside from all the patients was shown to be exclusively glucose by the glucose oxidase method (AGRANOFF et al., 1962). The sphingosine was all octadecene except for 3—4% octadecane. None of the fatty acids were hydroxylated. No elevation of the dihexoside, lac-cer, was found.

As described in an earlier section, BRADY et al. (1965a) have shown the presence in spleen of an enzyme which specifically hydrolyzes glc-cer to ceramide and glucose. A recent report by BRADY et al. (1965b) demonstrates that this enzyme is deficient in spleen tissue from patients with Gaucher's disease. An examination of spleens from three patients showed a glc-cer hydrolase level of 1.8 μmoles $\pm$ 0.36 SD hydrolyzed per hour per kg protein (calculated from a 14 hour incubation) which was compared with an average enzyme level of 12.7 $\pm$ 0.71 SD from four patients with several types of anemias. In the absences of data for spleens from normal people, it is difficult to know if this defect (in Gaucher's disease) is one of an enzyme deficiency *per se* or a failure of the host to respond to the challenge of an increased glycolipid level by inducing glc-cer hydrolase formation. The later possibility must be considered since the anemias studied are those due to increased hemolysis.

Cerebroside sulfatidoses (Infantile metachromatic leucodystrophy): JATZKE-WITZ (1958) first described the accumulation of cerebroside sulfate in tissues of patients with metachromatic leucodystrophy. A typical case of cerebroside sulfa-tidoses has been described thoroughly by HAGBERG et al. (1962). Lipid analysis of brain tissues have been reported by a number of workers including HAGBERG et al. (1960, 1961, 1962), SOURANDER and SVENNERHOLM (1962), LEES and MOSER (1962), and most recently by JATZKEWITZ et al. (1964). It has been found that cerebrosides, sphingomyelins (24: fatty acids), and cholesterol are all present in white matter at lower than normal amounts (JATZKEWITZ et al., 1964). Cere-broside sulfates levels are elevated. Thus there appears to be a general demyelina-tion coupled with cerebroside sulfate accumulation. Pathogenesis of the disease is not known. The lipid sulfate accumulations have been ascribed to a deficiency in cerebroside sulfatase (JATZKEWITZ et al., 1964). An enzyme has been described in normal tissue (kidney) which hydrolyzes cerebroside sulfate (MEHL and JATZKE-WITZ, 1964). Opposed to this interpretation, is the view of HAGBERG et al. (1962) which suggests a deficiency in a cerebroside synthetase — thus permitting an accumulation of precursors for the synthesis of cerebroside sulfate from a common intermediate (common to both cerebrosides and cerebroside sulfates). This would be compatable with the suggestion of O'BRIEN (1964) which pictures a defect in the fatty acid chain elongation system and hence in cerebroside metabolism, with an accommodation by cerebroside sulfates accumulation (of near normal fatty acid profile).

gal-gal-glc-ceramidosis (Fabry's disease): SWEELEY and KLIONSKY (1963) ex-tracted a glycolipid from pathological kidney tissue which has been identified as an acyl-sphingosine trihexoside whose structure appears to be gal-gal-glc-cer. The primary fatty acids present are 22:0-36%, 24:0-34%, and 24:1-12%. In addition, an acyl-sphingosine dihexoside, probably lac-cer or cytolipin-H, appears to be present in abnormal amounts.

Gangliosidosis (amaurotic familial idiocy; Tay-Sachs disease): The ganglioside family was discovered by KLENK (1939) in his studies on brain tissue of patients who died from Tay-Sachs disease. Subsequent studies on normally occuring gang-liosides have led to the structures B4 and C3 as the primary gangliosides of brain, with lesser amounts of C4. In Tay-Sachs disease, the ganglioside which accumu-lates has the structure B2 (SVENNERHOLM, 1962; KUHN and WEIGANDT, 1963a; KLENK et al., 1963 and MAKITA and YAMAKAWA, 1963). In addition, a neura-minic acid free glycolipid appears to accumulate (GATT and BERMAN, 1963, SVENNERHOLM, 1962, and MAKITA and YAMAKAWA, 1963). The structure of this latter glycolipid appears to be galNAc(1→4)gal(1→4)glc-cer (MAKITA and YAMA-KAWA, 1963). The nature of the enzymatic defect is unknown. It could be a lack of enzymes such as UDPgal(?): B2 transferase, CMPneuNAc : B3 transferase, and CMPneuNAc(?) or UDP gal(?):galNAc-gal-glc-cer transferase. Or the absence of hydrolases to remove the glycolipids accumulated, i. e. B2 and galNAc-gal-glc-cer. The presence of these hydrolases in normal tissues have been described (KOREY et al. 1963a and SANDHOFF, et al., 1964).

The multiple forms of the gangliosides which exist in brain and other tissues (see Table 1, page 214), suggests the potentiality for several varieties of Tay-Sachs disease, the differences being due to different inborn errors of metabolism and thus to the type of ganglioside and the locations (which organs) at which it accumulates. Such varients have recently been described by NORMAN, et al. (1959), LANDING et al. (1962, 1964), O'BRIEN and coworkers (1965), and JATZKEWITZ, et al. (1965). It should be empasized that chemical confirmation is essential to the diagnosis of the sphingolipidosis.

Sphingomyelinosis: A most interesting observation by HOLTZ et al. (1964) showed that cells from patients with Niemann-Pick's disease grown as monolayer tissue cultures (3—6 transfers) contained $18.4 \pm 3.4\%$ of the total lipid phosphorus as sphingomyelin whereas cells cultured from normal humans contained only $6.8 \pm 1.7\%$ as sphingomyelin. Even though the cells reverted to fibroblasts, the genetic defect persisted. A subsequent study was made using cells cultured from amnions of two infants from two sets of parents (who had children with Niemann-Pick's disease). Cells cultured from three normal controls gave a mean value of 7.4%. The cultured cells from one of the two babies (siblings with Niemann-Pick's disease) contained 7.9% of lipid phosphorus as sphingomyelin. This child has not developed this disease, as yet, whereas the second baby's cell culture showed 13.1—14.8% as sphingomyelin and subsequently was diagnosed as Niemann-Pick's.

References

AGRANOFF, B. W., N. RADIN, and W. SUOMI: Enzymic oxidation of cerebrosides: studies on Gaucher's disease. Biochim. biophys. Acta (Amst.) 57, 194 (1962).

AMINOFF, D., F. DODYK, and S. ROSEMAN: Enzymatic synthesis of colominic acid. J. biol. Chem. 238, 1177 (1963).

ARONSON, S. M., and B. W. VOLK: Cerebral Sphingolipidosis. New York: Academic Press, Inc. 1962.

BAKKE, J. E., and W. E. CORNATZER: Metabolism of brain and liver sulfatides. J. biol. Chem. 236, 653 (1961).

BANDURSKI, R. S., L. G. WILSON, and C. L. SQUIRES: The mechanism of "active sulfate" formation. J. Amer. chem. Soc. 78, 6408 (1956).

BARTSCH, G.: Incorporation of Acetate-1-C¹⁴ into Sphingolipids of the Rat Brain. VI. Int. Congress Biochem. Abst., p. 564, 1963.

BASU, S., and B. KAUFMAN: Ganglioside synthesis in embryonic chicken brain. Fed. Proc. 24, 479 (1965).

BLIX, G.: Zur Kenntnis der schwefelhaltigen Lipoidstoffe des Gehirns über Cerebronschwefelsäure. Hoppe-Seylers Z. physiol. Chem. 219, 82 (1933).

BOGOCH, S.: Aminoglycolipids and glycoproteins of human brain. III. Quantitative separation and determination of brain glycoproteins neuraminic acid, hexosamine, and hexoses by means of whole tissue emulsion-fractionation. Nature (Lond.) 190, 153 (1961).

BRADY, R. O.: Studies on the total enzymatic synthesis of cerebrosides. J. biol. Chem. 237, 2416 (1962).

— J. V. FORMICA, and G. J. KOVAL: The enzymatic synthesis of sphingosine. II. Further studies on the mechanism of the reaction. J. biol. Chem. 233, 1072 (1958b).

— J. N. KANFER, and D. SHAPIRO: The metabolism of glucocerebrosides. I. Purification and properties of a glucocerebroside cleaving enzyme from spleen tissue. J. biol. Chem 240, 39 (1964).

— — — Metabolism of glucocerebrosides. II. Evidence of an enzymatic deficiency in Gaucher's disease. Biochem. biophys. Res. Commun. 18, 221 (1965).

— and G. J. KOVAL: Biosynthesis of sphingosine in vitro. J. Amer. chem. Soc. 79, 2648 (1957)

— — The enzymatic synthesis of sphingosine. J. biol. Chem. 233, 26 (1958a).

Brande, G. in Folch-Pi (editor): Pathology of the nervous system, p. 57, London: Pergamon Press, 1961.

Burton, R. M.: Uridine nucleotides and the metabolism of nerve tissue. R. O. Brady, and D. Tower, editors, Neurochemistry of Nucleotides and Amino Acids, published by John Wiley and Sons, Inc. 1960.

— The action of neuraminidase from Clostridium perfringens on gangliosides. J. Neurochem. 10, 503 (1963).

— Y. M. Balfour, and J. M. Gibbons: Gangliosides and cerebrosides turnover rates in rat brain. Fed. Proc. 23, 230 (1964).

— L. Garcia-Bunuel, M. Golden, and Y. Balfour: Incorporation of radioactivity of D-glucosamine-1-C^{14}, D-glucose-1-C^{14}, D-galactose-1-C^{14}, and DL-serine-3-C^{14} into rat brain glycolipids. Biochemistry 2, 580 (1963).

— M. A. Sodd, and R. O. Brady: The incorporation of galactose into galactolipides. J. biol. Chem. 233, 1053 (1958).

— — — The involvement of uridine nucleotides in the biosynthesis of galactolipids in the central nervous system, in F. Brücke, editor, Fourth Int. Cong. of Biochem. Vol. III Biochemistry of the Central Nervous System 202 (1959).

— and E. R. Stadtman: The oxidation of acetaldehyde to acetyl coenzyme A. J. biol. Chem. 202, 873 (1953).

Cardini, C. E., and L. F. Leloir: Enzymatic formation of acetylgalactosamine. J. biol. Chem. 225, 317 (1957).

Carter, H. E., F. J. Glick, W. P. Norris, and G. E. Phillips: Biochemistry of the sphingolipids. III. Structure of sphingosine. J. biol. Chem. 170, 285 (1947).

— W. D. Celmer, W. E. M. Lands, K. L. Mueller, and H. H. Tomizawa: Biochemistry of the sphingolipids. VIII. Occurrence of a long chain base in plant phosphatides. J. biol. Chem. 206, 613 (1954).

— and Y. Fujino: Biochemistry of the sphingolipids. IX. Configuration of cerebrosides. J. biol. Chem. 221, 879 (1956).

— D. S. Galanos, and Y. Fujino: Chemistry of the sphingolipids. Canad. J. Biochem. 34, 320—331 (1956).

— R. A. Hendry, S. Nojima, N. Z. Stanacev, and K. Ohno: Biochemistry of the sphingolipids. XIII. Determination of the structure of cerebrosides from wheat flour. J. biol. Chem. 236, 1912 (1961).

— and C. G. Humiston: Biochemistry of the sphingolipids. V. The structure of sphingosine. J. biol. Chem. 191, 727 (1951).

— R. H. McCluer, and E. D. Slifer: Lipids of wheat flour. I. Characterization of galactosylglycerol components. J. Amer. chem. Soc. 78, 3735 (1956).

— W. P. Norris, F. J. Glick, G. E. Phillips, and R. Harris: Biochemistry of the sphingolipids II. Isolation of dihydrosphingosine from the cerebroside fractions of beef brain and spinal cord. J. biol. Chem. 170, 269 (1949).

— D. Shapiro, and J. B. Harrison: Synthesis and configuration of dihydrosphingosine. J. Amer. chem. Soc. 75, 1007 (1953).

Carubelli, R., R. E. Trucco, and R. Caputto: Neuraminidase activity in mammalian organs. Biochem. biophys. Acta (Amst.)60, 196 (1962).

Celmer, W. D., and H. E. Carter: Chemistry of phosphatides and cerebrosides. Physiol. Rev. 32, 167 (1952).

Chou, T. C., and M. Soodak: The acetylation of D-glucosamine by pigeon liver extracts. J. biol. Chem. 196, 105 (1952).

Christianson, O. O.: Experimental lesions produced by cerebrosides. Arch. Path. (Chic.) 32, 369 (1941).

Cleland, W. W., and E. P. Kennedy: The enzymatic synthesis of psychosine. J. biol. Chem. 235. 45 (1960).

Comb, D. G., and S. Roseman: Enzymatic synthesis of N-acetyl-D-mannosamine. Biochim. biophys. Acta (Amst.) 29, 653 (1958).

Crocker, A. C., and S. Farber: Niemann-Pick disease: A review of eighteen patients. Medicine (Baltimore) 37, 1 (1958).

Cumings, J. N., H. Goodwin, E. M. Woodward, and G. Curzon: Lipids in the brains of infants and children. J. Neurochem. 2, 289 (1958).

Davidson, E. A., H. J. Blumenthal, and S. Roseman: Glucosamine metabolism. II. Studies on glucosamine-6-phosphate N-acetylase. J. biol. Chem. 226, 125 (1957).

Davison, A. N., and M. Wajda: Metabolism of myelin lipids: Estimation and separation of brain lipids in the developing rabbit. J. Neurochem. 4, 353 (1959).

— and N. A. Gregson: The physiological role of cerebron sulphuric acid (sulphatide) in the brain. Biochem. J. 85, 558 (1962).

Deuel, H. J.: The lipids. Vol. I. New York: Chemistry Interscience Press, Inc. 1951.

FAIRBAIRN, D.: The phospholipase of the venom of the cotton-mouth moccasin (Agkistridon piscivorus L). J. biol. Chem. 157, 633 (1945).

FIELDS, M., and S. GATT: Absorption of 1-C^{14} lignoceric acid in the rat. Nature (Lond.) 198, 994 (1963).

FOLCH-PI, J.: Chemical Pathology of the Nervous System. London: Pergamon Press, 1961.

— and H. BAUER: Brain Lipids and Lipoproteins, and the Leucodystrophies. Amsterdam: Elsevier 1963.

— A. MEATH, and S. ARSOVE: Isolation of brain strandin, a new type of large molecule tissue component. J. biol. Chem. 191, 819 (1951).

— in M. WAELSCH: Biochemistry of the Developing Nervous System, p. 121. New York: Academic Press, Inc. 1955.

FUJINO, Y., and T. NEGISHI: Studies on the conjugated lipids. Part XI. Hydrolysis of cerebroside sulfate by shellfish liver enzyme. Bull. Agr. Chem. Soc. Japan, 21, 225 (1957).

— and I. ZABIN: Studies on conjugated lipids. Agricultural and Biological Chemistry 26, 267 (1962a).

— — The configuration of sphingosine synthesized in rat brain homogenates. J. biol. Chem. 237, 2069 (1962b).

GATT, S.: Enzymic hydrolysis and synthesis of ceramides. J. biol. Chem. 238, 3131 (1963a).

— Metabolism of (1-C^{14}) lignoceric acid in the rat. Biochim. biophys. Acta (Amst.) 70, 370 (1963b).

— and E. R. BERMAN: Studies on brain lipids in Tay-Sach's disease. I. Isolation of two sialic acid-free glycolipids. J. Neurochem. 10, 43 (1963).

— and B. SHAPIRO: Metabolism of 1-C^{14} C lignoceric acid in the rat. Nature (Lond.) 185,461 (1960).

GHOSH, S., and S. ROSEMAN: Enzyme phosphorylation of N-acetyl-D-mannosamine. Proc. nat. Acad. Sci. (Wash.) 47, 955 (1961).

— — Enzymatic interconversion of N-acetylglucosamine and N-acetylmannosamine. Fed. Proc. 21, 89 (1962).

GLASER, L.: Biosynthesis of deoxysugars. Physiol. Rev. 43, 215 (1963).

GOLDBERG, I. H.: Enzymatic sulfurylation mechanisms. Dissertation, Rockefeller Institute, New York 1960a.

— Parallels between enzymatic sulfurylation of N-acetyl sphingosine and chloramphemicol. Fed. Proc. 19, 220 (1960b).

— The sulfolipids. J. Lipid Res. 2, 103 (1961).

— and A. DELBRÜCK: Transfer of sulfate from 3'-phosphoadenosine-5'-phosphosulfate to lipids, mucopolysaccharides and aminoalkyl phenols. Fed. Proc. 18, 235 (1959).

GOULD, R. G., F. M. SINEX, I. N. ROSENBERG, A. K. SOLOMON, and A. B. HASTINGS: Excretion of radioactive carbon dioxide by rats after administration of isotopic bicarbonate, acetate, and succinate. J. biol. Chem. 177, 295 (1949).

GRAF, L., and M. M. RAPPORT: Immunochemical studies of organ and tumor lipids. VII. The reactivity of anti-human tumor sera with cytolipin H. cardiolipin, and forssman haptens. Cancer Res. 20, 546 (1960).

GREEN, J. P., and J. D. ROBINSON jr.: Cerebroside sulfate (sulfatide A) in some organs of the rat and in a mast cell tumor. J. biol. Chem. 235, 1621 (1960).

HAGBERG, B., P. SOURANDER, L. SVENNERHOLM, and H. VOSS: Late infantile metachromatic leucodystrophy of the genetic type. Acta paediat. (Uppsala) 49, 135 (1960).

— — — Clinical and laboratory diagnosis of metachromatic leucodystrophy. Cerebr. Palsy Bull. 3, 438 (1961).

— — — Sulfatide lipidoses in childhood. Amer. J. Dis. Childr. 104. 644 (1962).

— — — Diagnosis of Krabbe's infantile leucodystrophy. J. Neurol. Neurosurg. Psychiat. 26, 195 (1963).

HAJRA, A. K., and N. S. RADIN: Biosynthesis of the cerebroside odd-numbered fatty acids. J. Lipid Res. 3. 327 (1962).

— — Biosynthesis of odd- and even-numbered cerebroside fatty acids: Evidence for two routes. Biochim. biophys. Acta (Amst.) 70, 97 (1963a).

— — Isotopic studies of the biosynthesis of the cerebroside fatty acids in rats. J. Lipid Res. 4, 270 (1963b).

— — In vivo conversion of labeled fatty acids to the sphingolipid fatty acids in rat brain. J. Lipid Res. 4, 448 (1963c).

— — Cerebroside galactosidase of pig brain. Fed. Proc. 24, 360 (1965).

HAUSER, G.: Labeling of cerebrosides and sulfatides in rat brain. Biochim. biophys. Acta (Amst.) 84, 212 (1964).

HEALD, P. J., and M. A. ROBINSON: The metabolism of sulphatides in cerebral tissues. Biochem. J. 81, 157 (1961).

HELLER, M., and B. SHAPIRO: The hydrolysis of sphingomyelin by rat liver. Israel J. Chem. 1, No. 3a (1963).

HOLTZ, A. I., B. W. UHLENDORF, and D. S. FREDRICKSON: Persistence of a lipid defect in tissue cultures derived from patients with Niemann-Pick disease. Fed. Proc. 23, 128 (1964).

HUTCHENS, T. T., J. T. VAN BRUGGEN, and E. S. WEST: Fatty acid and cholesterol synthesis rates in the intact rat. Arch. Biochem. 52, 261 (1954).

IVEMARK, B. I., L. SVENNERHOLM, C. THROEN, and R. TUNELL: Niemann-Pick disease in infancy. Acta paediat. (Uppsala) 52, 391 (1963).

JATZKEWITZ, H.: Zwei Typen von Cerebrosid-Schwefelsäureestern als sogenannte „Prälipoide" und Speichersubstanzen bei der Leukodystrophie, Typ Scholz (metachromatische Form der diffusen Sklerose). Hoppe-Seylers Z. physiol. Chem. 311, 279 (1958).

— H. PILZ, u. H. HOLLÄNDER: Biochemische und vergleichende histochemische Untersuchungen in umschriebenen Gebieten des Gehirns bei Fällen von adulter und infantiler metachromatischer Leukodystrophie. Acta neuropath. (Berl.) 4, 75 (1964).

— — and K. SANDHOFF: The quantitative determination of gangliosides and their derivatives in different forms of amaurotic idiocy. J. Neurochem. 12, 135 (1965).

JENNY, E. F., and C. A. GROB: Die Synthese von Erythro-dihydrosphingosin aus Trans-2-octadecen-1-Säure. Helv. chim. Acta 36, 1936 (1953).

JOFFE, S., and M. M. RAPPORT: Identification of an organ specific lipid hapten in brain. Nature (Lond.) 197, 60 (1963).

JOURDIAN, G. W., D. M. CARLSON, and S. ROSEMAN: The enzymatic synthesis of sialyllactose. Biochem. biophys. Res. Commun. 10, 352 (1963).

KALCKAR, H. M., and E. S. MAXWELL: Biosynthesis and metabolic function of uridine diphosphoglucose in mammalian organisms and its revelance to certain inborn errors. Physiol. Rev. 38, 77 (1958).

KANFER, J. N., and R. O. BRADY: Studies on the structure of gangliosides. I. On the linkage of N-acetyl neuraminic acid in monosialoganglioside. Biochem. biophys. Res. Commun. 11, 267 (1963).

— R. S. BLACKLOW, L. WARREN, and R. O. BRADY: The enzymatic synthesis of gangliosides. Biochem. biophys. Res. Commun. 14, 287 (1964).

KARLSSON, K. Å.: Studies on sphingosines. 3. C_{20}-dihydrosphingosine, a hitherto unknown sphingosine. Acta chem. scand. 18, 565 (1964).

— Studies on sphingosines. 4. Composition of sphingomyelins from human plasma. Proc. biochem. Soc. 92, 39 (1964).

KATAOKA, T.: Sulfur metabolism of the nervous system. III. Incorporation of S^{35} into sulfur-containing lipids of the brain following intracisternal injection of sodium sulfate-S^{35}. Nara Igaku Zasshi 13, 7 (1962).

KISHIMOTO, Y., and N. S. RADIN: Structures of the 2-hydroxy unsaturated fatty acids of pig brain sphingolipids. J. Lipid Res. 5, 94 (1964).

KISS, J., G. FODOR, and D. BANFI: Zurückführung der Konfiguration des (natürlichen) Sphingosins auf die der D-erythro-2-amino-3,4-dioxy-Buttersäure. 12. Mitteilung über Sphingosin und Sphingolipoide. Helv. chim. Acta 37, 1471 (1954).

KLENK, E.: Über Sphingosin (10. Mitteilung über Cerebroside). Hoppe-Seylers Z. physiol. Chem. 185, 169 (1929).

— Beiträge zur Chemie der Lipoidosen. 3. Niemann-Picksche Krankheit und amaurotische Idiotie. Hoppe-Seylers Z. physiol. Chem. 262, 128 (1939).

— u. H. FAILLARD: Über Sphingosin. Hoppe-Seylers Z. physiol. Chem. 299, 48 (1955).

— u. W. GIELEN: Zur Kenntnis der Ganglioside des Gehirns. Hoppe-Seylers Z. physiol. Chem. 319, 283 (1960).

— — Über ein chromatographisch einheitliches hexosaminhaltiges Gangliosid aus Menschengehirn. Hoppe-Seylers Z. physiol. Chem. 326, 158 (1961).

— — and G. PADBERG, in S. M. ARONSON, and B. W. VOLK: Cerebral Sphingolipidoses, p. 301 New York: Academic Press, Inc. 1962.

— U. W. HENDRICKS, u. W. GIELEN: β-D-galaktosido-(1→3)-N-acetyl-D-Galaktosamine in kristallisiertem Disaccharid aus menschlichen Gehirngangliosiden. Hoppe-Seylers Z. physiol. Chem. 330, 140 (1963a).

— — — Über ein zweites hexosaminhaltiges Gangliosid aus Menschengehirn. Hoppe-Seylers Z. physiol. Chem. 330, 218 (1963b).

— U. LIEDTKE, u. W. GIELEN: Das Gangliosid des Gehirns bei der infantilen amaurotischen Idiotie vom Typ Tay-Sachs. Hoppe-Seylers Z. physiol. Chem. 334, 186 (1963).

— u. F. RENNKAMP: Über die Ganglioside und Cerebroside der Rindermilz. Hoppe-Seylers Z. physiol. Chem. 273, 253 (1942).

— in H. WAELSCH: Biochemistry of the Developing Nervous System. p. 397 New York: Academic Press Inc. 1961.

KOCHETKOV, N. K., I. G. ZHUKOVA, and I. S. GLUKGODED: Sphingoplasmalogens. A new type of sphingolipids. Biochim. biophys. Acta (Amst.) 70, 716 (1963).

— — — Sphingoplasmalogens, a new type of sphingolipid. Biokhima 29, 570 (1964).

Koch, W.: Zur Kenntnis der Schwefelverbindungen des Nervensystems. Hoppe-Seylers Z. physiol. Chem. 53, 496 (1907).

Kopaczyk, K. C., and N. S. Radin: Metabolic conversions of cerebroside by brain. Fed. Proc. 23, 230 (1964).

— — In vivo conversions of cerebroside and ceramide in rat brain. J. Lipid Res. 6, 140 (1965).

Korey, S. R., and A. Stein: A gangliosidase system. Fed. Proc. 21, 283 (1962).

— — A Gangliosidase System. Brain lipids and lipoproteins and the leucodystrophies, p. 71. Amsterdam: Elsevier 1963a.

— and J. Gonatas: Separation of human brain glycolipids. Life Sciences 5, 296 (1963b).

— — and A. Stein: Studies on Tay-Sachs disease. III. Biochemistry. A. Analytic and metabolic aspects. J. Neuropath. exp. Neurol. 22, 56 (1963c).

— and A. Stein: Studies in Tay-Sachs diseases. III. Biochemistry. Catabolism of gangliosides and related compounds. J. Neuropath. exp. Neurol. 22, 67 (1963d).

Kuhn, R., H. Egge, R. Brossmer, A. Gauche, P. Klesse, W. Lochinger, E. Röhm, u. H. Trischmann: Über die Ganglioside des Gehirns. Angew. Chemie 72, 805 (1960).

— — Über Ergebnisse der Permethylierung der Ganglioside G_I and G_{II}. Chem. Ber. 96, 3338 (1963c).

— u. H. Weigandt: Die Konstitution der Ganglio-N-Tetraose und des Gangliosids G_1. Chem. Ber. 96, 866 (1963a).

— — Die Konstitution der Ganglioside G_{II}, G_{III}, und G_{IV}. Z. Naturforsch. 18 b, 541 (1963).

— — Weitere Ganglioside aus Menschenhirn. Z. Naturforsch. 19 b, 256 (1964).

Kunan, W. H.: Über die Struktur von zwei hexosaminhaltigen Gangliosiden aus menschlichem Gehirn. Dissertation Köln 1964.

Landing, B. H.: Familial Neuroviceral Lipidosis. Amer. J. Dis. Child. 108, 503 (1964).

— and J. H. Rubenstein: Biopsy diagnosis of neurological diseases in childhood with emphasis on lipidosis. In S. M. Aronson and B. W. Volk (Editors): Cerebral Sphingolipidoses p. 1. New York: Academic Press 1962.

Landsteiner, K., and P. A. Levene: Observations on the specific part of the heterogenetic antigen. J. Immunol. 10, 731 (1925).

Lees, M. B., and H. W. Moser: The chemical pathology of Krabbe Disease and Metachromatic Leucodystrophy. In S. M. Aronson, and B. W. Volk (Editors): Cerebral Sphingolipidosis, p. 179. New York: Academic Press, 1962.

Leloir, L. F., and C. E. Cardini: Enzymes acting on glucosamine phosphates. Biochim. biophys. Acta (Amst.) 20, 33 (1956).

Levene, P. A., and C. J. West: On sphingosine. III. The oxidation of sphingosine and dihydrosphingosine. J. biol. Chem. 18, 481 (1914.)

Makita, A., and T. Yamakawa: The glycolipids of the brain of Tay-Sachs disease. The chemical structures of a globoside and main ganglioside. Jap. J. exp. Med. 33, 361 (1963).

Maley, G. F., and H. A. Lardy: The synthesis of α-D-glucosamine-1-phosphate and N-acetyl-α-D-glucosamine-1-phosphate. Enzymatic formation of uridine diphosphoglucosamine. J. Amer. chem. Soc. 78, 5303 (1956).

Marinetti, G., and E. Stotz: Studies on the structure of sphingomyelin IV. Configuration of the double bond in sphingomyelin and related lipids and a study of their infrared spectra. J. Amer. chem. Soc. 76, 1347 (1954).

McKhann, G. M., R. Levy, and W. Ho: Biosynthesis of Sulfatides in Rat Brain. Fed. Proc. 24, 360 (1965).

Mehl, E., u. H. Jatzkewitz: Über ein Cerebrosid-Schwefelsäureester spaltendes Enzym aus Schweineniere. Sonderdruck Hoppe-Seylers Z. physiol. Chem. 331, 292 (1963).

Mislow, K.: The geometry of sphingosine. J. Amer. chem. Soc. 74, 5155 (1953).

Morozova, M. S., and M. Promyslov: On the problem of enzymatic splitting of cerebrosides of the brain. Bull. exp. biol. Med. (USSR.) 50, 44 (1960).

Moser, H. W., and M. L. Karnovsky: Studies on the biosynthesis of glycolipids and other lipids of the brain. J. biol. Chem. 234, 1990 (1959).

Mueller, K. L.: Thesis, Master of Science, University of Illinois 1953.

Norman, R. M.: Tay-Sachs Disease with visceral involvement and its relationship to Niemann-Pick's disease. J. Path. Bact. 78, 409 (1959).

O'Brien, J. S.: A molecular defect of myelination. Biochem. biophys. Res. Commun. 15, 484 (1964).

— M. B. Stern, B. H. Landing, J. K. O'Brien, and G. N. Donnell: Generalized Gangliosidosis. Amer. J. Dis. Child. 109, 338 (1965).

Oda, T.: Components of penicillin-producing moulds. II. Fungus cerebrin. Pharm. Soc. jap. 72, 136, 139, 142 (1952).

Pilz,'H., u. H. Jatzkewitz: Dünnschichtchromatographische Bestimmungen von C-$_{18}$ und C$_{24}$-Sphingomyelin in normalen und pathologischen Gehirnen einschließlich eines Falles von Niemann-Pickscher Erkrankung. J. Neurochem. 11, 603 (1964).

POGELL, B. M., and R. GRYDER: Enzymatic synthesis of glucosamine 6-phosphate in rat liver. J. biol. Chem. **228**, 701 (1957).

PROSTENIK, M., and N. Z. STANACEV: Studies in the series of sphingolipids. X. The structure of yeast cerebrin base. Chem. Ber. **91**, 961 (1958).

— and B. MAJHOFER-ORESCANIN: Occurrence of a new sphingolipid base C_{20}-sphingosine in horse and beef brain. Naturwissenschaften **47**, 399 (1960).

PUTMAN, E. W., and W. Z. HASSID: Structure of galactosylglycerol from *Irideae laminarioides*. J. Amer. chem. Soc. **76**, 2221 (1954).

RADIN, N. S., F. B. LAVIN, and J. R. BROWN: Determination of cerebrosides. J. biol. Chem. **217**, 789 (1955).

— F. B. MARTIN, and J. R. BROWN: Galactolipid metabolism. J. biol. Chem. **224**, 499 (1957).

RAPPORT, M. M., L. GRAF, L. A. AUTILIO, and W. T. NORTON: Immunochemical studies of organ and tumor lipids: XIV. Galactocerebroside determinants in the myelin sheath of the central nervous system. J. Neurochem. **11**, 855 (1964).

— — and N. F. ALONZO: Immunochemical studies of organ and tumor lipids: VIII. Comparison of human tumor and ox spleen cytosides. J. Lipid Res. **1**, 301 (1960).

— — V. P. SKIPSKI, and N. F. ALONZO: Cytolipin H, a pure lipid hapten isolated from human carcinoma. Nature (Lond.) **181**, 1803 (1958).

— — and J. YARIV: Immunochemical studies of organ and tumor lipids: IX. Configuration of the carbohydrate residues in cytolipin H. Arch. Biochem. **92**, 438 (1961a).

— V. P. SKIPSKI, and C. C. SWEELEY: The lipid residues in cytolipin H. J. Lipid Res. **2**, 148 (1961b).

ROBBINS, P. W., and F. LIPMANN: The enzymatic sequence in the biosynthesis of active sulfate. J. Amer. chem. Soc. **78**, 6409 (1956).

— — Separation of the two enzymatic phases in active sulfate synthesis. J. biol. Chem. **233**, 681 (1958a).

— — Enzymatic synthesis of adenosine-5'-phosphosulfate. J. biol. Chem. **233**, 686 (1958b).

ROSEMAN, S.: Enzymatic synthesis of cytidine-5'-monophosphozialic acids. Proc. nat. Acad. Sci. (Wash.) **48**, 437 (1962).

ROSENBERG, A., and N. STERN: Changes in the lipid components of the gangliosides of developing brain. Fed. Proc. **24**, 360 (1965).

SAMBASIVARAO, K., and R. H. MCCLUER: Lipid components of gangliosides. J. Lipid Res. **5**, 103 (1964).

SAMMARTINO, V.: Über die Chemie der Lunge. I. Mitteilung. Biochem. Z. **124**, 234 (1921).

SANDHOFF, K., H. PILZ u. H. JATZKEWITZ: Über den enzymatischen Abbau von N-acetyl-neuraminsäurefreien Gangliosidresten (Ceramid-Oligosacchariden). Hoppe-Seylers Z. physiol. Chem. **338**, 281 (1964).

SCHEINBERG, L. C., M. W. KIES, and E. C. ALVORD jr.: Research in Demyelinating Diseases. Ann. N. Y. Acad. Sci. **122**, 1—570 (1965).

SCHMITZ, H., V. R. POTTER, R. B. HURLBERT, and D. M. WHITE: Alternative pathways of glucose metabolism. II. Nucleotides from the acid soluble fraction of normal and tumor tissues and studies on nucleic acid synthesis in tumors. Cancer Res. **14**, 66 (1954).

SODA, T.: in S. AKABORI, ed., Textbook of Enzymological Methods II. 73 (1956). Tokyo: Asakura Press.

SOMERS, J. E., J. N. KANFER, and R. O. BRADY: Immunochemical studies with gangliosides. II. Investigations of the structure of gangliosides by the hapten inhibition technique. Biochemistry **3**, 251 (1964).

SOURANDER, P., and L. SVENNERHOLM: Sulphatide lipidosis in the adult with the clinical picture of progressive organic dementia with epileptic seizures. Acta neuropath. (Berl.) **1**, 384 (1962).

SPRINSON, D. B., and A. COULON: The precursors of sphingosine in brain tissue. J. biol. Chem. **207**, 585 (1954).

SRIBNEY, M., and E. P. KENNEDY: The enzymatic synthesis of sphingomyelin. J. biol. Chem. **233**, 1315 (1958).

STANACEV, N. Z., and E. CHARGAFF: Icosisphingosine, a long chain base constituent of mucolipids. Biochem. biophys. Acta (Amst.) **59**, 733 (1962).

STANBURY, J. B., and D. S. FREDRICKSON: The metabolic basis of inherited disease. New York: McGraw Hill Book Co. 1960.

STODOLA, F. H., and L. J. WICKERHAM: Formation of extracellular sphingolipids by microorganisms. II. Structural studies on tetraacetylphytosphingosine from the yeast Hansenula ciferrii. J. biol. Chem. **235**, 2584 (1960).

— — C. R. SCHOLFIELD, and H. J. DUTTON: Formation of extracellular sphingolipids by microorganisms. II. Triacetyl dihydrosphingosine, a metabolic product of the yeast Hansenula ciferrii. Arch. Biochem. **98**, 176 (1962).

STOFFYN, P., and A. STOFFYN: Structure of sulfatides. Biochem. biophys. Acta (Amst.) 70, 218 (1963).

STROMINGER, J. L.: Uridine diphosphate acetylglucosamine phosphate and uridine diphosphate acetylglucosamine sulfate. Biochem. biophys. Acta (Amst.) 17, 283 (1955).

SUOMI, W. D., and B. W. AGRANOFF: Identification and estimation of glycolipids of the spleen in Gauchers' disease. Fed. Proc. 23, 375 (1964).

SUZUKI, K.: Incorporation of D-glucose-U-C^{14} into gangliosides in a cell-free system. Biochem. biophys. Res. Commun. 16, 88 (1964).

— and S. R. KOREY: Incorporation of D-(C^{14}) glucose into individual gangliosides. Biochem. biophys. Acta (Amst.) 78, 388 (1963).

SVENNERHOLM, L.: The chemical structure of normal human brain and Tay-Sachs gangliosides. Biochem. biophys. Res. Commun. 9, 436 (1962).

— Chromatographic separation of human brain gangliosides. J. Neurochem. 10, 613 (1963).

SWEELEY, C. C., and B. KLIONSKY: Fabry's disease: Classification as a sphingolipidosis and partial characterization of a novel glycolipid. J. biol. Chem. 238, 3148 (1963).

TAKETOMI, T., and T. YAMAKAWA: Immunochemical studies on lipids. I. Preparation and immunochemical properties of synthetic psychosine-protein antigens. J. Biochem. (Tokyo) 54, 444 (1963).

— — Further confirmation on the structure of brain cerebroside sulfuric ester. J. Biochem. (Tokyo) 55, 87 (1964).

— — Antigenic properties of synthetic protein complexes with glycolipids and related substances. Abstract, American Oil Chemists Society Symposium on Glycolipids and the Nervous System 1965.

THANNHAUSER, S. J., and M. REICHEL: Studies on animal lipids. X. The nature of cerebrosidase. Its relation to the splitting of polydiaminophosphatide by polydiaminophosphatase. J. biol. Chem. 113, 311 (1936).

THUDICUM, J. W. L.: A treatise on the chemical composition of the brain. London: Builliere, Tindall, and Cox 1884.

TRAMS, E. G., and C. J. LAUTER: On the isolation and characterization of gangliosides. Biochem. biophys. Acta (Amst.) 60, 350 (1962).

VAN BOGAERT, L., J. N. CUMMING, and A. LOWENTHAL (Editors): Cerebral Lipidosis. Springfield (Ill.): Thomas 1957.

VOLK, B. W., and W. D. SPERRY (Editors): Symposium on Amaurotic Family Idiocy. Amer. J. Dis. Child. 97, 655 (1959).

WARREN, L., and H. FELSENFELD: N-acetylmannosamine-6-phosphate on N-acetylneuraminic acid-9-phosphate as intermediates in sialic acid biosynthesis. Biochem. biophys. Res. Commun. 5, 185 (1961).

— — The biosynthesis of sialic acids. J. biol. Chem. 237, 1421 (1962).

WEISS, S. B., and E. P. KENNEDY: The function of cytidine coenzymes in the biosynthesis of phospholipids. J. biol. Chem. 222, 193 (1956).

WICKERHAM, L. J., and F. H. STODOLA: Formation of extracellular sphingolipids by microorganisms. J. Bact. 80, 484 (1960).

WILLIAMS, H. H., H. GALBRAITH, M. KANCHER, E. Z. MOYER, A. J. RICHARDS, and I. G. MACY: The effect of growth on the lipid composition of rat tissues. J. biol. Chem. 161, 475 (1945).

WILSON, L. G., and R. S. BANDURSKI: An enzymatic reaction involving adenosine triphosphate and selenate. Arch. Biochem. 62, 503 (1956).

— Enzymatic reactions involving sulfate, sulfite, selenate, and molybdate. J. biol. Chem. 233, 975 (1958).

WITTENBERG, J. B.: In S. R. KOREY (Editor): The Biology of Myelin, p. 296. New York: Hoeber-Harper Book 1959.

YAMAKAWA, T., N. KISO, S. HANDA, A. MAKITA, and S. YOKOYAMA: On the structure of brain cerebroside sulfuric ester and ceramide dihexoside of erythrocytes. J. Biochem. 52, 226 (1962).

YOKOYAMA, M., E. G. TRAMS, and R. O. BRADY: Sphingolipid antibodies in sera of animals and patients with central nervous system lesions. J. Immunol. 90, 372 (1963).

ZABIN, I.: Biosynthesis of ceramide by rat-brain homogenates. J. Amer. chem. Soc. 79, 5834 (1957).

— and J. F. MEAD: The biosynthesis of sphingosine. J. biol. Chem. 205, 271 (1953).

— — The biosynthesis of sphingosine. II. The utilization of methyl-labeled acetate, formate, and ethanolamine. J. biol. Chem. 211, 87 (1954).

Lipoproteins

By

David G. Cornwell

Introduction

Early investigators interested in lipid extraction and protein isolation recognized that protein-lipid complexes exist in plasma. Protein-lipid complexes were discussed in the classical extraction studies of SCHULZ (1897), NERKING (1901), and SHIMIDZU (1910). Protein chemists such as HARDY (1905), HASLAM (1913), CHICK (1914), and BANG (1918) accumulated considerable data on protein-lipid complexes. Subsequent investigators were more concerned with the properties of pure lipids and pure proteins than with the properties of heterogeneous protein-lipid complexes which were difficult to distinguish from isolation artifacts. Only a few significant studies were published in the decades between 1920 and 1940. A notable series of experiments on the isolation of pure lipoproteins was begun by MACHEBOEUF in 1929 (MACHEBOEUF and REBEYROTTE 1949). These studies demonstrated the feasibility of lipoprotein purification; however, biochemical techniques were not adequate for rigorous investigations of complex macromolecules such as lipoproteins.

Lipoprotein research was stimulated by the development and general availability since 1940 of ultracentrifugation, electrophoresis, and large scale fractionation procedures. An important ultracentrifugation technique was introduced by GOFMAN, LINDGREN, and ELLIOTT in 1949. These investigators showed that the anomalous schlieren patterns which had been obtained with whole serum (McFARLANE 1935, PEDERSEN 1945) were explained by an unusual Johnston-Ogston effect involving lipoproteins. Ultracentrifugal flotation in solutions of increased density eliminated the anomalous schlieren pattern. Flotation techniques are now the basis of many analytical and preparative methods.

Multi-variable or cold-ethanol precipitation techniques yielded plasma protein fractions rich in lipoprotein (ONCLEY et al. 1949). These isolation procedures were extremely important. They demonstrated that physical properties such as solubility could be studied with lipoproteins as well as other proteins. Electrophoretic mobilities and specific refractive increments of lipoproteins were shown to be measurable properties (ARMSTRONG et al. 1947a and 1947b). A detailed analysis of lipoprotein composition was undertaken (ONCLEY et al. 1950).

Analytical methods employing paper electrophoresis (for bibliography see PEZOLD 1961) have been used in lipoprotein research since the introduction of Sudan Black B as a lipid stain (SWAHN 1952). Paper electrophoresis is a deceptively simple technique. The analysis of electrophoretic data is more complex. While a number of important studies have been published, it has sometimes been difficult to interpret data showing arbitrary ratios between partially separated and poorly characterized serum lipoproteins whose concentrations were estimated by non-specific staining.

The isolation, composition, properties, and analysis of different plasma lipoprotein classes will be discussed in this chapter. Other reviews are suggested for information on the specialized topics of bonding forces and structure in protein-lipid complexes (SALEM 1962, BANGHAM 1963, VANDENHEUVEL 1963, CORNWELL and HORROCKS 1964, ELBERS 1964, THOMPSON 1964) and lipoprotein lipase (VAUGHN and KORN 1962, ROBINSON 1963, ZEMPLÉNYI 1964, RODBELL and SCOW 1964). A complete literature survey has not been included since a number of general reviews are available (LINDGREN and NICHOLS 1960, PEZOLD 1961, CORNWELL and KRUGER 1961a, DOLE and HAMLIN 1962, FREEMAN et al. 1963, ONCLEY 1963 and 1964).

Composition and Properties of Plasma Lipoproteins

1. Definition of a Lipoprotein Class. The most striking aspect of plasma lipoprotein preparations is their heterogeneity. Heterogeneity can be described by a number of physical parameters although the flotation rate (S_f) is the most readily determined parameter. The wide S_f distribution within a lipoprotein class reflects major variations in both size and density which render the exact definition of the lipoprotein class difficult. The usual criteria of purity and homogeneity are not applicable. With lipoproteins, purity generally means the absence of easily recognized plasma protein contaminants while the concept of homogeneity is replaced by the concept of similarity in structure, function, and the composition of protein components. It is highly probable that specific procedures will be developed for the isolation of lipoprotein molecules with many of the properties of a homogeneous protein preparation. These procedures are not available at the present time.

The following criteria are suggested for the definition of a lipoprotein class:

1. The lipoprotein class can be isolated by two different procedures.

2. The two fractions which are isolated have the same composition and properties.

3. Lipoprotein classes are not arbitrary segments of an S_f, density, or size continuum. Population distributions for at least two physical properties in one lipoprotein class are distinct from and not continuous with population distributions for the same physical properties in a different lipoprotein class.

4. Lipoprotein classes differ in their metabolism.

Four lipoprotein classes, chylomicrons ($\varrho = 0.94$), very low density lipoproteins ($\varrho = 0.98$), low density lipoproteins ($\varrho = 1.03$), and high density lipoproteins ($\varrho = 1.12$) satisfy these criteria. Lipoprotein classes with densities of 1.02 and 1.05 have also been suggested (ONCLEY 1963); however, their isolation, composition, and properties have not been studied in detail. A number of additional lipoprotein fractions such as S_f 12—20, S_f 20—100 and S_f 100—400 lipoproteins are frequently discussed in the literature (LINDGREN and NICHOLS 1960, CORNWELL and KRUGER 1961a, PEZOLD 1961, FASOLI 1963, HARLAN and BEISCHER 1963, GOFMAN and YOUNG 1963, BARCLAY et al. 1964). An S_f determined in the analytical ultracentrifuge is not sufficient evidence for the existence of a distinct lipoprotein class. In the normal human, these fractions probably represent segments of the S_f continuum within a plasma lipoprotein class. Procedures for estimating distributions in physical properties have not been generally applied to the analysis of lipoproteins in pathological states. The concentration of a minor lipoprotein class may be enhanced or new lipoprotein classes may be synthesized. The specific elevation of different segments of an S_f continuum suggests that new and as yet undefined lipoprotein classes are present in pathological states.

2. Homogeneity: Distribution in Size and Shape. In 1950, SHARP and BEARD demonstrated that Stokes' law could be used to determine the size of spherical latex particles of known density. Particles were sedimented in solvents with various densities and their size calculated from an equation relating the radius of the particle (r), the density of the particle (ϱ), the density of the solvent (ϱ_s), and the viscosity of the solvent (η).

$$4/3\,\pi\,r^3\,(\varrho-\varrho_s)\,\omega^2\chi = 6\,\pi\,\eta\,r\frac{d\chi}{dt} \tag{1}$$

Sedimentation velocity (S) is defined by the equation:

$$S = \frac{1}{\omega^2\chi}\frac{d\chi}{dt} \tag{2}$$

Equation (1) may then be expressed as a relationship between S, r, and $\varDelta\varrho$, the difference between particle and solvent densities.

$$2\,r^2\,(\varrho-\varrho_s) = 9\,\eta\,S \tag{3}$$

Good agreement was obtained between sedimentation velocity and other sizing measurements for particles 253 mμ in diameter. This diameter is in the same size range as the chylomicron particle.

DOLE and HAMLIN (1962) used Stokes' law to describe the lower limit of particle size for chylomicron fractions separated by ultracentrifugal flotation under carefully controlled conditions. They related the distance of flotation (χ) and the particle diameter (d) to $\varDelta\varrho/\eta$ and $\omega^2\chi\,\varDelta t$ or Gmin.

$$\frac{\chi}{d^2} = (3.27 \times 10^{-10})\left(\frac{\varDelta\varrho}{\eta}\right)(G\text{min}) \tag{4}$$

Two nomograms were prepared. The first calculated χ/d^2 as a function of $\varDelta\varrho/\eta$ and Gmin. The second calculated d as a function of χ. These nomograms are extremely important since they facilitate particle size calculations for the many different chylomicron fractions which have been described in the literature (CORNWELL and KRUGER 1961a, DOLE and HAMLIN 1962). DOLE and HAMLIN correctly emphasize that chylomicron preparations should be described by the Gmin. used and the particle size limit obtained.

The particle size limit is estimated by equation (4); however, this equation does not give the particle size distribution within the floating chylomicron fraction. PINTER and ZILVERSMIT (1962) and ZILVERSMIT (1963) have described an important and readily applied method for estimating the particle size distribution. They employed ultracentrifugal-flotation in concentrated sucrose gradients. Linear sucrose gradients were prepared so that density and viscosity at a point within the gradient were described by the equations:

$$\varrho_\chi = \alpha\,(\chi_0-\chi) + \varrho_0 \tag{5}$$

and

$$\eta_\chi = \beta\,(\chi_0-\chi) + \eta_0 \tag{6}$$

where χ_0 is the layer at which the sample was introduced, ϱ_0 and η_0. are the density and viscosity of the gradient at this layer, and α and β are constants characteristic of the gradient. The particle diameter in the layer at distance χ was estimated from the algebraic integration of equation (1) and the substitution of values for ϱ_χ, η_χ and Gmin. A population distribution was then obtained by the chemical analysis of gradient segments. Concentration effects were overcome in part by population distributions obtained with dilute solutions containing isotopically labeled chylomicrons. The sucrose gradient has a significant advantage in measuring the particle size distribution. Flotation rate is directly proportional to $\varDelta\varrho$ (equation 3). The variation in S obtained by small differences in particle density is less important where $\varDelta\varrho$ is large than where $\varDelta\varrho$ is small or particle and solvent are near the same density.

Chylomicron particles have very large S_f values which are difficult to measure in the analytical ultracentrifuge. The other lipoprotein classes have lower S_f values which reflect their smaller size and increased density. Homogeneity within these lipoprotein classes may be estimated by analytical ultracentrifugation. Several methods have been proposed for measuring the S distribution in a heterogeneous population from data on boundary spreading. WILLIAMS et al. (1952) described a procedure for estimating the weight fraction of material, $g(S)$, with sedimentation coefficients between S and dS. This distribution function is represented by the equation

$$g(S) = \frac{1}{|C^0|} \frac{dc}{ds} \tag{7}$$

where C^0 is the total concentration of the protein fraction. Boundary spreading caused by diffusion was eliminated from the $g(S)$ analysis which then indicated heterogeneity in size, shape, and density. The theoretical and practical limitations of this procedure have been discussed by SCHACHMAN (1959) and CLAESSON and MORING-CLAESSON (1961).

The $g(S)$ distribution within the S_f limits of a lipoprotein class was first measured by ONCLEY, WALTON, and CORNWELL (1957). The very low density lipoprotein class showed an S_f continuum between S_f 10 and S_f 80. Preliminary studies indicated that the S_f range for this lipoprotein class in hyperlipemic subjects with nephrosis extended beyond S_f 200 although the maximum for the $g(S)$ distribution function occurred in the S_f 40 to S_f 60 range (ONCLEY and CORNWELL, unpublished observations). The low density lipoprotein class showed an S_f continuum between S_f 3 and S_f 9. When this lipoprotein class was subfractionated in a density gradient (MANNICK 1955), a $g(S)$ distribution analysis demonstrated that the sub-fractions belonged to the same lipoprotein population even though there were small differences in the $g(S)$ maxima.

Since lipoproteins are nearly spherical in shape, boundary spreading tends to reflect variations in size and density. ONCLEY and his associates have estimated the variations in these parameters by detailed $g(S)$ distribution analyses. Heterogeneity in size was evaluated from flotation experiments in solvents which gave a large $\Delta \varrho$ term. Heterogeneity in density was evaluated from flotation experiments in solvents with a density near the mean density of the lipoprotein class which gave a small $\Delta \varrho$ term. Very low density (ONCLEY and NUMA, unpublished observations), low density (TORO-GOYCO 1958), and high density lipoproteins (ALLERTON 1962) have been examined. The results of these studies are summarized in two recent reviews (ONCLEY 1963 and 1964). They represent the only adequate physical description of lipoprotein homogeneity that is now available and should be extended to the lipoprotein classes isolated in pathological states.

3. Chylomicrons. These lipid particles are the vehicle for the transport of exogenous triglyceride from the alimentary tract to the blood via the chyle. A number of flotation procedures for their isolation have been described. The initial uncertainty in definition led to discrepancies in the literature. Thus "chylomicrons" isolated by flotation at 0.8×10^6 Gmin. reflected dietary lipid (BRAGDON and KARMEN 1960) while "chylomicrons" isolated at 3×10^6 Gmin. were not affected by dietary lipid (DOLE et al. 1959). These discrepancies were resolved with the definition of chylomicrons or "alimentary particles" by a Gmin. term or their size limit (DOLE and HAMLIN 1962), polyvinyl pyrrolidone flocculation (BURSTEIN and PRAWERMAN 1958, GORDIS 1962), and the distribution in a sucrose gradient (PINTER and ZILVERSMIT 1962). Plasma chylomicrons, 0.4×10^6 Gmin., approached alimentary lipid in composition while smaller particles, 3×10^6 Gmin., retained a fatty acid pattern more characteristic of endogenous lipid (BIERMAN

et al. 1962). The contribution of alimentary lipid to chylomicron composition was later confirmed with fat particles isolated from rat lymph, 1.8×10^6 Gmin., although the dilution of exogenous lipid with endogenous lipid was surprisingly large (KARMEN et al. 1963, WHYTE et al. 1963).

Representative data on the physical properties of chylomicron and very low density lipoprotein classes are compared in Table 1. It is apparent that chylomicrons are readily separated from very low density lipoproteins by ultracentrifugal flotation. The data suggest that a class of particulate lipid, secondary particles, which are distinct from primary particles or chylomicrons, exists in plasma

Table 1. *Physical properties of chylomicrons, secondary particles, and very low density lipoproteins*

	Chylomicrons	Secondary Particles	Very Low Density Lipoproteins		Reference
G min.	9×10^4 0.3×10^6 0.4×10^6	3×10^6	120×10^6		SCANU and PAGE 1959 CORNWELL et al. 1961 b BIERMAN et al. 1962
S_f	10,000 1000* $10,000 \pm 5,000$	400*	100 ± 60 30 ± 8		SCANU and PAGE 1959 BIERMAN et al. 1962 ONCLEY 1963
ϱ	0.94 0.93		0.96 0.99		PINTER and ZILVERSMIT 1963 ONCLEY 1963
$d\,(m\mu)$	200* 500 180—270** 1500—100	70*	20—70 54 27		BIERMAN et al. 1962 ONCLEY 1963 ZILVERSMIT 1963 FRENCH 1963

* Lower limit for the fraction.
** Diameter for most frequently occurring particle.

(BIERMAN et al. 1962). If ultracentrifugal flotation were the only evidence for this new class, it would be considered as an isolation artifact containing chylomicrons and very low density lipoproteins. However, secondary particles flocculate and sediment in a polyvinyl pyrrolidone (PVP) gradient while chylomicrons flocculate and float, and very low density lipoprotein are unchanged (BIERMAN et al. 1962). Furthermore, secondary particles migrate as β-globulins in free and starch block electrophoresis (BIERMAN et al. 1962, NYE 1964) while chylomicrons mirgate as α_2-globulins or albumin in free and starch block electrophoresis (CORNWELL and KRUGER 1961a, DOLE and HAMLIN 1962, NYE 1964) and very low density lipoproteins migrate as α_2-globulins in starch block electrophoresis (KUNKEL and TRAUTMAN 1956). There is some evidence that the lactescence observed in several types of hyperlipemia is caused by secondary particles. For example, secondary particles may explain the β-globulin component found in the chylomicron fraction of subjects with a nephrotic hyperlipemia (SWAHN 1953) and a subject with essential hyperlipemia (CARLSON and OLHAGEN 1954). Chylomicron composition differs significantly from the 1.3×10^6 Gmin. fraction isolated in essential hyperlipemia (JOBST and SCHETTLER 1956) and the 0.3×10^6 Gmin. fraction isolated in diabetic hyperlipemia (CORNWELL et al. 1961 b). Analyses reported for 0.3×10^6 Gmin. fractions suggest that ultracentrifugal flotation will not separate the two paticulate classes in hyperlipemic states. AHRENS and SPRITZ (1963) and NYE (1964) recently separated the chylomicrons of fat-induced lipemia from the secondary particles of carbohydrate-induced lipemia with a PVP gradient technique. This technique should be employed in the investigation of hyperlipemic states. Fractions which resemble chylomicrons and secondary particles have been isolated by flotation for 0.1×10^6 Gmin. and

0.6 X 10⁶ Gmin. (GUSTAFSON et al. 1965). These investigators describe the two
fractions as part of the heterogeneous very low density lipoprotein continuum;
however most workers consider chylomicrons a distinct class.

The chemical composition of human and dog chylomicrons is described in
Table 2. Significant variations in composition, especially protein content, were
obtained when chylomicrons were separated in sucrose gradients (YOKOYAMA and
ZILVERSMIT 1965). The origin and nature of chylomicron protein is an intriguing
and as yet unsolved problem. High density lipoproteins were first suggested as
components of the chylomicron molecule (RODBELL and FREDRICKSON 1959,

Table 2. *Composition of chylomicrons in weight percent*

Source	Particle Size mμ	Protein	T. G.	P. L.	Cholesterol Free	Cholesterol Ester	Reference
Human	—	2.0	84.0	7.0	2.0	5.0	ONCLEY 1963
Human	> 300	2.1	86.5	9.2	4.4		SCANU and PAGE 1959
Human	—	2.5	—	9.0	0.8	1.7	WOOD et al. 1964
Human	> 257	1.1	88.7	4.3	2.1	3.9	GUSTAFSON et al. 1965
Dog	> 60	2.4	86.4	8.5	0.8	1.7	HAVEL and FREDRICKSON 1956
Dog	> 200	0.6	95.3	3.8	0.6	0.5 ⎫	
	140—200	1.8	92.0	6.3	0.9	0.7 ⎬ YOKOYAMA and ZILVERSMIT 1965
	< 140	2.3	88.3	9.1	1.5	1.2 ⎭	

SCANU and PAGE 1959). Recent observations on the impaired transport of alimentary lipid in a hereditary low density lipoprotein deficiency (SALT et al. 1960,
POLONOVSKI et al. 1961, ISSELBACHER et al. 1964), normal fat transport in a high
density lipoprotein deficiency (FREDRICKSON 1961), and the inhibition of both
chylomicron (ISSELBACHER and BUDZ 1963) and low density lipoprotein (ROBIN-
SON and SEAKINS 1963) synthesis with puromycin all suggest that chylomicrons
and low density lipoproteins are closely related in their metabolism.

In metabolic studies, chylomicrons are generally isolated from the lymph after
cannulation of the thoracic duct. It should be remembered that chylomicron lipids
such as free cholesterol exchange with lipoprotein lipid when chylomicrons enter
the blood (GOODMAN 1962, LOSSOW et al. 1962). The free cholesterol content of
chylomicrons increases on incubation with serum (MINARI and ZILVERSMIT 1963,
CHEVALLIER and MATHE 1964). Phospholipids exhibit considerable exchange and
a net loss from chylomicrons through transfer to the high density lipoproteins
(MINARI and ZILVERSMIT 1963). Net lipid transfer may explain the appearance of
orally administered vitamin A ester and tocopherol in low density lipoproteins
(KRINSKY et al. 1958, McCORMICK et al. 1960, PELKONEN 1963). It is interesting
that β-carotene is either not transferred in the same manner or absorbed by a
different route (CORNWELL et al. 1962a).

4. Very Low Density and Low Density Lipoproteins. Although very low density
and low density lipoproteins represent two distinct lipoprotein classes, they share
several properties and are closely related in their metabolism. These two classes
will be discussed together. The very low density lipoproteins may contain two sub-
classes, S_f 100 ± 60 and S_f 30 ± 8 (Table 1), with different mean densities and
molecular weights estimated as 5 X 10⁷ and 6 X 10⁶ respectively (ONCLEY 1963).
These sub-classes have not been separated and analyzed as independent fractions.
Subfractions have been isolated by ultracentrifugal flotation (GUSTAFSON et al. 1965)
but these subfractions are probably arbitrary segments of the very low density
lipoprotein continuum. It may be possible to separate the sub-classes by selective

precipitation with solutions of varying ionic strength and PVP concentration (BUR-
STEIN and PRAWERMAN 1959). New separation methods will be important since
delipidization studies suggest that several different protein residues may exist
in the very low density lipoprotein class (GUSTAFSON et al. 1964). The presence of
both low and high density lipoproteins in the very low density fraction has recently
been confirmed (LEVY et al. 1965).

Low density lipoproteins represent a single lipoprotein class. The lipoproteins in
this class have the following properties: density, 1.0311 ± 0.0047; diameter,
19.6 ± 0.47 mμ; molecular weight, $2.55 \pm 0.17 \times 10^6$ (TORO-GOYCO 1958, ONCLEY
1963). Very low density and low density lipoproteins are precipitaded together in
cold-ethanol fractionation (BARR et al. 1951) and as molecular complexes with
sulfated polysaccharides (BURSTEIN 1961, CORNWELL and KRUGER 1961a). These
lipoprotein classes are not separated by chromatography on either glass powder
columns (CARLSON 1960) or hydroxylapatite columns (CRAMÉR 1961, CRAMÉR and
BRATTSTEN 1961). Very low density and low density lipoproteins are readily
separated by differential ultracentrifugal flotation (HAVEL et al. 1955, BRAGDON
et al. 1956) and ultracentrifugal flotation in a density gradient (MANNICK 1955,
ONCLEY et al. 1957, CORNWELL et al. 1961a and 1961b). Very low density lipoproteins migrate as α_2-globulins while low density lipoproteins migrate as β-globu-
lins on starch block electrophoresis (KUNKEL and TRAUTMAN 1956). Two low density lipoproteins were separated by electrophoresis on Reinagar (HOUTSMULLER
et al. 1964); however, electrophoretic procedures are difficult to employ in large
scale fractionation procedures. Selective precipitation techniques with heparin,
PVP, or phosphotungstate may be possible and should be investigated further
(BURSTEIN 1961, CORNWELL and KRUGER 1961a, BURSTEIN 1963). At the present
time, the ultracentrifugal flotation pattern, electrophoretic mobility, and metabolism are the criteria for differentiating between very low density and low density
lipoproteins.

Table 3. *Composition of very low density and low density lipoprotein classes in weight percent*

	Very Low Density	Low Density	Reference
Protein	8.0	21.0	
T.G.	50.0	11.0	
P.L.	18.0	22.0	ONCLEY 1963
Cholesterol			
Free	7.0	8.0	
Ester	12.0	37.0	
Total Chol./P.L. Ratio			
Normal	0.85	1.38	ONCLEY et al. 1957
Normal	0.90	1.3 — 1.4*	BRAGDON et al. 1956
Normal	0.68 ± 0.06**	1.41 ± 0.10**	
Hypercholesterolemia	0.70 ± 0.07**	1.43 ± 0.13**	CORNWELL et al. 1961a and 1961b
Hyperlipemia	0.60 — 1.30*	0.45—1.27*	

* Range.
** Mean ± standard deviation.

The composition of very low density and low density lipoproteins has been
studied by a number of investigators. Data, summarized by ONCLEY (1963), are
reported in Table 3. Values for the different components are in good agreement
even though conversion factors were used for protein and phospholipid, cholesterol
ester in weight percent was sometimes calculated from an assumed fatty acid

composition, and triglyceride was not always measured directly. The two lipoprotein classes are characterized by distinct total cholesterol/phospholipid ratios.
These ratios have been verified in many laboratories although DE GENNES et al.
(1964) recently reported much higher values than those summarized in Table 3.
The two lipoprotein classes are very similar in phospholipid composition (PHILLIPS
1959, NELSON and FREEMAN 1960). PHILLIPS reported 5 percent cephalin, 66 percent lecithin, 5 percent lysolecithin, and 24 percent sphingomyelin as percent of
total lipid phosphorus for both classes.

The lipid components of the different lipoprotein classes exhibit considerable
exchange. Free cholesterol (HAGERMAN and GOULD 1951, GOODMAN 1962, ROHEIM
et al. 1963), triglyceride (HAVEL et al. 1962), and phospholipid (KUNKEL and
BEARN 1954, ROWE 1960, POLONOVSKI and PAYSANT 1963) all exchange between
lipoprotein classes, erythrocytes, and other formed elements. Fatty acid analyses
have shown that only a part of the cellular and plasma phospholipids participate
in the exchange reaction (ROWE 1960). Lysolecithin appears to be the phospholipid
component which equilibrated most rapidly (POLONOVSKI and PAYSANT 1963).
Equilibration and exchange may explain similarities in fatty acid composition
between lipoprotein classes.

Equilibration and exchange suggest that lipids are loosely associated with the
low density lipoprotein molecular complex. However, only a part of the lipoprotein
lipid can be extracted with ether (AVIGAN 1957). Ether extractability was enhanced when the lipoprotein was subjected to limited proteolysis with trypsin and
chymotrypsin (BANASZAK and
McDONALD 1962, CANAL and
GIRARD 1962). BERNFELD and
KELLEY (1964) found that
proteolysis completely destroyed 20 percent of the lipoprotein molecules in a low density
lipoprotein solution. The lipid
from these molecules was
transferred to the remaining
lipoprotein molecules which
were less stable during storage
but resistant to proteolytic
enzyme attack. The additional
lipid associated with modified
lipoproteins may explain the
enhanced ether extractability
observed previously. These experiments indicate that lipid-
protein interactions contribute
to the stability of the molecular complex.

The fatty acid composition
of the low density and high
density lipoprotein classes is

Table 4.
Fatty acid composition of plasma lipoprotein classes

Fatty Acid	Very Low Density		Low Density		High Density	
	I*	II**	I*	II**	I*	II**
Cholesterol ester	Percent of total fatty acids					
16:0	13.6	21.0	12.0	10.5	11.6	10.3
18:0	1.5	5.6	1.1	1.5	1.3	1.2
18:1	26.9	34.9	23.9	18.2	23.6	18.5
18:2	48.2	25.3	52.1	50.7	52.5	51.0
20:4	5.2	1.8	7.6	5.6	7.0	6.3
Phospholipid						
16:0	35.5	33.2	37.2	30.1	32.7	29.6
18:0	14.6	19.0	14.3	15.1	14.4	15.5
18:1	11.9	13.4	11.2	12.1	12.0	12.6
18:2	17.7	16.0	16.4	19.3	19.1	18.9
20:4	15.1	4.9	15.2	7.5	17.2	9.5
Triglyceride						
16:0	28.8	23.3	25.0	23.1	24.2	23.5
18:0	2.8	3.5	3.4	4.1	4.1	4.0
18:1	44.6	36.5	44.4	35.4	40.4	35.3
18:2	14.1	21.8	14.3	15.6	13.6	15.7
20:4	3.5	1.0	7.1	1.4	12.0	1.6

* GOODMAN and SHIRATORI 1964a.
** LINDGREN, NICHOLS and WILLS 1961.

summarized in Table 4. The data which represent one subject (GOODMAN and
SHIRATORI 1964a) and mean values for 7 subjects (LINDGREN et al. 1961) are
in close agreement except for the fatty acid composition of the cholesteral ester
fraction in the very low density lipoproteins and the 20:4 acid content of the triglyceride and phospholipid fractions. Distinct differences in fatty acid patterns for

cholesterol ester, triglyceride, and phospholipid fractions indicate that a high degree of specificity exists in the synthesis of plasma lipids. Triglyceride and phospholipid patterns are duplicated in the three lipoprotein classes. The triglyceride fraction is very similar in composition to adipose tissue (see CORNWELL et al. 1962 b for a summary of data, KRUT and BRONTE-STEWART 1964). The triglyceride pattern is maintained even though free fatty acids, the precursors for liver triglycerides, contain a higher proportion of 18:0 and a lower proportion of 18:1 acids (CORNWELL et al. 1962 b).

Differences in the fatty acid analyses of the cholesterol ester fraction of the very low density lipoprotein class are difficult to explain. Cholesterol esters do not appear to exchange and equilibrate between lipoprotein classes (GOODMAN 1962, ROHEIM et al. 1963) except in the ruminant (EVANS and PATTON 1962). Inconsistencies exist between studies since cholesterol esters newly synthesized in plasma with fatty acid transferase do exchange (see High Density Lipoproteins). The cholesterol ester fraction in the very low density lipoproteins of the rat is not metabolized at the same rate as other plasma cholesterol ester fractions (GOODMAN and SHIRATORI 1964 b). In hyperlipemia, a condition where a markedly elevated very low density lipoprotein concentration and a markedly lowered low density lipoprotein concentration occur, plasma cholesterol esters approach the composition reported by LINDGREN et al. (1961) for the very low density lipoprotein class (CORNWELL et al. 1962 b). GOODMAN and SHIRATORI (1964) isolated very low density lipoproteins by flotation at density 1.019 while LINDGREN et al. (1961) isolated very low density lipoproteins by flotation at density 1.006. The discrepancy may be explained either by differences in the isolation procedure, by the influence of alimentary lipid on the cholesterol ester composition (KAYDEN et al. 1963), or by individual variations in fatty acid composition. If LINDGREN et al. (1961) are correct, two cholesterol ester pools may exist in plasma. Further study is needed to resolve this problem.

The protein components of very low density and low density lipoprotein classes have been investigated by a number of immunological procedures including precipitation, complement fixation, gel diffusion, and immuno-electrophoresis (for references see BRINER et al. 1959). Data from these studies and a more sensitive hemagglutination technique (BRINER et al. 1959, WALTON and DARKE 1963) demonstrated that the two lipoprotein classes had the same antigenic specificity. The observation of BRINER et al. (1959) that low density lipoproteins contained small amounts of an additional antigenic component was not confirmed (WALTON and DARKE 1963). The immunological properties of these lipoprotein classes may be more complex than the preceding discussion suggests. Recent studies have shown that the low density lipoproteins exist as two antigenically different and genetically determined forms (BLUMBERG et al. 1962 and 1964). It has not been possible to determine wheter these antigenic forms are caused by differences in protein or in the structure of lipoprotein molecules which differ in lipid composition. Indeed, both low and high density lipoprotein antigens have been found in delipidized very low density lipoproteins (GUSTAFSON et al. 1964).

It is now well established that very low density and low density lipoproteins are synthesized in the liver. Data supporting this conclusion have been obtained from studies on plasma triglyceride metabolism, the fatty liver and its origin, and protein biosynthesis in the liver. Many of the studies used animals which have a somewhat different lipoprotein pattern than the human. Metabolic sequences differ in detail between species and unique model systems are required (FARQUHAR et al. 1965). Nevertheless fundamental aspects of lipoprotein metabolism such as liver synthesis have been confirmed in several animals.

Plasma triglyceride metabolism has been reviewed recently by OLIVECRONA (1962), HAVEL (1963), and STEINBERG (1963). A number of investigations have shown that the endogenous triglyceride carried by very low density lipoproteins is synthesized in the liver. For example, hepatectomy diminished the conversion of labeled fatty acids to circulating triglycerides (HAVEL and GOLDFIEN 1960). Triglycerides were found in liver perfusates (STEIN and SHAPIRO 1959, KAY and ENTENMAN 1961). Hepatectomy reduced Triton hyperlipemia (BYERS and FRIED-MAN 1960), a condition caused by a block in the removal of circulating lipoproteins (SCANU and PAGE 1962). A precursor-product relationship exists between liver and plasma triglyceride (HAVEL et al. 1962, BAKER and SCHOTZ 1964, FARQUHAR et al. 1965). The relationship is complex and in the human only a small part of the newly synthesized triglyceride is secreted into the plasma (FARQUHAR et al. 1965). The tissue distribution and uptake of the triglyceride component from very low density lipoproteins is similar to distribution and uptake of chylomicron triglyceride (HAVEL et al. 1962, FRIEDBERG and ESTES 1964) and will be discussed elsewhere.

Indirect evidence from studies on various types of fatty liver supports the concept of hepatic lipoprotein synthesis. Thus carbon tetrachloride produced a fatty liver, prevented a Triton hyperlipemia (LOMBARDI and RECKNAGEL 1962) and diminished the conversion of labeled fatty acids to circulating triglycerides (MALING et al. 1962, SCHOTZ et al. 1964). Carbon tetrachloride, ethionine, and puromycin all produced a fatty liver and lowered the concentration of circulating lipid probably through the inhibition of protein synthesis (ROBINSON and SEAKINS 1963). The orotic acid fatty liver has also been related to decreased lipoprotein secretion from the liver (WINDMUELLER 1964); however, the inhibition of hepatic protein synthesis is more difficult to demonstrate in this pathological state (DEAMER et al. 1964). VIVIANI et al. (1964) recently found that the fatty acid composition of liver lipids was altered in the fatty liver developed with lysine and threonine deficient rats. It would be interesting to determine whether the lipo-protein molecule requires specific phospholipids for its synthesis in the liver.

Direct evidence for hepatic lipoprotein synthesis has been obtained from amino acid incorporation studies with liver slices (MARSH and WHEREAT 1959, RADDING and STEINBERG 1960), perfused livers (HAFT et al. 1962), and cell-free microsomal preparations (MARSH 1963). EDER et al. (1963) have shown that a "lipid acceptor proteins" is present in plasma. The "lipid acceptor protein" combines with lipid in the synthesis of very low density lipoproteins. This study is an important contribution to the elucidation of lipoprotein structure and synthesis. It suggests that the protein structure is altered in lipoprotein synthesis since no indication of a "lipid acceptor protein" in lipoprotein-free serum has been found by immunological techniques.

Evidence for a precursor-product relationship between very low density and low density lipoprotein classes has been obtained with lipoproteins labeled in their protein moieties with [131]-iodine (GITLIN et al. 1958, WALTON et al. 1963). Very low density lipoproteins were converted, *in vivo*, by an apparently unidirectional process to low density lipoproteins. The labeled protein moiety from very low density lipoproteins was found in the low density lipoprotein class. Labeled protein from low density lipoproteins was not re-cycled in the very low density lipoprotein class. High density lipoprotein was not involved in the metabolic sequence but this may only reflect selective labeling.

A simple precursor-product relationship was not readily demonstrated with labeled triglyceride (HAVEL 1963). Triglyceride studies did not differentiate be-tween very low density lipoprotein as the exclusive precursor or the direct synthesis of low density lipoprotein in the liver. Lipoprotein metabolism in hyperlipemia luggests that both metabolic sequences occur. In hyperlipemia, very low density sipoproteins are elevated and the low density lipoprotein class suppressed (CORN-WELL et al. 1961a and 1961b). Underutilization was suggested by the prolonged half-life of very low density lipoproteins in nephrotic hyperlipemia (GITLIN et al. 1958). In addition, the uptake of lipoprotein triglyceride by adipose tissue was impaired in aminonucleoside nephrosis (GUTMAN and SHAFRIR 1963). Underutilization may involve a deficiency in lipoprotein lipase or the inhibition of this enzyme reaction. Lipolysis, *in vitro*, with post-heparin plasma converted very low density lipoproteins to low density lipoproteins (LINDGREN et al. 1955, SHORE and SHORE 1962). Lipoprotein lipase inhibitors, *in vitro*, diminished the uptake of lipoprotein triglyceride by adipose tissue (MARKSCHEID and SHAFRIR 1963). Lipoproteins are first assimilated in a soluble adipose tissue compartment and the triglyceride is then shifted to the fat droplet (MARKSHEID and SHAFRIR 1965). The rate limiting step, triglyceride transfer to the fat droplet, probably involves intracellular lipoprotein lipase since partial transesterification has been demonstrated. These observations may be related to lipoprotein metabolism in some pathological states. Thus hyperlipemic subjects with deficient lipoprotein lipase activity have been described (HAVEL and GORDON 1960, FREDRICKSON et al. 1963). The lipoprotein lipase deficiency may be limited to conditions such as fat-induced hyperglyceridemia (FREDRICKSON et al. 1963) where chylomicrons are elevated specifically (AHRENS and SPRITZ 1963, NYE 1964). A lipoprotein lipase inhibitor was found in the serum of hyperlipemic subjects (KLEIN et al. 1959). The resistance of very low density lipoproteins (1.5×10^6 Gmin.) to lipolysis, may also contribute to underutilization (ANGERWALL et al. 1962). In contrast to adipose tissue, triglyceride uptake by rat liver apparently does not require lipolysis (OLIVECRONA and BELFRAGE 1965). Variations between tissues, and species variations mentioned previously, complicate the interpretation of lipolysis data.

Although a lipoprotein lipase deficiency has been described in essential hyperlipemia, nephrosis, and diabetes, normal lipoprotein lipase levels were also found in other subjects with these pathological states (for references see ROBINSON 1963, ZEMPLÉNYI 1964). The overproduction of very low density lipoproteins is suggested in diabetic acidosis where a high plasma FFA level was accompanied by elevated very low density lipoproteins, decreased low density lipoproteins, and no apparent deficiency in post-heparin lipolytic activity (HAMWI et al. 1962). Epinephrine elevates both the plasma FFA level and the liver triglyceride pool, and causes a delayed but nevertheless distinct elevation in circulating triglyceride (STEINBERG 1963). Liver perfusion experiments have shown that lipoprotein synthesis is proportional to the FFA level in the perfusate (NESTEL and STEINBERG 1963). WALTON et al. (1963) found that the half-life of labeled very low density and low density lipoproteins was normal in hyperlipemic subjects and suggested that Atromid (ethyl-β-p-chlorophenoxy-isobutyrate and androsterone) corrected hyperlipemia by reducing or altering triglyceride synthesis in the liver.

It has been difficult to evaluate both the quantitative importance in for example net protein transfer and the mechanism of the very low density-to-low density conversion process. This conversion is more complex than the simple removal of triglyceride by lipolysis. The low density lipoprotein class contains less triglyceride, more protein and cholesterol ester, and about the same relative amount of free cholesterol and phospholipid as the very low density lipoprotein class (Table 3). The free cholesterol/phospholipid ratio is the same for both lipoprotein classes. Indeed, the free cholesterol/lecithin mole ratios are 1.2 and 1.1 for very low density and low density lipoproteins respectively. Stable 1:1 complexes between cholesterol and phospholipid are possible (VANDENHEUVEL 1963). A cholesterol-phospholipid complex could form a portion of the lipoprotein surface which is lost together with the triglycerides moiety in the conversion process. On the other hand, the similarities in free cholesterol/phospholipid ratios may have little significance. In chylomicrons, free cholesterol and phospholipid do not exchange as a stable 1:1 complex (MINARI and ZILVERSMIT 1963). Heptane extraction studies with lipoprotein monolayers have shown that lipoprotein structure is important in the binding of cholesterol to the molecular complex. Thus heptane extracts almost all the cholesterol from a lipoprotein monolayer and very little cholesterol from a lipoprotein solution (ZILVERSMIT 1964). At the present time, it is not possible to assess the contributions of cholesterol-phospholipid, cholesterol-protein, and phospholipid-protein interactions to complex stability.

The composition of the very low density lipoprotein class isolated from hyperlipemic subjects is frequently quite different from the same class in normal subjects. A crude indication of the difference is obtained from cholesterol/phospholipid ratios (Table 3). It would be interesting to sub-fractionate very low density lipoproteins by controlled preparative ultracentrifugation, analyze their composition including the free cholesterol content, and study their metabolism. For example, triglyceride composition affects chylomicron metabolism (NESTEL and SCOW 1964) and physical properties (ZILVERSMIT 1964). ONCLEY (1963) has suggested ^{131}-iodine would tend to label only the very low density lipoproteins with a relatively high protein content, the lower end of the S_f spectrum for this class. Very low density lipoproteins in the higher S_f range may have different metabolic properties which would not be apparent in studies where the whole class was labeled. A thorough investigation of the composition and properties of the very low density lipoproteins present in pathological states is needed.

5. **High Density Lipoproteins.** There is considerable conflict in the literature about the properties of high density lipoproteins. Three high density lipoprotein sub-fractions — HDL_1, HDL_2, and HDL_3 — have been described (LINDGREN and NICHOLS 1960). Two of these sub-fractions, the HDL_2 and HDL_3 lipoproteins, were found in different concentrations in men and women (BARCLAY et al. 1963a) and in human neoplastic disease (BARCLAY et al. 1964). BARCLAY et al. (1963b) recently found two additional sub-fractions which were characterized as S_f 12—20 and S_f 4—12 by ultracentrifugal flotation in solvents at density 1.125. The existence of these new sub-fractions has been questioned (LINDGREN 1964). Indeed, a careful analysis of the high density lipoprotein class by density gradient flotation suggests that only one lipoprotein component in the density 1.12 ± 0.024 range exists (ALLERTON 1962, ONCLEY 1963 and 1964). Since cholesterol and phospholipid were distributed in the density gradient as a continuum, high density lipoproteins will be considered as a single lipoprotein class which varies somewhat in composition throughout a density continuum. The two high density lipoprotein fractions with densities of 1.08 and 1.15 probably represent different portions of this continuum (HILLYARD et al. 1955). This hypothesis is supported by studies which showed that density 1.063—1.125, 1.125—1.168, and 1.168—1.21 sub-fractions had the same amino acid composition and biological half-life (SCANU and HUGHES 1962). and immunological studies (see below) which showed the formation of a high density lipoprotein artifact (LEVY and FREDRICKSON 1965).

No consensus is available on the size and shape of high density lipoproteins. Molecular weights ranging from 165,000 to 450,000 have been reported (ONCLEY et al. 1947, SHORE 1957, HAZELWOOD 1958, SHORE and SHORE 1962). A molecular weight of 250,000 was found for lipoprotein molecules at the center of the density continuum (ALLERTON 1962).

High density lipoproteins which migrate as α-globulins (KUNKEL and TRAUTMAN 1956) can be separated into several components by disc electrophoresis on acrylimide-gels (Narayan et al. 1965). This lipoprotein class is separated in a different cold-ethanol fraction than low density lipoproteins (Barr et al. 1951) and is not precipitated by sulfated polysaccharides (Burstein 1961, Cornwell and Kruger 1961 a). A new precipitation technique for high density lipoproteins has been reported (Burstein 1962). The high density lipoprotein class is immunologically distinct from low density lipoproteins and other serum proteins (DeLalla et al. 1957, Scanu et al. 1958 a). Agar diffusion and immunoelectrophoresis show that two high density lipoprotein components are present in plasma and that one component is a lipid-poor artifact formed during aging or ultracentrifugation (Levy and Fred-rickson 1965).

The high density lipoprotein class was found to contain about 50 percent protein, 22 percent phospholipid, 3 percent free cholesterol, 14 percent cholesterol ester, and 8 percent triglyceride (data summarized by Oncley 1963). A phospholipid analysis showed 5 percent cephalin, 70 percent lecithin, 11 percent lysolecithin, and 14 percent sphingomyelin (Phillips 1959a). Less lysolecithin, 0.2 to 1.0 percent, and 3.5 percent phosphoinositol were reported in a recent study (Sanbar 1963). High density lipoproteins apparently contain less sphingomyelin than the two low density lipoprotein classes. It is interesting that chylomicrons which also contain less sphingomyelin (Wood et al. 1964) transfer phospholipid to the high density lipoprotein class (Minari and Zilversmit 1963). The lipid fractions of the high density lipoprotein class do not differ significantly from low density lipoproteins in fatty acid composition (Table 4).

A major advance in lipoprotein chemistry was achieved by the delipidation of high density lipoprotein with ethanol and ether at —25⁰ C (Scanu et al. 1958 b). The lipid-free protein residue recombined with lipid *in vitro* (Scanu and Hughes 1960) and *in vivo* (Scanu and Page 1961). Recombined lipoprotein was metabolized at the same rate as "native" lipoprotein (Sanbar et al. 1962). The protein moieties of both very low density and low density lipoproteins are denatured by similar delipidation techniques. However, a soluble phospholipid-protein complex has been obtained by extracting neutral lipid and some phospholipid with n-heptane at —12⁰ C. from a lyophilized very low density lipoprotein-potato starch mixture (Gustafson 1964). The high density lipoprotein contained threonine and aspartic acid in the C-terminal and N-terminal residues (Shore and Shore 1962). Sedimentation and diffusion data gave a molecular weight of 75,000 for the protein moiety (Scanu et al. 1958 b). This protein undergoes aggregation (Shore and Shore 1962, Sanbar and Alaupovic 1963). An amino acid analysis and sedimentation studies in the presence of detergent suggest that the minimum molecular weight for the protein is near 36,500 ± 1,000 (Shore and Shore 1962). The 75,000 unit may be a dimer and a trimer may actually exist in the lipoprotein which should have a protein moiety with a molecular weight near 110,000 (Shore and Shore 1962).

Lipid exchange between chylomicrons, high density lipoproteins, and cells, and the recombination of the lipid-free residue of the high density lipoprotein with lipid have been discussed previously. High density lipoprotein also binds cholesterol and palmitic acid, *in vitro*, (Ashworth and Green 1963) and transfers these bound lipids to cells in a somewhat different manner than the normal lipid components (Ashworth and Green 1964). Glycerides are also transferred from very low density lipoproteins to high density lipoproteins displacing cholesterol esters in the high density lipoprotein class (Nichols et al. 1964). Plasma fatty acid transferase catalizes the esterification of plasma cholesterol with fatty acids from lecithin (Glomset and Wright 1964). Newly synthesized cholesterol ester is bound to all lipoprotein fractions (Rehnborg and Nichols 1964) and there is a net transfer of cholesterol ester from low and high density lipoproteins to very low density lipoproteins (NICHOLS and SMITH 1965). Lipid exchange probably explains the reciprocal relationship frequently noted between very low density and high density lipoprotein concentrations (CORNWELL et al. 1961 b). Neutral lipid exchange may also explain decreased cholesterol/phospholipid ratios in hyperlipemia (Table 3, CORNWELL et al. 1961 b). Thus lipid transfer and exchange are important aspects of high density lipoprotein metabolism. Plasma contains a phospholipid-protein complex in the density 1.21 residue (HAVEL et al. 1955, HILLYARD et al. 1955, BRAGDON et al. 1956, FURMAN et al. 1961). SANBAR (1963) recently found that the protein moiety of the phospholipid-protein complex and the lipid-free residue from the high density lipoprotein class had similar ultracentrifugal and electrophoretic properties. Furthermore, [131]-iodine labeled protein from the high density lipoprotein class appeared in this residue. The phospholipid-protein complex may then represent high density lipoprotein which contains only part of its normal lipid components. The phospholipid-protein residue contained a large amount of lysolecithin (PHILLIPS 1959 b, SANBAR 1963), the phospholipid which exchanged most rapidly in plasma (POLONOVSKI and PAYSANT 1963). A recent study has shown that this residue is responsible for lysolecithin exchange (SAKAGAMI et al. 1965).

The metabolic function of the high density lipoprotein class has been difficult to elucidate. The concentration of this lipoprotein class does not appear to change significantly in disease states. It is interesting that triglyceride turnover in the high density lipoprotein class is more rapid than triglyceride turnover in low density lipoproteins (HAVEL 1963) even though the half-life of the protein moiety is longer for the high density lipoproteins (GITLIN et al. 1958, VOLWILER et al. 1955, LAMY et al. 1961). Triglyceride turnover may again reflect lipid exchange. Much of the physical, chemical, exchange, and metabolic data which has been obtained with high density lipoproteins should be re-examined and re-interpreted in relation to the formation of lipid-poor artifacts.

6. The Analysis of Chylomicrons and Lipoproteins. A simple and routine procedure for the separation of chylomicrons, very low density lipoproteins, low density lipoproteins, and high density lipoproteins is not available at this time. High density lipoproteins are readily separated by paper electrophoresis, ultracentrifugal flotation, or as the soluble supernatant fraction obtained with sulfated polysaccharide precipitation techniques. Significant variations are seldom found in the high density lipoprotein fraction (for recent studies see CORNWELL et al. 1961 a and 1961 b, VAN CAUWENBERGE et al. 1963, SPIGAI 1963, FELDMAN 1964, FRANZINI and SCHIVI 1964, TRAVIA 1964). A correlation between the β/α lipoprotein ratio and total lipid undoubtedly exists because the high density or α-lipoprotein class is relatively constant except in pronounced hyperlipemia.

Analytical methods employing immuno-precipitation (FELDMAN 1964) or flocculation with sulfated polysaccharides (BURSTEIN 1961, CORNWELL and KRUGER 1961) measure the total concentration of very low density and low density lipoproteins. These procedures do not distinguish between the two lipoprotein classes and probably do not yield more information than can be obtained from the estimation of triglyceride, total cholesterol, and phospholipid (ALBRINK 1961, SCHÖN and ZELLER 1962). However, flocculation procedures are less difficult to perform than chemical analyses. A specific flocculation procedure, the PVP gradient (BURSTEIN and PRAWERMAN 1958, GORDIS 1962, BIERMAN et al. 1962), has been developed for chylomicrons. A procedure that would distinguish between very low density and low density lipoproteins would be of real clinical significance. Analytical and preparative ultracentrifugal flotation procedures which may produced lipoprotein artifacts are the only methods now available for the quantitative esti-

mation of the major lipoprotein classes. Analytical ultracentrifugation has been
discussed in detail by DE LALLA and GOFMAN (1954) and BALTZER 1959). When the
plasma lipoproteins in 2 ml. of serum are first concentrated by preparative ultracentrifugation, the total lipoprotein pattern may be estimated by analytical ultracentrifugation in a sodium bromide solvent at density 1.20 (DEL GATTO et al. 1959).
Lipoprotein classes isolated by differential (HAVEL et al. 1955, BRAGDON et al. 1956)
or density gradient (CORNWELL et al. 1961a) ultracentrifugation are generally
estimated by the chemical analysis of the lipoprotein fractions. A procedure which
utilizes preparative ultracentrifugation and a physical property, the specific refractive increment, has been developed for the analysis of lipoprotein classes (LINDGREN
et al. 1964). Lipoproteins have also been pre-stained with Sudan Black B, separated
by ultracentrifugation, and then estimated by stain intensity in a qualitative
procedure (CORNWELL and KRUGER 1961b). The initial precipitation of very low
density and low density lipoproteins with sulfated polysaccharides yields a concentrated and partially purified lipoprotein fraction (CORNWELL and KRUGER 1961).
Precipitation techniques are therefore important in large-scale isolation and fractionation procedures.

References

AHRENS, E. H., and N. SPRITZ: Further studies on fat- and carbohydrate-induced lipemia in man: reduction of lipemia by feeding fat — p. 304—311. In: A. C. FRAZER: Biochemical Problems of Lipids. Amsterdam: Elsevier 1963.
ALBRINK, M. J.: Lipoprotein pattern as a function of total triglyceride concentration of serum. J. clin. Invest. 40, 536—544 (1961).
ALLERTON, S. E.: Ultracentrifugal studies on proteins. Ph. D. Thesis: Harvard University 1962.
ANGERWALL, G., P. BJÖRNTORP, and B. HOOD: Studies on the clearing phenomenon in essential hyperlipemia. Acta med. scand. 172, 5—14 (1962).
ARMSTRONG jr., S. H., M. J. E. BUDKA, and K. C. MORRISON: Preparation and properties of serum and plasma proteins. XI. Quantitative interpretation of electrophoretic schlieren diagrams of normal human plasma proteins. J. Amer. chem. Soc. 69, 416—429 (1947a).
— — — and M. HASSON: Preparation and properties of serum and plasma proteins. XII. The refractive properties of the proteins of human plasma and certain purified fractions. J. Amer. chem. Soc. 69, 1747—1753 (1947b).
ASHWORTH, L. A. E., and C. GREEN: The uptake of lipids by human α-lipoprotein. Biochem. biophys. Acta (Amst.) 70, 68—74 (1963).
— — The transfer of lipids between human α-lipoprotein and erythrocytes. Biochim. biophys. Acta (Amst.) 84, 182—187 (1964).
AVIGAN, J.: Modification of human serum lipoprotein fractions by lipide extraction. J. biol. Chem. 226, 957—964 (1957).
BAKER, N., and M. C. SCHOTZ: Use of multicompartmental models to measure rates of trigly-ceride metabolism in rats. J. Lipid Res. 5, 188—197 (1964).
BALTZER, V.: Untersuchungen über das physikalisch-chemische Verhalten der Lipoproteide humaner Seren. Bull. schweiz. Akad. med. Wiss. 15, 193—225 (1959).
BANASZAK, L. J., and H. J. MCDONALD: The proteolysis of human serum β-lipoproteins. Biochemistry 1, 344—349 (1962).
BANG, I.: Lipämie. Biochem. Z. 90, 383—387 (1918).
BANGHAM, A. D.: Physical structure and behavior of lipids and lipid enzymes. Advanc. Lipid Res. 1, 65—104 (1963).
BARCLAY, M., R. K. BARCLAY, and V. P. SKIPSKI: High density lipoprotein concentrations in men and women. Nature (Lond.) 200, 362—363 (1963a).
— — O. TEREBUS-KEKISH, E. B. SHAH, and V. P. SKIPSKI: Disclosure and characterization of new high-density lipoproteins in human serum. Clin. chim. Acta 8, 721—726 (1963b).
— G. C. ESCHER, R. J. KAUFMAN, O. TEREBUS-KEKISH, E. M. GREENE, and V. P. SKIPSKI: Serum lipoproteins in human neoplastic disease. Clin. chim. Acta 10, 39—47 (1964).
BARR, D. P., E. M. RUSS, and H. A. EDER: Protein-lipid relationships in human plasma. II. In atherosclerosis and related conditions. Amer. J. Med. 11, 480—493 (1951).
BERNFELD, P., and T. F. KELLEY: Proteolysis of human serum β-lipoprotein. J. biol. Chem. 239, 3341—3346 (1964).

BIERMAN, E. L., E. GORDIS, and J. T. HAMLIN: Heterogeneity of fat particles in plasma during alimentary lipemia. J. clin. Invest. 41, 2254—2260 (1962).

BLUMBERG, B. S., D. BERNANKE, and A. C. ALLISON: A human lipoprotein polymorphism. J. clin. Invest. 31, 1936—1944 (1962).

— P. L. WORKMAN, and J. HIRSCHFELD: Gamma-globulin, group specific, and lipoprotein groups in a U.S. white and negro population. Nature (Lond.) 202, 561—663 (1964).

BRAGDON, J. H., and A. KARMEN: The fatty acid composition of chylomicrons of chyle and serum following the ingestion of different oils. J. Lipid Res. 1, 167—170 (1960).

— R. J. HAVEL, and E. BOYLE: Human serum lipoproteins. I. Chemical composition of four fractions. J. Lab. clin. Med. 48, 36—42 (1956).

BRINER, W. W., J. W. RIDDLE. and D. G. CORNWELL: Studies on the immunochemistry of human low density lipoproteins utilizing an hemagglutination technique. J. exp. Med. 110, 113—122 (1959).

BURSTEIN, M.: Les lipoprotéines du plasma humain. Bull. schweiz. Akad. med. Wiss. 17, 92—110 (1961).

— Précipitation sélective d'une fraction des lipoprotéines sériques de densite élévée par le sulfate de dextrane en présence de chlorure de magnésium et de saccharose. Life Sci. 1, 739—744 (1962).

— Isolement des lipoprotéines sériques de faible densité apres floculation par le phosphotungstate de soude à pH neutre en présence de chlorure de magnésium. Rev. franc. Hémat. 3, 139—148 (1963).

— and A. PRAWERMAN: Sur la floculation des chylomicrons par le polyvinyl-pyrrolidone. Rev. Hémat. 13, 329—330 (1958).

— — Précipitation des β-lipoprotéines et des chylomicrons par le polyvinyl-pyrrolidone. Path. et Biol. 7, 1035—1038 (1959).

BYERS, S. O., and M. FRIEDMAN: Site of origin of plasma triglyceride. Amer. J. Physiol. 198, 629—631 (1960).

CANAL, J. R., and M. L. GIRARD: Modifications des lipoprotéines sériques sous ̄l'action des protéases pancréatiques. C.R. Acad. Sci. (Paris) 255, 2306—2308 (1962).

CARLSON, L. A.: Chromatographic separation of serum lipoproteins on glass powder columns. Description of the method and some applications. Clin. chim. Acta 5, 528—538 (1960).

— and B. OLHAGEN: The electrophoretic mobility of chylomicrons in a case of essential hyperlipemia. Scand. J. clin. Lab. Invest. 6, 70—73 (1954).

CHEVALLIER, F., and D. MATHE: Destinée du cholésterol des chylomicrons| chez le rat. III. Mouvements de cholésterol-4-^{14}C entre les chylomicrons et la lymphe ou le sérum, in vivo. Bull. Soc. Chim. biol. (Paris) 46, 509—527 (1964).

CHICK, H.: The apparent formation of euglobulin from pseudo-globulin and a suggestion as to the relationship between these two proteins in serum. Biochem. J. 8, 404—420 (1914).

CLAESSON, S., and I. MORING-CLEASSON: Ultracentrifugation — p. 121—171. In: P. ALEXANDER and R. J. BLOCK: Analytical Methods of Protein Chemistry, Vol. 3. London: Pergamon Press 1961.

CORNWELL, D. G., and L. A. HORROCKS: Protein-lipid complexes, p. 117—151. In: H. W. SCHULTZ and A. F. ANGELMIER: Proteins and Their Reactions. Westport (Conn.): Avi Publishing Co. 1964.

— and F. A. KRUGER: Molecular complexes in the isolation and characterization of plasma lipoproteins. J. Lipid Res. 2, 110—134 (1961).

— — Molecular complexes in the isolation and characterization of plasma lipoproteins. J. Lipid Res. 2, 110—134 (1961a).

— — Lipoprotein pre-staining and ultracentrifugal analysis in a density gradient. Proc. Soc. exp. Biol. (N. Y.) 107, 296—299 (1961b).

— — G. J. HAMWI, and J. B. BROWN: Studies on the characterization of human serum lipoproteins separated by ultracentrifugation in a density gradient. I. Serum lipoproteins in normal, hypothyroid and hypercholesterolemic subjects. Amer. J. clin. Nutr. 9, 24—40 (1961a).

— — — — Studies on the characterization of human serum lipoproteins separated by ultracentrifugation in a density gradient. II. Serum lipoproteins in hyperlipemic subjects. Amer. J. clin. Nutr. 9, 40—54 (1961b).

— — — — Correlations between lipoprotein concentration and fatty acid composition in serum of normal and hyperlipemic subjects: a review. Metabolism 11, 840—849 (1962b).

— — and H. B. ROBINSON: Studies on the absorption of beta-carotene and the distribution of total carotenoid in human serum lipoproteins after oral administration. J. Lipid Res. 3, 65—70 (1962a).

CRAMÉR, K.: Studies on human serum β-lipoproteins including their protein moiety. Acta med. scand. Suppl. 372 (1961).

— and I. BRATTSTEN: Characterization of β-lipoprotein isolated from hydroxylapatite columns. J. Atheroscler. Res. 1, 335—344 (1961).

DEAMER, D. W., F. A. KRUGER, and D. G. CORNWELL: Total liver protein and amino acid incorporation into liver protein in orotic acid induced fatty liver. Biochim. biophys. Acta (Amst.) **97**, 147—149 (1965).

DEGENNES, J. L., J. POLONOVSKI, M. AYRAULT-JARRIER, D. BARD, and G. LÉVY: Étude analytique des lipoprotéines par ultracentrifugation préparatrice dans 21 cas d'hyper-lipidémies majeures. Rev. franç. Étud. clin. biol. **9**, 273—286 (1964).

DELALLA, L., L. LEVENE, and R. K. BROWN: Immunologic studies of human high density lipoproteins. J. exp. Med. **106**, 261—271 (1957).

DELALLA, O. F., and J. W. GOFMAN: Ultracentrifugal analysis of serum lipoproteins. Meth. biochem. Anal. **1**, 459—478 (1954).

DEL GATTO, L., F. T. LINDGREN, and A. V. NICHOLS: Ultracentrifugal method for the deter-mination of serum lipoproteins. Anal. Chem. **31**, 1397—1399 (1959).

DOLE, V. P., and J. T. HAMLIN III: Particulate fat in lymph. and blood. Physiol. Rev. **42**, 674—701 (1962).

— A. T. JAMES, J. P. W. WEBB, M. A. RIZACK, and M. F. STURMAN: The fatty-acid patterns of plasma lipids during alimentary lipemia. J. clin. Invest. **38**, 1544—1554 (1959).

EDER, H. A., P. S. ROHEIM, L. I. GIDEZ, and S. SWITZER: Regulation of lipid transport in the liver, p. 202—209. In: H. C. MENG, J. G. CONIGLIO, V. S. LeQUIRE, G. V. MANN and J. M. MERRILL: Lipid Transport. Springfield (Ill.): Thomas 1963.

ELBERS, P. F.: The cell membrane: image and interpretation, p. 443—503. In: J. F. DANIELLI, K. G. A. PANKHURST and A. C. RIDDIFORD: Recent Progress in Surface Science, Vol. 2. New York: Academic Press 1964.

EVANS, L., and S. PATTON: Lipid exchange between bovine serum lipoproteins in vitro. J. Dairy Sci. **45**, 589—594 (1962).

FARQUHAR, J. W., R. C. GROSS, R. M. WAGNER, and G. M. REAVEN: Validation of an in-completely coupled two-compartment nonrecycling catenary model for turnover of liver and plasma triglyceride in man. J. Lipid Res. **6**, 119—134 (1965).

FASOLI, A.: Serum lipoprotein changes during fat absorption, p. 313—317. In: A. C. FRAZER: Biochemical Problems of Lipids. Amsterdam: Elsevier 1963.

FELDMAN, E. B.: Abnormalities of circulating lipids. An appraisal of current methods of study. Amer. J. Cardiol. **13**, 632—639 (1964).

FRANZINI, C., and T. SCHIVI: On the distribution of serum chelesterol between α- and β-lipoproteins. Clin. chim. Acta **9**, 87—89 (1964).

FREDRICKSON, D. S.: Tangier disease. Ann. intern. Med. **55**, 1016—1031 (1961).

— K. ONO, and L. L. DAVIS: Lipolytic activity of postheparin plasma in hyperglyceridemia. J. Lipid Res. **4**, 24—33 (1963).

FREEMAN, N. K., F. T. LINDGREN, and A. V. NICHOLS: The chemistry of serum lipoproteins. Progr. Chem. Fats Lipids **6**, 215—250 (1963).

FRENCH, J. E.: The behavior of chylomicrons in the circulation. Observations with the electron microscope, p. 296—302. In: A. C. FRAZER: Biochemical Problems of Lipids. Amsterdam: Elsevier 1963.

FRIEDBERG, S. J., and E. H. ESTES jr.: Tissue distribution and uptake of endogenous lipo-protein triglycerides in the rat. J. clin. Invest. **43**, 129—137 (1964).

FURMAN, R. H., R. P. HOWARD, K. LAKSHMI, and L. N. NORCIA: The serum lipids and lipo-proteins in normal and hyperlipidemic subjects as determined by preparative ultracentri-fugation. Amer. J. clin. Nutr. **9**, 73—102 (1961).

GITLIN, D., D. G. CORNWELL, D. NAKASATO, J. L. ONCLEY, W. L. HUGHES jr., and C. A. JANEWAY: Studies on the metabolism of plasma proteins in the nephrotic syndrome. II. The lipoproteins. J. clin. Invest. **37**, 172—184 (1958).

GLOMSET, J. A., and J. L. WRIGHT: Some properties of a cholesterol esterifying enzyme in human plasma. Biochim. biophys. Acta (Amst.) **89**, 266—276 (1964).

GOFMAN, J. W., F. T. LINDGREN, and H. ELLIOTT: Ultracentrifugal studies of lipoproteins of human serum. J. biol. Chem. **179**, 973—979 (1949).

— and W. YOUNG: The filtration concept of atherosclerosis and serum lipids in the diagnosis of atherosclerosis, p. 197—229. In: M. SANDLER and G. H. BOURNE: Atherosclerosis and its Origin. New York: Academic Press 1963.

GOODMAN, D. S.: Metabolism of chylomicron cholesterol ester in the rat. J. clin. Invest. **41**, 1886—1896 (1962).

— and T. SHIRATORI: Fatty acid composition of human plasma lipoprotein fractions. J. Lipid Res. **5**, 307—313 (1964a).

— — In vivo turnover of different cholesterol esters in rat liver and plasma. J. Lipid Res. **5**, 578—586 (1964b).

GORDIS, E.: Demonstration of two kinds of fat particles in alimentary lipemia with poly-vinylpyrrolidone gradient columns. Proc. Soc. exp. Biol. (N. Y.) **110**, 657—661 (1962).

GUSTAFSON, A.: A new method for partial delipidization of serum proteins. Biochim. biophys. Acta (Amst.) **84**, 223—225 (1964).

— P. ALAUPOVIC, and R. H. FURMAN: Studies on the composition and structure of serum lipoproteins: physical-chemical characterization of phospholipidprotein residues obtained from very-low density human serum lipoproteins. Biochim. biophys. Acta (Amst.) **84**, 767—769 (1964).

— — — Studies of the composition and structure of serum lipoproteins: isolation, purification, and characterization of very low density lipoproteins of human serum. Biochemistry **4**, 596—605 (1965).

GUTMAN, A., and E. SHAFRIR: Adipose tissue in experimental nephrotic syndrome. Amer. J. Physiol. **205**, 702—706 (1963).

HAFT, D. E., P. S. ROHEIM, A. WHITE, and H. A. EDER: Plasma lipoprotein metabolism in perfused rat livers. I. Protein synthesis and entry into the plasma. J. clin. Invest. **41**, 842—849 (1962).

HAGERMAN, J. S., and R. G. GOULD: The *in vitro* interchange of cholesterol between plasma and red cells. Proc. Soc. exp. Biol. (N. Y.) **78**, 329—332 (1951).

HAMWI, G. J., O. GARCIA, F. A. KRUGER, G. GWINUP, and D. G. CORNWELL: Hyperlipidemia in uncontrolled diabetes. Metabolism **11**, 850—862 (1962).

HARDY, W. B.: Colloidal solutions. The globulins. J. Physiol. (Lond.) **33**, 251—337 (1905).

HARLAN, W. R., and D. E. BEISCHER: Changes in serum lipoproteins after a large fat meal in normal individuals and in patients with ischemic heart disease. Amer. Heart J. **66**, 61—67 (1963).

HASLAM, H. C.: Separation of proteins. III. Globulins. Biochem. J. **7**, 492—516 (1913).

HAVEL, R. J.: Transport of fatty acids in the blood: pathways of transport and the role of catecholamines and the sympathetic nervous system, p. 43—65. In: E. C. HORNING and P. LINDGREN: First Intern. Pharmacol. Meeting, Vol. 2. New York: Macmillan 1963.

— H. A. EDER, and J. H. BRAGDON: The distribution and chemical composition of ultracentrifugally separated lipoproteins in human serum. J. clin. Invest. **34**, 1345—1353 (1955).

— J. M. FELTS, and C. M. VAN DUYNE: Formation and fate of endogenous triglycerides in blood plasma of rabbits. J. Lipid Res. **3**, 297—308 (1962).

— and D. S. FREDRICKSON: The metabolism of chylomicra. I. The removal of palmitic acid-1-C[14] labeled chylomicra from dog plasma. J. clin. Invest. **35**, 1025—1032 (1956.)

— and A. GOLDFIEN: Role of liver and extrahepatic tissues in plasma fatty acid metabolism. Clin. Res. Proc. 8, 141 (1960).

— and R. S. GORDON jr.: Idiopathic hyperlipemia: metabolic studies in an affected family. J. clin. Invest. **39**, 1777—1790 (1960).

HAZELWOOD, R. N.: Molecular weights and dimensions of some high density human serum lipoproteins. J. Amer. chem. Soc. **80**, 2152—2156 (1958).

HILLYARD, L. A., C. ENTENMAN, H. FEINBERG, and I. L. CHAIKOFF: Lipide and protein composition of four fractions accounting for total serum lipoproteins. J. biol. Chem. **214**, 79—90 (1955).

HOUTSMULLER, A. J., A. HUYSSON-HAASDYK, A. HUYSMAN, and E. RINKEL-VAN DRIEL: The application of Reinagar for the quantitative separation of α- and β-lipoproteins. Clin. chim. Acta 9, 497—499 (1964).

ISSELBACHER, K. J., and D. M. BUDZ: Synthesis of lipoproteins by rat intestinal mucosa. Nature (Lond.) **200**, 364—365 (1963).

— R. SCHEIG, G. R. PLOTKIN, and J. B. CAULFIELD: Congenital β-lipoprotein deficiency: an hereditary disorder involving a defect in the absorption and transport of lipids. Medicine (Baltimore) **43**, 347—361 (1964).

JOBST, H., and G. SCHETTLER: Über die chemische Zusammensetzung der Chylomicronen, p. 136—147. In: R. RUYSSEN: The Blood Lipids and the Clearing Factor. BRUSSELS: Koninkl. vlaam. Acad. Wetenschaup., Letter. en Schone Kunsten Belg., Kl. Wettenschaup. 1956.

KARMEN, A., M. WHYTE, and D. S. GOODMAN: Fatty acid esterification and chylomicron formation during fat absorption. 1. Triglycerides and cholesterol esters. J. Lipid Res. **4**, 312—321 (1963).

KAY, R. E., and C. ENTENMAN: The synthesis of „chylomicron-like" bodies and maintenance of normal blood sugar levels by the isolated perfused rat liver. J. biol. Chem. **236**, 1006—1012 (1961).

KAYDEN, H. J., A. KARMEN, and A. DUMONT: Alterations in the fatty acid composition of human lymph and serum lipoproteins by single feedings. J. clin. Invest. **42**, 1373—1381 (1963).

KLEIN, E., W. F. LEVER, and L. L. FEKETE: Defective lipemia clearing response to heparin in idiopathic hyperlipemia. J. invest. Derm. **33**, 91—97 (1959).

KRINSKY, N. I., D. G. CORNWELL, and J. L. ONCLEY: The transport of vitamin A and carotenoids in human plasma. Arch. Biochem. **73**, 233—246 (1958).
KRUT, L. H., and B. BRONTE-STEWART: The fatty acids of human depot fat. J. Lipid Res.
5, 343—351 (1964).
KUNKEL, H. G., and A. G. BEARN: Phospholipid studies of different serum lipoproteins
employing P^{32}. Proc. Soc. exp. Biol. (N. Y.) **86**, 887—891 (1954).
— and R. TRAUTMAN: The α_2-lipoproteins of human serum. Correlation of ultracentrifugal
and electrophoretic properties. J. clin. Invest. **35**, 641—648 (1956).
LAMY, M., J. FRÉZAL, J. POLONOVSKI, D. BARD, and J. REY: Mesure de la demi-vie des lipoprotéines plasmatiques. C.R. Acad. Sci. (Paris) **253**, 2135—2136 (1961).
LEVY, R. I., and D. S. FREDRICKSON: Heterogeneity of plasma high density lipoproteins.
J. clin. Invest. **44**, 426—441 (1965).
— R. S. LEES, and D. S. FREDRICKSON: A functional role for plasma alpha lipoprotein.
J. clin. Invest. **44**, 1068 (1965).
LINDGREN, F. T.: New high-density lipoproteins in human serum. Clin. chim. Acta **9**, 402—404
(1964).
— and A. V. NICHOLS: Structure and function of human serum lipoproteins, p. 2—58. In:
F. W. PUTNAM: The Plasma Proteins, Vol. 2. NewYork: Academic Press 1960.
— — and N. K. FREEMAN: Physical and chemical composition studies on the lipoproteins of
fasting and heparinized human sera. J. Phys. Chem. **59**, 930—938 (1955).
— — and R. D. WILLS: Fatty acid distributions in serum lipids and serum lipoproteins.
Amer. J. clin. Nutr. **9**, 13—23 (1961).
— — N. K. FREEMAN, R. D. WILLS, L. WING, and J. E. GULLBERG: Analysis of low-density
lipoproteins by preparative ultracentrifugation and refractometry. J. Lipid Res. **5**, 68—74
(1964).
LOMBARDI, G., and R. O. RECKNAGEL: Interference with secretion of triglycerides by the liver
as a common factor in toxic liver injury. Amer. J. Path. **40**, 571—586 (1962).
LOSSOW, W. J., N. BROT, and I. L. CHAIKOFF: Disposition of the cholesterol moiety of a chylo-
micron-containing lipoprotein fraction of chyle in the rat. J. Lipid Res. **3**, 207—215 (1962).
MACHEBOEUF, M., and P. REBEYROTTE: Studies on lipo-protein cenapses of horse serum.
Discussions Faraday Soc. **6**, 62—68 (1959).
MALING, H. M., A. FRANK, and M. G. HORNING: Effect of carbon tetrachloride on hepatic
synthesis and release of triglycerides. Biochim. biophys. Acta (Amst.) **64**, 540—545 (1962).
MANNICK, V. G.: Heterogeneity of human β-lipoprotein. Ph. D. Thesis: Radcliffe College
1955.
MARKSCHEID, L., and E. SHAFRIR: Assimilation of lipoprotein triglyceride (TG) in vitro:
Comparison of various adipose tissues and lipoproteins and effect of lipoprotein lipase (LL)
inhibitors. Israel J. Chem. **1**, 205—207 (1963).
— — Incorporation of lipoprotein-borne triglycerides by adipose tissue in vitro. J. Lipid.
Res. **6**, 247—257 (1965).
MARSH, J. B.: The incorporation of amino acids into soluble lipoproteins by cell-free prepara-
tions from rat liver. J. biol. Chem. **238**, 1752—1756 (1963).
— and A. F. WHEREAT: The synthesis of plasma lipoprotein by rat liver. J. biol. Chem. **234**,
3196—3200 (1959).
McCORMICK, E. C., D. G. CORNWELL, and J. B. BROWN: Studies on the distribution of tocopherol in human serum lipoproteins. J. Lipid. Res. **1**, 221—228 (1960).
McFARLANE, A. S.: Ultracentrifugal protein sedimentation diagram of normal human, cow
and horse serum. Biochem. J. **29**, 660—693 (1935).
MINARI, O., and D. B. ZILVERSMIT: Behavior of dog lymph chylomicron lipid constituents
during incubation with serum. J. Lipid Res. **4**, 424—436 (1963).
NARAYAN, K. A., S. NARAYAN, and F. A. KUMMEROW: Disc electrophoresis of human serum
lipoproteins. Nature (Lond.) **205**, 246—248 (1965).
NELSON, G. J., and N. K. FREEMAN: The phospholipid and phospholipid fatty acid compo-
sition of human serum lipoprotein fractions. J. biol. Chem. **235**, 578—583 (1960).
NERKING, J.: Über Fetteiweißverbindungen. Pflügers Arch. ges. Physiol. **85**, 330—344 (1901).
NESTEL, P. J., and D. STEINBERG: Fate of palmitate and of linoleate perfused through the
isolated rat liver at high concentrations. J. Lipid Res. **4**, 461—469 (1963).
— and R. O. SCOW: Metabolism of chylomicrons of differing triglyceride composition. J. Lipid
Res. **5**, 46—51 (1964).
NICHOLS, A. V., and L. SMITH: Effect of very low-density lipoproteins on lipid transfer in
incubated serum. J. Lipid Res. **6**, 206—210 (1965).
— — C. S. REHNBORG, and D. FRANCIS: Lipid transfer by high density lipoproteins of human
serum *in vitro*. Biochem. biophys. Res. Commun. **17**, 512—516 (1964).
NYE, W. H. R.: An assessment of the role of alpha and beta chylomicra in hyperlipemic states.
Proc. Soc. exp. Biol. (N. Y.) **116**, 350—354 (1964).

1177

.87

OLIVECRONA, T.: Kinetics of fatty acid transport. An experimental study in the rat. Thesis: University of Lund 1962.

— and P. BELFRAGE: Mechanisms for removal of chyle triglyceride from the circulating blood as studied with [^{14}C] glycerol and [^{3}H] palmitic acid-labeled chyle. Biochim. biophys. Acta (Amst.) 98, 81—93 (1965).

ONCLEY, J. L.: Lipid protein interactions, p. 1—17. In: J. FOLCH-PI and H. BAUER: Brain Lipids and Lipoproteins, and the Leucodystrophies. Amsterdam: Elsevier 1963.

— Lipoproteins, p. 70—91, p. 122—123. In: H. C. MENG, J. G. CONIGLIO, V. S. LeQUIRE, G. V. MANN, and J. M. MERRILL: Lipid Transport. Springfield (Ill.): Thomas 1964.

— F. R. N. GURD, and M. MELIN: Preparation and properties of serum and plasma proteins. XXV. Composition and properties of human serum beta-lipoprotein. J. Amer. chem. Soc. 72, 458—464 (1950).

— M. MELIN, D. A. RICHERT, J. W. CAMERON, and P. M. GROSS jr.: The separation of the antibodies, isoagglutimins, prothrombin, plasminogen and β_1-lipoprotein into subfractions of human plasma. J. Amer. Chem. Soc. 71, 541—550 (1949).

— G. SCATCHARD, and A. BROWN: Physical-chemical characteristics of certain of the proteins of normal human plasma. J. Phys. Colloid Chem. 51, 184—198 (1947).

— K. W. WALTON, and D. G. CORNWELL: A rapid method for the bulk isolation of β-lipoproteins from human plasma. J. Amer. chem. Soc. 79, 4666—4671 (1957).

PEDERSEN, K. O.: Ultracentrifugal studies of serum and serum fractions. Uppsala: Almqvist and Wiksell 1945.

PELKONEN, R.: Plasma vitamin A and E in the study of lipid and lipoprotein metabolism in coronary heart disease. Acta med. scand. 174, Suppl. 399 (1963).

PEZOLD, F. A.: Lipide und Lipoproteide im Blutplasma. Berlin-Göttingen-Heidelberg: Springer 1961.

PHILLIPS, G. B.: The phospholipid composition of human serum lipoprotein fraction separated by ultracentrifugation. J. clin. Invest. 38, 489—493 (1959a).

— Lipid composition of human serum lipoprotein fraction with density greater than 1.210. Proc. Soc. exp. Biol. (N. Y.) 100, 19—22 (1959b).

PINTER, G. G., and D. B. ZILVERSMIT: A gradient centrifugation method for the determination of particle size distribution of chylomicrons and of fat droplets in artificial fat emulsions. Biochim. biophys. Acta (Amst.) 59, 116—127 (1962).

POLONOVSKI, J., and M. PAYSANT: Métabolisme phospholipidique du sang. VIII. Échange des phospholipides marqués entre globules et plasma sanguin in vitro. Bull. Soc. Chim. biol. (Paris) 45, 339—347 (1963).

— J. REY, D. BARD, J. FRÉZAL, and M. LAMY: Modification des lipides plasmatiques apres ingestion d'huile chez trois enfants normaux et dans cas d'absence congénitale de β-lipoprotéines. Rev. franc. Étud. clin. biol. 10, 1006—1013 (1961).

RADDING, C. M., and D. STEINBERG: Studies on the synthesis and secretion of serum lipoproteins by rat liver slices. J. clin. Invest. 39, 1560—1569 (1960).

REHNBORG, C. S., and A. V. NICHOLS: The fate of cholesteryl esters in human serum incubated in vitro at 38°. Biochim. biophys. Acta (Amst.) 84, 596—603 (1964).

ROBINSON, D. S.: The clearing factor lipase and its action in the transport of fatty acids between the blood and the tissues. Advanc. Lipid Res 1, 133—182 (1963).

— and A. SEAKINS: Reduced plasma lipoprotein production as a factor in the development of fatty livers — p. 359—365. In: A. C. FRAZER: Biochemical Problems of Lipids. Amsterdam: Elsevier 1963.

RODBELL, M., and D. S. FREDRICKSON: Nature of the proteins associated with dog and human chylomicrons. J. biol. Chem. 234, 562—566 (1959).

— and R. O. SCOW: The removal and metabolism of triglycerides by perfused adipose tissue — p. 110—126. In: K. RODAHL, and B. ISSEKUTZ, jr.: Fat as a Tissue. New York: McGraw-Hill Book Co. 1964.

ROHEIM, P. S., D. E. HAFT, L. I. GIDEZ, A. WHITE, and H. A. EDER: Plasma lipoprotein metabolism in perfused rat livers. II. Transfer of free and esterified cholesterol into the plasma. J. clin. Invest. 42, 1277—1285 (1963).

ROWE, C. E.: The phospholipids of human blood plasma and their exchange with the cells. Biochem. J. 76, 471—475 (1960).

SAKAGAMI, T., O. MINARI, and T. ORII: Behavior of plasma lipoproteins during exchange of phospholipids between plasma and erythrocytes. Biochim. biophys. Acta (Amst.) 98, 111—116 (1965).

SALEM, L.: The role of long-range forces in the cohesion of lipoproteins. Canad. J. Biochem. 40, 1287—1298 (1962).

SALT, H., H. WOLFF, J. LLOYD, A. FOSBROOKE, A. CAMERON, and D. HUBBLE: On having no beta-lipoprotein. A syndrome comprising a beta-lipoptoteinemia, acanthocytosis, and steatorrhea. Lancet 1960/II, 325—329.

SANBAR, S. S.: Structure and metabolism of serum high density lipoproteins. Thesis: University of Oklahoma 1963.
— and P. ALAUPOVIC: Effect of urea on behavior of the protein moiety of human-serum α-lipoproteins in solution. Biochim. biophys. Acta (Amst.) **71**, 235—236 (1963).
— P. ALAUPOVIC, R. P. HOWARD, R. H. BRADFORD, and R. H. FURMAN: The metabolism of radioiodinated human alpha lipoprotein and its protein moiety in normal and hyperglyceridemic (hyperlipemic) subjects. J. Lab. clin. Med. **60**, 1014—1015 (1962).
SCANU, A., and W. L. HUGHES: Recombining capacity toward lipids of the protein moiety of human serum α-lipoprotein. J. biol. Chem. **235**, 2876—2883 (1960).
— — Further characterization of the human serum D 1.063—1.21α_1-lipoprotein. J. clin. Invest. **41**, 1681—1689 (1962).
— L. A. LEWIS, and I. H. PAGE: Studies on the antigenicity of β- and α_1-lipoproteins of human serum. J. exp. Med. **108**, 185—196 (1958a).
— — and F. M. BUMPUS: Separation and characterization of the protein moiety of human α_1-lipoprotein. Arch. Biochem. **74**, 390—397 (1958b).
— and I. H. PAGE: Separation and characterization of human serum chylomicrons. J. exp. Med. **109**, 239—256 (1959).
— — Recombination with lipids of the lipid-free protein from canine serum (d 1.063—1.21,α_1) lipoprotein. J. Lipid Res. **2**, 161—168 (1961).
— — Plasma transport of lipids and lipoprotein proteins in dogs treated with Triton WR—1339. J. clin. Invest. **41**, 495—504 (1962).
SCHACHMAN, H. K.: Ultracentrifugation in Biochemistry. New York: Academic Press 1959.
SCHÖN, H., and W. ZELLER: Über die Bedeutung erhöhter Serumlipidwerte für die Atherogenese. Behandlungsmöglichkeiten. Münch. med. Wschr. **104**, 2433—2440 (1962).
SCHOTZ, M. C., N. BAKER, and M. N. CHAVEZ: Effect of carbon tetrachloride ingestion on liver and plasma triglyceride turnover rates. J. Lipid Res. **5**, 569—577 (1964).
SCHULZ, F. N.: Über den Fettgehalt des Blutes beim Hunger. Pflügers Arch. ges. Physiol. **65**, 299—307 (1897).
SHARP, D. G., and J. W. BEARD: Size and density of polystyrene particles measured by ultracentrifugation. J. biol. Chem. **185**, 247—253 (1950).
SHIMIDZU, Y.: Ein Beitrag zur Kumagawa-Sutoschen Fettbestimmungsmethode. Biochem. Z. **28**, 237—273 (1910).
SHORE, B.: C- and N-terminal amino acids of human serum lipoproteins. Arch. Biochem. **71**, 1—10 (1957).
— and V. SHORE: Some physical and chemical properties of the lipoproteins produced by lipolysis of human serum S_f 20—400 lipoproteins by post-heparin plasma. J. Atheroscler. Res. **2**, 104—114 (1962a).
— — The protein subunit of human serum lipoproteins of density 1.125—1.200 gram/ml. Biochem. biophys. Res. Commun. **9**, 455—460 (1962b).
SPIGAI, C.: Studio critico sul ricambio lipidico nel divenire della malattia aterogenica. G. Gerant., Suppl. G. ital. Arterioscler. **1**, 81—112 (1963).
STEIN, Y., and B. SHAPIRO: Assimilation and dissimilation of fatty acids by the rat liver. Amer. J. Physiol. **196**, 1238—1241 (1959).
STEINBERG, D.: Fatty acid mobilization-mechanisms of regulation and metabolic consequences — p. 111—138. In: J. K. GRANT: The Control of Lipid Metabolism. London: Academic Press 1963.
SWAHN, B.: A method for localization and determination of serum lipids after electrophoretic separation on filter paper. Scand. J. clin. Lab. Invest. **4**, 98—103 (1952).
— Studies on blood lipids. Scand. J. clin. Lab. Invest. **5**, Suppl. 9 (1953).
THOMPSON, T. E.: The properties of bimolecular phospholipid membranes. In: M. LOCKE: Cellular Membranes and Development. New York: Academic Press 1964.
TORO-GOYCO, E.: Physical-chemical studies of the β_1-lipoproteins of human plasma. Ph. D. Thesis: Harvard University 1958.
TRAVIA, L.: Correlative variations of total lipemia, total cholesterolemia and the beta: alpha lipoprotein ratio in humans of excess weight due to hypernutrition. Nutr. et Dieta (Basel) **6**, 21—30 (1964).
VAN CAUWENBERGE, H., C. HEUSGHEM, N. BROUCHON, and G. P. LEFEBVRE: Quelques resultats de tests lipidiques chez des sujets normaux. Acta clin. belg. **18**, 495—510 (1963).
VANDENHEUVEL, F. A.: Study of biological structure at a molecular level with stereomodel projections. I. The lipids in the myelin sheath of nerve. J. Amer. Oil Chemists' Soc. **40**, 455—471 (1963).
VAUGHN, M., and E. D. KORN: Metabolic activity of adipose tissue — p. 173—235. In: L. W. KINSELL: Adipose Tissue as an Organ. Springfield (Ill.): Thomas 1962.
VIVIANI, R., A. M. SECHI, and G. LENAZ: Fatty acid composition of portal fatty liver in lysine- and threonine-deficient rats. J. Lipid Res. **5**, 52—56 (1964).

VOLWILER, W., P. D. GOLDSWORTHY, M. P. MacMARTIN, P. A. WOOD, I. R. MACKAY, and
K. FREMONT-SMITH: Biosynthestic determination with radioactive sulfur of turn-over rate
of various plasma proteins in normal and cirrhotic man. J. clin. Invest. **34**, 1126—1146
(1955).
WALTON, K. W., and S. J. DARKE: Immunological characteristics of human low-density lipoproteins and their relation to lipoproteins of other species — p. 146—148. In: H. PEETERS:
Protides of the Biological Fluids, Vol. 10. Amsterdam: Elsevier 1963.
— P. J. SCOTT, J. VERRIER JONES, R. F. FLETCHER, and T. WHITEHEAD: Studies on low-
density lipoprotein turnover in relation to atromid therapy. J. Atheroscler. Res. **3**, 396—414
(1963).
WHYTE, M., A. KARMEN, and D. S. GOODMAN: Fatty acid esterification and chylomicron
formation during fat absorption: 2. Phospholipids. J. Lipid Res. **4**, 322—329 (1963).
WILLIAMS, J. W., R. L. BALDWIN, W. M. SAUNDERS, and P. G. SQUIRE: Boundary spreading
in sedimentation velocity experiments. The degredation of serum globulin. J. Amer. Chem.
Soc. **74**, 1542—1548 (1952).
WINDMUELLER, H. G.: An orotic acid-induced, adenine-reversed inhibition of hepatic lipoprotein secretion in the rat. J. biol. Chem. **239**, 530—537 (1964).
WOOD, P., K. IMAICHI, J. KNOWLES, G. MICHAELS, and L. KINSELL: The lipid composition
of human plasma chylomicrons. J. Lipid Res. **5**, 225—231 (1964).
YOKOYAMA, A., and D. B. ZILVERSMIT: Particle size and composition of dog lymph chylo-
microns. J. Lipid Res. **6**, 241—246 (1965).
ZEMPLÉNYI, T.: The lipolytic and esterolytic activity of blood and tissues and problems of
atherosclerosis. Advanc. Lipid Res. **2**, 235—293 (1964).
ZILVERSMIT, D. B.: Centrifugation methods for the study of chylomicrons — p. 257—262.
In: A. C. FRAZER: Biochemical Problems of Lipids. Amsterdam: Elsevier 1963.
— Extraction of cholesterol from human serum lipoprotein films. J. Lipid. Res. **5**, 300—306
(1964).
— A comparison of cream and corn oil chylomicron stability and composition. Fed. Proc.
23, 501 (1964).

Methods for separation and determination of lipids

By

H. Wagener

Introduction

Lipids comprise a variety of substances with similar solubility properties but different chemical structures. Because of this heterogeneity, which in each lipid class is extended by different fatty acid compositions, a combination of preparative and chemical methods is needed for complete separation and specific determination of each fraction.

During the last decades methodological advances in the lipid field arose mainly from the introduction of chromatographic techniques. The combination of these with known procedures led to improvements which permit analyses to be performed faster and with considerably smaller amounts of material. In the following survey emphasis is laid on newer methods; older procedures which in many cases were shown to be less reliable are mentioned only briefly.

I. Isolation of Lipids

Quantitative isolation of lipids from tissues and plasma requires that the lipid-protein complexes occurring in biological materials are destroyed. For this purpose solvents have to be used which are sufficiently polar to split the complexes and denature the proteins. Complete extraction of lipids is achieved by addition of lipophilic solvents.

A suitable solvent mixture consists of chloroform-methanol (2:1) because this combination, according to THANNHAUSER and SETZ (1936), has the greatest solvent power for phospholipids, especially sphingomyelins. Ethanol-ether (3:1) as a solvent (BLOOR 1914) is feasible only if the lipids are composed predominantly of neutral lipids. For quantitative extraction of liquid samples at least 20 volumes of chloroform-methanol are required. Tissues are best homogenized and extracted with 100 volumes of solvent mixture for each gram of tissue. Heating, although unnecessary for complete extraction, is often employed. Moderate temperatures (30—50°C) and short heating periods should not be exceeded in order to avoid oxidative damage. After filtration for removal of precipitated proteins the lipid extracts are still contaminated with non-lipid material. For purification, according to FOLCH et al. (1951) the extracts are shaken with water or dilute salt solutions and the water phase is removed. This procedure should be preferred to evaporation and redissolution in lipophilic solvents. The purified extract may be concentrated by distillation in vacuo. An inert atmosphere (nitrogen) during solvent evaporation excludes oxidation and polymerization of unsaturated fatty acids. Samples may be taken to complete dryness only if no further operations are considered. Otherwise they should be stored in solvents such as benzene, hexane, chloroform, acetone at low temperature and under nitrogen.

Methanol and ethanol should not be used for storage because of transesterification resulting in the formation of fatty acid methyl and ethyl esters (LOUGH et al. 1962).

Extraction and purification of tissue lipids sometimes require special procedures to avoid loss of lipids such as gangliosides, sulfatides, and phosphoinositides.

The diffusion procedure for purification of chloroform-methanol solutions of lipids may be replaced by a method of shorter duration which consists of passing the extracts through columns of dextrane gel (sephadex) (WELLS and DITTMER 1963).

Plasma lipids may also be co-precipitated with proteins and extracted from the precipitate. Care should be taken not to use precipitating agents, which may alter the lipids, e.g. strongly acidic or basic materials. Suitable agents are colloidal iron (FOLCH and VAN SLYKE 1939), 5% trichloroacetic acid (ZILVERSMIT and DAVIS 1950), and zinc hydroxide (VAN SLYKE and PLAZIN 1965).

To exclude oxidation of unsaturated lipids during handling the addition of anti-oxidants (hydrochinone, butylated hydroxy toluene, butyl hydrochinone) is recommended (LEWIS 1958, NEUDOERFFER and LEA 1966).

II. Quantitative Determination of Total Lipids

The amounts of total lipids extracted from plasma or tissues are best determined by gravimetric or photometric procedures. These methods are superior to older procedures, e.g. bichromate oxidation according to BLOOR (1928), because they do not alter the material and permit further procedures to be performed or are less time consuming.

For gravimetry aliquots of purified extracts are evaporated and the residues dried and weighed. A detailed description of this technique was given by SPERRY (1955).

A photometric procedure which is based on the reaction of unsaturated fatty acids with concentrated sulfuric acid and a mixture of phosphoric acid and vanilline with development of a pink color was introduced by ZÖLLNER and KIRSCH (1962). Since in this reaction the various lipids show different extinction coefficients calibration is necessary according to gravimetric values. This method is also applicable directly to plasma samples without previous extraction.

Turbidity occurring after the addition of diluted sulfuric acid to lipid dioxane extracts permits measurement of total lipids from very small amounts of serum (SEARCY et al. 1963).

III. Separation of Lipid Classes

The choice of methods for separation of lipid classes depends on the desired degree of separation. Simpler methods permit concentration or separation of only a few fractions, whereas newer methods based mainly on chromatographic procedures permit fractionation into all main lipid classes. The selection is further dependent on the amounts of material available.

a) Fractionation into Polar and Unpolar Lipids

Fractionation of lipid mixtures into phosphorus containing polar constituents and non-polar neutral fats including cholesterol is frequently required and can be achieved by several procedures.

Since phospholipids are insoluble in acetone they may be precipitated from concentrated ethyl ether, petroleum ether or chloroform solutions by the addition of excess anhydrous acetone (ZUELZER 1899). Precipitation is completed by small amounts of magnesium sulfate (NERDING 1910) or calcium chloride (KATSURA et al. 1933). The concentrations of these salts are critical since greater amounts lead to incomplete precipitation and may cause irreversible alterations of the lipids.

Neutral fats and phospholipids can also be separated by dialysis (VAN BEERS et al. 1958, EBERHAGEN and BETZING 1962). Phosphatides aggregate in non-polar solvents whereas neutral lipids do not. Therefore only cholesterol esters, glycerides, free fatty acids, and free cholesterol pass through a rubber membrane in petroleum ether solution. The duration of dialysis depends on the pore size of the membrane. Contamination by soluble rubber components should be prevented by prewashing the membranes.

Separation of polar and non-polar lipids can also be achieved by column chromatography using heat-activated silica gel (BORGSTRÖM 1952). A chloroform solution of lipids is applied to such a column and the neutral lipids are eluted with chloroform. Phospholipids are obtained by elution with methanol and chloroform-methanol (1:1).

When chromatography on activated adsorbents is employed chemical alterations of lipids are possible. RENKONEN (1962) reported hydrolysis of lecithin on aluminium oxide columns. Because of the danger of isomerization and oxidation solvents have to be carefully purified.

b) Fractionation into Main Lipid Classes

Separation of a mixture of different lipids into its components can be achieved by several chromatographic procedures. Older methods, e.g. solvent fractionation,

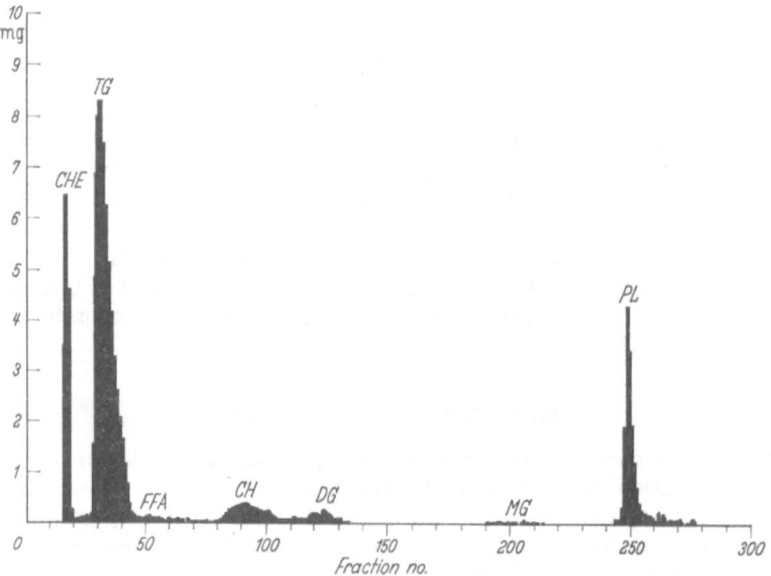

Figure 1. Fractionation of plasma lipids in a case of essential hyperlipemia by silicic acid column chromatography according to HIRSCH and AHRENS (1958): *CHE* = cholesterol esters, *TG* = triglycerides, *FFA* = free fatty acids, *CH* = cholesterol, *DG* = diglycerides, *MG* = monoglycerides, *PL* = phospholipids

usually do not result in clear separations. The quality of chromatographic methods depends mainly on the purity of the adsorbent and solvents, and the composition and amount of material to be processed. These aspects were discussed extensively by WREN (1960). With careful observation of these rules chromatography is a powerful tool, as was shown by WREN and MITCHELL (1958) who were able to separate plasma lipids into 20 different fractions. The efficiency of chromatography is illustrated by a microtechnique which requires only 200 mg of adsorbent for fractionation of the lipids from 1 mg wet tissue (LARRABEE and KLINGMAN 1963).

Silicic acid is the adsorbent most frequently used for column chromatography of lipids. It was introduced by BORGSTRÖM (1952) with hexane-benzene mixtures as eluting solvents. FILLERUP and MEAD (1953) used silicic acid with mixtures of diethyl ether-petroleum ether and hexane-benzene respectively. Reproducible results are obtained with the standardized method of HIRSCH and AHRENS (1958).

Separation of the lipids is achieved by either stepwise or gradient elution. With unpolar solvents such as petroleum ether or hexane hydrocarbons are first eluted. By addition of various amounts of ether or benzene cholesterol esters, triglycerides, free fatty acids, free cholesterol, di- and monoglycerides are eluted in this order. Phospholipids are adsorbed stronger and can be eluted with a polar solvent such as methanol (figure 1).

Fractionation of phospholipids by column chromatography is more difficult than the separation of neutral lipids. By using chloroform methanol mixtures and increasing the concentration of methanol up to 100% some fractionation is possible, although each fraction is still contaminated by other phospholipids (HIRSCH and AHRENS 1958, ZÖLLNER and KIRSCH 1960).

This overlapping of fractions shows the need for controlling the elution by qualitative or quantitative methods, such as phosphorus determination, total lipid determination, spot tests on silica thin-layers with subsequent sulfuric acid spray and charring,

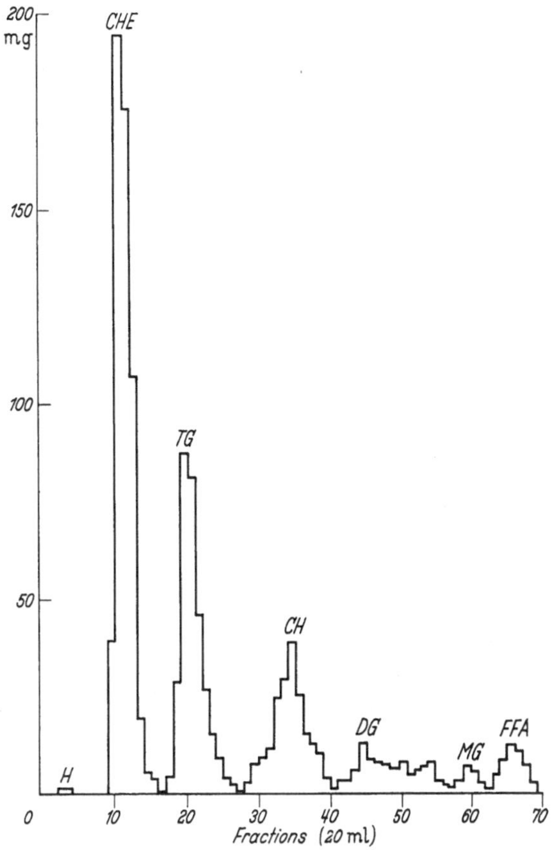

Figure 2. Fractionation of plasma lipids in a case of Refsum's syndrome by column chromatography using florisil (KAHLKE 1964): H = hydrocarbons, CHE = cholesterol esters, TG = triglycerides, CH = cholesterol, DG = diglycerides, MG = monoglycerides, FFA = free fatty acids

thin-layer chromatography of each fraction etc. Similar methods should also be used in checking the purity of the various neutral lipid fractions.

Neutral lipids can also be fractionated on columns of florisil (magnesium silicate) with ether-hexane mixtures as solvent (CARROLL 1961). Florisil columns have a higher capacity than silicic acid columns and usually allow faster flow rates. They are disadvantageous because phospholipids cannot be removed quantitatively from the column (figure 2).

Chromatographic separations can also be performed with thin-layers of silica gel or other adsorbents on glass plates (thin-layer chromatography). This method was standardized by STAHL (1958). WEICKER (1959) first applied this technique in the lipid field by separating serum lipids. A comprehensive survey of thin-layer chromatography of lipids was given by MANGOLD (1962). Thin-layer chromatography is superior to column chromatography with regard to speed of separation and quality of resolution. Furthermore, depending on the thickness of the adsorbent layer, analytical and preparative work is possible.

Thin-layers for separation of lipids are prepared by spreading a suspension of silica gel and calcium sulfate in water on carefully cleaned glass plates. The plates are dried at room temperature and activated at 100—110°C immediately before use and the lipids dissolved in chloroform, benzene or hexane are applied as spost or streaks. For development the plates are brought into glass chambers containing the liquid phase. When the solvent front has reached a certain height the plates are removed and dried. For visualization of separated lipids the chromatoplates may be sprayed with suitable dyes (rhodamin B, dichlorofluorescein) or reagents (phosphomolybdic acid etc.). Lipids may also be located under ultraviolet light without any pretreatment (WAGENER 1965). Detection of lipids with iodine vapor should be avoided if the fatty acid composition of the separated lipids is to be determined since there is some destruction of unsaturated lipids (NICHAMAN et al. 1963). Spraying with dilute sulfuric acid and subsequent charring reveals all organic materials present.

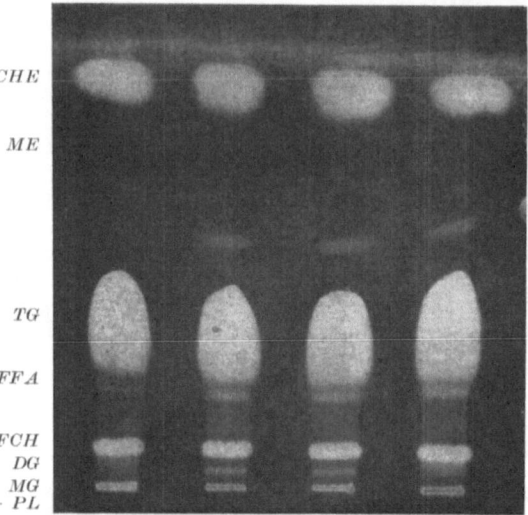

Figure 3. Fractionation of plasma lipids by thin-layer chromatography (WAGENER 1965): solvent = petroleum ether-diethyl ether-acetic acid 85 : 15 : 1 by volume, detection = ultraviolet light, CHE = cholesterol esters, ME = methyl esters, TG = triglycerides, FFA = free fatty acids, FCH = free cholesterol, DG = diglycerides, $MG + PL$ = monoglycerides and phospholipids

Solvents may be used singly or as mixtures for development of the thin-layer plates. Repeated development with the same or other solvents is also possible (WEICKER 1959). In this way a complete separation of neutral lipids (FREEMAN and WEST 1966) and also of neutral lipids plus phospholipids (VOGEL et al. 1962) on a single chromatoplate is possible.

AMENTA (1964) used this technique for subsequent quantification of separated lipids by reducing them with an acid dichromate solution.

Separation of total lipids is achieved by development with mixtures of hexane, petroleum ether, benzene, chloroform, or ethyl ether. The addition of small amounts of acetic acid is recommended for clear separation of fatty acids. The main lipid classes are thus separated as shown in figure 3. After visualization of the individual fractions by non-destructive treatment or after spraying only a small part of the chromatoplate corresponding areas can be scraped off the plate and the separated compounds eluted with chloroform or ether (neutral lipids), and methanol-chloroform, methanol, methanol-acetic acid-water (phospholipids). The eluted material can be processed further. Some chemical determinations are possible in the presence of silica gel.

The separation of bile acids in their physiological form as taurine and glycine conjugates from other lipids is very difficult. With silicic acid column chromatography according to HIRSCH and AHRENS (1958) bile acids are eluted in the monoglyceride region. Thin-layer chromatography with ethyl ether-petroleum ether-acetic acid yields a fraction consisting of phospholipids, monoglycerides and bile acids

(FROSCH and WAGENER 1965). Only countercurrent distribution permits almost complete separation of all substances present in bile (AHRENS and CRAIG 1952).

In contrast, free bile acids can be obtained more easily after alkaline hydrolysis of lipid mixtures, acidification, and extraction with ether. Contaminating lipids are removed from these extracts by distribution between 70% ethanol and petroleum ether (BERGSTRÖM and SJÖVALL 1954).

Fractionation with the use of filter and glass filter papers has been replaced by the chromatographic procedures described because they are more difficult to perform and the quality of resolution is poorer. If larger samples are to be separated column and thin-layer chromatography may be used as preparative methods.

IV. Separation of Individual Members of Lipid Classes

Lipid classes obtained by chromatographic techniques in many cases are not pure, e.g. phospholipids obtained by thin-layer chromatography using unpolar solvents are often contaminated with monoglycerides. Furthermore all lipid fractions with the exception of free cholesterol are mixtures of substances which differ in their fatty acid moieties. Procedures are now available for their further differentiation.

Cholesterol esters can be separated according to their degree of unsaturation. For preparative work a method was described by KLEIN and JANSSEN (1959) using silica gel chromatography. Since there is some overlapping of the fractions, the purity of each fraction should be checked by thin-layer chromatography.

In analytical work thin-layer chromatography should be preferred to chromatography on silicic acid impregnated paper and glassfiber paper. ZÖLLNER et al. (1960, 1962) developed a thin-layer method for separation of various serum cholesterol esters according to unsaturation which starts with a total lipid extract and uses repeated development with carbon tetrachloride or petroleum ether with 1% isopropyl ether. After spraying the plates with antimony trichloride solution and heating spots of red to violet color represent esters with saturated, mono-unsaturated, di-unsaturated, tri- and four-unsaturated, and higher unsaturated fatty acids (figure 4). The percentage composition of the cholesterol ester mixture can then be determined by photometry of the chromatoplates at 575 nm. A similar fractionation of cholesterol esters according to degree of unsaturation is achieved using silicic acid plates impregnated with silver nitrate (MORRIS 1963).

Separation of more complex cholesterol ester mixtures is possible by two-dimensional, reversed phase thin-layer chromatography (KAUFMANN et al. 1961).

The phospholipid fraction obtained by the methods mentioned above consists of various glycerophospholipids and sphingolipids with different fatty acid compositions.

Subfractionation of phospholipids is difficult because fractions overlap (HIRSCH and AHRENS 1958) and oxidation may lead to alteration of solubility properties. Compared with column chromatography preparative thin-layer chromatography usually gives better resolutions. For quantitative determination of the different phospholipids analytical chromatoplates have replaced silica impregnated papers (MARINETTI 1962). Separation is achieved by development in chloroform-methanol-water mixtures according to WAGNER (1960). HABERMANN et al. (1961) developed a method suitable for the separation of plasma phospholipids and subsequent determination of their phosphorus content. Figure 5 shows separation of plasma phospholipids into lysolecithin, sphingomyelin, lecithin, and cephalin fractions. For analytical work previous elimination of neutral lipids is not required.

One- and two-dimensional methods using chloroform-methanol-ammonium hydroxide mixtures permit the fractionation of more complex phospholipid mixtures (SKIPSKI et al. 1962, SKIDMORE and ENTENMAN 1962, ABRAMSON and BLECHER 1964).

Further separation of phospholipid fractions according to their fatty acid composition was demonstrated by ARVIDSON (1965) who subfractionated lecithin into

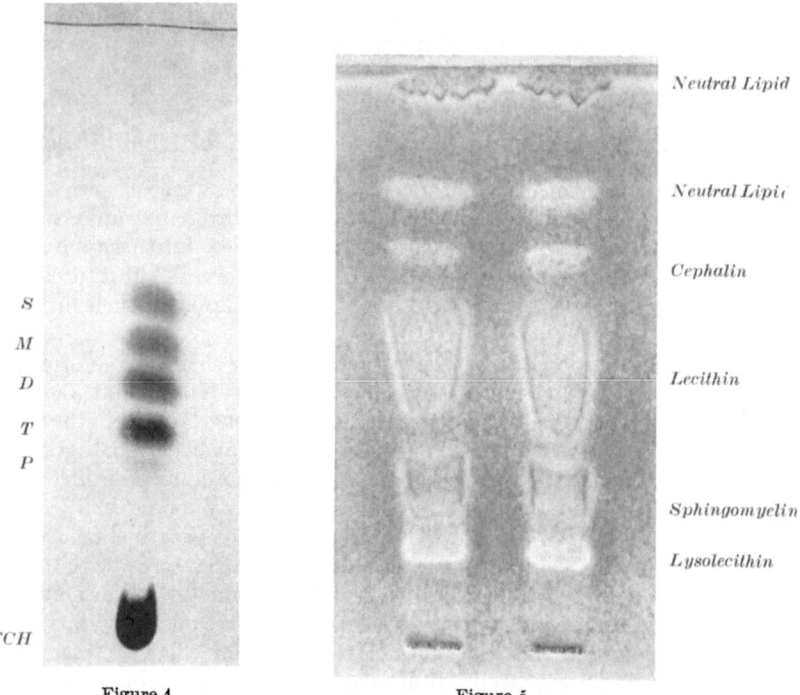

Figure 4   Figure 5

Figure 4. Fractionation of plasma cholesterol esters according to ZÖLLNER et al. (1962): S = saturated esters, M = monoenoic esters, D = dienoic esters, T = tri- and tetraenoic esters, P = polyenoic esters, FCH = free Cholesterol

Figure 5. Fractionation of plasma phospholipids according to HABERMANN et al. (1961): solvent = chloroform-methanol-water 65 : 25 : 4 by volume, detection = bromothymolblue spray

saturated and several unsaturated complexes on thin-layers of silica gel impregnated with silver nitrate. By thin-layer chromatography with chloroform-methanol-water plasma sphingomyelins are separated into two fractions which are mainly composed of palmitic acid and long-chain fatty acids (C_{20} and above) respectively (WOOD and HOLTON 1964).

Considerable difficulties are encountered in subfractionation of glycerides. Partial glycerides (mono- and diglycerides) may isomerize on silicic acid and florisil (MATTSON and VOLPENHEIM 1962). Triglycerides are more stable but comprise numerous isomers, the total separation of which has not been achieved.

Mono- and diglycerides can be separated from triglycerides by column chromatography on silica gel (HIRSCH and AHRENS 1958), florisil (CARROLL 1961), and polymerized soy bean oil according to HIRSCH (1963). Further resolution of triglycerides is possible on columns of silica gel impregnated with silver nitrate (DE VRIES 1962) and thin-layer plates prepared in the same way (BARRETT et al. 1962, 1963). Silver ions complex with olefinic double bonds with the cis-forms being more stable than the trans-forms. These compounds are then separated according to configuration and number of double bonds. Fractions obtained in this way are not pure.

Free fatty acids can be separated from other lipid classes by extracting total lipid solutions with dilute aqueous or alcoholic solutions of alkali hydroxides or with column and thin-layer chromatographic procedures. Fatty acids in ester or acid-amid linkages must be liberated by saponification.

Prior to introduction of gas-liquid chromatography, the resolution of fatty acid mixtures was tedious, and available methods required large amounts of material,

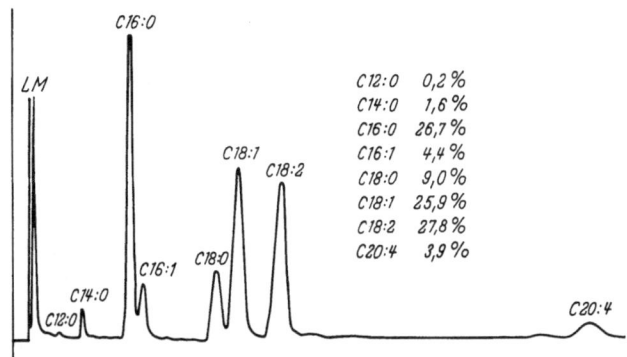

Figure 6. Separation of plasma total fatty acids by gas-liquid chromatography: chromatograph = Model 800 A Packard, column = 20 % diethylene glycol adipate on 60—80 mesh Chromosorb W, temperature = 180 °C, detector voltage = 725 V, argon pressure = 1,2 at., LM = solvent, C 12:0 = lauric acid, C 14:0 = myristic acid, C 16:0 = palmitic acid, C 16:1 = palmitoleic acid, C 18:0 = stearic acid, C 18:1 = oleic acid, C 18:2 = linoleic acid, C 20:4 = arachidonic acid

yielded incomplete resolution, and did not prevent structural changes especially of unsaturated acids (lead salt crystallization, bromination). Such changes were minimized by employing low temperature crystallization (SHINOWARA and BROWN 1940) and countercurrent distribution (CRAIG et al. 1944). Fractionation of mercury acetate adducts was a further improvement (JANTZEN and ANDREAS 1959, 1961). However, paper (KAUFMANN and NITSCH 1954) and thin-layer chromatography (MANGOLD 1959) replaced these methods mainly in handling small samples. Gas-liquid chromatography (JAMES and MARTIN 1952) is at present the most powerful tool for analytical separations. It can also be used for preparative purposes. A review of these methods was given by FONTELL et al. (1959/1960).

Separation of compounds by gas-chromatography is based on the partition of volatilized compounds between a liquid stationary phase on an inert support in a heated column and a mobile gas phase. Substances emerge with the gas stream from the column according to their partition coefficients in the two phases. Gas-liquid chromatography requires only microgram samples and yields a high degree of resolution. The separations depend on the stationary phases, supporting media, column dimensions, detection systems, operating temperatures etc.

As stationary phase for the resolution of fatty acid mixtures polar (polyesters of short chain dicarbonic acids and low molecular diols) and unpolar (hydrocarbons, silicones) substances can be used. Gas-chromatography under standardized conditions permits the tentative identification of separated fatty acids from the time elapsing between application of the sample and the emergence of the acid in question. Figure 6 shows the separation of serum fatty acid methyl esters using a polar stationary phase.

The percentage composition of a fatty acid mixture may be determined by planimetry of the fatty acid peaks. The essential requirements for quantitative gas-liquid chromatography were recently summarized by HORNING et al. (1964).

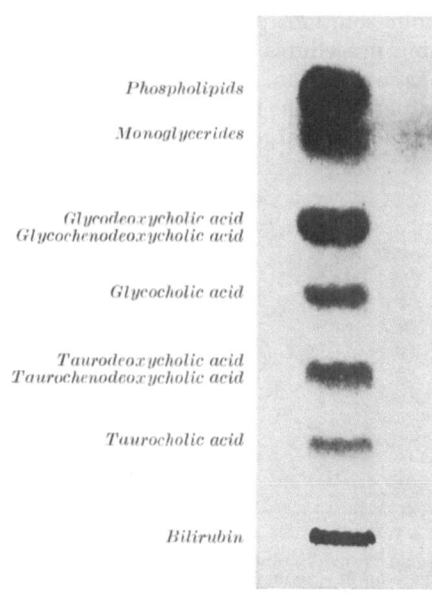

Phospholipids

Monoglycerides

Glycodeoxycholic acid
Glycochenodeoxycholic acid

Glycocholic acid

Taurodeoxycholic acid
Taurochenodeoxycholic acid

Taurocholic acid

Bilirubin

Figure 7. Separation of plasma conjugated bile acids according to FROSCH and WAGENER (1965): solvent = butanol-acetic acid-water 10 : 1 : 1 by volume, detection = phosphomolybic acid spray

Methods for separation of individual bile acids usually start with the free acids. WIELAND and SEIBERT (1936) performed separation by extraction of bile acids with varying concentrations of hydrochlorid acid from ether solutions. Better separation was obtained by column chromatography (NORMAN 1953, SJÖVALL 1953, MOSBACH et al. 1954, GÄNSHIRT et al. 1960). Paper chromatography with various solvent mixtures enabled separation of free and conjugated bile acids (SJÖVALL 1959).

Thin-layer chromatography of bile acids was introduced by GÄNSHIRT et al. (1960) and modifiedfor separation of isomeric dihydroxy cholanic acids (deoxy- and chenodeoxy cholic acid) by several authors (HOFMAN 1962, ENEROTH 1963, HAMILTON 1963, WAGENER and FROSCH 1963). Gas-liquid chromatography of bile acid methyl esters was described by VAN DEN HEUVEL (1960) and SJÖVALL (1961) but is as yet applicable only to free bile acids.

V. Quantitative Determination of Lipid Classes

Most lipid classes can be quantitated without previous separation on the basis of characteristic constituents or specific properties. If quantitative determination is preceded by preparative procedures specificity and sensitivity of the assays may be increased. Direct quantitative determinations in plasma, without prior extraction of total lipids frequently may yield erroneously high values.

a) Cholesterol and Cholesterol Esters

Cholesterol occurs in most biological materials in both the free and esterified forms. Quantitative determination of cholesterol is based on color reactions, which are not absolutely specific but suffice since cholesterol is the predominating sterol in most materials. The color reactions include the Liebermann-Burchard reaction with sulfuric acid and acetic acid anhydride, the Tschugaeff reaction with zinc chloride and acetyl chloride in acetic acid, or the Lifschütz reaction with ferric chloride in acetic acid and sulfuric acid. Both free and esterified cholesterol participate in these reactions. Methods for the determination of cholesterol which are commonly used are those of SCHOENHEIMER and SPERRY (1934), SPERRY and WEBB (1950), ZAK et al. (1951), ZLATKIS et al. (1953). They were recently reviewed by VANZETTI (1964).

Because of their high sensitivity methods using ferric chloride are recommended. This reagent permits determination of nanogram amounts of cholesterol in microgram quantities of tissues or microliter volumes of serum (GLICK et al. 1964).

Ferrous sulfate may be used instead of ferric chloride (SEARCY and BERGQUIST 1960).

Free cholesterol is determined after precipitation by digitonin. The difference between total and free cholesterol corresponds to the esterified fraction. For estimation of cholesterol esters the value for ester cholesterol is multiplied by the factor 1.67 which is derived from the mean molecular weight of cholesterol ester fatty acids (BRAGDON et al. 1956).

In addition to digitonin, agents such as tomatine have been used for precipitation (KABARA et al. 1961, RINEHART et al. 1962).

Quantitation of total cholesterol is also possible with gas-liquid chromatography (AWLEY et al. 1963).

b) Phospholipids

Total phospholipids are quantitated by determination of the phosphorus content of lipid extracts from which non-lipid phosphorus has been removed by purification procedures. For this purpose chloroform-methanol extracts subjected to diffusion purification (FOLCH et al. 1951, SPERRY 1955) are suitable. Lipid phosphorus is determined in aliquots of these extracts after digestion. Most procedures for determination of phosphorus are based on the method of FISKE and SUBBAROW (1925) which utilizes conversion of phosphate to phosphomolybdate and its subsequent reduction to molybdic blue. Modifications of this method were reviewed by LINDBERG and ERNSTER (1956). A very convenient phosphorus assay was described by BARTLETT (1959). Total phospholipids are calculated by multiplication of the lipid phosphorus values with 25. These values are only approximations since phosphorus does not represent exactly 4% of each phospholipid molecule.

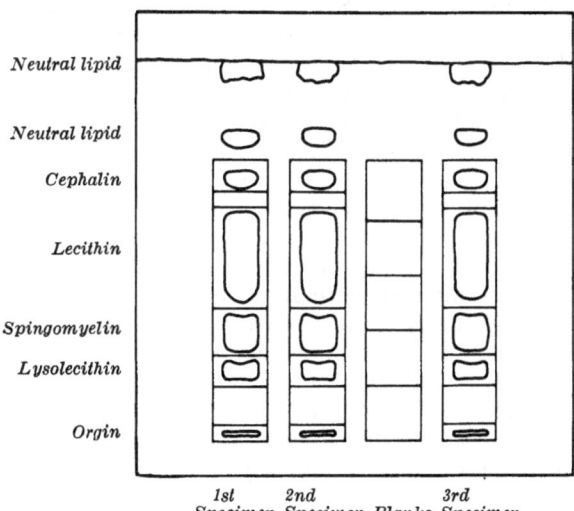

Figure 8. Division of silica gel thin-layer for quantitative determination of plasma phospholipids (WAGENER et al. 1964)

Individual phospholipids are conveniently determined after thin-layer chromatographic separation. After development of the chromatoplates phospholipids are localized by iodine vapor, fluorescent dyes, or bromothymol blue. The areas containing the separated phospholipids are scraped off. This material is used either directly for digestion or otherwise extracted with methanol and digested. Determinations should be performed in duplicate. The estimation of blank values from corresponding silica gel areas and correction of the test areas is necessary. A convenient arrangement of specimens and blanks may be seen from figure 8. Serum phospholipid concentrations determined by thin-layer chromatography agree well with those obtained by column and paper chromatography (table 1). A semimicro method for the analysis of serum phospholipids by the use of column chromatographic fractionation and infrared absorption measurement has been developed by NELSON and FREEMAN (1959).

Table 1.
Percentage composition of serum phospholipids from normals as determined by different methods (CC = column chromatography, PC = paper chromatography, TLC = thin-layer chromatography)

Author	Method	Cephalin (+ un-identified substances)	Lecithin	Sphingo-myelin	Lyso-lecithin
GJONE et al. (1959)	CC	6	66	18	9
VOGEL et al. (1962)	PC	2	66	23	9
PHILLIPS (1958)	PC	5	69	19	7
MARINETTI et al. (1959)	PC	3	67	21	9
WAGENER et al. (1964)	TLC	3	66	21	9

c) Glycerides

Previously glycerides were usually calculated from values for total lipids, lipid phosphorus, free and esterified cholesterol. The difference between total lipids and the sum of phospholipids, free cholesterol and cholesterol esters was regarded as representing neutral lipids. For satisfactory results, non-lipid material has to be removed carefully from the lipid extracts. Since substances such as hydrocarbons, free fatty acids, fat-soluble vitamins etc. are also contained in the total lipids, they contribute to the calculated neutral fat values. Instead of total lipids, total fatty acids and total esterified fatty acids have been used.

These indirect methods have been replaced by specific procedures for glyceride determination which require either isolation of the glyceride fraction or measurement of specific components. A batch elution technique using florisil was described by MICHAELS (1962) for isolation of plasma glycerides. The glyceride fraction which in addition to triglycerides contains diglycerides and most of the monoglycerides is subsequently determined quantitatively by colorimetry of the ferric hydroxamates.

A more specific method uses thin-layer chromatography for selective isolation of triglycerides and infrared photometry for quantitation (KRELL and HASHIM 1963). Quantitative determination of plasma triglycerides by spot size measurement after thin-layer chromatography has been described by SCHLIERF and WOOD (1965).

The most specific component of glycerides is glycerol. Several methods for quantitation of glycerides are therefore based on the determination of the amount of glycerol which is liberated by alkaline hydrolysis. Pertinent methods were published by VAN HANDEL and ZILVERSMIT (1957), CARLSON and WADSTRÖM (1959), RANDRUP (1960), and BLANKENHORN et al. (1961). In these procedures glycerol is oxidized with periodate to formaldehyde which is measured colorimetrically after reaction with chromotropic acid or phenylhydrazine. The chromotropic acid procedure was modified by LOFLAND (1964) for semi-automated determination of serum glycerides. The liberated glycerol can also be condensed with o-amino-phenol which in turn is oxidized to yield 8-hydroxyquinoline which can be measured fluorimetrically (MENDELSOHN and ANTONIS 1961).

Since the elimination of phospholipids is necessary in these methods a more specific procedure was developed by EGGSTEIN and KREUTZ (1966) which is based upon enzymatic determination of free glycerol (KREUTZ 1962). After alkaline hydrolysis without extraction of lipids or isolation of glycerides glycerol liberated only from glycerides is assayed with glycerokinase. This procedure is applicable to glyceride determination in serum, homogenates, incubation mixtures etc. A similar method using the enzymatic estimation of glycerol according to WIELAND (1957) was described by SPINELLA and MAGER (1966).

d) Total Fatty Acids

For determination of total fatty acids lipids must be split by alkaline hydrolysis. Hydrolysis of lipids from purified lipid extracts is preferable to hydrolysis of tissues or serum directly. After extraction of unsaponifiable matter fatty acids are recovered from their soaps by treatment with acids and can subsequently be assayed by titration. During hydrolysis high concentrations of alkali must be avoided to prevent isomerization of unsaturated fatty acids. A suitable method for quantitation of plasma total fatty acids was described by ALBRINK (1959/1960).

e) Free Fatty Acids

Free fatty acids occur only in small amounts in biological materials. They can be recovered from ether or petroleum ether extracts by extraction with diluted aqueous or alcoholic alkaline solutions as the corresponding alkaline salts and reconverted to free acids by treatment with acids. The use of diluted alkaline solutions prevents hydrolytic cleavage of glycerides and glycerophospholipids. Free fatty acids may also be isolated by adsorption to basic ion exchange resins (CARLSON and WADSTRÖM 1958, HORNSTEIN et al. 1960). Because of a tendency of polyunsaturated fatty acids to isomerization BIEGLER et al. (1960) recommend the use of weak basic adsorbents. After isolation free fatty acids are assayed by titration.

A convenient method for quantitation of free fatty acids in plasma, incubation mixtures, tissue homogenates etc. was introduced by DOLE (1956), according to which the free fatty acids are extracted directly with an isopropanol-heptane mixture from acidified samples. Further addition of heptane and water results in formation of a two-phase system. Aliquots of the upper heptane phase containing the free fatty acids are titrated with a dilute solution of aqueous sodium hydroxide.

For elimination of dicarbonic acids and phospholipids which interfere with titration washing of the final heptane extracts with dilute sulfuric acid is recommended (TROUT et al. 1960, FRIEDBERG et al. 1960). For the same reasons GORDON and CHERKES (1956) and GORDON et al. (1957) used extraction of lyophilized plasma with isooctane and acetic acid. Lyophilization is unnecessary if extraction is performed with isooctane-acetic acid anhydride-acetic acid-sulfuric acid mixture (SHAFRIR 1958, SHAFRIR and STEINBERG 1960).

Difficulties arising from titration in the two-phase system of heptane and aqueous sodium hydroxide may be overcome by using a non-aqueous titration mixture (tetrabutylammonium hydroxide) according to KELLEY (1965).

The Dole method was adapted to colorimetry using either the copper salts (ITAYA and UI 1965) or color changes of phenol red (MOSINGER 1965). ANTONIS proposed a semi-automated method (1965).

f) Bile Acids

The quantitative determination of both conjugated and free bile acids must be preceded by elimination of other lipids and the separation of individual bile acids. This can be achieved with the use of chromatographic procedures as already described.

Since free and conjugated dihydroxy cholanic acids cannot be separated completely by paper and thin-layer chromatography they must be differentiated by specific reactions. The following procedures are suitable for quantitative determination of free bile acids: reaction with concentrated sulfuric acid for determination of cholic acid (Hammarsten 1925), reaction with salicylic aldehyde and sulfuric acid for determination of deoxycholic acid (Szalkowski and Mader 1952), reaction with ethyl acetate, concentrated sulfuric acid and acetic acid anhydride for chenodeoxycholic acid (Isaksson 1954).

All these reactions are also applicable to conjugated bile acids (Frosch et al. 1964). Quantitative methods based on these reactions were developed for bile (Frosch and Wagener 1964) and serum (Frosch 1965) extending the paper and thin-layer chromatographic procedures of Sjövall (1959) and Gänshirt et al. (1960).

Using reference compounds Sandberg et al. (1956) were able to quantitate hydrolyzed serum bile acids by means of gas-liquid chromatography.

g) Other Lipids

Methods concerning isolation and quantitative determination of lipid classes occurring in minor amounts, in certain tissues only, and in various pathological conditions are outlined in the appropriate chapters of this book. Further information may be obtained from papers and monographs by Deuel 1951/1957, Lettré, Inhoffen and Tschesche 1954, Hanahan 1960, Fieser and Fieser 1961, Stahl 1962, Zöllner and Eberhagen 1965.

The importance of reliable methods is illustrated by the example of determining the concentration of cerebrosides in plasma. By measuring the increase in reducing power of a serum lipid extract before and after hydrolysis which was believed to be due to sugar released from cerebrosides Kirk (1938) found concentrations between 0 and 167 mg per 100 ml. With the use of purification procedures and specific reactions for sugars Svennerholm and Svennerholm (1958) were able to demonstrate a mean cerebroside content of 4.36 $\pm$ 0.18 mg per 100 ml of plasma.

VI. Determination of Lipoproteins

At present no simple routine method is available for separation, identification and quantitation of lipoproteins. Accurate procedures are based on preparative or analytical ultracentrifugation, reviews of which were given by de Lalla and Gofman (1954), Jahnke and Scholtan (1960), Furman et al. (1961), Pezold (1961).

Separation by precipitation fractionation (Cohn 1950) is as complicated as free and zone electrophoresis (Kunkel and Slater 1952, Dietrich 1955). More convenient methods are based upon flocculation with sulfated polysaccharides (Burstein 1961, Cornwall and Kruger 1961) and immunoprecipitation (Burstein and Samaille 1958, Heiskell et al. 1961, Feldman 1964). Paper-electrophoretic separation of lipoproteins with the use of buffer containing albumin has proved valuable for differentiation of hyperlipoproteinemias (Fredrickson and Lees 1965).

VII. Determination of Lipoprotein Lipase Activity

Lipoprotein lipase catalyzes the hydrolysis of lipoprotein-bound triglycerides (chylomicrons, low-density lipoproteins) to di- and monoglycerides, free fatty acids, and free glycerol. This cleavage is accompanied by a decrease in turbidity of the lipoprotein mixtures. Increased lipoprotein lipase activity in blood occurs after intravenous injection of heparin. The physiological role of lipoprotein lipase is still incompletely understood.

Lipoprotein lipase also acts on emulsions prepared from natural fats (coconut fat, cotton-seed oil), if these are pre-incubated with plasma or serum.

Several procedures are available for determination of the activity of this enzyme in plasma and tissues.

One of them consists of measuring the decrease in turbidity of incubated lipoproteins or fat emulsions at 650 nm after addition of small amounts of plasma. A more specific and reliable method is based on determination of the reaction products, either by assay of liberated glycerol or free fatty acids. Simple methods for quantitation of both substances are available. The liberation of fatty acids is studied using the original or modified Dole's procedure for determination of free fatty acids. It is essential to observe the incubating conditions carefully, in particular substrate concentration, pH, ionic strength, presence of an acceptor substance for liberated fatty acids (albumin), and temperature. Methodological details were given by KORN (1959), KERN et al. (1961), FREDRICKSON et al. (1963) and SCHÖLL and KOPITZKI (1964).

VIII. Normal Lipid Concentrations

Normal values for the various lipid classes are derived from determinations in populations composed of "normal" subjects. In doing so it is essential to define normality by careful medical examination, and to include a sufficient number of subjects for statistical evaluation.

Values obtained in such a way comprise a range of concentrations which is characterized by its mean value and the standard deviation. If the determined values follow a normal distribution 95% of all values fall within the mean value $\pm$ 2 standard deviations. 5% of values not covered by this calculation may be regarded as pathological values. The mean value $\pm$ 3 standard deviations would comprise 97% of the normal values, but at the same time includes a significant number of pathological values in view of the overlapping of normal and pathological ranges.

Cumulative distribution curves may be used for defining "normal" ranges if the values do not correspond to a normal distribution.

In determination of tissue concentrations values can be related to various factors, e.g. wet weight, dry weight, total protein etc. Sometimes simultaneous estimation of deoxyribonucleic acid is used for comparison as a measure of total cell number. Nevertheless care should be taken to receive material for control examinations in each case. Plasma lipids are generally related to 100 ml of plasma.

An additional difficulty in defining normal plasma lipid values results from the influence of various factors on plasma lipid concentrations. Cholesterol and phospholipid concentrations vary with age and show an increase from the third to the sixth decade followed by a slight decrease thereafter (ADLERSBERG et al. 1956, LEWIS et al. 1957, SCHAEFER et al. 1958). In higher decades values may be influenced by the inclusion of persons with clinically silent disease. Furthermore, alimentary influences result from the total amount of ingested fat and the composition of dietary fatty acids. Therefore, blood samples should not only be taken in the fasting state, but in many instances after a period of controlled dietary intake.

The following tables give normal ranges for plasma lipids expressed as mean values $\pm$ 2 standard deviations.

Table 2. *Normal ranges of plasma lipid concentrations (mean values ± 2 standard deviations)*

Lipid	Concentration	Author
Total lipids	400 —900 mg/100 ml	(WAGENER et al. 1964)
Total cholesterol	140 —330 mg/100 ml	(LEWIS et al. 1957)
Free cholesterol	25 — 30% of total	
Phospholipids	150 —250 mg/100 ml	(WAGENER et al. 1964)
Glycerides	25 —220 mg/100 ml	(EGGSTEIN 1966)
Total fatty acids	5 — 19 meq/l = 150 —520 mg/100 ml	(PETERS and MAN 1943)
Free fatty acids	0.1— 1.1 meq/l = 3 — 30 mg/100 ml	(STUHLFAUTH and ZÖLLNER 1959)
Cerebrosides	4.0— 4.7 mg/100 ml	(SVENNERHOLM and SVENNERHOLM 1958)
Carotenoids	0.1— 0.2 mg/100 ml	(BLANKENHORN 1957)

Table 3. *Percentage composition of plasma cholesterol ester fraction from normals (mean values ± 2 standard deviations) (ZÖLLNER et al. 1962)*

Cholesterol esters	Per cent of total fraction
Saturated	16.1 ± 4.0
Monoenoic	23.6 ± 3.4
Dienoic	46.7 ± 4.8
Tri- and tetraenoic	11.8 ± 3.4
Polyenoic	2.0 ± 1.0

Table 4. *Concentrations and percentage composition of plasma phospholipids from normals (mean values ± 2 standard deviations) (WAGENER et al. 1964)*

Phospholipid	mg/100 ml plasma	Per cent of total phospholipids
Lecithin	132 ± 38	66 ± 9
Sphingomyelin	43 ± 12	22 ± 5
Lysolecithin	19 ± 12	9 ± 7
Cephalin	6 ± 2	3 ± 1

Table 5. *Percentage composition of fatty acids of plasma total lipids and lipid fractions in normals (SCHRADE et al. 1960)*

Fatty acid	Total lipids	Cholesterol esters	Phospholipids	Glycerides	Free fatty acids
Lauric	0.3				
Myristic	1.5	1.1	0.9	1.6	2.0
Palmitic	27.5	12.1	30.7	28.1	27.9
Palmitoleic	6.8	6.8	3.3	7.6	7.2
Stearic	6.6	2.6	11.9	3.7	14.9
Oleic	25.3	18.9	15.1	36.8	25.5
Linoleic	23.9	47.1	21.5	12.2	13.1
Linolenic	0.8				
Arachidonic	4.3	5.0	3.1	3.1	2.4

References

ABRAMSON, D., and M. BLECHER: Quantitative two-dimensional thin-layer chromatography of naturally occurring phospholipids. J. Lipid Res. **5**, 628 (1964).

AHRENS, E. H., and L. C. CRAIG: The extraction and separation of bile acids. J. biol. Chem. **195**, 763 (1952).

ALBRINK, M. J.: The microtitration of total fatty acids of serum, with notes on the estimation of triglycerides. J. Lipid Res. 1, 53 (1959/1960).

AMENTA, J. S.: A rapid chemical method for quantification of lipids separated by thin-layer chromatography. J. Lipid Res. 5, 270 (1964).

ANTONIS, A.: Semiautomated method for the colorimetric determination of plasma free fatty acids. J. Lipid Res. 6, 307 (1965).

ARVIDSON, G. A. E.: Fractionation of naturally occuring lecithins according to degree of unsaturation by thin-layer chromatography. J. Lipid Res. 6, 574 (1965).

BARRETT, C. B., M. S. J. DALLAS, and F. B. PADLEY: The separation of glycerides by thin-layer chromatography on silica impregnated with silver nitrate. Chem. & Ind. 1962,1050.

— — — The quantitative analysis of triglyceride mixtures by thin layer chromatography on silica impregnated with silver nitrate. J. Amer. Oil Chem. Soc. 40, 580 (1963).

BARTLETT, G. R.: Phosphorus assay in column chromatography. J. biol. Chem. 234, 466 (1959).

BEERS, G. J. VAN, H. DE JONGH, and J. BOLDINGH: Isolation of phospholipids by dialysis through a rubber membrane. In: H. M. Sinclair: Essential fatty acids, p. 43. London: Butterworths Sci. Publ. 1958.

BERGSTRÖM, S., and J. SJÖVALL: Occurrence and metabolism of chenodesoxycholic acid in the rat. Bile acids and steroids 13. Acta chem. Scand. 8, 611 (1954).

BIEGLER, R., E. BÖHLE, W. SCHRADE u. W. ABT: Eine säulenchromatographische Methode zur Darstellung der unveresterten Fettsäuren des Blutes. Klin. Wschr. 38, 532 (1960).

BLANKENHORN, D. H.: Carotenoids in man. II. Fractions obtained from atherosclerotic and normal aortas, serum, and depot fat by separation on alumina. J. biol. Chem. 227, 963 (1957).

— G. ROUSER, and T. J. WEIMER: A method for the estimation of blood glycerides employing florisil. J. Lipid Res. 2, 281 (1961).

BLOOR, W. R.: A method for the determination of fat in small amounts of blood. J. biol. Chem. 17, 377 (1914).

— The determination of small amounts of lipid in blood plasma. J. biol. Chem. 77, 53 (1928).

BORGSTRÖM, B.: Investigation on lipid separation methods. Separation of phospholipids from neutral fat and fatty acids. Acta physiol. scand. 25, 101 (1952).

— Investigation on lipid separation methods. Separation of cholesterol esters, glycerides and free fatty acids. Acta physiol. scand. 25, 111 (1952).

BRAGDON, J. H., H. A. EDER, R. G. GOULD, and R. J. HAVEL: Lipide momenclature. Recommendations regarding the reporting of serum lipids and lipoproteins made by the committee on lipid and lipoprotein nomenclature of the American Society for the Study of Atherosclerosis. Circulat. Res. 4, 129 (1956).

BURSTEIN, M.: Les lipoprotéines du plasma humain. Bull. schweiz. Akad. med. Wiss. 17, 92 (1961).

— J. SAMAILLE: Sur le dosage immunologique des β-lipoprotéines. Rev. franç. Étud. clin. biol. 3, 780 (1958).

CARLSON, L. A., and L. B. WADSTRÖM: On the occurrence of tri-, di-, and monoglycerides in human serum. In: The blood lipids and the clearing-factor. IIIrd Int. Conf. Biochem. Probl. Lipids, 1956, p. 123.

— — A colorimetric method of determining unesterified fatty acids in plasma. Scand. J. clin. Lab. Invest. 10, 407 (1958).

CARROLL, K. K.: Separation of lipid classes by chromatography on florisil. J. Lipid Res. 2, 135 (1961).

CAWLEY, L. P., B. O. MUSSER, S. CAMPBELL, and W. FAUCETTE: Analysis of total serum cholesterol by means of gas-liquid chromatography. Amer. J. clin. Path. 39, 450 (1963).

COHN, E. J., F. R. N. GURD, D. M. SURGENOR, B. A. BARNES, R. K. BROWN, G. DEROUAUX, J. M. GILLESPIE, F. W. KAHNT, W. F. LEVER, C. H. LIU, D. MITTLEMAN, R. F. MOUTON, K. SCHMID, and E. UROMA: A system for separation of the components of human blood: Quantitative procedures for the separation of the protein components of human plasma. J. Amer. chem. Soc. 72, 465 (1950).

CORNWELL, D. G., and F. A. KRUGER: Molecular complexes in the isolation and characterization of plasma lipoproteins. J. Lipid Res. 2, 110 (1961).

CRAIG, L. C.: Identification of small amounts of organic compounds by distribution studies. II. Separation by countercurrent distribution. J. biol. Chem. 155, 519 (1944).

DE LALLA, O. F., and J. W. GOFMAN: Ultracentrifugal analysis of serum lipoproteins. In: Methods of biochemical analysis, Vol. 1, p. 459. Ed.: D. Glick. New York: Interscience Publishers 1954.

DEUEL, H.: The lipids. Vol. 1—3. New York: Interscience Publishers 1951—1957.

DIETRICH, F.: Zur Differenzierung der Lipoproteide des Serums mittels präparativer Elektrophoresemethoden. Hoppe-Seylers Z. physiol. Chem. 302, 227 (1955).

DOLE, V. P.: A relation between non-esterified fatty acids in plasma and the metabolism of glucose. J. clin. Invest. 35, 150 (1956).

Eberhagen, D., and H. Betzing: An improved technique for dialysis of lipids. J. Lipid Res.
  3, 382 (1962).
Eggstein, M.: Eine neue Bestimmung der Neutralfette im Blutserum und Gewebe. II. Mitt.
  Zuverlässigkeit der Methode, andere Neutralfettbestimmungen, Normalwerte für Tri-
  glyceride und Glycerin im menschlichen Blut. Klin. Wschr. **44**, 267 (1966).
— u. F. H. Kreutz: Eine neue Bestimmung der Neutralfette im Blutserum und Gewebe.
  I. Mitt. Prinzip, Durchführung und Besprechung der Methode. Klin. Wschr. **44**, 262
  (1966).
Eneroth, P.: Thin-layer chromatography of bile acids. J. Lipid Res. **4**, 11 (1963).
Feldman, E. B.: Abnormalities of circulating lipids. An appraisal of current methods of study.
  Amer. J. Cardiol. **13**, 632 (1964).
Fieser, L. F., u. M. Fieser: Steroide. Verlag Chemie, Weinheim (Bergstraße) 1961.
Fillerup, D. L., and J. F. Mead: Chromatographic separation of the plasma lipids. Proc. Soc.
  exp. Biol. (N.Y.) **83**, 574 (1953).
Fiske, C. H., and Y. Subbarow: The colorimetric determination of phosphorus. J. biol. Chem.
  66, 375 (1925).
Folch, J., and D. D. van Slyke: Preparation of blood lipid extracts free from non-lipid
  extractives. Proc. Soc. exp. Biol. (N.Y.) **41**, 514 (1939).
— I. Ascoli, M. Lees, J. A. Meath, and F. N. Lebaron: Preparation of lipide extracts from
  brain tissue. J. biol. Chem. **191**, 833 (1951).
— M. Lees, and G. H. Sloane-Stanley: A simple method for the isolation and purification
  of total lipids from animal tissues. J. biol. Chem. **226**, 497 (1957).
Fontell, K., R. T. Holman, and G. Lambertsen: Some new methods for separation and
  analysis of fatty acids and other lipids. J. Lipid Res. **1**, 391 (1959/60).
Fredrickson, D. S., and R. S. Lees: A system for phenotyping hyperlipoproteinemia.
  Circulation **31**, 321 (1965).
— K. Ono, and L. L. Davis: Lipolytic activity of post-heparin plasma in hyperglyceridemia.
  J. Lipid Res. **4**, 24 (1963).
Freeman, C. P., and D. West: Complete separation of lipid classes on a single thin-layer plate.
  J. Lipid Res. **7**, 324 (1966).
Friedberg, S. J., W. R. Harlan, D. L. Trout, and E. H. Estes: The effect of exercise on the
  concentration and turnover of plasma nonesterified fatty acids. J. clin. Invest. **39**, 215
  (1960).
Frosch, B.: Die quantitative Bestimmung der durch alkalische Hydrolyse freigesetzten
  Gallensäuren des Serums nach dünnschichtchromatographischer Trennung. Klin. Wschr.
  43, 262 (1965).
— Die quantitative Bestimmung der konjugierten Gallensäuren des Serums nach dünnschicht-
  chromatographischer Trennung. Arzneimittel-Forsch. **15**, 178 (1965).
— E. Hennig u. H. Wagener: Zur quantitativen Bestimmung der mit Glycin oder Taurin
  konjugierten Desoxycholsäure. Z. Naturforsch. **19**, 481 (1964).
— u. H. Wagener: Methode zur quantitativen Bestimmung von Gallensäuren aus Menschen-
  galle. Klin. Wschr. **42**, 901 (1964).
— — Dünnschichtchromatographische Trennung konjugierter Serumgallensäuren. Z. klin.
  Chem. **3**, 84 (1965).
— H. Wagener u. E. Hennig: Zur quantitativen Bestimmung der mit Glycin oder Taurin
  konjugierten Chenodesoxycholsäure. Mikrochim. Acta 5, 620 (1964).
Furman, R. H., R. P. Howard, K. Lakshmi, and L. N. Norcia: The serum lipids and lipo-
  proteins in normal and hyperlipidemic subjects as determined by preparative ultracentri-
  fugation. Amer. J. clin. Nutr. **9**, 73 (1961).
Gänshirt, H., F. W. Koss u. K. Morianz: Untersuchung zur quantitativen Auswertung der
  Dünnschichtchromatographie. Arzneimittel-Forsch. **10**, 943 (1960).
Gjone, E., J. F. Berry, and D. A. Turner: The isolation and identification of lysolecithin
  from lipid extracts of normal human serum. J. Lipid Res. **1**, 66 (1959/60).
Glick, D., B. F. Fell, and K. Sjølin: Spectrophotometric determination of nanogram
  amounts of total cholesterol in microgram quantities of tissue or microliter volumes of
  serum. Analyt. Chem. **36**, 1119 (1964).
Gordon, R. S., and A. Cherkes: Unesterified fatty acid in human blood plasma. J. clin.
  Invest. **35**, 206 (1956).
— — and H. Gates: Unesterified fatty acid in human blood plasma. II. The transport func-
  tion of unesterified fatty acid. J. clin. Invest. **36**, 810 (1957).
Habermann, E., G. Bandtlow u. B. Krusche: Bestimmung von Plasma-Phospholipiden
  nach Dünnschichtchromatographie. Klin. Wschr. **39**, 816 (1961).
Hamilton, J. G.: Glass fiber paper and thin-layer chromatography. Gas-Chrom Newsletter 4,
  Nr. 1, Febr. 1963.
Hanahan, D. J.: Lipide chemistry. New York-London: John Wiley & Sons, Inc. 1960.

HEISKELL, C. L., R. T. FISK, W. H. FLORSHEIM, A. YACHI, J. R. GOODMAN, and C. M. CAR-
PENTER: A simple method for quantitation of serum beta-lipoproteins by means of immuno-
crit. Amer. J. clin. Path. **35**, 222 (1961).
HIRSCH, J.: Factice chromatography: An automatically monitored, liquid-gel system for the
separation of nonpolar lipids. J. Lipid Res. **4**, 1 (1963).
— and E. H. AHRENS: The separation of complex lipide mixtures by the use of silicic acid
chromatography. J. biol. Chem. **233**, 311 (1958).
HOFMAN, A. F.: Thin-layer adsorption chromatography of free and conjugated bile acids
on silicic acid. J. Lipid Res. **3**, 127 (1962).
HORNING, E. C., E. H. AHRENS, S. R. LIPSKY, F. H. MATTSON, J. F. MEAD, D. A. TURNER,
and W. H. GOLDWATER: Quantitative analysis of fatty acids by gas-liquid chromatography.
J. Lipid Res. **5**, 20 (1964).
HORNSTEIN, I., J. A. ALFORD, L. E. ELLIOT, and P. F. CROWE: Determination of free fatty
acids in fat. Analyt. Chem. **32**, 540 (1960).
ITAYA, K., and M. ÚI: Colorimetric determination of free fatty acids in biological fluids.
J. Lipid Res. **6**, 16 (1965).
JAMES, A. T., and A. J. P. MARTIN: Gas-liquid partition chromatography: The separation
and microestimation of volatile fatty acids from formic acid to dodecanoic acid. Biochem.
J. **50**, 679 (1952).
JANTZEN, E., u. H. ANDREAS: Reaktion ungesättigter Fettsäuren mit Quecksilber (II)-acetat.
Anwendung für präparative Trennungen, I. Chem. Ber. **92**, 1427 (1959).
— — Reaktion ungesättigter Fettsäuren mit Quecksilber (II)-acetat. Anwendung für prä-
parative Trennungen, II. Chem. Ber. **94**, 628 (1961).
JATZKEWITZ, H.: Cerebron- und Kerasinschwefelsäureester als Speichersubstanzen bei der
Leukodystrophie, Typ Scholz (metachromatische Form der diffusen Sklerose). Hoppe-
Seylers Z. physiol. Chem. **320**, 134 (1960).
KABARA, J. J., J. T. MCLAUGHLIN, and C. A. RIEGEL: Quantitative microdetermination of
cholesterol using tomatine as precipitating agent. Analyt. Chem. **33**, 305 (1961).
KAHLKE, W.: Refsum-Syndrom. — Lipoidchemische Untersuchungen bei 9 Fällen. Klin.
Wschr. **42**, 1011 (1964).
KATSURA, S., T. HATAKEYAMA, and K. TAJIMA: Eine titrimetrische Bestimmungsmethode für
sehr kleine Mengen Blutphosphatide. Biochem. Z. **257**, 22 (1933).
KAUFMANN, H. P., u. W. H. NITSCH: Die Papier-Chromatographie auf dem Fettgebiet. XVI.
Weitere Versuche zur Trennung von Fettsäuren. Fette, Seifen, Anstrichmittel **56**, 154 (1954).
— Z. MAKUS u. F. DEICKE: Die Dünnschicht-Chromatographie auf dem Fettgebiet. II. Tren-
nung der Cholesterin-Fettsäureester. Fette, Seifen, Anstrichmittel **63**, 235 (1961).
KELLEY, T. F.: Improved method for microtitration of fatty acids. Analyt. Chem. **37**, 1078
(1965).
KERN, F., L. STEINMANN, and B. B. SANDERS: Measurement of lipoprotein lipase activity
in post heparin plasma: description of technique. J. Lipid Res. **2**, 51 (1961).
KIRK, E.: The concentration of lecithin, cephalin, etherinsoluble phosphatide and cerebrosides
in plasma and red blood cells of normal adults. J. biol. Chem. **123**, 637 (1938).
KLEIN, P. D., and E. T. JANSSEN: The fractionation of cholesterol esters by silicic acid
chromatography. J. biol. Chem. **234**, 1417 (1959).
KORN, E. D.: The assay of lipoprotein lipase in vivo and in vitro. In: Methods of biochemical
analysis, Vol. 7, p. 145. Ed.: D. Glick. New York: Interscience Publishers 1959.
KRELL, K., and S. A. HASHIM: Measurement of serum triglycerides by thin-layer chromato-
graphy and infrared spectrophotometry. J. Lipid Res. **4**, 407 (1963).
KREUTZ, F. H.: Enzymatische Glycerinbestimmung. Klin. Wschr. **40**, 362 (1962).
KUNKEL, H. G., and R. J. SLATER: Lipoprotein patterns of serum obtained by zone electro-
phoresis. J. clin. Invest. **31**, 677 (1952).
LARRABEE, M. G., and J. D. KLINGMAN: A silicic acid microcolumn for continuous gradient elu-
tion of lipids, used in studies on sympathetic ganglia of rats. Analyt. Biochem. **6**, 111 (1963).
LETTRÉ, H., H. H. INHOFFEN u. R. TSCHESCHE: Über Sterine, Gallensäuren und verwandte
Naturstoffe, Bd. 1. Stuttgart: Encke 1954.
LEWIS, B.: Composition of plasma cholesterol ester in relation to coronary-artery disease
and dietary fat. Lancet **1958/II**, 71.
LEWIS, L. A., F. OLMSTED, I. H. PAGE, E. Y. LAWRY, G. V. MANN, F. J. STARE, M. HANIG,
M. A. LAUFFER, T. GORDON, and F. E. MOORE: Serum lipid levels in normal persons. Findings
of a cooperative study of lipoproteins and atherosclerosis. Circulation **16**, 227 (1957).
LINDBERG, O., and L. ERNSTER: Determination of organic phosphorus compounds by phos-
phate analysis. In: Methods of biochemical analysis, Vol. 3, p. 1. Ed.: D. Glick. New York:
Interscience Publishers 1956.
LOFLAND, H. B.: A semiautomated procedure for the determination of triglycerides in serum.
Analyt. Biochem. **9**, 393 (1964).

Lough, A. K., L. Felinsky, and G. A. Garton: The production of methyl esters of fatty acids as artifacts during the extraction or storage of tissue lipids in the presence of methanol. J. Lipid Res. 3, 478 (1962).

Mangold, H. K.: Zur Analyse von Lipiden mit Hilfe der Radioreagenzmethode. Fette, Seifen, Anstrichmittel 61, 877 (1959).

— Aliphatische Lipide, S. 141. In E. Stahl: Dünnschichtchromatographie. Berlin-Göttingen-Heidelberg: Springer 1962.

Marinetti, G. V.: Chromatographic separation, identification, and analysis of phosphatides. J. Lipid Res. 3, 1 (1962).

— M. Albrecht, T. Ford, and E. Stotz: Analysis of human plasma phosphatides by paper chromatography. Biochem. biophys. Acta (Amst.) 36, 4 (1959).

Mattson, F. H., and R. A. Volpenhein: Synthesis and properties of glycerides. J. Lipid Res. 3, 281 (1962).

Mendelsohn, D., and A. Antonis: A fluorimetric micro glycerol method and its application to the determination of serum triglycerides. J. Lipid Res. 2, 45 (1961).

Michaels, G.: A method for the determination of plasma glycerides and free fatty acids. Metabolism 11, 833 (1962).

Morris, L. J.: Fractionation of cholesterol esters by thin-layer chromatography. J. Lipid Res. 4, 357 (1963).

Mosbach, E. H., C. Zomzely, and F. E. Kendall: Separation of bile acids by column-partition chromatography. Arch. Biochem. 48, 95 (1954).

Mosinger, F.: Photometric adaptation of Dole's microdetermination of free fatty acids. J. Lipid Res. 6, 157 (1965).

Nelson, G. J., and N. K. Freeman: Serum phospholipide analysis by chromatography and infrared spectrophotometry. J. biol. Chem. 234, 1375 (1959).

Nerking, J.: Zur Methodik der Lecithinbestimmung. Biochem. Z. 23, 262 (1910).

Neudoerffer, T. S., and C. H. Lea: Antioxidants for the (thin-layer) chromatography of lipids. J. Chromat. 21, 138 (1966).

Nichaman, M. Z., C. C. Sweeley, N. M. Oldham, and R. E. Olson: Changes in fatty acid composition during preparative thin-layer chromatography. J. Lipid Res. 4, 484 (1963).

Norman, A.: Separation of conjugated bile acids by partition chromatography. Bile acids and steroids 6. Acta chem. scand. 7, 1413 (1953).

Peters, J. P., and E. B. Man: The interrelations of serum lipids in normal persons. J. clin. Invest. 22, 707 (1943).

Pezold, F. A.: Lipide und Lipoproteide im Blutplasma. Berlin-Göttingen-Heidelberg: Springer 1961.

Phillips, G. B.: The isolation and quantitation of the principle phospholipid components of human serum using chromatography on silicic acid. Biochim. biophys. Acta (Amst.) 29, 594 (1958).

Randrup, A.: A specific and reasonably accurate method for routine determination of plasma triglyceride. Scand. J. clin. Lab. Invest. 12, 1 (1960).

Renkonen, O.: Breakdown of lecithin on aluminium oxide columns. J. Lipid Res. 3, 181 (1962).

Rinehart, R. K., S. E. Delaney, and H. Sheppard: Determination of cholesterol as the tomatinide using the iron reagent. J. Lipid Res. 3, 383 (1962).

Sandberg, D. H., J. Sjövall, K. Sjövall, and D. A. Turner: Measurement of human serum bile acids by gas-liquid chromatography. J. Lipid Res. 6, 182 (1965).

Schlierf, G., and P. Wood: Quantitative determination of plasma free fatty acids and triglycerides by thin-layer chromatography. J. Lipid Res. 6, 317 (1965).

Schöll, H., u. F. Kopitzki: Antilipämische Wirkung von saurem Natrium-Heparin bei sublingualer oder rectaler Verabreichung. Klin. Wschr. 42, 699 (1964).

Schoenheimer, R., and W. M. Sperry: A micromethod for the determination of free and combined cholesterol. J. biol. Chem. 106, 745 (1934).

Schrade, W., E. Böhle, R. Biegler, V. Meder u. R. Teicke: Gaschromatographische Untersuchungen der Serumfettsäuren des Menschen. I. Mitt. Über die Fettsäurenzusammensetzung des Serumfettes beim Gesunden, Arteriosklerotiker und Diabetiker. Klin. Wschr. 38, 126 (1960).

— — — — — Gaschromatographische Untersuchungen der Serumfettsäuren des Menschen. III. Mitt. Die Fettsäuren der Cholesterinester, Phospholipoide und Triglyceride, sowie die unveresterten Fettsäuren bei Gesunden und Arteriosklerosekranken. Klin. Wschr. 38, 739 (1960).

Searcy, R. L., and L. M. Bergquist: A new color reaction for the quantitation of serum cholesterol. Clin. chim. Acta 5, 192 (1960).

— J. L. Korotzer, and L. M. Bergquist: Micro measurement of serum total lipids. Clin. chim. Acta 8, 376 (1963).

SHAFRIR, E.: Partition of unesterified fatty acids in normal and nephrotic syndrome serum and its effect on serum electrophoretic pattern. J. clin. Invest. **37**, 1775 (1958).

— and D. STEINBERG: The essential role of the adrenal cortex in the response of plasma free fatty acids, cholesterol, and phospholipids to epinephrine injection. J. clin. Invest. **39**, 310 (1960).

SHINOWARA, G. Y., and J. B. BROWN: Studies on the chemistry of the fatty acids. VI. The application of crystallization methods to the isolation of arachidonic acid, with a comparison of the properties of this acid prepared by crystallization and by debromination. Observations on the structure of arachidonic acid. J. biol. Chem. **134**, 331 (1940).

SJÖVALL, J.: On the separation of bile acids by partition chromatography. Bile acids and steroids 4. Acta physiol. scand. **29**, 232 (1953).

— The determination of bile acids in bile and duodenal contents by quantitative paper chromatography. Clin. chim. Acta **4**, 652 (1959).

— C. R. MELONI, and D. A. TURNER: A study of the separation of substituted cholanic acids by gas-liquid chromatography. J. Lipid Res. **2**, 317 (1961).

SKIDMORE, W. D., and C. ENTENMAN: Two-dimensional thin-layer chromatography of rat liver phosphatides. J. Lipid Res. **3**, 471 (1962).

SKIPSKI, V. P., R. F. PETERSON, and M. BARCLAY: Separation of phosphatidyl ethanolamine, phosphatidyl serine, and other phospholipids by thin-layer chromatography. J. Lipid Res. **3**, 467 (1962).

SPERRY, W. M.: Lipide analyses, Vol. 2, p. 83. In: Methods of biochemical analysis. Ed.: D. Glick. New York: Interscience Publishers 1955.

— M. WEBB: A revision of the Schoenheimer-Sperry method for cholesterol determination. J. biol. Chem. **187**, 97 (1950).

SPINELLA, C. J., and M. MAGER: Modified enzymatic procedure for the routine determination of glycerol and triglycerides in plasma. J. Lipid Res. **7**, 167 (1966).

STAHL, E.: Dünnschicht-Chromatographie. II. Standardisierung, Sichtbarmachung, Dokumentation und Anwendung. Chemiker-Ztg. **82**, 323 (1958).

— Dünnschicht-Chromatographie. Berlin-Göttingen-Heidelberg: Springer 1962.

STUHLFAUTH, K., u. N. ZÖLLNER: Der Einfluß von Fructose auf den Gehalt des Serums an nicht veresterten Fettsäuren. Klin. Wschr. **37**, 1162 (1959).

SVENNERHOLM, E., and L. SVENNERHOLM: Quantitative estimation of cerebrosides in plasma. Scand. J. clin. Lab. Invest. **10**, 97 (1958).

THANNHAUSER, S. J., and P. SETZ: Studies on animal lipids. XII. A method for quantitative determination of diaminophosphatide in organs and fluids. Application to stromata of red blood cells and serum. J. biol. Chem. **116**, 533 (1936).

TROUT, D. L., E. H. ESTES, and S. J. FRIEDBERG: Titration of free fatty acids of plasma: a study of current methods and a new modification. J. Lipid Res. **1**, 199 (1959/1960).

VANDEN HEUVEL, W. J. A., C. C. SWEELEY, and E. C. HORNING: Microanalytical separations by gas chromatography in the sex hormone and bile acid series. Biochem. biophys. Res. Commun. **3**, 33 (1960).

VAN SLYKE, D. D., and J. PLAZIN: The preparation of extracts of plasma lipids free from water-soluble contaminants. Clin. chim. Acta **12**, 46 (1965).

VANZETTI, G.: Méthodes photométriques de dosage du cholestérol dans le sérum. Clin. chim. Acta **10**, 389 (1964).

VOGEL, W. C., W. M. DOIZAKI, and L. ZIEVE: Rapid thin-layer chromatographic separation of phospholipids and neutral lipids of serum. J. Lipid Res. **3**, 138 (1962).

— L. ZIEVE, and R. O. CARLETON: Measurement of serum lecithin, lysolecithin, and sphingomyelin by a simplified chromatographic technique. J. Lab. clin. Med. **59**, 335 (1962).

VRIES, B. DE: Quantitative separations of lipid materials by column chromatography on silica impregnated with silver nitrate. Chem. & Ind. **1962**, 1049.

WAGENER, H.: Detection and documentation of lipids after thin-layer chromatography. Nature (Lond.) **205**, 386 (1965).

— u. B. FROSCH: Zweidimensionale dünnschichtchromatographische Trennung von Gallensäuren. Klin. Wschr. **41**, 1094 (1963).

— D. LANG u. B. FROSCH: Dünnschichtchromatographische Untersuchungen über die Phosphatide des Blutserums Gesunder und Arteriosklerosekranker. Z. ges. exp. Med. **138**, 425 (1964).

WAGNER, H.: Neuere Ergebnisse auf dem Gebiet der Isolierung und Analytik von Phosphatiden und Glykolipiden. Fette, Seifen, Anstrichmittel **62**, 1115 (1960).

WEICKER, H.: Adsorptionschromatographische Untersuchung von Serumlipiden auf Kieselgelplatten. Klin. Wschr. **37**, 763 (1959).

WELLS, M. A., and J. C. DITTMER: The use of sephadex for the removal of nonlipid contaminants from lipid extracts. Biochemistry **2**, 1259 (1963).

WIELAND, O.: Eine enzymatische Methode zur Bestimmung von Glycerin. Biochem. Z. **329**, 313 (1957).

WOOD, P. D. S., and S. HOLTON: Human plasma sphingomyelins. Proc. Soc. exp. Biol. (N.Y.) **115**, 990 (1964).

WREN, J. J.: Chromatography of lipids on silicic acid. J. Chromat. **4**, 173 (1960).

— and H. K. MITCHELL: Silicic acid chromatography of lipids of whole human blood. Proc. Soc. exp. Biol. (N. Y.) **99**, 431 (1958).

ZAK, B., R. C. DICKENMAN, E. G. WHITE, H. BURNETT, and P. J. CHERNEY: Rapid estimation of free and total cholesterol. Amer. J. clin. Path. **24**, 1307 (1954).

ZILVERSMIT, D. B., and A. K. DAVIS: Microdetermination of plasma phospholipids by trichloroacetic acid precipitation. J. Lab. clin. Med. **35**, 155 (1950).

ZLATKIS, A., B. ZAK, and A. J. BOYLE: A new method for the direct determination of serum cholesterol. J. Lab. clin. Med. **41**, 486 (1953).

ZÖLLNER, N., u. D. EBERHAGEN: Untersuchung und Bestimmung der Lipoide im Blut. Berlin-Heidelberg-New York: Springer 1965.

— u. K. KIRSCH: Die säulenchromatographische Trennung der Plasmalipoide. I. Mitt. Methodik und Identifizierung der Fraktionen. Z. ges. exp. Med. **134**, 10 (1960).

— — Über die quantitative Bestimmung von Lipoiden (Mikromethode) mittels der vielen natürlichen Lipoiden (allen bekannten Plasmalipoiden) gemeinsamen Sulfophosphovanillin-Reaktion. Z. ges. exp. Med. **135**, 545 (1962).

— — u. G. AMIN: Über die chromatographische Trennung der Cholesterinester des Plasmas. Verh. dtsch. Ges. inn. Med. **66**, 677 (1960).

— G. WOLFRAM u. G. AMIN: Über die quantitative Auswertung von Dünnschichtchromatogrammen der Cholesterinester. Klin. Wschr. **40**, 273 (1962).

ZUELZER, G.: Über Darstellung von Lecithin und anderen Myelinsubstanzen aus Gehirn- und Eigelbextracten. Hoppe-Seylers Z. physiol. Chem. **27**, 255 (1899).

Part II

Lipidoses

Clinic, Pathology, Pathophysiology, Genetics

Gangliosidoses

By

G. Schettler and W. Kahlke

Introduction

The term gangliosides* was introduced by KLENK for neuraminic acid-containing glycolipids which he found (1939—1942) in the brains of subjects with infantile amaurotic family idiocy. The neuraminic acid content of gangliosides permitted differentiation from other carbohydrate-containing lipids such as cerebrosides which accumulate in Gaucher's disease.

A number of subgroups of amaurotic family idiocy (AFI) have been described which differ with regard to time of onset, symptomatology, course and morbid anatomy. By far the most common is the *infantile form = type Tay-Sachs (TSD)*. A *congenital form* (NORMAN and WOOD 1941, BROWN et al. 1954, HAGBERG et al. 1965) is characterized by the presence of symptoms at birth, and is lethal within weeks. Patients with the *late-infantile form = type Jansky-Bielschowsky* (BATTEN 1903, HADDENBROCK 1950, SEITELBERGER et al. 1957, SCHNECK et al. 1965b) differ from subjects with TSD in that their disease runs a longer course, there is no racial prevalence, and eye findings are variable. The *juvenile form = type Spielmeyer-Vogt* becomes manifest in children of school age (GREENFIELD and HOLMES 1925, VAN BAGH and HORTLING 1948, RAYNER 1952, DIEZEL 1957, JERVIS 1959). Finally, a late form, *adult amaurotic family idiocy = type Kufs-Hallervorden* (KUFS 1925, HALLERVORDEN 1938, DIEZEL 1954a) begins during puberty or thereafter and can be differentiated from the other forms by the lack of eye changes, the chronic course and the typical neurologic symptoms.

With the exception of TSD, lipid data are scarce in the literature for the various forms of amaurotic family idiocies, and the subclassification as outlined is mainly based on clinical and histochemical differences. Since tinctorial properties of a chemical compound are much more dependent on the physico-chemical state than on the concentration (HAGBERG et al. 1965), histochemistry is limited to qualitative studies and does not allow a quantitation of lipid storage.

There is no question that there is ganglioside storage in TSD. In addition, recent analyses have shown that gangliosides are also increased in the late-infantile amaurotic family idiocy. Variable findings have been reported for the juvenile form, and increased gangliosides have not yet been found in the adult variety.

While visceral ganglioside storage is not a typical feature of the various forms of AFI noted above, there have been reports on disorders which, in addition to an abnormal ganglioside pattern in the central nervous system, exhibited evidence of lipid storage in other organs. These "neurovisceral lipidoses" were discussed by CRAIG et al. (1959), NORMAN et al. (1959, 1964), LANDING and RUBINSTEIN (1962), LANDING et al. (1964), GONATAS and GONATAS (1965) and others. Although their differentiation from Gaucher's disease and Niemann-Pick disease could be achieved, more information is required for their further classification.

---

* The nomenclature of gangliosides is outlined in table 1 page 214. See also table of the chapter by STOFFEL (pg. 22).

Table 1. *Terminology of gangliosides as used by various authors*

Structure (short hand designation)	KUHN and WIEGANDT (1963, 1964) WIEGANDT (1965)	SVENNERHOLM (1964)	KLENK (1963, 1964, 1965)	KOREY and GONATAS (1963)	BURTON*
FA—Sph—0^1 ← 1 Glc 4 ←$^\beta$ 1 Gal 3 ← 2 NANA	G_{LACT}	G_{M3}	B_2	G_6	B_1
FA—Sph—0^1 ← 1 Glc 4 ←$^\beta$ 1 Gal 4 ←$^\beta$ 1 GalNac; 3 ← 2 NANA	G_{GNTrII}	G_{M2}	A_1	G_5	B_2
FA—Sph—0^1 ← 1 Glc 4 ←$^\beta$ 1 Gal 4 ←$^\beta$ 1 GalNac 3 ←$^\beta$ 1 Gal; 3 ← 2 NANA	G_{GNTI}	G_{M1}	A_2	G_4	B_3
FA—Sph—0^1 ← 1 Glc 4 ←$^\beta$ 1 Gal 4 ←$^\beta$ 1 GalNac 3 ←$^\beta$ 1 Gal 3 ← 2 NANA; 3 ← 2 NANA	G_{GNTII}	G_{D1a}	B_1	G_3	B_4
FA—Sph—0^1 ← 1 Glc 4 ←$^\beta$ 1 Gal 4 ←$^\beta$ 1 GalNac 3 ←$^\beta$ 1 Gal; 3 ← 2 NANA; 2 NANA 8 ← 2 NANA	G_{GNTIII}	G_{D1b}	C_1	G_2	C_3
FA—Sph—0^1 ← 1 Glc 4 ←$^\beta$ 1 Gal 4 ←$^\beta$ 1 GalNac 3 ←$^\beta$ 1 Gal 3 ←$^\beta$ 2 NANA; 3 ← 2 NANA; 2 NANA 8 ← 2 NANA	G_{GNTIV}	G_{T1}	C_3	G_1	C_4
FA—Sph—0^1 ← 1 Glc 4 ←$^\beta$ 1 Gal 4 ←$^\beta$ 1 GalNac 3 ←$^\beta$ 1 Gal 3 ← 2 NANA; 8 ←? NANA 2; 3 ← 2 NANA; 2 NANA 8 ← 2 NANA	G_{GNTV}				

* See page 22 and page 122.

Since ganglioside storage is observed in gargoylism (Pfaundler-Hurler syndrome), this disease will be considered under the heading of gangliosidoses, although the complex disturbance of lipid and mucopolysaccharide metabolism in gargoylism is still poorly understood.

In addition to the disorders mentioned, accumulation of certain gangliosides has been observed in various other diseases with involvement of the central nervous system, such as Niemann-Pick disease, infantile Gaucher's disease, metachromatic and 'globoid cell' leucodystrophy, subacute encephalitis. Accumulation of gangliosides may also be found in tumors; an example is the isolation of the ganglioside G_{LACT}* (a ceramide lactoside) by SEIFERT and UHLENBRUCK (1965) from meningeomas.

From the foregoing it is apparent that a discussion of the various gangliosidoses cannot yet be based on a biochemical basis according to the prevailing ganglioside. With the understanding that clinical entities may have to be modified in the light of future information on their lipid chemistry, the gangliosidoses will be discussed in the following order:

1. Congenital AFI.
2. Infantile AFI = Tay-Sachs disease.
3. Late-infantile AFI.
4. Juvenile AFI.
5. Adult AFI.
6. Neurovisceral gangliosidoses.
7. Hurler's disease (Gargoylism).

I. Congenital Amaurotic Family Idiocy

Definition and Introduction

This group is composed of infants who exhibit the symptomatology of Tay-Sachs disease (TSD) either at birth or during the immediate neonatal period. In the case of EPSTEIN (1917) symptoms appeared during the second week and in that of SCHICK (1941) during the fourth week of life. Two out of 108 patients with TSD reviewed by KANOF et al. (1959) had signs referable to the disease at birth, two others developed them during the first months. Two siblings with microcephaly from a large family (NORMAN and WOOD 1941, BROWN et al. 1954) developed symptoms of AFI immediately after birth and died after 18 and 42 days, respectively.

A separate consideration of congenital amaurotic family idiocy (CAFI) is supported by findings of HAGBERG et al. (1965) in an affected infant who was not of Jewish ancestry. In this patient the ganglioside pattern differed from that of TSD. Gangliosides were not analysed in the remaining "congenital" cases, and it is possible that such studies might have revealed different types of gangliosides.

Clinical Manifestations

The earliest signs consist of irregular respiration with bouts of apnea and cyanosis, and impairment of the sucking and swallowing mechanism with episodes of vomiting. They are associated with progressive muscular rigidity which is followed by the appearance of clonic, focal or generalized seizures occurring upon minimal stimulation (noise) and accompanied by a shrill cry. A burnt-out stage of decerebrate rigidity persists until progressive neurologic deterioration leads to the death of the affected infants.

---

* Nomenclature of KUHN and WIEGANDT (1963, 1964) and of WIEGANDT (1965).

Atrophy of the optic nerve appears to be a consistent finding. Pigmented macular protrusions have been observed by HAGBERG et al. (1965). The spinal fluid was found to be clear and colorless (BROWN et al. 1954), and cells were not increased. Spinal fluid protein was initially elevated (480 mg%) and later normal (51.3 mg%) in the case of HAGBERG et al. The electroencephalogram in this patient showed lack of the normal basal rythmic activity and cortical activity. Ventriculography revealed marked dilatation of the ventricles with paper-thin walls and signs of underdevelopment of the cerebellum. Routine laboratory examinations were normal. Vacuolized lymphocytes were not seen.

Pathology

Marked hydrocephalus appears to be the most striking finding. In the cases of BROWN et al. there was hydrocephalus externus, with the small brain lying "like a shrunken walnut within its shell", while in HAGBERG's case the remaining brain tissue consisted of a cyst-like formation, the walls of which were extremely thin (1—2 mm) and were pushed against the skull by approximately 700 ml of straw colored fluid. The brain stem appears grossly normal, the cerebellum is atrophic, and shows signs of delayed myelination.

Histologic findings are quite similar to those found in TSD, although they were more markedly abnormal in the cases of BROWN et al. (1954). In the patient of HAGBERG, nerve cells could not be identified in the cerebral hemispheres and glial proliferation was less than in BROWN's material. The general morphologic picture gives the impression of pronounced immaturity of the brain tissue.

Cells which appear to be of reticuloendothelial origin and which contain sudanophilic material, may be found in spleen, liver, lungs, thymus, kidneys and adrenal medulla.

Results of Lipid Analyses

In the cases of BROWN et al., and NORMAN and WOOD, only cholesterol and total phospholipids were analysed in the brain. The cholesterol content was increased almost four-fold while phospholipids were significantly decreased.

A diminution of total brain lipids was evident in the case of HAGBERG. Decreased concentration of myelin lipids such as cerebrosides in the cerebral hemispheres was in accordance with morphologic findings. In the cerebellum, glycerophosphatides were also decreased, and only traces of triglycerides were found. The total cholesterol concentration was normal with a significant proportion of ester cholesterol. Of particular interest was the finding of a decrease in total gangliosides as estimated from the hexosamine and N-acetyl-neuraminic acid (NANA) concentrations. It was similar to or even more marked than the lowering of other lipid classes. This does not, of course, exclude localized intracellular accumulation of gangliosides in certain areas as suggested by histochemical findings.

Results of visceral lipid analyses were less abnormal. A low phospholipid content, with normal or slightly increased cholesterol, was reflected in low values for total lipids.

Analyses of the gangliosides in CAFI (HAGBERG et al. 1965) have yielded evidence for the presence of an hitherto unknown compound. By use of thin-layer chromatography significant amounts of a neuraminic acid-containing component have been found with an Rf-value between that of mono- and disialogangliosides from normal brain. Results of enzymatic hydrolysis suggested that this was a disialoganglioside containing two hexose units, which was named G_{D3}.

A ganglioside with identical chromatographic characteristics was found in traces in spleen, liver and white matter of normal brains. The ganglioside G_{M2}

$(=G_{GNTrII})$ (see table 1), which is characteristic of Tay-Sachs disease, was not increased.

Discussion

In retrospect it is not possible to determine whether all cases which are considered CAFI on clinical grounds, result from a common metabolic error. Only the case of HAGBERG, with evidence for storage of an atypical or extra-cerebral type ganglioside, meets the criteria for a lipidosis. It is likely that the ganglioside G_{D3} of CAFI is actually a component of normal brain just like the ganglioside G_{GNTrII} $(=G_{M2})$ which is stored in Tay-Sachs disease, but that normally it is not found without special precautions due to its very low concentration. More cases must be carefully studied before it can be decided whether or not the case of HAGBERG et al. (1965) can be considered the prototype of CAFI.

Diagnosis

The diagnosis of CAFI should be considered when the symptomatology of amaurotic family idiocy develops immediately at birth or during the first weeks thereafter. Biopsies from brain and rectum permit recognition of the histologic abnormalities of amaurotic family idiocy.

Chromatographic methods will result in the identification of the ganglioside G_{D3}, if this component is present in increased amounts. The finding of low total brain lipids and phospholipids with normal values for cholesterol and increase of the ester fraction may support the diagnosis.

II. Infantile Amaurotic Family Idiocy (Tay-Sachs Disease)

Definition and Introduction

Tay-Sachs disease (TSD), the infantile amaurotic family idiocy, is the commonest type of this group of lipidoses and the prototype of the gangliosidoses. It is an hereditary disorder which is characterized by a typical symptomatology consisting of regression of mental and somatic functions and progressive impairment of vision. Biochemically, there is accumulation in brain of a ganglioside which occurs normally only in trace amounts. Morphologic changes of the central nervous system result from lipid storage in ganglion cells, glial proliferation and demyelination.

Historical Review

In 1881 the British ophthalmologist W. TAY observed in a child the bilateral occurrence of a cherry-red spot in place of the fovea centralis and three years later described similar changes in two other siblings from the same family. The American neurologist SACHS, in 1887, reported on clinical and pathologic findings in a child with dementia and blindness. During the course of the following years he added eight patients with similar abnormalities and introduced the term "amaurotic family idiocy" for this syndrome (SACHS 1896, 1898, SACHS and HAUSMAN 1926). Since then numerous reviews on the subject have been published (ROTH-STEIN and WELT 1941, GLOBUS 1942, SCHETTLER 1955, DIEZEL 1957, THANN-HAUSER 1958, FREDRICKSON 1960, KOREY et al. 1963, FREDRICKSON and TRAMS 1966). ARONSON's group (1964) has observed the majority (over 300) of the 500 to 600 cases which have been reported to date (ARONSON et al. 1955, 1958—1962, KANOF et al. 1959, ARONSON and VOLK 1962).

The similarity of the central nervous system pathology and the occurrence of eye lesions in both TSD and Niemann-Pick disease (Baumann et al. 1936) have suggested to some (Pick 1926, Pick and Bielschowsky 1927, Bielschowsky 1928, 1936, Spielmeyer 1929, Kufs 1930, van Bogaert and Bertrand 1934) that both disorders were different forms of the same disease. Reports on the occurrence of foam cells in the spleen and other tissues of Tay-Sachs children (Davison and Jacobson 1936, Brouwer 1936) supported this theory. Even Gaucher's disease and gargoylism were at one time thought possibly to share a common metabolic abnormality with TSD. Although Schaffer (1926, 1930a, 1930b) had already emphasized the difference between TSD and Niemann-Pick disease by pointing out the involvement of ectodermal tissues only in amaurotic family idiocy as compared to the ecto- and mesodermal involvement in Niemann-Pick disease, it was not until 1939 that Klenk showed that in TSD a neuraminic acid-containing glycolipid was stored, rather than the sphingomyelin of Niemann-Pick disease. In spite of a moderate increase in gangliosides which may be found in the Niemann-Pick brain (Klenk 1957, Jatzkewitz et al. 1965) and in spite of the occurrence of both disorders in the same family (van Bogaert and Klein 1955) a different etiology for both sphingolipidoses appears certain.

In recent studies Aronson's group (see page 220) examined the activities of various enzymes in serum and cerebrospinal fluid and found among other abnormalities a lack of fructose-1-phosphate aldolase in children with TSD. This is a unique finding among the lipidoses and may be useful for detection of heterozygotes for the disease (see below).

Incidence (Age, Sex, Race)

In general, the first symptoms of TSD appear between the third and seventh months of life with an average age of the patients at the time of disease onset of $5\frac{1}{2}$ months. Rarely is the onset earlier, but in approximately 20% of cases it is later, between the eighth and tenth months. The siblings of Norman and Wood (1941) and Brown et al. (1954), with symptoms of TSD soon after birth, will be considered under a separate category according to the classification outlined on page 215, since a similar patient (Hagberg et al. 1965) showed storage of a ganglioside which was different from that of TSD. The same may apply to subjects with disease onset after ten months, for example the patient described by Hassin and Parmelee (1928). Since frequently recognition of the first symptoms depends on the attentiveness of the parents, exact timing of the disease onset is often difficult. Environmental influences during pregnancy and delivery are unlikely to affect the development of TSD.

It is now well established that great majority of cases of TSD occur in Jewish families. Exceptions were reported by Falkenheim (1901), Starck (1920), Catel (1943), Aronson et al. (1960). Probably, the incidence of TSD in races other than the Jewish would actually be even smaller than reported with more complete knowledge of the type of amaurotic family idiocy in some subjects and of the ancestry in others. 90% of 219 Tay-Sachs children of Aronson and Volk (1962) belonged to the Jewish race as jugded by their religion. TSD in Japanese families was reported by Cordes and Horner (1929) and Murakami (1957). From epidemiologic studies on the frequency of a deficiency of fructose-1-phosphate aldolase (Volk et al. 1964), the incidence of TSD in Jews is 100 times that of non-Jews. This is discussed in more detail in the chapter by Fuhrmann.

The disease shows no sexual prevalence. A review by Aronson and Volk (1962) of their own cases and of those of Slome (1933), Goldschmidt et al. (1956) and

Kozinn et al. (1957) showed that from a total of 434 patients, 49.5% were males and 50.5% were females.

Clinical Manifestations

The symptomatology of TSD is typical as regards both the order of appearance of the various signs and symptoms as well as their progression. In general, behavioural changes become evident first with apathy and increasing disinterest of affected infants toward their surroundings. They are followed by loss of muscle tone and progressive inanition with ensuing retardation and regression of mental and somatic development. A lack of facial expression is accentuated by the deterioration of vision. Irritability of the central nervous system leads to startle reactions towards noise, and hyperacusis was the initial symptom in 37 out of 73 cases examined by Kanof et al. (1959). Other stimuli are less potent in eliciting the hyperactive responses. Next is impairment of motor activity, with inability to sit up, to maintain the position of the head, or to crawl. Development of spasticity and rigidity of the musculature results in contractures and finally quadriplegia. Excessive drooling of salivary secretions seems frequent (Schneck 1964). Brief bouts of unmotivated laughter (Schneck 1965) usually appear several months before the onset of focal or generalized convulsions and may represent seizure phenomena. Extrapyramidal signs like athetosis and chorea are infrequent. Deep tendon reflexes tend to be hyperactive; a positive Babinski and Hoffmann sign may be only unilateral. The progression of central nervous system changes in association with impairment of growth and periods of weight loss (Kanof et al. 1959) result in a state of idiocy with immobility and all signs of a decerebrate vegetative existence.

The incipient visual disturbance usually becomes evident by a lack of attentiveness and by disorderly ocular movements. The macula may then assume a greyish-white, edematous appearance due to lipid storage and degeneration of ganglion cells, and the fovea, with no overlying ganglion cells, may be seen as a cherry-red spot in its center. Secondary degeneration of the optic nerves is common (van Bogaert and Bertrand 1934, Didion 1950) and loss of pupillary reaction to light and blindness follow.

Increasing attention has recently been paid to the megencephaly which, in general, develops 1½ years after onset of the disease. In the patients of Kanof et al. (1959) the head size after two years of the disease was generally 10%—25% above the average for normals. The increase in size and weight of the brain is in accordance with these cranial measurements (Kanof et al. 1959). After 50 months the cranial volume ceases to increase (Aronson and Volk 1962), probably secondary to progressive glial proliferation.

Precocious puberty has been observed in some cases; in one child (Kanof et al. 1959) growth of pubic hair was noted at the age of 2½ years.

Electroencephalography

There is no agreement on the significance of the observed patterns. While some authors consider certain changes specific for the disease (Cobb et al. 1952), this is doubted by Watson and Denny-Brown (1953), Morrell and Torres (1960), Schneck (1965) and others. In six patients examined by Korey and Terry (1963) a variety of patterns, from normal to clearly pathologic ones, were observed, but there was no evidence for any specific changes. According to the most recent studies in 14 patients (Schneck 1965) EEG abnormalities are rare during the first year of life. During the second year the EEG is characterized by high voltage, slow activity with single and multiple spike potentials. After two years of age there is a decrease in both voltage amplitude and number of spike potentials.

A normal *electroretinogram* was seen in one of the six subjects examined by Korey and Terry (1963), but the cortical response was absent even in this case.

Cerebrospinal Fluid

There is no specific abnormality of the cerebrospinal fluid (Aronson et al. 1958, Spiegel-Adolf et al. 1959, Saifer and Gerstenfield 1962, Korey and Terry 1963). The protein content may be increased, but sugar and cell count are normal.

The occurrence in the liquor of foam cells measuring from 20—40 μ has been described by Tourtelotte et al. (1965). They are similar to those which may occasionally be found in normal subjects, and their identity with lipomacrophages and a possible role in lipid transport via the Virchow-Robin spaces into the liquor has been discussed, since their number was correlated with abnormalities in the lipid profile of the liquor.

In some Tay-Sachs patients the lipid content of the cerebrospinal fluid was increased from the normal 1.25 mg per 100 ml to 2 mg per 100 ml or more. The excess lipid may result from degeneration of myelin since cholesterol, cerebrosides, sphingomyelin and plasmalogens prevail. Photometric determination of N-acetyl-neuraminic acid (NANA) in the cerebrospinal fluid (Saifer and Gerstenfield 1962) gave borderline results. Since NANA may be increased in other neurologic disorders the test is of no value for the diagnosis of TSD.

Serum

There are no significant abnormalities of the main serum lipid classes in TSD. An increased NANA content (Saifer and Gerstenfield 1962) is found in a variety of diseases, but an elevated globulin neuraminic acid to globulin protein ratio was found to be a good statistical indicator for biochemical distinction of amaurotic family idiocy from other disease groups.

The finding by Barclay et al. (1959) in an affected girl of increased plasma Sf 0—400 lipoproteins and a slightly abnormal distribution of phospholipids among alpha and beta lipoproteins (34 and 61% as compared with the ratio of 46:52 in normal infants) were largely reversible upon controlled intake of a balanced diet.

Enzymes in Plasma and Cerebrospinal Fluid

Alterations in the activities of various serum enzymes in TSD have been discovered during the last few years (Aronson et al. 1961).

SGOT levels were consistently elevated in 30 patients with TSD, with values up to five times normal. A slow decline of the enzyme activity after the first 20 to 24 months towards a normal level occurred concomitantly with the beginning of the protracted stage of the disease. SGOT-elevation appears to precede neurologic signs and may be indicative of the disease in children who are still asymptomatic. There is a similar time course of GOT activity in the cerebrospinal fluid.

Lactic acid dehydrogenase and malic acid dehydrogenase are also increased with a maximum for both enzymes after two years and a decrease thereafter.

Of great interest is the discovery of a deficiency or absence of fructose-1-phosphate aldolase in TSD serum (Volk et al. 1964). The enzyme, which normally catalyzes the splitting of fructose-1-phosphate into two three-carbon compounds which then gain access to the glycolytic pathway, was determined by a modi-

fication of the Sibley and Lehninger method by SCHAPIRA et. al. (1957), and by the
UV spectrophotometric procedure of WOLF (1962), which allowed distinction from
fructose-1-6-diphosphate aldolase. It is also absent in mothers and fathers of patients with TSD. In addition, in the study of VOLK et al. (1964), approximately
50% of paternal and maternal grandparents had no serum fructose-1-phosphate
aldolase activities, and the same was the case in about 25% of unaffected siblings.
The frequency of a lack of fructose-1-phosphate aldolase is ten times greater in
Jews than in non-Jews, and is indicative of the incidence of carriers of the disease.

   In contrast to hereditary fructose intolerance where lack of fructose-1-phos-
phate aldolase (LEVIN et al. 1963) in serum and liver is a prominent feature, liver
fructose-1-phosphate aldolase activity in TSD is only reduced to approximately
60%, and fructose tolerance is not impaired in the latter disorder (SCHNECK et al.
1965), while in the former accumulation of fructose-1-phosphate and hypoglycemia
occur.

Pathology

   As a rule, typical morphologic abnormalities in TSD are restricted to the central
nervous system. Ganglioside storage in other organs may occasionally be found
in the congenital form of amaurotic family idiocy and in the late infantile form,
but is actually a feature of the neurovisceral gangliosidoses to be discussed
separately. There are a number of reports on visceral lipid storage in TSD (BROUWER
1936, DAVISON and JACOBSON 1936, MARBURG 1942, 1943, TURBAN 1944, FISCHER
1955, DIEZEL 1957, NORMAN et al. 1959, 1964). In all these cases with the exception of the last one no information is available on the structure of the stored brain
gangliosides; likewise, the visceral lipids have not been identified as glycolipids
by chemical analysis. One can therefore not be sure whether such cases may not
belong to the category of neurovisceral gangliosidoses or gargoylism.

Brain

   The abnormal macroscopic findings in TSD concern size, weight and consistency
of the central organ and may depend on the duration of disease. The meninges
may be thickened and fibrotic, or, after prolonged illness, may have a gelatinous
appearance and contain numerous foam cells. In children who succumb early to
their disease, the brain is atrophic and underweight and has a leathery consistency.
The gyri are shrunken, the sulci wide. Autopsies during the second year yield
different findings. Here the weight of the brain is increased with an average
of 15% above normal (KANOF et al. 1959) and the hemispheres are enlarged, while
the dimensions of the ventricles are still normal. In contrast to the increasing
mass of the hemispheres, there is progressive atrophy of the phylogenetically
older parts of the brain like cerebellum and brain stem. With survival over two years
the changes become more marked, and the brain weight may increase to 50%
above normal with documented weights exceeding 2000 gm. Compression of the
ventricles can now be observed, but hydrocephalus, in contrast to other types,
has never been seen in this age group. From cranial measurements it appears
that growth of the brain ceases after 50 months.

   Cross-sections clearly show that the increase in brain size is entirely due to
swelling of the white matter which has a particular mucoid texture and appears
confluent with the cerebral grey which is firmer than normal. Located within the
white matter are irregularly outlined, edematous areas of cystic degeneration
measuring up to 1 cm in diameter and occurring particularly in the deep layers
of the frontal and parietal white matter (ARONSON and VOLK 1962). With
duration of the disease over two years the discrepancy becomes more marked

between atrophy of the infratentorial parts on one hand, and progressive increase of the supratentorial parts on the other. Intravascular thrombi have been observed and may result from desquamation of lipid-storing endothelial cells into the vessel lumen.

The cerebellum has a rubbery consistency, its cortical layers are shrunken. The roof nuclei are grossly visible and minimally implicated. Necrotic areas have not been described.

Eye

The "cherry-red" spot in TSD results from changes of ganglion cells and nerve fibers of the retina comparable to those of the brain. There is swelling and necrosis of the ganglion cells in the macula, where they are particularly numerous, leading to a greyish-white appearance of this area, in the center of which the fovea appears dark-red due to the transparency of chorioideal vessels. Atrophy of the optic nerve with demyelination is secondary.

Other Organs

Results of rectum biopsies show that nerve cell lesions in TSD occur outside the central nervous system. Involvement of cells other than nerve cells will be discussed in the chapter on neurovisceral gangliosidoses.

Histology

There is ubiquity of neurocellular involvement and of progressive reactive gliosis, although the degree of involvement varies considerably in certain areas. In addition to the findings in the central nervous system, retina and nerve cells of the myenteric plexus (Leistyna 1962) show changes.

Ganglion cells are swollen and rounded with widening or ballooning of the dendritic processes. The nuclei are displaced to the periphery and may show signs of disintegration (see fig. 1). With the electronmicroscope infoldings and other irregularities of their surface may be seen which impart to such nuclei a lobulated appearance. Deposition of abnormal material within the nucleus has not been observed; the nucleoli are normal (Terry and Weiss 1963).

The typical ultrastructural ganglion cell abnormalities consist of "membranous cytoplasmic bodies" (MCB) (see fig. 3) which are round or oval, measure 0.5 to 2.0 μ in diameter and may occupy a considerable portion of the cytoplasm (Terry and Weiss 1963, Korey et al. 1963a, b, Samuels et al. 1962, 1963, 1965, Terry and Korey 1960, 1963). They are also found in the axis cylinders, glial cells and perivascular cells. Their composition and pathogenesis is discussed in detail below. Other intracellular components appear diminished in number. Vacuoles and small channels may be seen which impinge on the Golgi apparatus. The mitochondria appear normal, even in highly abnormal cells, and ribosomes are plentiful.

The intensity of glial proliferation varies according to location. Microglial elements show hyperplasia and hypertrophy and may form colonies (Fischer 1955, Diezel 1957, 1962). Lipid deposits in these cells are rare. Microglial proliferation is particularly marked in the neighbourhood of distended ganglion cells (see fig. 2); its degree depends on the duration of the disease and may be extensive in some cases. The participation of the microglial cells in the disease process is reflected in their transformation to granule cells. With the electronmicroscope less affected glial cells are seen to contain clusters of vesicles and granules, while more severely involved ones show compact, well outlined structures which are round or oval and measure 1 μ in diameter. MCB can also occur in glial cells.

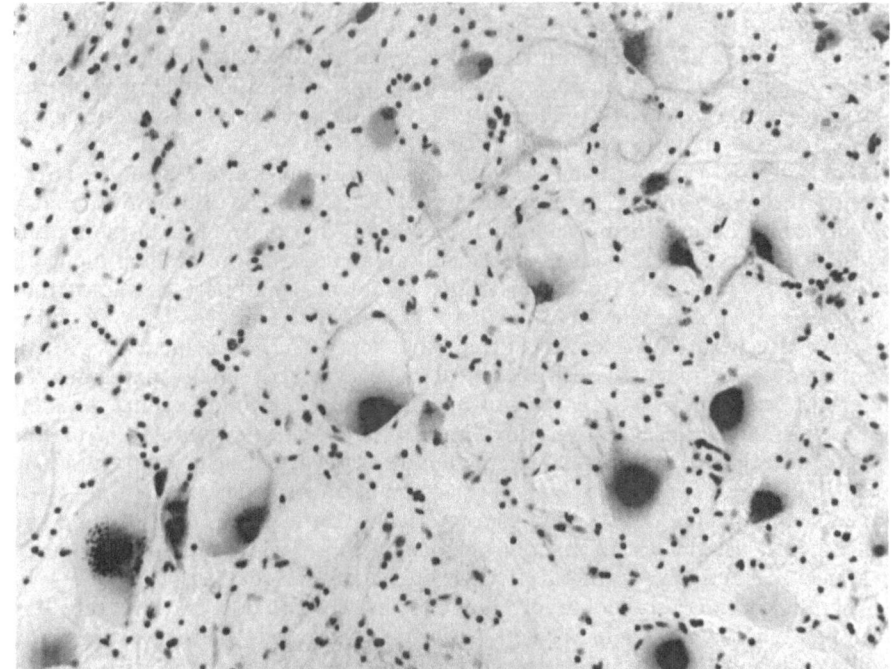

Fig. 1. Infantile amaurotic family idiocy. HE-stain. Enlargement 230-fold. Ballooned motor ganglion cell of the brain stem. (Reproduced by courtesy of Prof. P. B. DIEZEL)

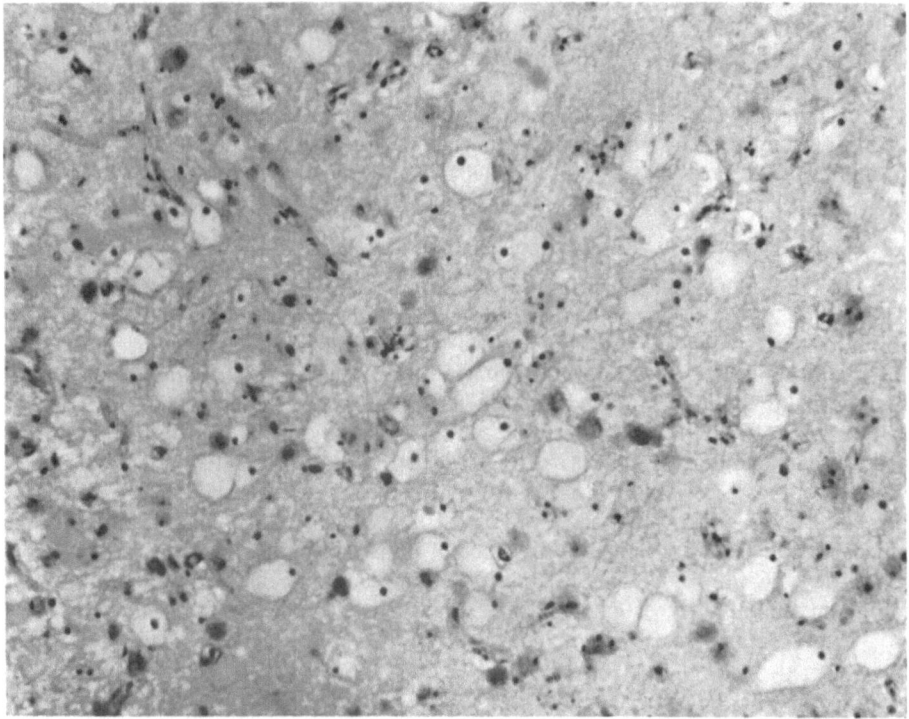

Fig. 2. Infantile amaurotic family idiocy. Cerebral cortex. HE-stain. Enlargement 150-fold. All ganglion cells are ballooned and store gangliosides. Small dark glial cells surround ganglion cells and contain the storage substance bound to protein. (Reproduced by courtesy of Prof. P. B. DIEZEL)

Demyelination is usually diffuse, but normal myelin sheaths can be found. The pyramidal tract may be intact through brain stem and medulla, with demyelination of its lower portions (Fischer 1955). Significant demyelination in the spinal cord may be more typical in adult cases.

A detailed description of microscopic changes of the white matter in TSD is that by Aronson and Volk (1962) and by Volk (1964). The diffuse white matter atrophy which occurs during the first 18 months is due to decrease in the number of visible axis cylinders. Occasionally small areas of fusiform swelling along the axons may be observed. Up to this time, before megencephaly develops, there is hardly any glial proliferation. In later stages of the disease there is diffuse intensive degeneration of axons and massive demyelination coincident with the manifest acceleration of cerebral cortical neurocytolysis, finally exceeding the phagocytic capacity of the reactive microglia. Isolated, swollen axonal remnants may persist and in place of the myelin sheaths there is accumulation of fluid and congregation of proliferating microglia and astrocytes. The latter are predominant; connected with their cell membranes are granules which measure 1—2 μ in diameter and display the staining characteristics of the axonal cytoplasmic substance. At the height of this reaction the deep cerebral white matter is converted to a mass of actively proliferating, multinucleated astrocytes.

There is considerably less involvement of the white matter in the cerebellum. Even in advanced cases some myelin can be demonstrated. There is no segmental swelling of axons except in the case of the Purkinje cell ramifications within the cortical molecular layer (Aronson and Volk 1962). A major microglial reaction is missing and the astrocytes, although increased in number, are unremarkable. It appears that, since neurocytolysis is only moderate, microglial scavenger activity is of sufficient magnitude to prevent deposition of products in the interstitium with its undesirable consequences (Aronson et al. 1961).

With the electronmicroscope the axoplasm may appear coarsely granulated and peripherally displaced. In the presence of structurally intact myelin this is strongly reminiscent of very early Wallerian degeneration (Vial 1958, Terry and Harkin 1959, Terry and Weiss 1963).

Membranous Cytoplasmic Bodies

These peculiar formations have been exhaustively studied by Samuels et al. (1962, 1963, 1965), with the use of electronmicroscopy, of chemical analyses and of in vitro experiments. From this work it appears that the MCB are not lysosomes nor are they derived from normal cell components, but they seem to consist of aggregates of lipids (90%) and protein (10%) (Samuels et al. 1962). One third to one half of the lipid consists of gangliosides, about 20% of phospholipids and 40% of cholesterol. The ratio of N-acetyl-neuraminic acid : phospholipids : cholesterol was 1 : 1 : 3.8 in the study of Samuels et al. (1965). From in vitro experiments it seems that the formation of MCB is due to a high ganglioside concentration in neurons in the presence of phospholipids and cholesterol. Apropos is the report by Diezel (1957) of storage in ganglion cells of cholesterol esters, sphingomyelin and glycerophosphatides in addition to acidic glycolipids.

Histochemistry

Although combinations of different stains allow a general classification of stored matter, it is still difficult by these methods to differentiate storage cells which in different diseases (TSD, gargoylism, etc.) contain similar compounds. Diezel

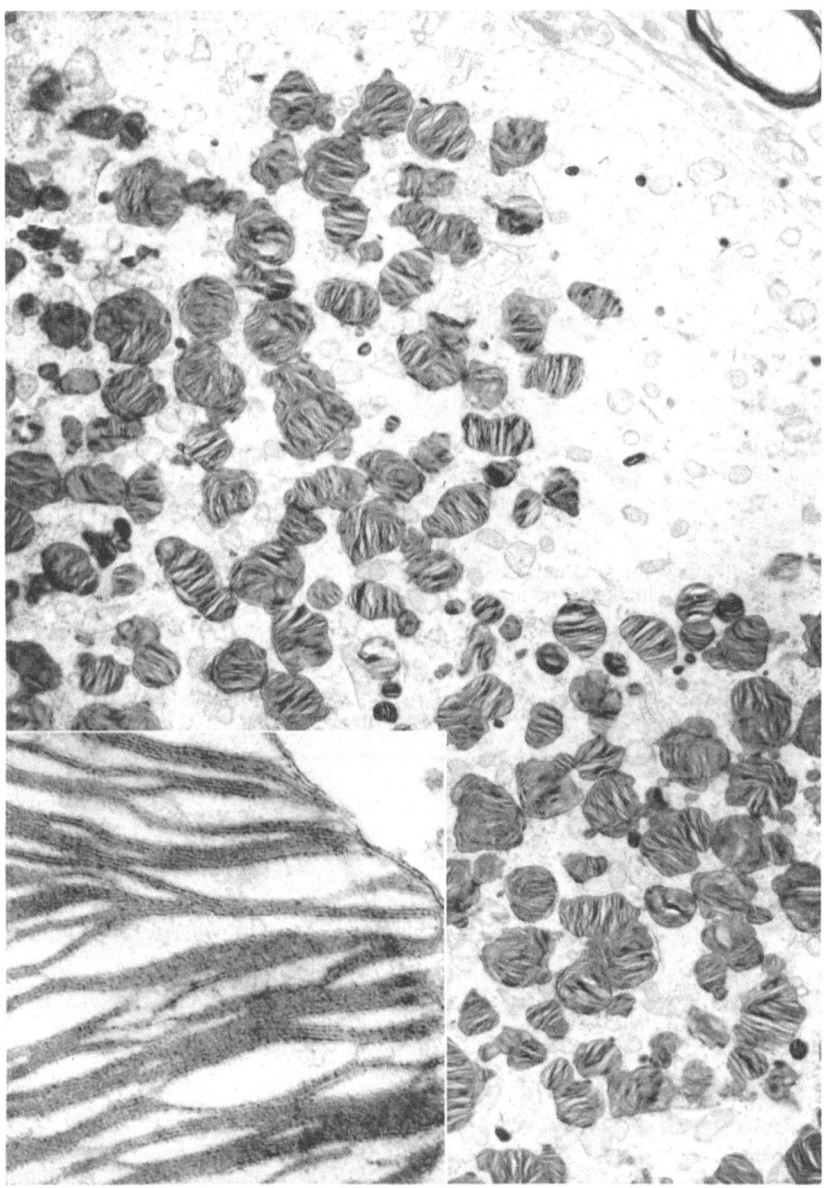

Fig. 3. Amaurotic Idiocy. Anterior horn cell, lamellated bodies (LB). These bodies represent the smallest morphologic units formed by the stored material. Larger, "composed bodies" may be formed from LB. Enlargement 1800:1. Section at the left is with higher magnification (33400:1). Reproduced by courtesy of Prof. P. B. DIEZEL)

(1954b, 1955) has employed a modified Bial-reaction for histochemical identification of neuraminic acid, and deduced the presence of gangliosides from a positive reaction (see table 2 and 3). On the basis of his studies, neuraminic acid-containing lipids occur mainly in the granule cells, microglial cells and interstitial spaces, while the majority of ganglion cells react Bial-negative. He concluded that ganglion cells in TSD store a lipid which does not contain neuraminic acid, and

Table 2. *Histochemical differentiation of the stored lipids in several disturbances of lipid metabolism*

	Amaurotic idiocy, infantile type	Niemann-Pick, infantile type	Gargoylism, infantile type	Metachromatic leukodystrophy, infantile type
PAS-reaction	++	(+)	+	+
CP-reaction*	((+)) only in some cases	+	((+))	+
Cresyl-violet	metachromatic red	faintly metachromatic red	metachromatic red	metachromatic brown
Bial's test**	+	((+))	+	negative; sometimes weakly positive
Evans' blue	metachromatic red	blue, sometimes faintly met. red	faintly metachromatic red	light blue; in some cells the lipids are faintly red
Birefringent lipids	++	+	+	(+)
Sudan black in pol. light	red	black and faintly red	faintly red	black and faintly red
Primary fluorescence	blue-green	negative	green-yellow	faintly blue-green

* Copper-phthalocyanin reaction (Pearse, Diezel).
** Bial's test for proving neuraminic acid (Diezel 1955).

Source: Diezel (1960)

Table 3. *Histochemical characteristics of different forms of amaurotic idiocy*

	Infantile	Late infantile	Juvenile	Adult
Beginning of the disease (age)	0—2.	1.—5. (80% 2.—4.)	5.—9.	20.—40.
Increase in volume of the ganglion cells	6—10 times	2—3 times (some cells to 10 times)	1—2 times	Hardly enlarged
Protein linkage of the storage material in ganglion cells	No linkage to protein	Only in some ganglion cells protein bound material	All lipids bound to proteins	All lipids bound to proteins
Birefringent lipids in ganglion cells	In all ganglion cells	Sometimes many, sometimes only a few ganglion cells contain birefringent material	No birefringence	No birefringence
Evans' blue	Only the birefringent lipids appear metachromatically red	Only the birefringent lipids are metachromatic red, the others appear light blue	Light blue	Light blue
Primary fluorescence	Light blue, the stored substance shows nearly no fluorescence	Only in the small ganglion cells with protein bound material yellow-green fluorescence; some yellow granula	Yellow fluorescence of the storage cells with some yellow-brown granula	Yellow to yellow-brown fluorescence of the granular storage substance

Source: Diezel (1960)

which becomes Bial-positive after modification in other cellular elements. Accordingly, the main lipid of TSD would not be a typical ganglioside, but rather an acidic glycolipid which may be related to cerebrosides, since it is easily extractable with 100% alcohol.

Several comments may be made to these interpretations. On one hand, SVEN-NERHOLM (1957c) has pointed out that neuraminic acid occurring in tissues is not necessarily a component of gangliosides. On the other hand, conclusions drawn from solubility properties of an isolated compound may not be valid when the same material occurs as a component of a tissue; furthermore, staining properties may be modified depending on the physical state of a substance within the cells. Therefore, the advantage of histochemical methods lies more in the localization of a given compound than in its structural determination. Differentiation of various gangliosides still depends on chemical analysis.

Results of Lipid Analyses

Brain

Early determinations in cerebral grey matter of neuraminic acid showed levels which, in TSD, were 10 to 20 times normal (KLENK 1939, 1942a, b). Neuraminic acid was also increased in the cerebellum and the dentate nucleus suggestive of accumulation in all these tissues of gangliosides (KLENK 1947, 1955). These findings have been confirmed in every case of TSD, but data reported for the ganglioside content of Tay-Sachs brains vary considerably, the discrepancy being caused in part by the different origins and methods of conservation of examined tissues (CUMINGS 1957, FOLCH-PI and LEES 1959, BOGOCH 1962, BERMAN and GATT 1962, SVENNERHOLM 1962, KOREY and STEIN 1963, KOREY et al. 1963b, JATZKEWITZ et al. 1965, ROUSER et al. 1965). Comparable data are given in tables 4 and 5.

Recent analyses with the use of a micromethod of samples of 15—50 mg wet material (JATZKEWITZ 1964) show a content of total gangliosides and derived compounds of 4—10 times normal (JATZKEWITZ et al. 1965). Lower figures have been reported by KOREY et al. (1963). In their material total gangliosides were twice normal (related to the dry weight). The gangliosides as a fraction of total lipids were 9% and 4% in their three year-old and 1½ month-old patients, respectively. The calculated ganglioside content of neurons was 5% of the dry weight in TSD as compared to 2.5% normally. The apparent discrepancy between the relatively small increase in gangliosides on one hand, and the massive morphologic abnormalities on the other, point in the direction of qualitative ganglioside abnormalities.

Gangliosides are also increased in the white matter (KLENK 1947, 1955). The degree of increase above the normal content is greater than the increase observed in the cortical grey. While normally the ganglioside content of the white matter is about one tenth to one fourth that of grey matter (FOLCH-PI and LEES 1959), in TSD this ratio is much higher (FOLCH-PI and LEES 1959, TINGEY 1959, TERRY and KOREY 1960, KOREY et al. 1963b, SAIFER 1964).

Increase of gangliosides is associated with elevation of the concentration of asialo-derivatives (JATZKEWITZ et al. 1965), which is particularly marked in the white matter (KOREY et al. 1963b) and reflected in the increase in brain hexosamine which is typically found in TSD (KOREY et al. 1963b, KOREY and STEIN 1963).

The concentration of all lipid classes, with the exception of gangliosides, is lowered. Total brain phospholipids were 19.68 mg % (normal 25—30 mg %) in the material of THANNHAUSER et al. (1939) and lipid phosphorus in a four year-old patient (BOGOCH 1962) was distinctly low with 0.81 mg/gm (wet weight) (normal: 1.15 at 8 months, 1.27 at 5½ years and 1.24 in adults). A relative decrease has been reported for sphingomyelin; on the other hand, with progressive enlargement of the brain, there may be an absolute increase of this lipid (EDGAR 1962). A low concentration of glycerophosphatides has already been found by KLENK (1939). Recent studies of ROUSER et al. (1965) show that lecithin in TSD is relatively and absolutely diminished.

The cerebroside content of the brain is very low and comparable to that of the infantile brain (ROUSER et al. 1965). There is no increase with progression of the disease. Since cerebrosides and sphingomyelin are the main components of the myelin-lipids, a decrease of these classes is in accordance with the histologic finding of demyelination (BRANTE 1949, JOHNSON et al. 1949). Similar changes occur in Niemann-Pick disease with central nervous system involvement, in meta-chromatic leucodystrophy and in Alzheimer's disease (ROUSER et al. 1965). The case of WILDI (1950) which has been reported as a mixed type of TSD and Gaucher's disease is an exception since here cerebrosides were increased in addition to gangliosides.

The Gangliosides in TSD

Upon differentiation of Tay-Sachs gangliosides (see table 4 and 5) it became apparent that these consisted mainly (80—90%) of a fraction which occurs normally only in trace amounts (KLENK et al. 1957, ROSENBERG and CHARGAFF 1959, KLENK and GIELEN 1961a, b, BERMAN and GATT 1962, SVENNERHOLM 1962, WAGNER et al. 1963, GATT and BERMAN 1963a—c, KUHN and WIEGANDT 1963, and others).

Table 4. *Brain gangliosides in case of Tay-Sachs disease*

	Normal infantile brain	Tay-Sachs brain
	(Values expressed as per cent of dry weight)	
Total gangliosides	1	8.9
Total gangliosides without Tay-Sachs-ganglioside (G$_{GNTrII}$)	1	1.1
	(Values expressed as per cent of total gangliosides)	
G$_{GNT}$IV	12	1.8
G$_{GNT}$III	21	2.8
G$_{GNT}$II	28	2.6
G$_{GNT}$I	24	3.9
G$_{GNTrII}$ (Tay-Sachs)	—	86.2
Incompletely separated residue (mainly G$_{GNT}$II, G$_{GNT}$III, and G$_{GNT}$IV)	15	2.7
Recovery:	79.5	87.0

Source: WAGNER (1966)

Thus, separation of gangliosides by thin-layer chromatography showed that the Rf-value for the main portion of Tay-Sachs gangliosides was considerably higher than that of the prevailing fraction in normals (MÜLDNER et al. 1962, KLENK et al. 1963), and a different solubility of normal and Tay-Sachs gangliosides has been reported by BERMAN and GATT (1962), GATT and BERMAN (1963b), and KLENK et al. (1962, 1963), with a greater affinity of the latter for the chloroform

Table 5. *Ganglioside patterns in gray matter of patients with Tay-Sachs disease*

Gangliosides	Cases				Normal control (range)
	1	2	3	4	
	(Values expressed as per cent of NANA)				
G_0	1	0.8	1.3	0.9	3.0— 4.8
G_1 (GGNTIV)	1.6	1.3	1.9	1.4	12.4—19.3
G_2 (GGNTIII)	3.2	1.1	1.0	4.2	11.1—20.0
G_3 (GGNTII)	8.1	4.5	4.4	5.2	39.6—48.0
G_4 (GGNTI)	2.1	1.3	1.4	1.6	14.6—21.4
G_5 (GGNTrII)	83.4	88.4	87.9	84.1	1.5— 4.4
G_6 (GLACT)	1.3	2.7	2.1	2.7	1

Source: SUZUKI (1966)

Average of six normal control brains, ages 2.5 months to 8 years. Values given for G_2 include G_2A and those for G_4 include G_3A, two minor sialic acid-containing components with chromatographic mobilities between G_2 and G_3, and between G_3 and G_4, respectively (SUZUKI 1966).

phase in a diphasic chloroform-alcohol-water system. Both the chromatographic and solubility properties of the Tay-Sachs ganglioside are shared by a ganglioside which occurs in small amounts in normal brain tissue.

Pioneer studies on the structure of this Tay-Sachs ganglioside, with the use of partial acid hydrolysis, periodate oxidation and exhaustive methylation, have been performed simultaneously by SVENNERHOLM (1962, 1963), KLENK et al. (1963), KUHN and WIEGANDT (1963), KUNAU (1964), and KLENK and KUNAU (1964). They showed that it consists of one mol each of ceramide, glucose, galactose, N-acetyl-galactosamine and NANA according to the following formula (see fig. 4).

The diminution of normal gangliosides in TSD, which is apparent on thin-layer chromatography, has been confirmed with microanalytical methods (JATZKEWITZ et al. 1965). Here, the instability of gangliosides towards acids (formalin fixation) needs to be considered, which results in loss of neuraminic acid and decrease of normal multisialo-gangliosides (KLENK et al. 1957, SUZUKI 1965). Since KLENK et al. (1963) used freeze-dried material for isolation of gangliosides, a formalin effect can be excluded. The sphingosine of the Tay-Sachs ganglioside is mainly the normal C-18 sphingosine. From oxidative ozonization of triacetylsphingosine it appears that there is, in addition, a significant amount of

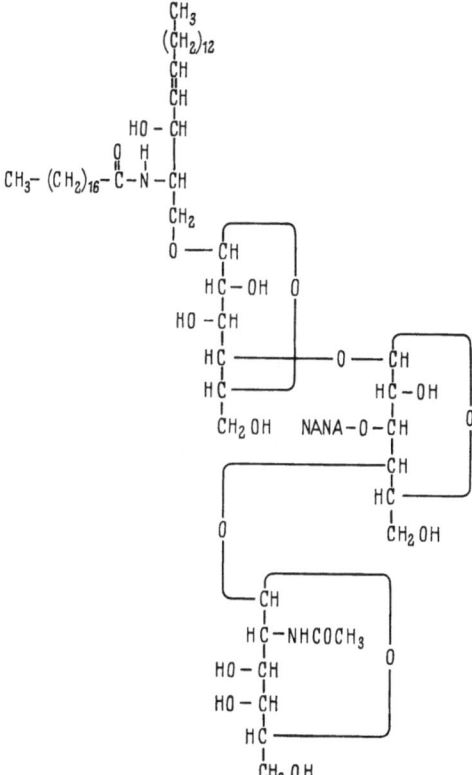

Fig. 4. Structure of Tay-Sachs ganglioside GGNTrII (GM 2)

C-20 sphingosine (Proštenik and Mahjofer-Oreščanin 1960) which is found in large amounts in cattle brain (Klenk and Gielen 1961c, Klenk et al. 1962, Stanacev and Chargaff 1963, Erlaçin 1963). Traces of a C-20 dihydrosphingosine (Sambasivarao and McCluer 1964, Karlsson 1964a—c) probably occur.

The ganglioside fatty acids in TSD consist of 85% stearic acid, 4.5% myristic acid, 6.6% arachidonic acid, and 1.6% behenic acid (Klenk et al. 1963). The nomenclature of gangliosides is outlined in table 1.

Diagnosis

TSD is a possibility in infants who exhibit neurologic symptoms during the first year of life. The diagnosis is supported by the typical ophthalmologic changes. Limitation of the disease process to the central nervous system in the absence of hepatosplenomegaly aid in exclusion of Niemann-Pick disease and Gaucher's disease. Of serum enzyme studies, deficiency or lack of fructose-1-phosphate aldolase is typical for TSD, and a normal response to exogenous fructose aids in differentiation from hereditary fructose intolerance.

Histologic and histochemical properties of material from brain biopsy or rectum biopsy render further evidence for the diagnosis, and secure to some degree the differentiation of TSD from other types of amaurotic family idiocy. Lipid analyses from brain tissue with the demonstration of the increase in Tay-Sachs ganglioside finally provide conclusive evidence for the diagnosis.

Pathogenetic Considerations

The discovery by Klenk (1939) of ganglioside storage in TSD has ended the discussion whether that disease might not be a variety of Niemann-Pick disease. The various theories on the pathogenesis of amaurotic family idiocy center around potential abnormalities of the metabolism of gangliosides, although other metabolic abnormalities of TSD tissues have been found. Korey et al. (1963b), for instance, measuring O_2-consumption and lactate production in biopsy specimens of Tay-Sachs brains, found a respiratory depression of about 50% in advanced cases which was correlated with the neuronal changes. In addition, upon anaerobic incubation of Tay-Sachs brain homogenates, asialo-derivatives of gangliosides appeared (Korey and Stein 1963). A further finding concerned a low free amino acid content of the cerebral cortex in TSD which might result in decreased protein synthesis (Korey et al. 1963b).

As regards the origin of the accumulated ganglioside, it seems certain that it is formed in the affected ganglion cells themselves. Deposition of gangliosides on the basis of an elevated blood level, as discussed for the storage of cerebrosides by the reticuloendothelial cells in Gaucher's disease, has no experimental support and seems unlikely. An increased serum content of neuraminic acid is found in many diseases with and without central nervous system involvement (Saifer et al. 1959) and, like the increased ratio of globulin sialic acid to globulin protein in TSD, appears to be the result rather than the cause of the storage in brain. Morphologic observation suggests that ganglioside storage occurs primarily in ganglion cells and is secondary in phagocytic elements.

The following discussion summarizes available information on structure and metabolism of the Tay-Sachs gangliosides. Pathogenetic discussions center once more on two questions:

1. is the stored ganglioside of TSD different from normal gangliosides, either with regard to its components, its structure, the binding to protein or polymerization; and/or

2. is there evidence for an (enzymatic?) abnormality in the metabolism of a "normal" ganglioside.

Extensive studies on the chemical structure of the Tay-Sachs ganglioside have not shown a significant abnormality. As mentioned earlier, a compound with identical structure has been found among brain gangliosides of normal subjects. However, the sensitivity of these complex molecules toward treatment with alkali or acid, the possibility of spontaneous hydrolysis during handling and the complicated methods of structural identification render definite clarification of this point difficult.

Ganglioside fatty acids were analyzed repeatedly in TSD (KLENK 1942, 1955, SVENNERHOLM 1957b, KLENK and GIELEN 1961a, b, SVENNERHOLM and RAAL 1961, KLENK et al. 1963) and no significant differences from the normal pattern were observed (ROUSER et al. 1965).

The sphingosine base, according to available information, is identical with the normal 1,3-dihydroxy-2-amino-4-octadecene and is present in the D-erythro-configuration.

Small amounts of dihydrosphingosine (CARTER 1958) and C-20 sphingosine are found in TSD as well as in normals (KLENK et al. 1963).

While all gangliosides contain ceramide, they differ with respect to the amounts and binding of hexose units, hexosamines and NANA.

Several studies have shown that in this regard, too, no difference could be found between the Tay-Sachs ganglioside (formula see fig. 4) and a hexosamine-containing monosialoganglioside (G_{GNTrII} in table 1) (KLENK et al. 1962, SVENNERHOLM 1962, 1963) which normally makes up 1—5% of total brain gangliosides. From these findings it is unlikely that an abnormal ganglioside molecule is the cause of intracellular accumulation. It is, however, possible that the Tay-Sachs ganglioside occurs in a form which prevents the normal action of catabolic enzymes. One of the physical properties of gangliosides is the formation of molecular aggregates in aqueous solution with a molecular weight of at least 250.000 (FOLCH-PI and LEES 1959) and of the MCB with their high ganglioside content (SAMUELS et al. 1963, TERRY and WEISS 1963, SAMUELS 1965). If gangliosides of nerve cells occur as components of polymers (mucolipids, ROSENBERG and CHARGAFF 1959), an abnormal product may result from abnormal binding or from an atypical sequence of the components. It is then possible that storage results from inability of (normal) enzymes to degrade these substances. An increase in the polymeric mucolipid content associated with a low monomeric ganglioside fraction in TSD has been discussed by ROSENBERG and CHARGAFF (1959). They showed that through the action of receptor-destroying enzyme of V. cholera on mucolipids of TSD, only one fifth of the sialic acid was liberated which could be split from "normal" brain gangliosides, and suggested that a peptide necessary for the action of the enzyme may be missing in TSD, so that a biologically useless mucolipid accumulates. The finding of KUHN and WIEGANDT (1963) that neuraminidase did not split sialic acid from the ganglioside $G_{GNT}IV$ and $G_{GNT}I$ (see table 1) is relevant here.

BOGOCH (1962), using emulsion fractionation of gray matter in TSD, found a significant deviation from normal, with an accumulation of aminoglycolipids which did not have the molar ratios of NANA to hexose to hexosamine found in normal brains. Increase of a fraction with a higher hexosamine: phosphate ratio could be the result of a disturbance in the uridine-diphospho-hexosamine-transferase system whereby hexosamine rather than hexosamine-phosphate is exchanged. Increased amounts of non-phosphorylated hexosamine might favor synthesis of excess neuraminic acid via the NANA-aldolase reaction and thus induce increased formation or decreased destruction of gangliosides in TSD (BOGOCH 1962). All these theories are based upon findings and observations on mucolipids or amino-glycolipids that have not yet been completely defined. The possibility of abnormalities in their structure cannot yet be assessed. The increased content of polymerized glycolipids could be related to the occurrence of MCB, but the finding of their formation in vitro from "normal" components (see page 224) indicates that they are the result rather than the cause of storage.

Korey and Stein (1963) have examined the hexose-binding of normal and Tay-Sachs gangliosides by incubation with enzyme fractions from normal and Tay-Sachs brains. They could show that Tay-Sachs enzymes degraded the internal hexose chain of Tay-Sachs gangliosides less efficiently than that of normal gangliosides, and concluded that abnormal hexose-hexose binding in Tay-Sachs gangliosides inhibits enzymatic degradation. In addition, it was shown that homogenates from rat brain catabolize Tay-Sachs gangliosides faster than normal human or cattle brain gangliosides, again indicating structural differences between the normal and Tay-Sachs ganglioside (Korey and Stein 1963).

If there is no structural ganglioside abnormality in TSD, an enzymatic lesion along the degradative pathway must be considered. The alternate possibility, namely overproduction of sphingolipids, appears to be unlikely (see chapter of Burton, page 159).

It is now generally accepted that gangliosides are precursors of sphingolipids which do not contain neuraminic acid (Klenk 1955, Svennerholm 1957b, Fredrickson 1960). Klenk, in this context, emphasized the similarity of the ganglioside and sphingomyelin fatty acid patterns, stearic acid being the main component. Since Svennerholm (1957a—c) could demonstrate gangliosides with longer-chain and unsaturated fatty acids like those found in cerebrosides, it is not unlikely that there is also a precursor-product relationship between gangliosides and cerebrosides, which would explain a number of observations in Gaucher's disease (Philippart and Menkes 1964, see page 260).

The possibility that in TSD there is a block of the pathway from gangliosides to cerebrosides is supported by the marked increases in gangliosides in places where myelin lipids (cerebrosides and sphingomyelin) normally prevail, namely the white matter (Folch-Pi and Lees 1959, Korey et al. 1963b). A similar pathogenesis may underly the ganglioside accumulation which is found in other demyelinating diseases. The "advantage" of this somewhat complicated pathway, from a more complex compound to a simpler one, may be that ceramide is made available for the synthesis of myelin lipids in a more hydrophilic vehicle (Fredrickson 1960).

A defect between gangliosides and cerebrosides can be located at each of a number of enzymatic steps.

One possibility is impaired liberation of N-acetyl-galactosamine as proposed by Svennerholm (1957b). A defective removal of a carbohydrate moiety from a monosialoganglioside is also assumed by Rouser et al. (1965), since other gangliosides can be degraded to the Tay-Sachs ganglioside by neuraminidase.

The isolation (Gatt and Berman 1963a, Makita and Yamakawa 1964) and increased content in TSD (Korey et al. 1963, Jatzkewitz et al. 1965) of the asialoglycolipid, which corresponds to the Tay-Sachs ganglioside, make an impairment of liberation of N-acetyl-neuraminic acid unlikely as a cause of TSD, and support the thesis that the galactosamine-galactose bond cannot be split in TSD (Rouser et al. 1965). Thus, the degradation of various gangliosides would proceed up to the Tay-Sachs ganglioside, which then accumulates. The enzymes which are potentially involved are reviewed by Burton (page 123). A further potential site for the block resides with hydrolases which split glycolipids and which have been found in normal brain tissue (KOREY and STEIN 1963, SANDHOFF, PILZ and JATZKEWITZ 1964). Still another pathogenetic possibility is faulty control of the rates of synthesis and/or degradation. Thus, steady state conditions may not be reached following the initial increase after birth and the subsequent decrease in synthesis rates of gangliosides and cerebrosides which occurs normally (BURTON et al. 1958, BURTON 1963).

Finally, the possibility of immunologic reactions should be mentioned. It has repeatedly been shown (see chapter by BURTON) that glycolipids can participate in antigen-antibody reactions. Thus SOMERS et al. (1964) prepared rabbit antisera against the gangliosides $G_{GNT}II$ and $G_{GNT}III$ and against the corresponding asialo-gangliosides. The antiganglioside-antibodies were specific and did not crossreact with asialo-gangliosides. It is likely that the antigenicity of gangliosides resides with the carbohydrate units. Although the possibility of antigen-antibody reaction in TSD is remote, auto-immune mechanisms may well play a part in other demyelinating diseases.

A summary of present (incomplete) knowledge of the pathogenesis in TSD follows: The basic defect which leads to ganglioside storage in ganglion cells and secondary changes in other cells appears to reside with the metabolism of the nerve cells. From the selective accumulation of a specific ganglioside ($G_{GNTr}II$) it can be tentatively concluded that degradation of this particular ganglioside is impaired. Although an atypical structure cannot be excluded, it is more likely that there is an enzymatic defect in the catabolic pathway, which is most probably located at the point of liberation of N-acetyl-galactosamine.

III. Late-Infantile Amaurotic Family Idiocy
Definition and Introduction

There has been some controversy regarding differentiation of late-infantile amaurotic family idiocy (LIAFI) from other forms of amaurotic family idiocy, and some authors classed the LIAFI either as Tay-Sachs disease (TSD) or as an early variant of the juvenile form (WYBURN-MASON 1943, SEITELBERGER 1957, NORMAN 1958). However, distinguishing features exist. The onset of LIAFI is, in general, later than that of TSD and in most cases the disease becomes manifest between the ages of two and four years, occasionally after five years. The progression of LIAFI is generally slower than that of TSD and depends on the age of the patient at the time of disease onset. Since cases during the first months of life have been seen (SCHNECK et al. 1965b), differentiation of LIAFI from TSD is not always possible on the basis of the patient's age.

Although LIAFI can usually be distinguished from other amaurotic family idiocies on the basis of clinical and pathologic findings, the neurologic symptomatology and even histologic and histochemical features in some cases may be similar to TSD and to juvenile amaurotic family idiocy, type Spielmeyer-Vogt. In these cases only chemical analyses which, in LIAFI, fail to show the typical Tay-Sachs ganglioside, justify the distinction. In addition, contrary to TSD, there is no racial predisposition towards LIAFI.

Reports suggest that there is localized intracellular storage of gangliosides in LIAFI (SCHNECK et al. 1965b, JATZKEWITZ et al. 1965, GONATAS and GONATAS 1965), but further analyses are necessary to see whether these cases, which share common features, are also characterized by storage of the same ganglioside.

In a review by SEITELBERGER et al. (1957) a total of 34 cases of LIAFI have been collected. This number is now closer to 40 (DIEZEL 1957, GONATAS and

4

Gonatas 1965, Schneck et al. 1965b, Klinken-Rasmussen and Dyggve 1965, Ledeen et al. 1965) although in some cases uncertainties exist as to the correct classification. Whether some cases of myoclonic epilepsy (Unverricht-Lundberg) belong in the category of LIAFI, remains to be proved by chemical analyses.

Clinical Manifestations

There are many signs and symptoms common to LIAFI as well as TSD, such as hyperacusis, muscular twitching, irritability and decreasing response to the environment. However, bouts of screaming or laughter are rare and, in contrast to TSD, initial symptoms include loss of intellectual capacity and impairment of speech rather than progressive motor weakness and impaired mobility. In general, the symptoms resemble more those of the juvenile type of amaurotic family idiocy.

Neurologic findings include cerebellar ataxia and extrapyramidal rigidity which are not as common in TSD. A cherry-red spot is rarely seen, but retinitis pigmentosa as well as abnormal pupillary reactions are frequent. Cases without ophthalmologic abnormalities have been reported (Corberi 1926, Liebers 1927, Schneck et al. 1965b).

The clinical course of LIAFI is more protracted than that of TSD. We found only four cases where the disease lasted for less than two years, the shortest course was one year and the longest nine years with an average duration of three years and seven months. The later stages are characterized by progressive loss of intelligence and finally idiocy. Undifferentiated speech, imbalance or inability to walk are further late signs of the disease. Somnolence, syncopal attacks, grand mal seizures and general loss of body tone indicate the prefinal stage.

Pathology

In almost all cases reported as LIAFI there is atrophy of the brain and spinal cord and occasionally hydrocephalus externus. The brain weight is low and there may be thickening of the meninges. Spongy cortical atrophy has been described by Bielschowsky (1914) in two cases.

The gyri are narrowed, the sulci widened and there is compensatory enlargement of the ventricles. Klinken-Rasmussen and Dyggve (1965) saw a greatly enlarged foramen Magendi resulting from aplasia of cerebellar vermis and tonsils. However, although cerebellar atrophy appears to be a common finding, it is not pathognomonic and may be lacking (Schob 1912, Jansky and Myslivecek 1918, Greenfield and Nevin 1933, Seitelberger et al. 1957).

On cross sectioning the brain, cystic areas like those observed in TSD are rarely seen. The white matter appears firmer than normal, the grey matter is softer (Klinken-Rasmussen and Dyggve 1965), and the cerebellum is quite hard.

Regional differences in the intensity of the disease process are more marked than in TSD. Typical histologic changes of cortical cells may be found only in certain areas, for instance in the frontal and occipital regions. Basal nuclei are involved in most cases. Occasionally the disease is limited to the cerebellum. The spinal cord is frequently involved. In the cases of Seitelberger et al. (1957) there were marked changes of the anterior horn cells, the area striata, corpus geniculatum laterale, thalamus, and degeneration of the structures of the optic system. Thalamic involvement has also been described by Wildi (1950) and Lemieux (1954).

The phylogenetic age of different regions and the sequence of maturation of different areas may determine to some degree the non-homogenous distribution of the lesions. Since storage is considerably less as compared to TSD, part of the ganglion cells may continue to function normally.

As in TSD there is accumulation of lipid mainly in ganglion cells; however, in LIAFI, they are considerably less swollen (see table 3). Enlargement may be two- or three-fold; rarely, ganglion cells which are ten times the normal size may be seen (DIEZEL 1960) and there are always cells which appear normal. SCHNECK et al. (1965b), upon electronmicroscopic examination of brain biopsy specimens, found in about two-thirds of the neurons marked swelling caused by the accumulation in each cell of 40 or more cytoplasmic bodies. Only approximately 1% of ganglion cells appeared completely normal by their standards. However, classification of this case appears uncertain since the symptomatology of amaurotic family idiocy began a few weeks after birth.

The morphologic changes of storing ganglion cells are, in general, similar to those observed in TSD. The deposited matter appears to be non-uniform (SEITELBERGER et al. 1957, DIEZEL 1957, KLINKEN-RASMUSSEN and DYGGVE 1965); it may be fine-granular or homogenous with the granular material prevailing in moderately enlarged cells and missing in ballooned ones (SEITELBERGER et al. 1957). Dendritic swelling can be seen in the latter. DIEZEL (1957) found a substance in the extremely enlarged ganglion cells of his cases which was PAS-positive, easily soluble in alcohol, gave a positive Bial-reaction and was metachromatic with thio-reagents; in addition, there was material which was extracted with difficulty. Rather large lipid granules in the ganglion cells of the thalamus were already described by GREENFIELD and HOLMES (1925), later by SJÖVALL and ERICSSON (1933), WILDI (1950), LEMIEUX (1954), and by KLINKEN-RASMUSSEN and DYGGVE (1965).

Involvement of the glia varies in different areas. Granule cells may be absent. The microglial elements accumulate in the neighbourhood of ganglion cells undergoing swelling and necrosis. They may contain a PAS-positive, red-metachromatic material (DIEZEL 1957) which stains brighter red with Sudan III than the granules of ganglion cells (KLINKEN-RASMUSSEN and DYGGVE 1965). Astrocytes and cells of the oligodendroglia may also be increased in number.

Not all glial cells of the white matter participate in the storage process and glial changes, as in TSD, depend on the extent of myelin breakdown. Involvement of the white matter is generally less in LIAFI than in TSD, and also appears to be somewhat focal, like the changes of ganglion cells. There may be no evidence of demyelination in some cases (DIEZEL 1957) while others show pronounced granular degeneration and deposition of droplets besides lipid-filled macrophages (KLINKEN-RASMUSSEN and DYGGVE 1965). In areas with major involvement, i.e. thalamus, hypothalamus and corpus striatum, foci of glial tissue may replace the myelin sheaths. A marked sclerosis can be seen in the cerebellum.

Intensive *histochemical studies* by DIEZEL (1957), SEITELBERGER et al. (1957), KLINKEN-RASMUSSEN and DYGGVE (1965) have resulted in the demonstration of a significant accumulation in degenerated ganglion cells of neuraminic acid-containing glycolipids which appear to exist partly free, partly bound to protein. According to these workers it is possible to differentiate TSD and LIAFI unequivocally with a combination of the Bial-reaction and the coupled tetrazonium reaction (DIEZEL 1957, 1960) (see table 2). In the latter author's opinion the stored material is histochemically a glycolipid which in LIAFI, contrary to findings in TSD, combines with NANA within the storage cells. The stored product is therefore not the genuine LIAFI ganglioside, but rather the result of an additional intracellular reaction.

Storage of sphingomyelin is also suggested by histochemical findings (DIEZEL 1957, SEITELBERGER et al. 1957).

Results of Lipid Analyses

Chemical analyses in LIAFI were performed in only a few cases. Schneck et al. (1965b) analyzing biopsy specimens, found the normal monosialo-ganglioside $G_{GNT}I$ (see figure 5) or the disialoganglioside $G_{GNT}II$ increased, but not the Tay-Sachs ganglioside G_{GNTrII} (see table 1). In the case of Gonatas and Gonatas (1965) of a 25 months-old child with "systemic late infantile lipidosis" there were various peculiar features, such as marked involvement of spleen, lymph nodes, bone marrow and lungs, and similarities to TSD as well as gargoylism. Here, too, the ganglioside $G_{GNT}I$ made up the bulk of the total gangliosides which were increased four-fold. The other normally occurring fractions $G_{GNT}I$ to $G_{GNT}IV$ and G_{LACT} were present in trace amounts. Another example of LIAFI may be a case studied by Jatzkewitz and Sandhoff (1963). They isolated from brain tissue which had been stored in formalin for 26 years, major amounts of the gangliosides $G_{GNT}I$ while the Tay-Sachs ganglioside was present only in trace amounts and its non-neuraminic acid containing derivative not at all. $G_{GNT}I$ amounted to $10.59 \pm .132\%$ of total lipids as compared to $3—3.5\%$ normally. The value for the non-neuraminic acid containing derivative was 7.5% (normal less than 0.3%). Exact classification of this case is impossible because of the prolonged formalin fixation. There is the possibility of an artefact in that increasing amounts of $G_{GNT}I$ may be formed from multisialo-gangliosides through the action of formalin. According to Suzuki (1965) after four to five years of fixation no other ganglioside can be identified. This matter is controversial; Klenk et al. (1957, 1963) and Jatzkewitz et al. (1965) have not come to similar results.

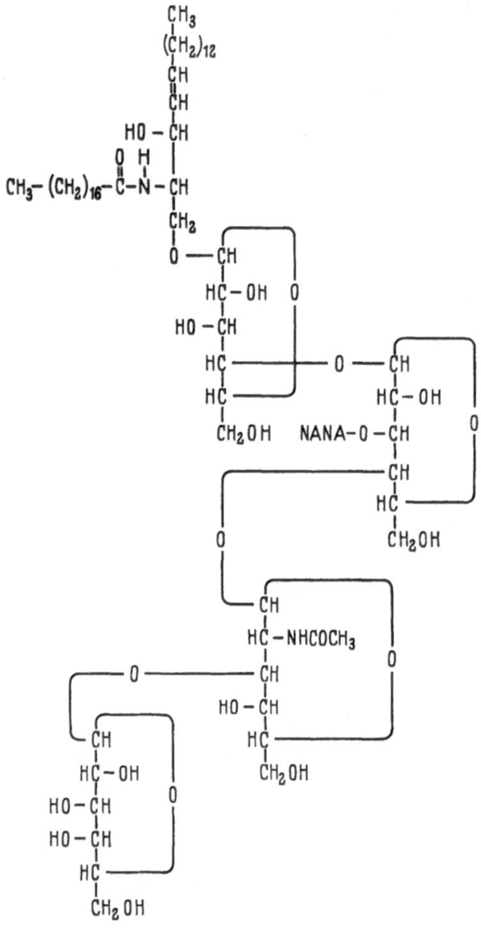

Fig. 5. Structure of monosialo-ganglioside $G_{GNT}I$ (G_{M1})

Since the stored lipid in neurovisceral gangliosidoses (see page 242) also seems to be the ganglioside $G_{GNT}I$ (Norman et al. 1959 and 1964, Landing et al. 1964, O'Brien et al. 1965, and others), some of the cases described above (Jatzkewitz and Sandhoff 1963, Gonatas and Gonatas 1965, Schneck et al. 1965b) should consequently be classed as neurovisceral gangliosidoses.

IV. Juvenile Amaurotic Family Idiocy

Definition and Introduction

Juvenile amaurotic family idiocy (JAFI) is distinguished from the other types of amaurotic family idiocy by the time of onset, by ophthalmologic, neurologic and pathologic findings, by the protracted clinical course, and by the fact that it does not occur in members of the Jewish race. In 1826, the Norwegian physician STENGEL observed the first cases of the disease in four siblings (see NISSEN 1954) and 80 years later, VOGT (1906) distinguished JAFI from Tay-Sachs disease on the basis of extensive clinical studies. Several years earlier, BATTEN (1903) had called attention to a familial disorder characterized by cerebral degeneration with symmetrical macular changes, which was later confirmed as JAFI. SPIELMEYER, in 1906—1908, published cases of JAFI in whom he demonstrated the so-called "Schaffer cell changes" which were considered pathognomonic for JAFI by SJÖGREN (1931). Subsequently, case reports of JAFI were given by ROGALSKI (1910), SCHOB (1912, 1919), KUFFLER (1912), BERGER (1913), HARBITZ (1913), RÖNNE (1916), DIDE et al. (1920), GLOBUS (1923), GREENFIELD and HOLMES (1925), LEVY and LITTLE (1940) and others. In 1919, SCHOB reviewed the pathologic anatomy of the disease and in 1924 its clinical manifestations. The most comprehensive review of 115 cases from 59 families, and a description of five additional cases of JAFI has been given by SJÖGREN (1931) in Sweden. His studies were facilitated by the fact that in this country the visit of schools for the blind was obligatory already in the last century. A particular vacuolation of lymphocytes in six cases from Sweden was described in 1948 by BAGH and HORTLING, and the possibility of using this finding as a test for the detection of heterozygotes for the disease was discussed by RAYNER (1952) who reported seven additional cases of JAFI. Ten more cases were described by NISSEN (1954), and others (VAN BOGAERT and KLEIN 1955, HOFFMAN 1956, CRAWLEY 1957, DIEZEL 1957, JEEFERSON and RUTTER 1958). A recent review containing the description of nine cases of JAFI from the U.S.A. is that by JERVIS (1959). Hematologic and electroencephalographic studies in ten members of a Norwegian family, two of whom showed the typical symptoms of JAFI, were performed by HARLEM (1960). A possible case of JAFI is that by KOREY et al. (1963) which was reported as "juvenile lipidosis". The association of cerebral and ophthalmologic findings has prompted terms such as "maculocerebral degeneration" (BATTEN 1903) or "juvenile cerebroretinal degeneration" (HARLEM 1960), which should be avoided in favor of the term JAFI, when this disorder is meant.

Incidence (Age, Sex, Race)

The onset of the disease occurs usually between the ages of five and seven years and coincides with the time of second dentification (SJÖGREN 1931). Rarely does the disease become manifest before the fourth or after the tenth years of life. Therefore, the first intellectual and visual changes become apparent towards the end of the first year of school, while at its beginning the children may be completely asymptomatic. When the disease occurred in siblings it became manifest at similar ages (SJÖGREN 1931).

The incidence is similar in male and female children. In the material of SJÖGREN, the proportion of males to females was 64:56.

In contrast to the infantile type of amaurotic family idiocy (Tay-Sachs disease), none of the patients with JAFI came from Jewish families (JERVIS 1959, DIEZEL 1962). JAFI in a Negro girl could be confirmed at autopsy. Familial occurrence was observed in the majority of reported cases. Details on the heredity of JAFI are given by FUHRMANN in a separate chapter.

Clinical Manifestations

The first signs consist of mental deterioration and decrease of visual acuity, both of which may be difficult to substantiate in this particular age group. Progressive deterioration of vision was the first symptom in most cases reviewed by Sjögren (1931). It occurred rarely before the age of six or after the age of ten. Progression is rapid; after a couple of years vision has usually deteriorated to perception of contours only from a close distance. Finally, complete blindness ensues.

Upon fundoscopy in the initial stage the optic disc has a yellowish-grey color and its vessels are narrowed. The changes are symmetrical and their progression results in the appearance of typical degenerative lesions consisting of small, confluent yellow foci of the entire fundus and retinitic atrophy of the optic discs, which had developed in all cases of Jervis (1959) by the age of ten years. The picture resembles typical pigmentary retinitis, whereby the pigmentation is most marked peripherally but may cover the entire fundus. Posterior cortical cataracts may be additional findings (Sjögren 1931). Initially, pupillary reactions are normal, and are lost after the establishment of amaurosis (Sjögren 1931, Jervis 1959). In the final stage nystagmus and strabismus develop. When fundoscopy was normal but amaurosis was already present, typical retinal lesions developed eventually (Sjögren 1931). Mental changes usually appear simultaneously with visual ones. They, too, are progressive and result in complete idiocy, the development of which has been described in detail by Sjögren (1931).

The first neurologic symptoms are referable to the extrapyramidal motor system (Spielmeyer 1906, Berger 1913). Their progression results in stuttering, mumbling and explosive articulation with a tendency for iteration of words and syllables which prevents the formation of normal sentences. Athetosis and abnormalities of posture are further findings (Vogt 1906, Rogalski 1910, Greenfield and Holmes 1925), and walking finally becomes impossible (Frenkel and Dide 1913, Schob 1930, Sjögren 1931). Cerebellar ataxia as described by Frenkel and Dide (1913) is rare (Sjögren 1931, Jervis 1959).

The musculature is hypertonic and rigid and later becomes atrophic. Contractures of knees, elbows and hips are late signs. There are no typical reflex abnormalities; deep tendon reflexes are brisk and symmetrical, later in the disease Romberg's sign is usually positive. Vegetative disturbances are manifested as progressive acrocyanosis of hands and feet.

Grand mal epileptic seizures are observed in most cases. They start usually between the ages of ten and 12 years and last until death. In the material of Sjögren, 102 out of 120 patients had typical epileptic seizures.

Cerebrospinal Fluid

There are no typical abnormalities of the cerebrospinal fluid. The protein concentration is increased in the majority of cases.

Electroencephalography

The electroencephalogram is usually markedly abnormal, although findings are not characteristic for JAFI. They correspond to abnormalities seen in other convulsive disorders and are suggestive of a progressive degenerative brain lesion. (Crawley 1957). Abnormalities of brain potentials were described by Cobb et al. (1952) and by Jervis (1959). Pathologic EEG findings in healthy appearing relatives (Hoffman 1956, Crawley 1957, Jervis 1959) of patients may be preclinical manifestations of JAFI (Harlem 1960).

Hematology

A rather typical finding is that of vacuolated lymphocytes, first detected by
BAGH and HORTLING (1948) and confirmed by a number of others (RAYNER 1952,
NISSEN 1954, STUBBE-TEGLBJAERG and PLUM 1955, GILJE and NISSEN 1956,
JULIAO et al. 1957, FRIEDRICH 1957, HARLEM 1960). However, vacuolation of
lymphocytes was not seen in any of the ten cases from the U.S.A. (JERVIS 1959),
and in another case (HOFFMANN 1957) which likewise was not from Scandinavia.

The first describers of this phenomenon saw vacuolation of the cytoplasm of
otherwise normal appearing lymphocytes of blood and bone marrow. They could
not identify the content of these vacuoles with the use of lipid stains and there
were no birefringent substances. The percentage of vacuolated lymphocytes ranges
from 5 to 60% in different cases and concerns mainly small lymphocytes. The
higher values are found in older patients. Although vacuolated lymphocytes were
also seen in parents and siblings of affected subjects (RAYNER 1952, HARLEM 1960),
the test is not suitable for the detection of heterozygotes, since the finding is not
specific, and similar lymphocytes are found in Niemann-Pick disease (BLACKFAN et al.
1944, CROCKER and FARBER 1958), Tay-Sachs disease (SPIEGEL-ADOLF et al. 1959)
and in the neurovisceral gangliosidoses (CRAIG et al. 1959, SANFILIPPO et al. 1962,
LANDING and RUBINSTEIN 1962, LANDING et al. 1964, O'BRIEN et al. 1965). Furthermore, there may be similarities with hematologic abnormalities occurring in Hurler's
disease. Interesting is the finding by SPIEGEL-ADOLF et al. (1959) of a greater proportion of vacuolated lymphocytes in the fathers of male patients with JAFI than
in the mothers while the opposite was found in Tay-Sachs disease, namely a higher
proportion of altered lymphocytes in the mothers as compared to the fathers.

Serum

Serum lipids are found to be normal when generally employed methods are
used. The same applies to phosphatases, transaminases, lactic acid dehydrogenase
and aldolases.

Pathology

Neuropathologic changes are principally similar to those found in Tay-Sachs
disease, except that they are usually less marked. Skull and brain are unremarkable
on gross examination.

Histologically, ganglion cells are enlarged two- to four-fold (DIEZEL 1957).
Different areas may be involved to a different extent, but there is no predilection
for certain parts of the brain (JERVIS 1959). Changes of the basal ganglia and
of the thalamus are qualitatively similar to those of the cortex, but generally
less marked (JERVIS 1959). Nerve cell necroses may be seen, particularly in the
fifth cortical layer (JERVIS 1959). The dendritic processes are little altered and
the axis cylinders are only slightly swollen or not at all. There is some lipid storage
in the cerebellum, mainly by ganglion cells of the dentate nucleus and by the
Purkinje cells. Degeneration of the cerebellofugal type was seen in two out of
ten cases by JERVIS (1959). Involvement of the motor cells of the spinal cord
is insignificant (JERVIS 1959).

Histochemical studies show storage in ganglion cells of a hyaline, acidic glycolipid (DIEZEL 1957). There is no birefringence with polarized light (see table 2 and 3).

The white matter is well myelinated (DIEZEL 1957), and thus distinctly different
from Tay-Sachs disease, where extensive demyelination occurs.

Involvement of the microglia may be lacking (DIEZEL 1957) or else result in
the formation of large hypertrophic cells in response to destruction of brain tissue
(JERVIS 1959, GONATAS et al. 1963). The macroglial elements show hypertrophy

and hyperplasia, the material contained in their cytoplasm has identical histochemical properties as enlarged ganglion cells (Jervis 1959). The oligodendroglia
is not involved in the process of lipid storage or degradation.

Examination of ganglion cells in a case of "juvenile lipidosis" (Gonatas et al.
1963) with the electronmicroscope showed a great number of lipofuscin-containing
granules which resembled lysosomes (lysosome-like bodies). These were also seen
in involved cells of the microglia. Diezel et al. (1965) saw similar bodies in the
brains of dogs with a type of amaurotic idiocy which resembles the juvenile form.

The Stored Material

The substance contained in swollen ganglion cells of JAFI has the histochemical
properties of a lipid and stains with Sudan III and IV as well as with other fat
stains (Scarlet-red, Nile-blue). A positive PAS reaction suggests the presence of
polysaccharides and points to the presence of glycolipids, as in Tay-Sachs disease.
A positive Bial-reaction (Diezel 1957) is indicative of neuraminic acid. According
to the latter author binding of the glycolipid to neuraminic acid occurs within the
storing cells. From a positive reaction with phosphomolybdic acid stannous
hematoxyline, Jervis (1959) concludes to the presence of sphingomyelin the
choline moiety of which is responsible for the reaction. While histochemistry
permits of identification of ganglioside storage in JAFI, it does not allow differentiation of the gangliosides.

Quantitative lipid analyses fail to show increased brain ganglioside concentrations in most cases. The content of other lipids is not significantly altered, with the
exception in one case of a decreased concentration of cerebrosides in the white
matter (Folch-Pi and Lees 1959). In the same case gangliosides seemed to be
increased in the white matter rather than in the cerebral cortex. Jervis (1959),
measuring the neuraminic acid content with the method of Klenk and Langerbeins (1941), found no significant increase. In the case of Jatzkewitz et al. (1965)
there was a 1.3-fold increase of the ganglioside concentration, but this was less
than that found in a brain from a patient with Niemann-Pick disease, which was
studied at the same time. Gonatas et al. (1963) analyzing brain material from
their case of "juvenile lipidosis" found normal total lipids and increased concentrations in the cortex of total cholesterol, cholesterol esters and cerebrosides. The
ganglioside concentration was at the upper limit of normal or slightly elevated.
In the white matter there was a decreased concentration of cholesterol and cerebrosides. Differentiation of gangliosides was not carried out.

We are not aware of analyses aimed at the structural identification of the
stored material in JAFI. Even thin-layer chromatographic studies are hampered
by the fact that the total ganglioside content of the brain, being increased only
slightly or not at all, is very small. Svennerholm (1963), using this method for
analysis of gangliosides in a case of JAFI, did not find any qualitative difference
of the various fractions as compared to normals. Jatzkewitz et al. (1965) found
a slight increase in the concentration of the Tay-Sachs ganglioside to 1.11% of
the total lipids (normally less than 0.3%), however, the brain so studied was
exposed to formalin for 30 years.

In contrast, therefore, to Tay-Sachs disease, to some cases of late-infantile
amaurotic family idiocy and to one case of congenital amaurotic family idiocy,
there is no evidence of storage of a specific ganglioside in JAFI. The solution to
yet unanswered questions may come from analyses of particularly involved areas
instead of unselected parts, since, in contrast to Tay-Sachs disease, the biochemical lesion responsible for the development of JAFI, does not result in ganglioside
storage which is as impressive as that observed in Tay-Sachs disease.

V. Adult Amaurotic Family Idiocy

Definition and Introduction

The adult amaurotic idiocy (type Kufs-Hallervorden) is considered with the amaurotic idiocies on the basis of typical pathologic findings in the central nervous system. Biochemical studies in this type are very scarce.

This late form of the amaurotic idiocies has been described for the first time by Kufs (1925, 1929, 1930), and its clinical features were defined in detail by Hallervorden (1938, 1939). Subsequently, various other authors have contributed to the knowledge about the disorder (van Bogaert and Borremanns 1937, Bird 1948, van Bogaert 1952, Diezel 1954a, 1957, 1962, Moschel 1954, Allegranza 1956, Jatzkewitz et al. 1965).

First clinical manifestations appear after puberty, between the 15th and 25th years of life. They consist mainly of symptoms of mental involution. Neurologic signs result from involvement of the extrapyramidal system, in addition, cerebral seizures are observed. Visual disturbances, pigmentary retinitis and optic atrophy occur rarely, and blindness does not develop. The disease runs a chronic course, which may last for decades and end up with the picture of pseudobulbar palsy or marasm.

Difficulties in differential diagnosis result from the chronic course. According to Hallervorden (1938), distinction from late infantile and juvenile cases is not always possible if these progress slowly. A relationship of these three types of amaurotic idiocy is also suggested by the observation of Zeman and Hoffmann (1962) who saw cases of juvenile and adult amaurotic idiocy in one family. Morphologically, differentiation from Alzheimer's disease may be difficult (Diezel 1962).

Main pathologic findings consist of typical ganglion cell changes, although extreme ballooning is rare. In contrast to the more acute types, involvement of the brain is less uniform in adult amaurotic idiocy, where the amygdaloid nucleus and the striate body are usually involved to a greater extent than the cerebral cortex. In addition to ganglion cell changes, deposition of a lipid-containing pigment has been described (Moschel 1954, Diezel 1957, 1962). A similar pigment had been found by Jervis (1952) in a Jewish boy who became symptomatic at the age of five months and died at the age of 11 years. The pigment is found mainly in the meninges and the plexus. In these areas many epithelial cells are transformed to foam cells. The pattern of distribution of pigmented cells does not allow recognition of a relationship between deposition of pigments and distension of ganglion cells (Moschel 1954). A sign of the protracted storage process is the appearance of fibrillar changes as in Alzheimer's disease (Diezel 1962), or of so-called amyloid structures.

Results of Lipid Analyses

Analyses of the ganglioside pattern in adult amaurotic idiocy have been performed by Jatzkewitz et al. (1965) in two brains, which had been stored in formalin for six and for 26 years respectively. He found a concentration of the Tay-Sachs ganglioside which was 1.6 to two times normal. In addition to storage of the ganglioside, there was an increased concentration of a derivative which did not contain neuraminic acid. The authors conclude from the similarity of the abnormal ganglioside pattern in one of their adult cases to that of the infantile type, that biochemically the former can be termed a "delayed early case" as suggested by Hallervorden (1938). Because of possible changes of gangliosides by prolonged formalin action (Suzuki 1965) conclusive statements on the ganglioside abnormalities in adult amaurotic idiocy are not possible before fresh brain tissue can be analyzed. Since histologic changes are restricted to certain areas of the central nervous system, material for analyses should be taken from these.

VI. Neurovisceral Gangliosidoses
Definition and Introduction

Neurovisceral gangliosidoses (NVG) are characterized by storage of gangliosides in the central nervous system and in visceral organs. Thus, the distribution of lipid storage serves for distinction from Tay-Sachs disease, and the fact that a ganglioside is stored differentiates NVG from Niemann-Pick disease and Gaucher's disease. In contrast to the Hurler-Pfaundler syndrome (gargoylism) there is no accumulation of acid mucopolysaccharides in NVG.

The stored ganglioside differs from the Tay-Sachs ganglioside G_{GNTrII} and from the ganglioside G_{D3} of congenital amaurotic family idiocy (HAGBERG et al. 1965). Chemical analyses in NVG suggest the storage of the major ganglioside $G_{GNT}I$ in the central nervous system and involved organs.

Case Reports

The literature contains a number of cases reported as Tay-Sachs disease, late-infantile amaurotic family idiocy, congenital amaurotic family idiocy and gargoylism with foam cells in various visceral organs. While storage of gangliosides was demonstrated for a fraction of these cases the ganglioside was identified in only a few.

Since the homogeneity of this particular class of amaurotic family idiocy is not yet established, a brief review of reported cases seems justified (see table 6).

Lipid storage or foam cells in visceral organs were described by BIELSCHOWSKY (1928), BROUWER (1936), DAVIDSON and JACOBSON (1936), NORMAN and WOOD (1941), and BROWN et al. (1954). MARBURG (1942) reported for the liver lipids of his case staining properties similar to those of the stored material in neurons. The case of a non-Jewish child who died at the age of two was reported by TURBAN (1944) as TSD, and tissues were analysed by KLENK (1955), who found the ganglioside content of the cerebral cortex elevated five-fold. Foam cells were found in liver and alveoli of the lungs. Hepatomegaly with foam cells in liver, spleen, lymph nodes, thymus, intestine, bone marrow and lungs was also a feature of the case described by NORMAN et al. in 1959; the same authors published a similar observation in 1964. The 11 affected families reported by VAN BOGAERT and KLEIN (1955) also harbour cases of amaurotic family idiocy with visceral involvement. A patient considered as a possible variant of gargoylism was that of CRAIG et al. (1959). Similarly SANFILIPPO et al. (1962) described an "unusual storage disease resembling the Hurler-Pfaundler syndrome". A young Negro patient who was described by MINKOWITZ (1964) presented with a new form of visceral histiocytic glycolipidosis with mental retardation and did not fit the criteria of amaurotic family idiocy. Eight patients of six families were described by LANDING et al. (1964); four of them had been published two years earlier as "pseudo-Hurler disease" (LANDING and RUBINSTEIN 1962). While, in these patients, clinical and radiological findings were suggestive of gargoylism, pathologic and hematologic features resembled Niemann-Pick disease and ballooning of glomeruli was similar to that seen in Fabry's disease. Upon histochemical analyses it could be shown that the stored material was not an acid mucopolysaccharide, but rather resembled

Table 6. *Clinical data and histological findings in 13 cases of neurovisceral gangliosidosis*

Case*	1	2	3	4	5	6	7	8	9	10	11	12	13
Sex (m = male, f = female)	f	f	m	m	f	m	f	m	f		f	m	m
Age at death (months)	3.5	16	4	7	4.5	10	15	21	3½	**	24	25	8
Mental and/or motor retardation	+	+	+	+	+	+	+	+	+	+	+	+	+
Abnormal facies	+			+	+			+					
Large tongue		+			+			+				—	
Cherry-red spot		+	—	—		—	+						
Peripheral edema	+	+	+	+	?							+	
Ascites	+		+						+				
Hepatomegaly	+	+	+	+	+	+	+	+	+		—	+	+
Splenomegaly	+	+	+	+		+		+	+		—	—	—
X-ray changes													
Skeleton	+	+	+	+	+	+	+	+	+	+		—	+
Vertebrae	+	+	+	+			+		+			+***	+
Pelvis	+		+	+					+				
Long bones	+	+	+	+		+	+		+			—	
Short bones							+						
Vacuolated lymphocytes/ monocytes	+	+	+	+		+		+	+	+			+
Alder's anomaly of white cells			+	+	+					—			
Foam cells:													
Bone marrow	+	—	+	—	+	+	+	+		+		+	+
Spleen	+	+	+									+	+
Lymph nodes	+					+	+			+		+	
Liver	+	+		+	—	+	+		+	+		+	+
Lungs	+	+		+		+	+				+	+	
Glomerular epithelial lesion	+	+	+	+	+	+	+		+				+
Ballooned neurons in CNS	+	+			—	+	+		+		+	+	+

*   1—8 from Landing et al. (1964)
    9 from Craig et al. (1959)
    10 from Sanfilippo et al. (1962)
    11 from Norman et al. (1964)
    12 from Gonatas and Gonatas (1965)
    13 from O'Brien et al. (1965)
** 6 year old when examined (1962). No increase in urinary acid mucopolysaccharides.
*** Diagnosed at autopsy (no X-ray examination of vertebrae)

gangliosides. Gonatas and Gonatas in 1965 described a patient with "systemic late infantile lipidosis with relationship to Tay-Sachs disease and gargoylism" who died at the age of 25 months and can, therefore, hardly be classed as late-infantile amaurotic family idiocy. The case of O'Brien et al. (1965) with ganglioside storage in brain, liver and spleen, fulfills all the essential criteria for familial neurovisceral lipidosis or generalized gangliosidosis which were established by Landing et al. (1964). In particular, involvement of the glomeruli was present. According to the review of Landing et al. (1964) on familial NVL, the cases of Norman et al. (1959), Craig et al. (1959) and O'Brien et al. (1965), in addition to their own cases, belong in this class of gangliosidoses.

From a study of these cases the following conclusions emerge:

1. The disease affects non-Jewish infants during the first year of life, usually in its first half It is lethal around the age of two years.

2. The symptomatology is characterized by progressive mental and motor retardation, skeletal changes similar to those of gargoylism, and occasionally hepatosplenomegaly or isolated enlargement of the liver.

3. Pathologic features are progressive cerebral degeneration with swollen, ballooned ganglion cells and storage of glycolipids as in Tay-Sachs disease. A cherry-red spot is occasionally seen in the macula. Glycolipid-storing histiocytes are found in liver, spleen, glomeruli and in other visceral organs.

4. Differential diagnosis from Tay-Sachs disease is possible on the basis of visceral storage, from Niemann-Pick disease and Gaucher's disease through the identification of the stored lipid and from Hurler's syndrome by the storage and excretion of acid mucopolysaccharides in the latter.

Results of Lipid Analyses

Most publications on NVG contain incomplete lipid analyses or none. Craig et al. (1959) examined only some fractions of the liver lipids but not the brain. No chemical analyses were performed in the eight cases of Landing et al. (1964). In the case of Norman et al. (1959) with a cherry-red spot in the macula and hepatomegaly the spleen and liver hexosamine content was increased several-fold, while no neuraminic acid was present. Liver phospholipids but not total lipids were increased.

A detailed description is available of the case of O'Brien et al. (1965). Here total lipids of grey matter, spleen and liver were increased, while those of white matter were low. The gangliosides of the brain grey matter were increased to three to four times normal. The main component (84%) had the same Rf-value on thin-layer chromatography as the ganglioside $G_{GNT}I$ which, in the normal newborn, makes up 25% of total gangliosides. Other gangliosides were present with normal ratios, and the Tay-Sachs ganglioside $G_{GNTr}II$ could not be demonstrated. Further analysis of the main ganglioside fraction showed a molar ratio of ceramide : hexosamine : hexose : N-acetyl-neuraminic acid = 1 : 1 : 3 : 1; the galactose-glucose ratio being 2 : 1. There was no abnormality of the normal ganglioside fatty acid pattern. All these findings strongly support the identity of the stored ganglioside with the normal ganglioside $G_{GNT}I$ (see fig. 5). The ganglioside which was isolated from spleen and liver had the same Rf-value as $G_{GNT}I$, while in normals no gangliosides can be found in these organs.

The ganglioside pattern of grey and white matter in a case of "late infantile systemic lipidosis" as reported by Suzuki (1966) is given in table 7.

Gangliosides of white matter in the case of Norman et al. (1964) were increased ten-fold, and the major portion according to these authors migrated on thin-layer chromatography like the Tay-Sachs ganglioside $G_{GNTr}II$. Further characterization of this fraction and analyses of organ lipids were not attempted. From the figure in their paper it seems possible that the major portion of the gangliosides was actually $G_{GNT}I$. In this case determinations of fructose-1-phosphate aldolase would have been of value to exclude Tay-Sachs disease. When storage of $G_{GNT}I$ is considered typical for NVG, the case of systemic late infantile lipidosis (Gonatas and Gonatas 1965) quite certainly belongs in this category. The symptomatology was largely in agreement, and a four-fold increase in brain gangliosides was mainly due to an accumulation of a ganglioside with the properties of $G_{GNT}I$.

In the publication by Jatzkewitz and Sandhoff (1963) (see page 236) of a possible case of late-infantile amaurotic family idiocy with storage of $G_{GNT}I$ there was also evidence of lipid storage in spleen, thymus and liver.

In summary, available data on the type of stored ganglioside in NVG do not yet permit of a definite statement with regard to the homogeneity of syndromes

Table 7.
Ganglioside pattern in case of late infantile systemic lipidosis (neurovisceral gangliosidosis)

Gangliosides	Gray matter		White matter	
	Case	Normal control (range)	Case	Normal control (range)
(Values expressed as per cent of NANA)				
G_0	2.5	3.0— 4.8	4.8	5.9—10.4
G_1 ($G_{GNT}IV$)	3.4	12.4—19.3	6.1	16.0—20.3
G_2 ($G_{GNT}III$)	3.9	11.1—20.0	9.8	12.0—13.9
G_3 ($G_{GNT}II$)	9.5	39.6—48.0	8.9	34.0—42.9
G_4 ($G_{GNT}I$)	74.5	14.6—21.4	65.6	18.0—21.2
G_5 ($G_{GNT}rII$)	2.5	1.5— 4.4	2.4	1.3— 1.7
G_6 (G_{LACT})	3.7	1	2.5	1
(Values expressed as µg/g wet weight)				
Total NANA	4760	635—827	850	64—73

Source: Suzuki (1966)

Values given for G_2 include G_2A and those for G_4 include G_3A, two minor sialic acid-containing components with chromatographic mobilities between G_2 and G_3, and between G_3 and G_4, respectively, (Suzuki 1966).

like "familial neurovisceral lipidosis" (Landing et al. 1964), "Tay-Sachs disease with visceral involvement" (Norman et al. 1959, 1964), "generalized gangliosidosis" (O'Brien 1965), "systemic late-infantile lipidosis" (Gonatas and Gonatas 1965), and "biochemically special form of infantile amaurotic idiocy" (Jatzkewitz and Sandhoff 1963, Jatzkewitz et al. 1965). Of particular interest is the question whether in late-infantile amaurotic family idiocy there is also accumulation of the ganglioside $G_{GNT}I$.

If it can be confirmed that all NVG is characterized by storage of $G_{GNT}I$, differentiation from other gangliosidoses will be possible: from Tay-Sachs disease with its prevailing $G_{GNT}rII$ ganglioside, and from gargoylism where in brain there is a normal content of $G_{GNT}I$, but increase of $G_{GNT}rII$ and G_{LACT} and decrease of $G_{GNT}IV$ and $G_{GNT}III$ (Gonatas and Gonatas 1965).

Towards this goal complete ganglioside analyses of all involved organs are necessary. They are possible with available techniques.

VII. Hurler's Disease (Gargoylism)

Definition and Introduction

Gargoylism*, which has been classified as a mucopolysaccharidosis (table 8) with storage of acid mucopolysaccharides (Brante 1951, 1952), requires discussion under the aspect of a gangliosidosis on the basis of recent findings of an abnormal brain ganglioside pattern, and the demonstration by electronmicroscopy of membranous cytoplasmic bodies resembling those observed in Tay-Sachs disease (Aleu et al. 1965, Gonatas and Gonatas 1965). A relationship between gargoylism on the one hand and gangliosidoses on the other is also suggested by the similarity to gargoylism of a number of cases of neurovisceral gangliosidosis, occasionally described as pseudo-Hurler's disease (Landing and Rubinstein 1962) and of cases

---

* The term gargoylism, from gargouille (French), denotes the resemblance of the faces of patients with those of the grotesque face-like spouts of Gothic cathedrals.

of Tay-Sachs disease (Norman et al. 1964). Possibly, abnormal ganglioside patterns will eventually also be found in other types of mucopolysaccharidosis.

Recently, the term gargoylism (Ellis et al. 1936) has been restricted to the most common mucopolysaccharidosis type I (see table 8), which is the autosomal recessive Hurler-Pfaundler-syndrome (Hurler 1919). In contrast, the mucopolysaccharidosis type II represents about one-third (Maroteaux and Lamy 1965) of cases of Hurler's disease (HD), is sex-linked and also known as Hunter's syndrome (Hunter 1917, Gills et al. 1965, Goldberg et al. 1965). Its signs and symptoms are less pronounced; there is lack of corneal cloudiness, less impairment of intelligence and greater life expectancy. These patients may reach adulthood (Gills et al. 1965).

In addition to Hurler's description, a great number of reports and reviews are available, such as those by Ellis et al. (1936), Hallervorden (1953), Hienz (1953, 1960), Marie et al. (1955), Lamy et al. (1958), McKusick (1960), Burke (1962), Seitelberger and Simma (1962), Maroteaux and Lamy (1965), Gills et al. (1965), Goldberg et al. (1965), Melchior (1965), Doss and Matiar-Vahar (1965).

Clinical Manifestations

Typical signs of HD do not rarely exist at birth. They are noticeable before the third year of life in all cases. At an early stage, differentiation from Morquio's disease may be difficult. Among the striking features are the grotesque gargouille face with thick lips, a large tongue, irregular teeth, flattened nose, thick ears and prominence of the forehead (see fig. 6). The head appears too large for the dwarfed body. As a rule, a number of other skeletal abnormalities are found, such as lumbar kyphosis, gibbus, deformities of elbows, knees and hips with limitation of motion and claw hands and feet (see figs. 7 and 8). Roentgenograms of the

Table 8. *Classification of mucopolysaccharidoses*

Type*	Mucopolysaccharidosis Name	Genetics	Clinical features	Mucopolysaccharides in the urine
I	Hurler's disease	Autosomal recessive	Dwarfism, gargoyle facies, mental retardation, early death	Chondroitin sulfate B and heparitin sulfate
II	Hunter's disease	X-linked recessive	Dwarfism, gargoyle facies (less severe than in Hurler's disease)	Chondroitin sulfate B and heparitin sulfate
III	Polydystrophic oligophrenia, Sanfilippo's disease	Autosomal recessive	Minor somatic changes, severe mental retardation	Heparitin sulfate
IV	Osteochondrodystrophy, Morquio-Brailsford disease	Autosomal recessive	Dwarfism, distinctive skeletal features (emerging with aging)	Keratosulfate
V	Polydystrophic dwarfism, Scheie's disease	Autosomal recessive	Dwarfism, coarse facies, normal mental development	Chondroitin sulfate B

* According to McKusick (1966).
Source: Maroteaux and Lamy (1965); Goldberg et al. (1965); Gills et al. (1965).

spine reveal abnormalities of vertebrae, such as block vertebra formation involving the 12th thoracic and the first and second lumbar vertebrae. The diaphyses of long bones and the metacarpals are broad and short, the epiphyses are narrowed. Other findings, such as hepatosplenomegaly, umbilical and inguinal hernias, deafness, heart lesions, corneal opacities, ptosis, hypertelorism, and increase of body

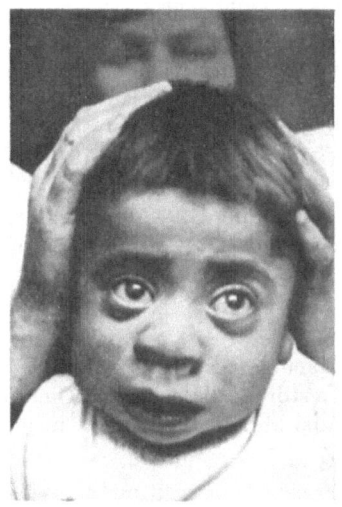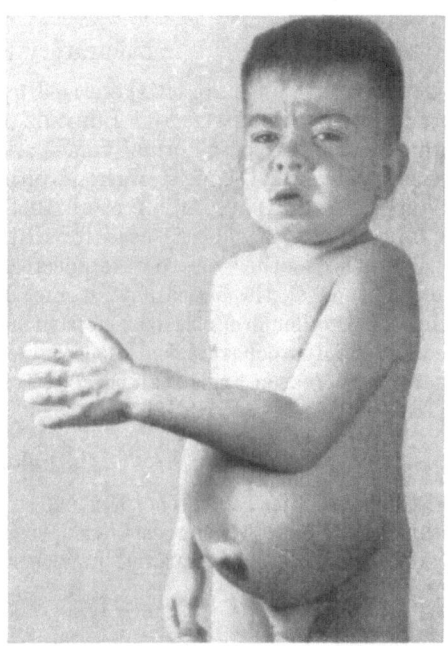

Fig. 6   Fig. 7

Fig. 6. Hurler's disease. Typical gargoyle facies. (From JACOBI and WAARDENBURG 1940)

Fig. 7. A seven year old boy with Hurler's disease. (From CATEL 1951)

hair are not consistently found. Hematologic findings consist of various morphologic abnormalities of white blood cells (REILLY 1941, ULLRICH 1943, ADLER 1950,

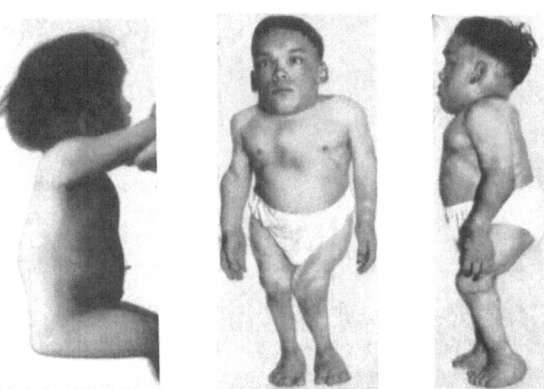

a   b   c

Fig. 8. Hurler's disease. a. Four year old boy with kyphosis of the upper lumbar spine. b. and c. The same patient measuring 92 cm at the age of 22 years. (From SCHINZ and FURTWÄNGLER 1928)

GASSER 1950, GRIFFITH and FINDLAY 1958, MITTWOCH 1959, 1961, LAMY et al. 1959, ROYER 1959). Mental development is retarded early, and learning of speech is incomplete.

The prognosis is poor. Most patients die before puberty, usually from inter-current pulmonary infections, the development of which is favored by deformities of the thorax causing respiratory difficulties, and by cardiac involvement. Rarely do affected subjects reach the 20th year (MAROTEAUX and LAMY 1965).

Laboratory Findings

Laboratory findings are characterized by increased urinary excretion of muco-polysaccharides (DORFMAN and LORINCZ 1957), with values of 60 mg per liter and more as compared to normal values of 5—10 mg per liter. The urinary muco-polysaccharides in HD consist of chondroitinsulfate B and heparitin sulfate (DORF-MAN and LORINCZ 1957, MEYER et al. 1958) with a 2 : 1 ratio. The occurrence of both mucopolysaccharides is used for distinction of HD from other mucopoly-saccharidoses or other disorders associated with increased mucopolysaccharide excretion, such as the Marfan syndrome (BERENSON and DALFERES 1965). The finding of a smaller proportion of heparitinsulfate in HD as compared to the sex-linked mucopolysaccharidosis II (see table 8) (TERRY and LINKER 1964) is not obligatory. Increased arylsulfatase B activity was found in the urine of patients with HD by AUSTIN et al. (1964).

Pathology

Histologic studies reveal the presence of large vacuolated cells in many tissues and this finding has early suggested the presence of a storage disease. Histochemical properties of the stored material in visceral organs and in the central nervous

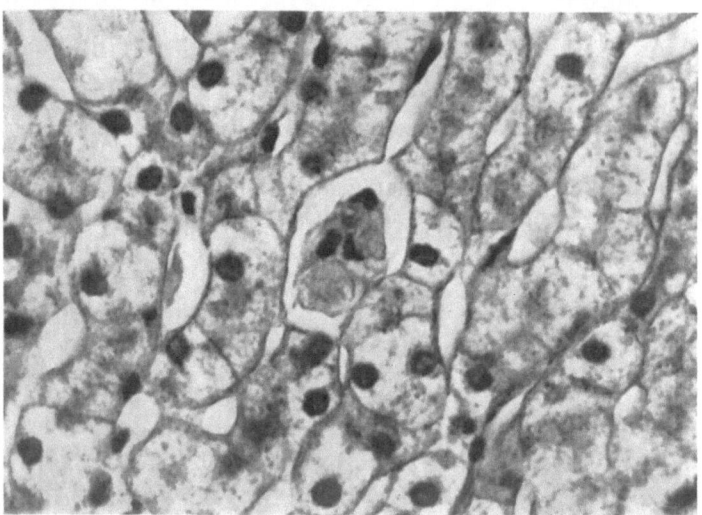

Fig. 9. Pfaundler-Hurler disease. Liver. Enlargement 210-fold. Liver cells store glycogen and show a light, slightly ballooned cytoplasm. Kupffer cells (middle) store a glycolipid which is PAS-positive. (Reproduced by courtesy of Prof. P. B. DIEZEL)

system are compatible with those of acid mucopolysaccharides (see fig. 9). The cerebral cortex shows loss of neurons (see fig. 10) and distortion of the normal architecture. The remaining neurons are markedly swollen and are filled with a PAS- positive material, similar to findings in Tay-Sachs disease (DIEZEL 1960, HIENZ 1960). Electronmicroscopic studies also show similarities with Tay-Sachs disease, particularly as regards the appearance of typical membranous cytoplasmic bodies (ALEU et al. 1965, GONATAS and GONATAS 1965). Likewise, changes in the cerebellum are similar to those occurring in Tay-Sachs disease and also in late-infantile amaurotic idiocy (WALLACE et al. 1965).

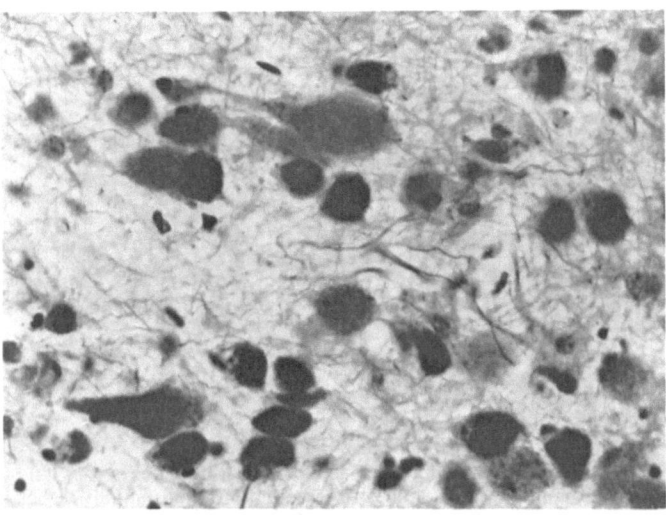

Fig. 10. Pfaundler-Hurler disease, infantile form. Ballooning of the ganglion cells of the cerebrum and storage of protein-bound gangliosides. (Reproduced by courtesy of Prof. P. B. DIEZEL)

Results of Lipid Analyses

Analyses of glycolipids, particularly of gangliosides, in the central nervous system and in visceral organs in HD have been performed by JERVIS (1942), KUTZIM (1946), KLENK (1955), KLENK and LÖHR (1955), BRANTE (1952, 1957), TINGEY (1959), TAGHAVY et al. (1964), LEDEEN et al. (1965), GONATAS and GONATAS (1965). Evidence for increased concentrations of gangliosides in the central nervous system has first been found by JERVIS (1942). Later, but independently, KUTZIM (1946), from Klenk's institute, examined two brains of HD patients, only one of which showed the typical pathologic changes and a significant increase in the ganglioside concentration to values which were four to five times normal. Similar were findings by KLENK and LÖHR (1955) in another case. BRANTE (1952, 1957) also found increased amounts of gangliosides in the nerve cells of three cases of Pfaundler-Hurler disease. In these cases, the concentrations of cerebrosides were diminished and those of phospholipids and cholesterol normal.

In contrast to other gangliosidoses, the alteration of ganglioside concentration is not caused by one specific ganglioside, but involves a number of normally occurring gangliosides the proportions of which are abnormal (see table 9).

A significant increase was found for G_{LACT}, and to a lesser degree, for G_{GNTrII} and $G_{GNT}I$ (TAGHAVY et al. 1964, LEDEEN et al. 1965, GONATAS and GONATAS 1965). The content of $G_{GNT}IV$ and $G_{GNT}III$ was diminished, that of $G_{GNT}II$ normal. These findings allow distinction from the ganglioside pattern in Tay-Sachs disease where G_{GNTrII} amounts to approximately 90% of total brain gangliosides, and from neurovisceral gangliosidoses, where only $G_{GNT}I$ seems to be increased.

It is unlikely, although not impossible that there are structural abnormalities of gangliosides in HD. This aspect has been studied particularly for the ganglioside $G_{GNT}I$ (LEDEEN et al. 1965).

The relationship between the increase of ganglioside content and storage of acid mucopolysaccharides is not known. Both groups of compounds share hexose

Table 9. *Ganglioside patterns in gray and white matter of two cases of gargoylism*

Gangliosides	Gray matter			White matter		
	Cases		Normal control* (range)	Cases		Normal control* (range)
	1	2		1	2	
	(Values expressed as per cent of NANA)					
G_0	4.6	8.5	3.0— 4.8	3.3	11.6	5.9—10.4
G_1 (GGNTIV)	12.8	9.9	12.4—19.3	11.2	11.6	16.0—20.3
G_2 (GGNTIII)	11.8	17.7	8.3—15.4	10.8	17.4	11.0—12.1
G_2A	3.6	4.4	2.8— 4.6	2.8	2.9	1.0-- 1.8
G_3 (GGNTII)	24.6	20.1	39.6—48.0	23.3	16.9	34.0—42.9
G_3A	3.5	1.4	3.1— 4.8	1.4	1.1	2.0—4.8
G_4 (GGNTI)	18.5	33.0	11.5—16.6	31.3	32.6	16.0—16.4
G_5 (GGNTrII)	7.4	3.4	1.5— 4.4	6.1	4.0	1.3 — 1.7
G_6 (GLACT)	13.2	1.4	1	9.8	1.7	1
	(Values expressed as µg/g wet weight)					
Total NANA	1268	493	635—827	667	521	46—73

Source: Suzuki (1966), cases 1 and 3.

* Average of six normal control brains, ages 2.5 months to 8 years. G_2A and G_3A are two minor sialic acid-containing components with chromatographic mobilities between G_2 and G_3, and between G_3 and G_4, respectively (Suzuki 1966).

units and N-acetyl hexosamine, but common metabolic pathways have not been established.

One theory (Doss and Matiar-Vahar 1965) states that gangliosides accumulate in the brain of HD patients, because the ganglion cell has no other way to metabolize polysaccharide fragments except using them for ganglioside synthesis. However, it is unlikely that increased formation of gangliosides would lead to their accumulation in the absence of a simultaneous disturbance of the degrading system or of impairment of a feedback mechanism.

On the basis of quantitative and qualitative abnormalities of the amino acids of urinary chondroitinsulfate B in gargoylism, Dorfman (1963, 1966) suspects a deficiency of its protein binding with the result that chondroitinsulfate is not retained properly in connective tissues, leading to increased concentrations in serum, organs, and urine. Studies on mucopolysaccharides are limited by methodological difficulties, and artefacts may result from their complexity and their particular physicochemical state.

Therapy of Gangliosidoses

There is no causal treatment of gangliosidoses. In cases where lipid storage is not limited to the central nervous system, involvement of visceral organs usually does not result in impairment of organ function, and symptomatic treatment does not become necessary, in contrast to the bleeding tendency observed in some cases of Gaucher's disease which may necessitate therapeutic intervention.

In the chronic types of gangliosidoses which in general have a favorable prognosis as to longevity complications should be treated as indicated in the individual case. In Tay-Sachs disease, therapy directed against intercurrent infections only slows down the relentless course. Details of the care of lipidosis patients have been given by Crocker and Farber (1962).

References

ADLER, A.: Konstitutionell bedingte Granulationsveränderungen der Leukocyten und Knochenveränderungen. Schweiz. med. Wschr. 80, 1095 (1950).

ALEU, F. P., R. D. TERRY, and H. ZELLWEGER: Electron microscopy of two cerebral biopsies in gargoylism. J. Neuropath. exp. Neurol. 24, 304 (1965).

ALLEGRANZA, A.: Studio istologico et istochemico di un caso di idiozia amaurotica dell'adulto (tipo Kufs). Acta neurol. (Napoli) 11, 596 (1956).

ARONSON, S. M.: Epidemiology. In: Tay-Sachs Disease. Ed.: B. W. Volk, p. 118. New York: Grune and Stratton 1964.

— B. E. ARONSON, and B. W. VOLK: A genetic profile of infantile amaurotic family idiocy. Amer. J. Dis. Child. 98, 50 (1959).

— G. PERLE, A. SAIFER, and B. W. VOLK: Biochemical identification of the carrier state in Tay-Sachs disease. Proc. Soc. exp. Biol. (N.Y.) 111, 664 (1962).

— A. SAIFER, A. KANOF, and B. W. VOLK: Progression of amaurotic family idiocy as reflected by serum and cerebrospinal fluid changes. Amer. J. Med. 24, 390 (1958).

— — G. PERLE, and B. W. VOLK: Studies on enzyme alterations in the infantile sphingolipidoses. Amer. J. clin. Nutr. 9, 103 (1961).

— M. P. VALSAMIS, and B. W. VOLK: Infantile amaurotic family idiocy. Occurrence, genetic considerations, and pathophysiology in the non-Jewish infant. Pediatrics 26, 229 (1960).

— and B. W. VOLK: Genetic and demographic considerations concerning Tay-Sachs disease. In: Cerebral Sphingolipidoses. Eds.: S. M. Aronson and B. W. Volk. New York: Academic Press 1962.

— — and N. EPSTEIN: Morphologic evolution of amaurotic family idiocy. Amer. J. Path. 31, 609 (1955).

AUSTIN, J., D. McAFEE, D. ARMSTRONG, M. O'ROURKE, L. SHEARER, and B. BACHHAWAT: Abnormal sulfatase activities in two human diseases (metachromatic leucodystrophy and gargoylism). Biochem. J. 93, 15c (1964).

BAGH, K. VAN, and H. HORTLING: Blodfynd vid juvenil amaurotisk idioti. Nord. Med. 38, 1072 (1948).

BARCLAY, M., D. N. CALATHES, and H. W. DARGEON: Plasma lipoproteins in the lipidoses. Amer. J. Dis. Child. 97, 719 (1959).

BATTEN, F. E.: Cerebral degeneration with symmetrical changes in the maculae in two members of a family. Trans. opthal. Soc. U. K. 23, 386 (1903).

BAUMANN, T., E. KLENK u. S. SCHEIDEGGER: Niemann-Pick'sche Krankheit: eine klinische, chemische und histopathologische Studie. Ergebn. allg. Path. path. Anat. 30, 183 (1936).

BERENSON, G. S., and E. R. DALFERES: Urinary excretion of mucopoly saccharides in normal individuals and in the Marfan syndrome. Biochim. biophys. Acta (Amst.) 101, 183 (1965).

BERGER, H.: Über zwei Fälle der juvenilen Form der familiären amaurotischen Idiotie. Z. ges. Neurol. Psychiat. 15, 435 (1913).

BERMAN, E. R., and S. GATT: Chemical pathology of glycolipids in brain tissue of Tay-Sachs disease. In: Cerebral Sphingolipidoses. Eds.: S. M. Aronson and B. W. Volk, p. 237. New York: Academic Press 1962.

BIELSCHOWSKY, M.: Über spätinfantile familiäre amaurotische Idiotie mit Kleinhirnsymptomen. Dtsch. Z. Nervenkr. 50, 7 (1914).

— Amaurotische Idiotie und lipoidzellige Splenohepatomegalie. J. Psychol. Neurol. (Lpz.) 36, 103 (1928).

— Über eine bisher unbekannte Form von infantiler amaurotischer Idiotie. Z. ges. Neurol. Psychiat. 155, 321 (1936).

BIRD, A.: The lipidoses and the central nervous system. Brain 71, 434 (1948).

BLACKFAN, K. D., L. K. DIAMOND, and M. LEISTER: Atlas of the blood in children. New York: The Commonwealth Fund 1944.

BOGAERT, L. VAN: Sur une form familiale très tardive de l'idiotie amaurotique. (Deuxième observation de la famille Al . . .). Dtsch. Z. Nervenheilk. 168, 267 (1952).

— et I. BERTRAND: Étude généalogique, clinique et histopathologique sur la forme infantile de l'idiotie amaurotique. Encéphale 29, 505 (1934).

— et P. BORREMANS: Sur une forme adulte de l'idiotie amaurotique familiale s'étendant jusqu' à la période précédant de la vieillesse. Z. ges. Neurol. Psychiat. 159, 136 (1937).

— et D. KLEIN: Observations sur l'hérédité des idiotes amaurotiques et de la spléno-hepatomégalie lipidienne (11 familles). J. Génét. hum. 4, 23 (1955).

BOGOCH, S.: Aminoglycolipids and glycoproteins of human brain. New methods for their extraction and further study in the sphingolipidoses. In: Cerebral Sphingolipidoses. Eds.: S. M. Aronson and B. W. Volk, p. 249. New York: Academic Press 1962.

BRANTE, G.: Studies in the nervous system with special reference to quantitative chemical determination and topical distribution. Acta physiol. scand. 18 (Suppl. 63) 1 (1949).

BRANTE, G.: Gargoylismus als Lipoidose. Fette und Seifen **53**, 457 (1951).
— Gargoylism – a mucopolysaccharidosis. Scand. J. clin. Lab. Invest. **4**, 43 (1952).
— Chemical pathology in gargoylism. In: Cerebral lipidoses, p. 164. Eds.: J. M. Cumings and
  M. Lowenthal. Oxford: Blackwell 1957.
BROUWER, B.: The spleen, the liver and the brain. Proc. roy. Soc. Med. **29**, 579 (1936).
BROWN, N. J., B. D. CORNER, and M. C. H. DODGSON: A second case in the same family of
  congenital familial cerebral lipidosis resembling amaurotic family idiocy. Arch. Dis. Child.
  29, 48 (1954).
BURKE, E. C.: The clinical spectrum in gargoylism. Proc. Mayo Clin. **37**, 241 (1962).
BURTON, R. M.: The action of neuraminidase from Clostridium perfringens on gangliosides.
  J. Neurochem. **10**, 503 (1963).
— Biochemistry of sphingosine containing lipids. In: Lipids and Lipidoses. Ed.: G. Schettler.
  Berlin-Heidelberg-New York: Springer 1967.
— M. A. SODD, and R. O. BRADY: The incorporation of galactose into galactolipides. J. biol.
  Chem. **233**, 1053 (1958).
CARTER, H. E.: Sphingolipids. In: Chemistry of lipids as related to atherosclerosis. Ed.:
  I. H. Page, p. 82. Springfield (Ill.): Thomas 1958.
CATEL, W.: Amaurotische Idiotie (Typ Tay-Sachs) bei etwa einjährigem nichtjüdischen Kind.
  (Verhandlungsbericht.) Dtsch. med. Wschr. **69**, 860 (1943).
— Differentialdiagnostische Symptomatologie von Krankheiten des Kindesalters. Leipzig:
  Thieme 1944. 2. Aufl. Stuttgart: Georg Thieme 1951.
COBB, W., F. MARTIN, and G. PAMPIGLIONE: Cerebral lipidoses: electroencephalographic study.
  Brain **75**, 343 (1952).
CORBERI, G.: Suble regressione mentali nell età infantile e nell età giovanile. Riv. sper.
  Freniat. **50**, 566 (1926).
CORDES, F. C., and W. D. HORNER: Infantile amaurotic idiocy in two Japanese families.
  Amer. J. Ophthal. **52**, 558 (1929).
CRAIG, J. M., J. T. CLARKE, and B. Q. BANKER: Metabolic neurovisceral disorder with accumulation
  of unidentified substance: variant of Hurler's Syndrome? Amer. J. Dis. Child. **98**, 577 (1959).
CRAIG, W. S.: Gargoylism in a twin brother and sister. Arch. Dis. Child. **29**, 293 (1954).
CRAWLEY, J. W.: Three cases of the juvenile form of amaurotic family idiocy (Vogt-Spielmeyer
  disease) with electroencephalographic findings. J. Pediat. **51**, 571 (1957).
CROCKER, A. C., and S. FARBER: Niemann-Pick disease; a review of 18 patients. Medicine
  (Baltimore) **37**, 1 (1958).
CUMINGS, J. N.: The diagnostic value of lipid estimations in the cerebral lipidoses. In: Cerebral
  Lipidoses, ed. by L. van Bogaert, p. 112. Oxford: Blackwell 1957.
DAVISON, C.: The role of the globus pallidus and substantia nigra in the production of
  rigidity and tremor. Res. Publ. Ass. nerv. ment. Dis. **21**, 267 (1942).
— and S. A. JACOBSON: Generalized lipidosis in a case of amaurotic familial idiocy. Amer. J.
  Dis. Child. **52**, 345 (1936).
DIDE, M., P. GUIRAUD, et R. MICHEL: Lésions nerveuses dans un cas de maladie de Tay-Sachs
  juvénile. Encéphale **15**, 303 (1920).
DIDION, H.: Die amaurotischen Veränderungen des Augenhintergrundes bei Niemann-Pick-
  scher Krankheit. Klin. Mbl. Augenheilk. **116**, 131 (1950).
DIEZEL, P. B.: Histochemische Untersuchungen an primären Lipoidosen: Amaurotische Idiotie,
  Gargoylismus, Niemann-Picksche Krankheit, Gauchersche Krankheit, mit besonderer Be-
  rücksichtigung des Zentralnervensystems. Virchows Arch. path. Anat. **326**, 89 (1954a).
— Histochemischer Nachweis des Gangliosids in Ganglien- und Gliazellen bei Amaurotischer
  Idiotie und Isolierung der lipoidspeichernden Zellen nach der Methode von M. Behrens.
  Dtsch. Z. Nervenheilk. **171**, 344 (1954b).
— Bestimmung der Neuraminsäure im histologischen Schnittpräparat. Naturwissenschaften
  42, 487 (1955).
— Die Stoffwechselstörungen der Sphingolipoide; eine histochemische Studie an den primären
  Lipoidosen und den Entmarkungskrankheiten des Nervensystems, S. 74. Berlin-Göttingen-
  Heidelberg: Springer 1957.
— Lipidoses of the central nervous system. In: Modern Scientific Aspects of Neurology, p. 98.
  London: Edward Arnold 1960.
— Disturbances in lipid and carbohydrate metabolism in relation to the brain. In: Mental
  retardation, p. 277. Eds.: P. W. Bowman and H. V. Mantuer. New York-London: Grune
  and Stratton 1960.
— Die angeborenen Störungen des Lipoidstoffwechsels. In: Med. Grundlagenforschung,
  Bd. IV, S. 239. Stuttgart: Thieme 1962.
— N. KOPPANG u. J. A. ROSSNER: Fermenthistochemische und elektronenmikroskopische
  Untersuchungen an der juvenilen amaurotischen Idiotie des Hundes. Dtsch. Z. Nervenheilk.
  187, 720 (1965).

DORFMAN, A.: The Hurler syndrome. In: Congenital defects, p. 41. Philadelphia: Lippincott 1963.
— Heritable diseases of connective tissues: The Hurler syndrome. In: The metabolic basis of inherited disease, p. 963. Eds.: J. B. Stanbury, J. B. Wyngaarden and D. S. Fredrickson. New York: McGraw-Hill Book Company 1966.
— and A. E. LORINCZ: Occurrence of urinary acid mucopolysaccharides in the Hurler syndrome. Proc. nat. Acad. Sci. **43**, 443 (1957).
DOSS, M., u. H. MATIAR-VAHAR: Neurolipidosen und angeborene Entmarkungskrankheiten. Fortschr. Neurol. Psychiat. **33**, 671 (1965).
EDGAR, G. W. F.: Alkali-stable choline phospholipids ("sphingomyelin") in tissue of amaurotic idiocies. In: Cerebral Sphingolipidoses. Ed.: S. M. Aronson, and B. W. Volk, p. 165. New York: Academic Press 1962.
ELLIS, R. W. B., W. SHELDON, and N. B. CAPON: Gargoylism (Chondro-osteo-dystrophy, corneal opacities, hepatosplenomegaly, and mental deficiency). Quart. J. Med. **5**, 119 (1936).
EPSTEIN, J.: Amaurotic family idiocy. New York Med. J. **106**, 887 (1917).
ERLAÇIN, S.: Über das Vorkommen des Sphingosins und seiner Homologen in den Sphingolipoidosen des Gehirns. Dissertation Köln 1963.
FALKENHEIM, K.: Über familiäre amaurotische Idiotie. Jb. Kinderheilk. **54**, 123 (1901).
FISCHER, R.: Über Tay-Sachs'sche amaurotische Idiotie mit Organbeteiligung. Dissertation Frankfurt 1955.
FOLCH-PI, J., and M. LEES: Studies on the brain ganglioside strand in normal brain and in Tay-Sachs disease. Amer. J. Dis. Child. **97**, 730 (1959).
FREDRICKSON, D. S.: Infantile amaurotic family idiocy. In: The metabolic basis of inherited disease. Eds.: J. B. Stanbury, J. B. Wyngaarden and D. S. Fredrickson, p. 553. New York: McGraw-Hill Book Co. 1960.
— and E. G. TRAMS: Ganglioside lipidosis: Tay-Sachs' disease. In: The metabolic basis of inherited disease. Eds.: J. B. Stanbury, J. B. Wyngaarden and D. S. Fredrickson, p. 523. New York: McGraw-Hill Book Co. 1966.
FRENKEL, H., et M. DIDE: Rétinite pigmentaire avec atrophie papillaire et ataxie cérébelleuse familiales. Rev. neurol. **25**, 729 (1913).
FRIEDRICH, G.: Familiäre amaurotische Idiotie. In: Handbuch der speziellen path. Anat. Histologie, Bd. 13, 1. Teil, Bandteil A, S. 540. Hrsg.: Lubarsch-Henke-Rössle. Berlin-Göttingen-Heidelberg: Springer 1957.
GASSER, C.: Discussion de l'article de Adler. Schweiz. med. Wschr. **80**, 1097 (1950).
GATT, S., and E. R. BERMAN: Studies on brain lipids in Tay-Sachs disease. I. Isolation of two sialic acid-free glycolipids. J. Neurochem. **10**, 43 (1963a).
— — Studies on brain lipids in Tay-Sachs disease. II. Solubility properties of gangliosides. J. Neurochem. **10**, 65 (1963b).
— — Studies on brain lipids in Tay-Sachs disease. III. Incorporation of tritiated water into brain lipids. J. Neurochem. **10**, 73 (1963c).
GILJE, K., and A. J. NISSEN: Tidlig diagnose av juvenil amaurotisk idioti. T. norske laegefor. **76**, 855 (1956).
GILLS, J. P., R. HOBSON, W. B. HANLEY, and V. A. McKUSICK: Electroretinography and fundus oculi findings in Hurler's disease and allied mucopolysaccharidoses. Arch. Ophthal. **74**, 596 (1965).
GLOBUS, J. H.: Ein Beitrag zur Histopathologie der amaurotischen Idiotie. Z. ges. Neurol. Psychiat. **85**, 424 (1923).
— Amaurotic family idiocy. J. Mt Sinai Hosp. **9**, 451 (1942).
GOLDBERG, M. F., A. E. MAUMENEE, and V. A. McKUSICK: Corneal dystrophies associated with abnormalities of mucopolysaccharide metabolism. Arch. Ophthal. **74**, 516 (1965).
GOLDSCHMIDT, E., R. LENZ, S. MARIN, A. RONEN, and I. RONEN: Frequency of the Tay-Sachs gene in the Jewish communities of Israel (abstract). In: Proceedings of 25th Annual Meeting of Genetics Society of America, August 27, 1956.
GONATAS, N. K., and J. GONATAS: Ultrastructural and biochemical observations on a case of systemic late infantile lipidosis and its relationship to Tay-Sachs disease and Gargoylismus. J. Neuropath. exp. Neurol. **24**, 341 (1965).
— R. D. TERRY, R. WINKLER, S. R. KOREY, C. J. GOMEZ, and A. STEIN: A case of juvenile lipidosis: The significance of electron microscopic and biochemical observations of a cerebral biopsy. J. Neuropath. exp. Neurol. **22**, 557 (1963).
GREENFIELD, J. G., and G. HOLMES: The histology of juvenile amaurotic idiocy. Brain **48**, 183 (1925).
GREENFIELD, J. H., and S. NEVIN: Amaurotic family idiocy. Study of a late case. Trans. ophthal. Soc. U.K. **53**, 170 (1933).
GRIFFITH, S. B., and M. FINDLAY: Gargoylism: clinical, radiological and haematological features in two siblings. Arch. Dis. Childh. **33**, 229 (1958).

G. Schettler and W. Kahlke:

Haddenbrock, S.: Zur Pathogenese systematischer Bahndegenerationen bei amaurotischer Idiotie und zur Frage der Beziehungen dieses Leidens zur Myoklonusepilepsie. Arch. Psychiat. Nervenkr. **185**, 129 (1950).

Hagberg, B., G. Holtquist, R. Öhman, and L. Svennerholm: Congenital Amaurotic Idiocy. Acta paediat. scand. **54**, 116 (1965).

Hallervorden, J.: Spätform der amaurotischen Idiotie unter dem Bilde der Paralysis agitans. Mschr. Psychiat. Neurol. **99**, 74 (1938).

— Spätfälle von amaurotischer Idiotie. Verh. dtsch. Ges. Verdauungs- u. Stoffwechselkr. **14**, 103 (1939).

— Dysostosis multiplex. In: G. v. Bergmann, W. Frey u. H. Schwiegk: Handb. d. Inn. Med. Bd. V/3, S. 979. Berlin-Göttingen-Heidelberg: Springer 1953.

Harbitz, F.: Familiäre amaurotische Idiotie. Arch. Augenheilk. **73**, 140 (1913).

Harlem, O. K.: Juvenile cerebroretinal degeneration (Spielmeyer-Vogt): Blood and EEG findings in a family of 10 members. Amer. J. Dis. Child. **100**, 918 (1960).

Hassin, G. B., and A. H. Parmelee: Amaurotic family idiocy (Tay-Sachs type). A case with a protracted course. Amer. J. Dis. Child. **33**, 87 (1928).

Hienz, A.: Beitrag zur pathologischen Anatomie der enchondralen Dysostosen. Dissertation Heidelberg 1953.

— Die Pfaundler-Hurlersche Krankheit. Ergebn. allg. Path. path. Anat. **40**, 1 (1960).

Higier, H.: Über die seltenen Formen der hereditären und familiären Gehirn- und Rückenmarkskrankheiten. Dtsch. Z. Nervenheilk. **9**, 1 (1896).

Hoffman, J.: Pigmentary retinal lipoid neuronal heredodegeneration (Spielmeyer Vogt disease). Electroenceph. clin. Neurophysiol. **8**, 506 (1956).

Hunter, Ch.: A rare disease in two brothers. Proc. roy. Soc. Med. **10**, 104 (1917).

Hurler, G.: Über einen Typ multipler Abartungen, vorwiegend am Skelettsystem. Z. Kinderheilk. **24**, 220 (1919).

Jacobi, M. L., and P. J. Waardenburg: Een geval van dysostosis multiplex van Hurler. Mschr. Kindergeneesk. **9**, 175 (1940).

Janský, J., and Z. Mysliveček: Beitrag zur familiären amaurotischen Idiotie. Arch. Psychiatr. **59**, 668 (1918).

Jatzkewitz, H.: Eine neue Methode zur quantitativen Ultramikrobestimmung der Sphingolipoide aus Gehirn. Hoppe-Seylers Z. physiol. Chem. **336**, 25 (1964).

— and K. Sandhoff: On a biochemically special form of infantile amaurotic idiocy. Biochim. biophys. Acta (Amst.) **70**, 354 (1963).

— H. Pilz u. K. Sandhoff: Quantitative Bestimmungen von Gangliosiden und ihren neuraminosäurefreien Derivaten bei infantilen, juvenilen und adulten Formen der amaurotischen Idiotie und einer spätinfantilen biochemischen Sonderform. J. Neurochem. **12**, 135 (1965).

Jefferson, M., and M. L. Rutter: A report of two cases of the juvenile form of amaurotic familial idiocy (cerebromacular degeneration). J. Neurol. Neurosurg. Psychiat. **21**, 31 (1958).

Jervis, G. A.: Familial mental deficiency akin to amaurotic idiocy and gargoylism. A apparently new type. Arch. Neurol. Psychiat. (Chic.) **47**, 943 (1942).

— Hallervorden-Spatz-disease associated with atypical amaurotic idiocy. J. Neuropath. exp. Neurol. **11**, 4 (1952).

— Juvenile amaurotic Idiocy. Amer. J. Dis. Child. **97**, 663 (1959).

Johnson, A. C., A. R. McNabb, and R. J. Rossiter: Chemical studies of peripheral nerve during Wallerian degeneration. Biochem. J. **45**, 500 (1949).

Juliao, V. T., H. M. Canelas, and N. A. Longo: Juvenile form of familial amaurotic idiocy; clinical and laboratory studies of the cases. Arq. neuropsiquiat. **14**, 136 (1957). Cited after Spiegel-Adolf et al. (1959).

Kanof, A., S. M. Aronson, and B. W. Volk: Clinical progression of amaurotic family idiocy. Amer. J. Dis. Child. **97**, 656 (1959).

Karlsson, K. A.: Studies on sphingosines. 3. C_{20}-dihydrosphingosine, a hitherto unknown sphingosine. Acta. chem. scand. **18**, 565 (1964a).

— Studies on sphingosines. 4. Composition of sphingomyelins from human plasma. Proc. biochem. Soc. **92**, 39 (1964b).

— Studies on sphingosines. 6. C_{16}- and C_{17}-sphingosines hitherto unknown sphingosines. Acta chem. scand. **18**, 2395 (1964c).

Klenk, E.: Beiträge zur Chemie der Lipoidosen. Niemann-Pick'sche Krankheit und amaurotische Idiotie. Hoppe-Seylers Z. physiol. Chem. **262**, 128 (1939/1940).

— Neuraminsäure, das Spaltprodukt eines neuen Gehirnlipoids. Hoppe-Seylers Z. physiol. Chem. **268**, 50 (1941).

— Über die Ganglioside des Gehirns bei der infantilen amaurotischen Idiotie vom Typ Tay-Sachs. Ber. dtsch. chem. Ges. **75**, 1632 (1942a).

— Über die Ganglioside, eine neue Gruppe von zuckerhaltigen Gehirnlipoiden. Hoppe-Seylers Z. physiol. Chem. **273**, 76 (1942b).

KLENK E.: Über die Verteilung der Neuraminsäure im Gehirn bei der familiären amaurotischen Idiotie und bei der Niemann-Pick'schen Krankheit (Beiträge zur Chemie der Lipidosen, 6. Mitteilung). Hoppe-Seylers Z. physiol. Chem. **282**, 84 (1947).
— The pathological chemistry of the developing brain. In: Biochemistry of the developing nervous system. E. Waelsch (Ed.). New York: Academic Press Inc. 1955.
— Die Chemie der Lipoidosen und der Entmarkungskrankheiten. Wien. Z. Nervenheilk. **13**, 309 (1957).
— u. W. GIELEN: Das Gangliosid des Gehirns bei der infantilen amaurotischen Idiotie vom Typ Tay-Sachs. Hoppe-Seylers Z. physiol. Chem. **323**, 126 (1961a).
— — Das Gangliosid des Gehirns bei der infantilen amaurotischen Idiotie vom Typ Tay-Sachs. Hoppe-Seylers Z. Physiol. Chem. **326**, 144 (1961b).
— — Über ein chromatographisch einheitliches hexosaminhaltiges Gangliosid aus Menschengehirn. Hoppe-Seylers Z. physiol. Chem. **326**, 158 (1961c).
— — and G. PADBERG: The structure of the gangliosides. In: Cerebral Sphingolipidoses. Eds.: S. M. Aronson and B. W. Volk, p. 301. New York: Academic Press 1962.
— u. W. KUNAU: Beitrag zur Konstitution der Ganglioside. Hoppe-Seylers Z. physiol. Chem. **335**, 275 (1964).
— u. H. LANGERBEINS: Über die Verteilung der Neuraminsäure im Gehirn. Hoppe-Seylers Z. physiol. Chem. **270**, 185 (1941).
— U. LIEDTKE u. W. GIELEN: Das Gangliosid des Gehirns bei der infantilen amaurotischen Idiotie vom Typ Tay-Sachs. Hoppe-Seylers Z. physiol. Chem. **334**, 186 (1963).
— and H. LÖHR: Unpublished results; cit. by KLENK (1955), ref. [44].
— W. VATER, and G. BARTSCH: Storage of gangliosides in nervous tissue in Tay-Sachs disease and changes in material preserved in formalin. J. Neurochem. **1**, 203 (1957).
KLINKEN-RASMUSSEN, L., and H. DYGGVE: A case of late infantile amaurotic idiocy of the myoclonus type. Acta neurol. scand. **41**, 172 (1965).
KOREY, S. R., C. J. GOMEZ, A. STEIN, J. GONATAS, K. SUZUKI, R. D. TERRY, and M. WEISS: Studies in Tay-Sachs disease. I. A. Methods. 1. Biochemical, 2. Electron microscopic. J. Neuropath. exp. Neurol. **22**, 2 (1963a).
— J. GONATAS, and A. STEIN: Studies on Tay-Sachs disease. III. Biochemistry. A. Analytic and metabolic aspects. J. Neuropath. exp. Neurol. **22**, 56 (1963b).
— and A. STEIN: Studies in Tay Sachs disease. III. Biochemistry. B. Catabolism of gangliosides and related compounds. J. Neuropath. exp. Neurol. **22**, 67 (1963).
— and R. D. TERRY: Studies in Tay-Sachs' disease. I. B. Clinical and pathologic descriptions. J. neuropath. exp. Neurol. **22**, 10 (1963).
KOZINN, P. J., H. WIENER, and P. COHEN: Infantile amaurotic family idiocy. J. Pediat. **51**, 58 (1957).
KUFFLER, O.: Beitrag zur Kenntnis vom juvenilen (Vogtschen) Typ der amaurotischen Idiotie. Beitr. Augenheilk. 8 (1912).
KUFS, H.: Über eine Spätform der amaurotischen Idiotie und ihre heredofamiliären Grundlagen. Z. ges. Neurol. Psychiat. **95**, 169 (1925).
— Über einen Fall von Spätform der amaurotischen Idiotie mit atypischem Verlauf und mit terminalen schweren Störungen des Fettstoffwechsels im Gesamtorganismus. Z. ges. Neurol. Psychiat. **122**, 395 (1929).
— Sind die familiäre amaurotische Idiotie (Tay-Sachs) und die Splenohepatomegalie (Niemann-Pick) in ihrer Pathogenese identisch? Arch. Psychiatr. **91**, 101 (1930).
KUHN, R., u. H. WIEGANDT: Die Konstitution der Ganglio-N-tetraose und des Gangliosids G 1. Chem. Ber. **96**, 866 (1963).
— — Weitere Ganglioside aus Menschenhirn. Z. Naturforsch. **19b**, 256 (1964).
KUNAU, W.: Über die Struktur von zwei hexosaminhaltigen Gangliosiden aus menschlichem Gehirn. Diss. Köln 1964.
KUTZIM, H.: Chemische Untersuchungen des Gehirns bei zwei Fällen von Hurlerscher Erkrankung. Diss. Köln 1946.
LAMY, M., J. P. BADER, and P. MAROTEAUX: La maladie de Hurler-Gargoylisme, dysostosis multiplex. Sem. Hôp. Paris **34**, 1735 (1958).
— P. MAROTEAUX et J. FRÉZAL: Les chondrodystrophies génotypiques: Definition et limities. Sem. Hôp. Paris **34**, 1675 (1958).
— P. ROYER et C. NEZELOF: Présence d'inclusions cellulaires dans la moelle osseuse chez des sujets atteints de gargoylisme. Presse méd. **67**, 1058 (1959).
LANDING, B. H., and J. H. RUBINSTEIN: Biopsy diagnosis of neurologic diseases in children, with emphasis on the lipidoses. In: Cerebral Sphingolipidoses. Eds.: S. M. Aronson and B. W. Volk, p. 1. New York: Academic Press 1962.
— F. N. SILVERMAN, J. M. CRAIG, M. D. JACOBY, M. D. LAHEY, and D. L. CHADWICK: Familial neurovisceral lipidoses. Amer. J. Dis. Child. **108**, 503 (1964).

Ledeen, R., K. Salzman, J. Gonatas, and A. Taghavy: Structure comparison of the major monosialogangliosides from brains of normal human, gargoylism, and late infantile systemic lipidosis. Part I. J. Neuropath. exp. Neurol. 24, 341 (1965).

Leistyna, J. A.: Lipid storage disorders of the central nervous system. Amer. J. Dis. Child. 104, 680 (1962).

Lemieux, L.: Thalamic pathology of amaurotic family idiocy: contribution of cytology of thalamus. J. Neuropath. exp. Neurol. 13, 343 (1954).

Levin, B., V. G. Oberholzer, G. J. A. I. Snodgrass, L. Stimmler, and H. J. Wilmers: Fructosaemia: an inborn error of fructose metabolism. Arch. Dis. Childh. 38, 220 (1963).

Levy, S., and A. O. G. Little: Juvenile familial amaurotic idiocy (Vogt-Spielmeyer disease). Review of literature and clinical report of a case. Arch. Neurol. Psychiat. (Chic.) 44, 1274 (1940).

Liebers, M.: Zur Histopathologie der amaurotischen Idiotie und Myoklonusepilepsie. Z. ges. Neurol. Psychiat. 111, 465 (1927).

Makita, A., and T. Yamakawa: The glycolipids of the brain of Tay-Sachs disease. The chemical structures of a globoside and main ganglioside. Jap. J. exp. Med. 33, 361 (1963).

Marburg, G. O.: Studies on the pathology and pathogenesis of amaurotic family idiocy (Tay-Sachs disease). Amer. J. ment. Defic. 46, 312 (1942).

Marburg, O.: Inclusion bodies and late fate of ganglion cells in infantile amaurotic family idiocy. Arch. Neurol. Psychiat. (Chic.) 49, 708 (1943).

Marie, J. L., L. Marchand, J. Borel, J. Laroche et I. F. Foucin: Considerations anatomo-cliniques sur la polydystrophie de Hurler. A propos un case. Encéphale 44, 201 (1955).

Maroteaux, P., and M. Lamy: Hurler's disease, Morquio's disease, and related mucopolysaccharidoses. J. Pediat. 67, 312 (1965).

McKusick, V. A.: Veritable disorders of connective tissue. Ed. 2. St. Louis: Mosby Co. 1960.

— The genetic mucopolysaccharidoses. (1966) In press. Cited after Gills et al. 1965.

Melchior, J. C., J. Clausen, and H. V. Dyggve: The mucopolysaccharidoses. A clinical and biochemical survey. Clin. Pediat. 4, 468 (1965).

Meyer, K., M. M. Grumbach, A. Linker, and P. Hoffman: Excretion of sulfated mucopolysaccharides in gargoylism (Hurlers syndrome). Proc. Soc. exp. Biol. (N.Y.) 97, 275 (1958).

Minkowitz, S.: A new form of visceral histiocytic glycolipidosis with mental retardation. Amer. J. Med. 37, 623 (1964).

Mittwoch, U.: Inclusion of mucopolysaccharides in the patients with gargoylism. Nature (Lond.) 191, 1315 (1961).

— Abnormal lymphocytes in gargoylism. Brit. J. Haemat. 5, 365 (1959).

Morrell, F., and F. Torres: Electrophysiological analysis of a case of Tay-Sachs disease. Brain 83, 213 (1960).

Moschel, R.: Amaurotic Idiotie mit einer besonderen Form von Pigmentablagerung. Dtsch. Z. Nervenheilk. 172, 102 (1954).

Müldner, H. G., J. R. Wherret, and J. N. Cumings: Some applications of thin layer chromatography in the study of cerebral lipids. J. Neurochem. 9, 607 (1962).

Murakami, O.: Folia psychiat. neurol. jap. Suppl. 1, 1 (1957). Cit. by Aronson and Volk, 1962.

Nissen, A. J.: Juvenil amaurotisk idioti i Norge. Nord. Med. 52, 1542 (1954).

Norman, R. M.: The neuronal storage diseases. In: Neuropathology, p. 383, ed. by J. G. Greenfield. London: Arnold & Co. 1958.

— A. H. Tingey, C. G. H. Newman, and S. P. Ward: Tay-Sachs disease with visceral involvement and its relation to gargoylism. Arch. Dis. Child. 39, 634 (1964).

— H. Urich, A. H. Tingey and R. A. Goodbody: Tay-Sachs disease with visceral involvement and its relationship to Niemann-Pick disease. J. Path. Bact. 78, 409 (1959).

— and N. Wood: A congenital form of amaurotic family idiocy. J. Neurol. Psychiat. 4, 175 (1941).

Norman, S. J., and E. P. Benditt: Function of the reticuloendothelial system. I. Study on the phenomen of carbon clearance inhibition. J. exp. Med. 122, 693 (1965).

— — Function of the reticuloendothelial system. II. Participation of a serum factor in carbon clearance. J. exp. Med. 122, 709 (1965).

O'Brien, J. S., M. B. Stern, B. H. Landing, J. K. O'Brien, and G. N. Donnell: Generalized gangliosidosis. Amer. J. Dis. Child. 109, 338 (1965).

Philippart, M., and J. Menkes: Isolation and characterization of main splenic gangliosides in Gaucher's disease: Evidence for site of metabolic Block. Biochem. biophys. Res. Commun. 15, 551 (1964).

Pick, L.: Der Morbus Gaucher und die ihm ähnlichen Krankheiten. Exp. inn. Med. 29, 519 (1926).

— u. M. Bielschowsky: Über lipoidzellige Splenomegalie (Typus Niemann Pick) und amaurotische Idiotie. Klin. Wschr. 6, 1631 (1927).

PROŠTENIK, M., and B. MAJHOFER-OREŠČANIN: Occurance of a new sphingolipid base C$_{20}$-sphingosine in horse and beef brain. Naturwissenschaften **47**, 399 (1960).

RAYNER,S.: Juvenile amaurotic idiocy: diagnosis of heterocygotes. Acta genet. (Basel)**3**,1 (1952).

REILLY, W.: The granules in the leucocytes in Gargoylism. Amer. J. Dis. Child. **62**, 489 (1941).

RÖNNE, H.: Zur pathologischen Anatomie der Augenleiden bei juveniler familiärer amaurotischer Idiotie (Spielmeyer-Stocksche Form). Klin. Mbl. Augenheilk. **56**, 497 (1916).

ROGALSKI, T.: Zur Kasuistik der juvenilen Form der amaurotischen Idiotie. Arch. Psychiatr. **47**, 1195 (1910).

ROSENBERG, A., and E. CHARGAFF: Some observations on the mucolipids of normal and Tay-Sachs disease brain tissue. Amer. J. Dis. Child. **97**, 739 (1959).

ROTHSTEIN, J. L., and S. WELT: Infantile amaurotic family idiocy. Amer. J. Dis. Child. **62**, 801 (1941).

ROUSER, G., G. KRITCHEVSKY, C. GALLI, and D. HELLER: Determination of polar lipids: quantitative column and thin layer chromatography. J. Amer. Oil. Chem. Soc. **42**, 215 (1965).

ROYER, P.: La cellule de Buhot et le diagnostic de gargoylisme Sang. **30**, 37 (1959).

SACHS, B.: On arrested cerebral developement with special reference to its cortical pathology. J. nerv. ment. Dis. **14**, 541 (1887).

— A family form of idiocy, generally fatal, associated with early blindness. J. nerv. ment. Dis. **21**, 475 (1896).

— A family form of idiocy. N.Y. St. J. Med. **63**, 697 (1898).

— and L. HAUSMAN: Nervous and mental disorders from birth through adolescence. New York: Hoeber 1926.

SAIFER, A.: The biochemistry of Tay-Sachs disease. In: Tay-Sachs Disease, p. 68. Ed.: B. W. Volk. New York: Grune and Stratton 1964.

— and S. GERSTENFIELD: Photometric determination of sialic acid in serum and in cerebrospinal fluid with the thiobarbituric acid method. Clin. chim. Acta **7**, 467 (1962).

— B. W. VOLK, and S. M. ARONSON: Neuraminic (sialic) acid studies of biological fluids in amaurotic family idiocy and related disorders. Amer. J. Dis. Child. **97**, 745 (1959).

SAMBASIVARAO, K., and R. H. McCLUER: Lipid components of gangliosides. J. Lipid Res. **5**, 103 (1964).

SAMUELS, S., N. K. GONATAS, and M. WEISS: Formation of the membranous cytoplasmic bodies in Tay-Sachs disease: an in vitro study. J. Neuropath. exp. Neurol. **24**, 256 (1965).

— S. R. KOREY, J. GONATAS, R. TERRY, and M. WEISS: The membranous granules in Tay-Sachs disease. In: Cerebral Sphingolipidoses: a symposium on Tay-Sachs disease and allied disorders. p. 309. Eds.: S. M. Aronson and B. W. Volk. New York: Academic Press 1962.

— — — — Studies in Tay-Sachs disease. IV. Membranous cytoplasmic bodies. 1. Biochemistry. 2. Ultrastructure. J. Neuropath. exp. Neurol. **22**, 81 (1963).

SANDHOFF, K., H. PILZ u. H. JATZKEWITZ: Über den enzymatischen Abbau von N-acetyl-neuraminsäurefreien Gangliosidresten (Ceramid-oligosaccheriden). Hoppe-Seylers Z. physiol. Chem. **328**, 281 (1964).

SANFILIPPO, S. J., J. YUNIS, and H. G. WORTHEN: An unusual storage disease resembling the Hunter-Hurler-Syndrome. Amer. J. Dis. Child. **104**, 553 (1962).

SCHAFFER, K.: Über das morphologische Wesen und die Histopathologie der hereditären Nervenkrankheiten. Berlin: Springer 1926.

— The pathogenesis of amaurotic idiocy. Arch. Neurol. (Chic.) **24**, 765 (1930a).

— Sind die familiäre amaurotische Idiotie und die Splenohepatomegalie in ihrer Pathogenese identisch? Arch. Psychiatr. **89**, 814 (1930b).

SCHAPIRA, F., J. C. DREYFUSS et G. SCHAPIRA: Presence de deux aldolases de type different dans le serum. C. R. Acad. Sci. (Paris) **245**, 808 (1957).

SCHETTLER, G.: Lipidosen. 3. Gangliosidosen. In: Handb. d. Inn. Med., Eds.: G. v. Bergmann, W. Frey, H. Schwiegk, S. 657. Berlin-Göttingen-Heidelberg: Springer 1955.

SCHICK, B.: Personal communication to ROTHSTEIN and WELT, 1941.

SCHINZ, H. R., u. A. FURTWAENGLER: Zur Kenntnis einer hereditären Osteoarthropathie mit recessivem Erbgang. Dtsch. Z. Chir. **207**, 398 (1928).

SCHNECK, L.: The clinical aspects of Tay-Sachs' disease. In: Tay-Sachs' disease. Ed.: B. W. Volk, p. 16. New York: Grune and Stratton 1964.

— The early electroencephalopathic and seizure characteristics of Tay-Sachs disease. Acta neurol. scand. **41**, 163 (1965).

— G. PERLE, and B. W. VOLK: Fructose tolerance in Tay-Sachs disease. Pediatrics **36**, 272 (1965a).

— J.B. WALLACE, A. SAIFER, and B. W. VOLK: A clinical biochemical and electron microscopic study of late infantile amaurotic family idiocy. Amer. J. Med. **39**, 285 (1965b).

SCHOB, F. G. K.: Über die amaurotische Idiotie. Fortschr. Med. **28** (1912).

— Zur pathologischen Anatomie der juvenilen Form der amaurotischen Idiotie. Z. ges. Neurol. Psychiat. **10**, 303 (1912); **46** (1919).

SCHOB, F. G. K.: Congenitale, früh erworbene und heredofamiliäre organische Nervenkrankheiten. In: Spezielle Pathologie und Therapie der inneren Krankheiten. Herausgeb.: F. Kraus
u. T. Brugsch. Bd. X, Teil 3: Nervenkrankheiten III. Berlin-Wien: Urban & Schwarzenberg
1924.
— Pathologische Anatomie der Idiotie. In: Handbuch der Geisteskrankheiten. Herausgeb.: O.
Bumke. Bd. XI. Berlin: Springer 1930.
SEIFERT, H., and G. UHLENBRUCK: Über Ganglioside in Hirntumoren. Naturwissenschaften
52, 190 (1965).
SEITELBERGER, F.: Zur Morphologie und Histochemie der degenerativen Axonveränderungen
im Zentralen Nervensystem. I. Congrès international des sciences neurologiques. Bruxelles
1957, Vol 3, p. 127.
— and K. SIMMA: On the pigment variant of amaurotic idiocy. In: Cerebral sphingolipidoses.
Eds.: S. M. Aronson and B. W. Volk. New York: Academic Press 1962.
— G. VOGEL u. H. STEPAN: Spätinfantile amaurotische Idiotie. Arch. Psychiat. Nervenkr.
196, 154 (1957).
SJÖGREN, T.: Die juvenile amaurotische Idiotie „Klinische und erblichkeitsmedizinische
Untersuchungen". Hereditas (Lund) 14, 197 (1931).
SJÖVALL, E., and E. ERICSSON: Anatomical type in Swedish cases of juvenile amaurotic
idiocy. Acta path. microbiol. scand. Supp. 16, 460 (1933).
SLOME, D.: The genetic basis of amaurotic family idiocy. J. Genet. 27, 363 (1933).
SOMERS, J. E., J. N. KANFER, and R. O. BRADY: Immunochemical studies with gangliosides,
II. Investigations of the structure of gangliosides by the hapten inhibition technique.
Biochemistry 3, 251 (1964).
SPIEGEL-ADOLF, M., H. W. BAIRD, D. KOLLIAS, and G. SZEKELY: Cerebrospinal fluid, serum
and blood investigations in amaurotic idiocy. J. Amer. Dis. Child. 97, 676 (1959).
SPIELMEYER, W.: Über eine besondere Form von familiärer amaurotischer Idiotie. Neurol.
Cbl. 25, 51 (1906).
— Klinische und anatomische Untersuchungen über eine besondere Form von familiärer
amaurotischer Idiotie. Habil.-Schrift, Freiburg 1907.
— Histologische und histopathologische Arbeiten über die Großhirnrinde. Klinische und
anatomische Untersuchungen über eine besondere Form von familiärer amaurotischer
Idiotie. Nissl. Arbeit. 2, 193 (1908).
— Über den amaurotischen Prozeß bei der amaurotischen Idiotie. Z. Psychiat. Neurol. 38
120 (1929).
STANACEV, N. Z., and E. CHARGAFF: Icosisphingosine, a long-chain base constituent of mucolipids. Biochem. biophys. Acta (Amst.) 59, 733 (1963).
STARCK, V.: Zur Kasuistik der familiären amaurotischen Idiotie. Mschr. Kinderheilk. 18, 139
(1920).
STENGEL, C.: reprinted in: A. J. NISSEN: Juvenil amaurotisk idioti i Norge. Nord. Med. 52,
1542 (1954).
STUBBE-TEGLBJAERG, H. P., and C. M. PLUM: Vacuolized lymphocytes in lipidosis. Acta neurol.
scand. 30, 327 (1955).
SUZUKI, K.: The pattern of mammalian brain gangliosides — II. Evaluation of the extraction
procedures, post mortem changes and the effect of formalin preservation. J. Neurochem.
12, 629 (1965).
— Ganglioside patterns of normal and pathological brains. In: Sphingolipidoses. The 3rd
international symposium on sphingolipidoses, 1965. Eds.: S. M. Aronson and B. W. Volk.
New York: Pergamon Press 1966.
SVENNERHOLM, L.: Quantitative estimation of gangliosides in senile human brains. Acta Soc.
Med. upsalien. 62, 1 (1957a).
— The nature of the gangliosides in Tay-Sachs disease. In: Cerebral Lipidosis. Eds.: L. van
Bogaert, J. N. Cumings, and A. Lowenthal. Oxford: Blackwell 1957b.
— Determination of gangliosides in nervous tissue. In: Cerebral Lipidoses, p. 122. Eds.:
L. van Bogaert, J. N. Cumings, and A. Lowenthal. Oxford: Blackwell 1957c.
— The chemical structure of normal human brain and Tay-Sachs gangliosides. Biochem.
biophys. Res. Commun. 9, 436 (1962).
— Chromatographic separation of human brain gangliosides. J. Neurochem. 10, 613 (1963).
— The distribution of lipids in the human nervous system — I. Analytical procedure. Lipids
of foetal and newborn brain. J. Neurochem. 11, 839 (1964).
— The gangliosides. J. Lipid Res. 5, 145 (1964).
— and Å. RAAL: Composition of brain gangliosides. Biochem. biophys. Acta (Amst.) 53, 422
(1961).
TAGHAVY, A., K. SALSMAN, and R. LEDEEN: An abnormal ganglioside pattern from a gargoyle
brain. (Abstract) Fed. Proc. 23, 128 (1964).

TAY, W.: Symmetrical changes in the region of the yellow spot in each eye of an infant. Trans. ophthal. Soc. U.K. **1**, 55 (1881).

TERRY, R. D., and J. C. HARKIN: Wallerian degeneration and regeneration of peripheral nerves, p. 303. In: S. R. Korey, (Ed.). The biology of myelin. New York: Hoeber 1959.

— and S. R. KOREY: Membranous cytoplasmic granules in infantile amaurotic idiocy. Nature (Lond.) **188**, 1000 (1960).

— — Studies in Tay-Sachs disease. V. The membrane of the membranous cytoplasmic body. J. Neuropath. exp. Neurol. **22**, 98 (1963).

— and A. LINKER: Distinction among four forms of Hurler's syndrome. Proc. Soc. exp. Biol. (N.Y.) **115**, 394 (1964).

— and M. WEISS: Studies in Tay-Sachs disease. II. Ultrastructure of the cerebrum. J. Neuropath. exp. Neurol. **22**, 18 (1963).

THANNHAUSER, S. J.: Infantile amaurotic idiocy. In: Lipidoses. Diseases of the intracellular lipid metabolism, p. 573. 3rd Ed. New York: Grune and Stratton 1958.

— J. BENOTTI, and H. REINSTEIN: Studies on animal lipids: the determination of lecithin, cephalin and sphingomyelin in body fluids and tissues; with analyses of normal human sera. J. biol. Chem. **129**, 709 (1939).

TINGEY, A.: Results of glycolipid analysis in certain types of lipidosis and leukodystrophy. J. Neurochem. **3**, 230 (1959).

TOURTELLOTTE, W. W., R. J. ALLEN, A. F. HAERER, and E. R. BRAIN: Study of lipids in cerebrospinal fluid and serum. Arch. Neurol. **12**, 300 (1965).

TURBAN, H.: Über einen Fall familiärer amaurotischer Idiotie vom Typ Tay-Sachs. Diss. Freiburg 1944.

ULLRICH, O.: Die Pfaundler-Hurler'sche Krankheit. Ergebn. inn. Med. Kinderheilk. **62**, 929 (1943).

VIAL, J. D.: Early changes in the axoplasm during Wallerian degeneration. J. biophys. biochem. Cytol. **4**, 551 (1958).

VOGT, H.: Über familiäre amaurotische Idiotie und verwandte Krankheitsbilder. Mschr. Psychiat. Neurol. **18**, 161 u. 310 (1906).

VOLK, B. W.: Pathologic anatomy. In: Tay-Sachs Disease, p. 36. Ed.: B. W. Volk, New-York: Grune and Stratton 1964.

— S. M. ARONSON, and S. M. SAIFER: Fructose-1-phosphate aldolase deficiency in Tay-Sachs disease. Amer. J. Med. **36**, 481 (1964).

WAGNER, A.: Über Hirnganglioside bei Tay-Sachsscher Erkrankung. Klin. Wschr. **44**, 398 (1966).

— I. D. DAIN, and G. SCHMIDT: Accumulation of an abnormal brain ganglioside in Tay-Sachs disease. (Abstract) Fed. Proc. **22**, 234 (1963).

WALLACE, B. J., L. SCHNECK, H. KAPLAN, and B. W. VOLK: Fine structure of the cerebellum of children with lipidoses. Arch. Path. **80**, 466 (1965).

WATSON, S. W., and D. DENNY-BROWN: Myoclonus epilepsy as a symptom of diffuse neuronal disease. Arch. Neurol. Psychiat. (Chic.) **70**, 151 (1953).

WIEGANDT, H.: Ganglioside. In: Untersuchung und Bestimmung der Lipoide im Blut, S. 19. Eds.: N. Zöllner and D. Eberhagen. Berlin-Heidelberg-New York: Springer 1965.

WILDI, E.: Contribution a l'étude anatomopathologique et clinique de la maladie de Tay-Sachs. Thèse de Genève **1978** (1950).

WOLF, H. P.: 1-Phosphofructaldolase. In: Methoden der enzymatischen Analyse, S. 732. Weinheim: Verlag Chemie 1962.

WYBURN-MASON, R.: On some anomalous forms of amaurotic idiocy and their bearing on relationship of various types. Brit. J. Ophthal. **27**, 145 and 193 (1943).

ZEMAN, W., and J. HOFFMANN: Juvenile and late forms of amaurotic idiocy in one family. J. Neurol. Neurosurg. Psychiat. **25**, 352 (1962).

Gaucher's Disease

By

G. Schettler and W. Kahlke

Synonyms: Cerebroside lipidosis, cerebrosidosis.

Definition and Introduction

Gaucher's disease (GD) is an hereditary disorder of which over 350 cases have been described to date. The main clinical finding is hepatosplenomegaly. Typical histologic changes consist of the appearance of cerebroside-containing cells (Gaucher cells) in the reticuloendothelial system (RES), mainly in spleen, liver, bone marrow and lymphatic tissues. Symptoms and signs of the disease may appear at any age. An acute picture is observed in infants, with evidence of central nervous system involvement. A chronic course is typical for adults. Reviews of GD have been published by PICK (1926/1933), OBERLING and WORINGER (1927), ATKINSON (1938), KLENK et al. (1938), REICH et al. (1951), VAN CREFELD (1953), SCHETTLER (1955), THANNHAUSER (1958), FREDRICKSON and HOFMANN (1960/66), DOSS and MATIAR-VAHAR (1965) and others.

Historical Review

In 1882, PHILLIPE C. E. GAUCHER described a disease which was characterized by hepatosplenomegaly, skin pigmentations and a chronic progressive course. Abnormal cells which he found in the spleen and which were later to bear his name were considered by him to result from a primary neoplasm of this organ, with secondary changes in liver and other tissues. Like COLLIER (1895) who described the disease in a 6 year-old boy, GAUCHER did not appreciate the systemic nature of the disease. This was first recognized 25 years after his first description by SCHLAGENHAUFER (1907) who thought that he was dealing with a proliferative disorder of connective tissue with accompanying enlargement of parenchymal cells in affected organs. Consecutively, it was thought that chronic infection or toxic or neoplastic processes were responsible for the development of the observed abnormalities (BOVAIRD and MANDLEBAUM, cit. by MARCHAND, 1907). The proper avenue for further studies was pointed out by MARCHAND (1907) who showed storage of foreign material by RES cells of affected subjects. In 1920, EPPINGER, under the influence of ASCHOFF and on the basis of the findings up to this time, classified GD as a disorder of the RES in liver and spleen. Detailed studies by PICK (1922/26) on histology and morbid anatomy of GD resulted in the differentiation of the Gaucher cells from morphologically similar foam cells which occur in Niemann-Pick disease. In addition, PICK pointed out that endothelial cells do not participate in the storage of lipid. Opinions with regard to the origin of the stored material were already divided at that time and uptake from the bloodstream or formation within the storing cells were subjects of controversy. Following MARCHAND (1907) who had emphasized the firm, hyaline consistency of the stored material, its lipid-like nature was suggested by several studies. In 1924, EPSTEIN isolated from the Gaucher spleen significant amounts of a substance which was soluble in alcohol and insoluble in acetone, and in the same year LIEB (1924/27) identified the material obtained from a variety of Gaucher tissues as the cerebroside kerasin which had been found long before as a component of brain tissue by THU-DICHUM (1882/1901). Storage of cerebrosides in GD has been found consistently since. In 1934 AGHION showed that the cerebroside stored in visceral organs was a glucocerebroside, which occurs there normally only in traces. Nevertheless, the question of the sugar component in the cerebroside of GD — whether glucose or galactose — has come up again and again and has only recently been unequivo-cally settled in favor of glucose (see pg. 278). More than 40 years after the discovery of cerebroside storage in GD, improved methodology led to the recognition of accumulation of gangliosides in addition to cerebrosides (THANNHAUSER 1953). Isolation and characterization of the splenic glycolipids in GD by PHILIPPART and MENKES (1964) showed them to contain two major components one of which was similar to the ganglioside G_{M3} (G_{LACT}) isolated by SVENNERHOLM (1963a). It is probably identical with the hexosamine-free ganglioside recovered recently from the brains of individuals with gargoylism (TAGHAVY et al. 1964). The composition of gangliosides and glycolipids from post-mortem cases of infantile Gaucher's disease, as reported recently by SVENNERHOLM (1966), indicates that the neuro-logical manifestations are caused by a disturbance in the metabolism of brain gangliosides. The minor gangliosides G_{M2} (G_{GNTrII}) and G_{M3} (G_{LACT}) were mod-erately increased and, to a larger extent, ceramide lactosides and glucocerebrosides accumulated with a similar ceramide composition as the gangliosides (SVENNER-HOLM 1966).

An additional feature of GD, namely elevated serum levels of an acid phos-phatase, has been found during the last 10 years (TUCHMAN et al. 1956, CROCKER and LANDING 1960). However, even though GD is the "oldest" lipidosis and has now been known for over 80 years, its pathogenesis has not yet been clarified.

Incidence (Age, Sex, Race)

The disease may become manifest at any age. The youngest patient described was a one-week-old infant (OBERLING and WORINGER 1927), while the patients of greatest age at the time of diagnosis were 79 (PETIT and SCHLEICHER 1943), 80 (GÖTT and PEXA 1964) and 86 (BRINN and GLABMAN 1962) years old. Only about one third of all cases are diagnosed during infancy and childhood. In the majority the disease becomes manifest later, and the frequency decreases again with advancing age.

Significant differences in the clinical picture, as observed in infants on one hand, and adults on the other, suggested to some the existence of different forms of GD. However, it is likely that a single biochemical lesion can result in different clinical and pathologic findings depending on the stage of development of the affected subjects.

Initially an increased incidence of the disease in females was reported, with a ratio of 4:1 according to RUSCA (1921) and EPSTEIN (1924). PICK in 1926 found 25 females and 14 males among 39 cases of GD, and GÄNSSLEN (1940) still empha-sized the higher incidence in females. However, in THANNHAUSER's experience the rate of occurrence is the same for both sexes. This was confirmed by HSIA et al. (1959) with 74 affected males and 69 affected females. A preponderance of GD in the Jewish race has been observed by several authors (PICK 1926, HOFFMAN and MAKLER 1929), and, inspite of the dissenting voice of HANHART (1954), seems firmly established. Negro patients with GD have been described by HERNDON and BENDER (1950) and CHOISSER and MONTGOMERY (1949). A case from China was reported by CHUNG et al. (1948). THANNHAUSER (1958) mentioned three affected Japanese siblings, and another Japanese patient was described by MASAI and KATURADA (1960).

The familial nature of the disease had already been recognized by COLLIER (1895) and by BOVAIRD (1900). Quite soon it became apparent that affected family members could be found in about one third of cases (BRILL 1901/05, PICK 1926). BRILL et al. (1905/09) described four affected siblings in a family with six children, and JOSSELIN, DE JONG and VAN HEUKELOM (1910) observed three patients with GD among 11 siblings. Since then, many cases have been found in siblings from affected families (lit. see HSIA et al. 1959).

GD in more than one generation was observed by GÖTT and PEXA (1964) with an affected mother and two affected children, by GERKEN and WIEDEMANN (1964) who found Gaucher cells in the bone marrow of an asymptomatic sibling and the asymptomatic parents of a patient, and by HSIA et al. (1959) who described GD in a Jewish father and his son. Skipping of a generation was seen by MATOTH and FRIED (1965). Here, grandfather and grandson were affected.

The genetics of the disease are discussed in the chapter by FUHRMANN (page 503).

Clinical Manifestations

As mentioned earlier, signs, symptoms and course depend to a considerable degree on the *time of appearance* of the disease. In adults, *splenomegaly* develops slowly, remains asymptomatic until late and not infrequently is detected only during a routine examination. The Gaucher cells which appear in tissues of the RES and occasionally other tissues as well do not impair organ function until late. Finally, splenomegaly and sometimes *hepatomegaly* result in symptoms of abdominal pressure, and at that time enlarged *lymph nodes* may be found on physical examination. Bone pain can occur, or *pathologic fractures* may point to the underlying disease. Occasionally a tendency to bleeding is the first symptom but, in general, *anemia, leukopenia* and *thrombopenia* appear late und may lead to fatigue, decreased resistance to infections or hemorrhage respectively.

Signs in children — with onset of the disease after the age of 6 months — develop much faster, and include crying, inanition, weight loss, fever and the findings in various viscera to be described. Occasionally, *involvement of the central nervous system* becomes symptomatic, while, in contrast, mental changes are never observed in adults. The patients described by HERRLIN and HILLBORG (1962), with onset of GD between 6 and 12 months, had intelligence quotients below 74, and some developed psychoses, progressive mental deterioration ($5 \times$) and epilepsy ($3 \times$). A juvenile patient (WEINSCHENK 1964), initially with normal intelligence, slowly progressed into a psychotic state with increasing impairment of intellectual capacity during his school age.

In infants up to the age of 6 months GD is characterized by sudden onset and a dramatic course. Progressive *neurologic symptoms* which result apparently from extensive cell damage through lipid deposition dominate the clinical course. Feeding difficulties appear during the first weeks, and weight loss is rapid. Somatic and mental development are greatly impaired, with appearance of strabismus, opisthotonus, trismus, jactations and development of generalized spasticity. Signs of neurovegetative dysfunction such as laryngospasm, crises of dysphagia and dyspnea, vomiting, and hyperthermia contribute decisively to the downhill course, and the final state of the little patients is one of cachexia and idiocy, usually terminated by intercurrent infections. Prevention of the latter with antibiotic treatment now allows for the preservation over some time of these vegetating infants.

Interference by the disease with the process of maturation and myelinization of the infantile brain is probably the basis for these extensive neurologic disturbances, and explains also the lack of neurologic symptoms in affected adults. An additional interpretation has been offered by PICK (1926/33). From studies on the phagocytosis of iron pigments and fat it appears that the RES cells of brain and some other tissues lose their ability for phagocytosis after the first year of life, and GD would therefore be severe when it begins before this time, and would also affect more tissues than in the "adult" form. It is of interest that the possibility of a deterioration of the central nervous system status by splenectomy has been discussed (HERRLIN and HILLBORG 1962). Here the loss of the main storage organ may play a role.

Retinal abnormalities like those which are consistently observed in Tay-Sachs disease, and which occur frequently in Niemann-Pick disease, are not a feature of GD. Here, *pinguecula-like formations* are frequent which consist of yellowish proliferations of the bulbar conjunctiva near the sclero-corneal junction, usually on the nasal side. These changes which may be seen normally in elderly people, occur more frequently in Gaucher patients, where they have a dark-yellow to brownish color which deepens with increasing age. In this form they have been considered pathognomonic for GD by some authors (PICK 1926, SCHETTLER 1955) and were described as early as 1901 in two siblings by BRILL. A bilateral occurrence is found in about ¼ of patients with the disease (FREDRICKSON and HOFMANN 1960/66).

Pingueculae are considered to result from hyaline degeneration of subepithelial layers of the conjunctiva with concomitant overgrowth of elastic fibers. Although typical Gaucher cell (GC) have not been found in these lesions, EAST and SAVIN (1940) saw large epitheloid cells with a foamy cytoplasm the histochemical properties of which were those of GC. The pingueculae of GD remain asymptomatic.

Most Gaucher patients exhibit brownish-yellow or bronzy *skin pigmentations* which resemble chloasma gravidarum and which become more intensely colored with advancing age. The pigmentation is darker on surfaces which are exposed to light (PICK 1926), may be quite localized, and, in the cases of MANDELBAUM et al. (1942), involve only one or both lower legs, or the face. Mucous membranes are usually normal. Skin pigmentations have not been observed in infants and small children (PICK 1926, WORINGER 1934, GIAMPALMO 1949).

Not all pigments have been identified histochemically. Hemosiderin is usually present; in addition, melanin has been found by WECHSLER and GUSTAFSON (1940). The pigmentations were therefore spoken of as "hemochromatosis" of Gaucher's disease (PICK), and indeed, the deposits of hemosiderin in various visceral organs resemble those of hemochromatosis (HEILMEYER 1954). On the other hand, the similarity with the pigmentation of Addison's disease suggests a causal role of the adrenals (EPSTEIN 1924), although GC have only rarely been found in the adrenal glands (BANKER et al. 1962). Since, in chronic cases, the adrenal cortex contains a large amount of iron, a disturbance of adrenal function may result therefrom (ZEHNDER 1938, THANNHAUSER 1950). Addison's disease developing from a complicating tuberculosis (THANNHAUSER 1950) may also have resulted in hyperpigmentation in a number of cases which were reported early. This mechanism should now be rare. In some cases the skin pigmentation was thought to diminish after splenectomy (MANDELBAUM et al. 1942).

Course and Prognosis: As mentioned earlier, the course of GD is determined mainly by the age of the patients when the disease becomes manifest. The infantile or "malignant" (DE LANGE 1939) form progresses rapidly, is usually fatal within a few months and the first year is never survived. The decisive prognostic factor is the extent to which the central nervous system is involved.

A more protracted course is observed in subjects who exhibit the first manifestations between the age of 6 and 12 months, and GIAMPALMO (1953) and DE LANGE (1939) therefore distinguished a subacute form from the acute form of very young infants. Children in the subacute category may live for 2 years or longer.

Children who are asymptomatic during their first year of life have a good chance of reaching adulthood. The later the first manifestations make their appearance in older children and in adults, the better, in general, will be the outlook. The inability in many adults to accurately time the onset of the disease hampers more detailed prognostic predictions for this age group. Asymptomatic periods may be followed after years by exacerbations. The size of spleen or liver and the finding of involvement of bones and other organs are not necessarily indicative of the severity or prognostic of the course of the disease. It is not possible to divide the course into an initial "splenic" stage with subsequent attack of liver and skeleton.

In the chronic, "adult" form the extent to which the hematopoetic system is involved, usually determines the prognosis. Signs of a slowly progressing anemia may be followed by the findings of thrombopenia and leukopenia, and cases with fatal outcome from panmyelopathy have been reported. The first place among intercurrent infections was occupied for years by tuberculosis, which at one time was considered to play a role in the etiology of the disease (SCHLAGENHAUFER 1907). Although this theory could not be confirmed (MARCHAND 1907, PICK 1926), the interest in the combination GD and tuberculosis remained, since GAUCHER's original patient suffered from pulmonary tuberculosis as well as tuberculous pleurisy and peritonitis. Case reports of GD with tuberculous pericarditis were given by SCHLAGENHAUFER (1907), RISEL (1909), BARÀT (1921) and ZADEK (1924); tuberculous peritonitis existed in subjects described by EPSTEIN (1924), MIENZIL (1924) and PICK (1926). Occasionally, tubercles were observed in the spleen (SCHLAGENHAUFER 1907) or in spleen and liver (EPSTEIN 1924b) of patients with GD, and adrenal tuberculosis was described by THANNHAUSER (1958). Today an increased incidence of tuberculosis in patients with GD is no longer found.

Other complications which adversely affect prognosis are thromboses of portal and splenic veins, and spontaneous or traumatic rupture of the spleen. The latter occurrence has been described in a subject who up to that time was asymptomatic for the disease.

Whenever pulmonary infiltration by Gaucher cells is visible on X-ray examination, recurrent bronchopneumonias may complicate the disease. In the chronic form of GD the use of chemotherapy and antibiotics significantly improves the prognosis.

Hematology

The kind and extent of hematologic changes depend on the duration of the disease. Acutely ill infants usually do not exhibit the hematologic abnormalities which occur in the chronic cases, but a bleeding tendency may be occasionally observed in children (HERNDON and BENDER 1950). Hematologic changes in adults include anemia, leukopenia and thrombopenia, all of which may become very severe during the course of the disease.

A normocytic or microcytic, hypochromic anemia is most frequently observed, but macrocytosis has been seen in the final stages of GD (FEINBERG and QUIGLEY 1946, REICH et al. 1951). The life span of the red cells has been found shortened in the few cases so examined (MOTULSKY et al. 1958). Usually osmotic resistance is normal (PICK 1933, BÜRGER 1934), but a hemolytic component with increased red cell fragility may exist (SOBEL and KAYE 1942). Hemoglobinuria was observed in one case of GD (CARLING et al. 1933). Areas of the bone marrow which are unaffected by GC infiltration may then contain an increased number of reticulocytes (SCHETTLER 1955). Rarely have nucleated red cells bcen found in circulating blood. The anemia can become so severe as to decisively contribute to a lethal outcome, particularly with additional hemorrhage from thrombopenia.

Leukopenia can similarly be of prognostic significance. It may be associated with a shift to the left with appearance of myelocytes, or, more frequently, may progress toward agranulocytosis favoring the development of intercurrent infections. Myeloid metaplasia has been found in the liver (PICK 1926, MELAMED and CHESTER 1929/38, LETTERER 1939).

The thrombocytes are diminished in adult patients who have not undergone splenectomy, and a hemorrhagic tendency may lead to epistaxis, bleeding into skin and mucous membranes (gastrointestinal tract) and metrorrhagia. In addition, hemorrhagic infarctions in a variety of organs with subsequent development of extensive hemosiderosis may ensue. Clinically, the Rumpel-Leede test is positive, while clotting time and prothrombin time are usually normal. An exceptional case with prolongation of the prothrombin time, hypofibrinogenemia and a deficiency of accelerin and convertin has been reported by KAPLAN et al. (1953). Morphologically, thrombocytes and megacaryocytes are normal.

The main cause for the hematologic abnormalities appears to be the Gaucher spleen; bone marrow involvement probably plays a minor role (MATOTH and FRIED 1965). Splenic bone marrow inhibition and increased destruction of red cells in addition to impairment of hematogenesis in the infiltrated bone marrow will result in the changes described. Phagocytosis of thrombocytes by GC (DANOPOULOS and LOGOTHETOPOULOS 1954) is not likely to contribute significantly to the thrombocytopenia. BÜRGER (1934) makes the interesting suggestion that the supply of thrombocytes may become exhausted as a result of continuous capillary hemorrhage within the RES.

Splenectomy in GD shows the typical sequelae of this procedure. The transient elevation of the thrombocyte count may, however, last longer than that observed after splenectomy for other reasons. Elimination of thrombopenia by splenectomy is independent of associated bone marrow disease and occurs even with marked infiltration by GC (PICK 1926, DAVIDSOHN 1928, BONTA 1929, HUNTER and EVANS 1929, CARLING et al. 1933, LOGAN 1941). An increase in circulating white cells may persist for months with counts up to 30000. HERRLIN and HILLBORG (1962) saw recurring leukocytosis 4—5 years after splenectomy. There is also some improvement of anemia after splenectomy.

Other Laboratory Findings

A consistent finding in GD is elevation of acid phosphatase activity of the serum. This chance observation by TUCHMAN et al. (1956) has subsequently been confirmed by the same author in 17 additional Gaucher patients (TUCHMAN and SWICK 1957, TUCHMAN et al. 1959). Others have reported similar findings. The increase was two- to threefold (7—14 Gutman units instead of 4—5 found in normals). (Lit. see CROCKER and LANDING 1960, ESTBORN and HILLBORG 1960). Recent studies on this subject have been published by TYSON et al. (1964), by HILLBORG and ESTBORN (1964), and by CZITOBER et al. (1964).

A comparison with the acid phosphatase(s) which may be increased in carcinoma of the prostate, Paget's disease, certain liver diseases, and hyperparathyroidism showed that the acid phosphatase of Gaucher's disease can be differentiated from the former with the use of various activators and inhibitors (GRÜNDIG et al. 1965). In contrast to prostatic phosphatases it is not inhibited by L-tartrate

(Abul-Fadl and King 1949, Tuchman et al. 1959). While normally a fraction of serum phosphatase activity can result from thrombocytes and red cells, this source has been excluded for the hyperphosphatasia of GD by demonstration of different reactions to inhibitors (Hillborg and Estborn 1964). The same authors even found decreased activity of the acid phosphatase in red cells of Gaucher patients.

A high phosphatase activity in the GC, in excess of that normally found in histiocytes, was demonstrated by Crocker and Landing (1960). These authors as well as others (Hillborg and Estborn 1964) considered the GC to be the source of the increased serum phosphatase, which would be liberated when GC undergo necrosis. The observed decrease of the serum phosphatase after splenectomy (Crocker and Landing 1960) and the increase later, while GC continue to accumulate in other organs, would tend to support this theory. Thus the elevation of acid phosphatase in the serum of Gaucher patients would represent a secondary phenomenon, and, while being of diagnostic value, would have no meaning as regards the pathogenesis of GD.

Another potential source of the enzyme is the central nervous system which normally contains not only the greatest amount of cerebrosides, but also large quantities of acid phosphatase. The significance of this association for the pathogenesis of GD deserves further study.

A search for elevated serum phosphatase in healthy relatives of Gaucher patients has been unsuccessful; neither parents nor siblings of affected subjects had abnormal values (Hillborg and Estborn 1964). Measurement of the acid phosphatase is therefore not a potential test for heterozygous subjects.

Pathology
Gaucher cells

The Gaucher cells (GC) are the histologic earmark of GD. The average diameter of this large reticulum cell was 84 μ in the series of Pick (1922/26) with a range from 20 to 100 μ. The fresh cells appear homogenous and their hyaline content resembles amyloid. One cell may possess several nuclei, the number of which appears to be related to the size of the cells. As many as 21 nuclei have been described in a giant GC (Pick 1926). The nuclei have an average diameter which is $^1/_4$—$^1/_6$ that of the cell, they are usually round to oval (Fisher and Reidbord 1962), but may be irregularly shaped, and their location within the cell is excentric (Mandlebaum and Downey 1916). The chromatin appears more dense at the rim of the nucleus (Fisher and Reidbord 1962), the nucleoli are inconspicuous. The question of cell division, previously the subject of controversy (Epstein 1924b, Rusca 1921), has now been settled in favor of a preponderance of amitosis (Pittaluga and Goyanes 1933, Cazal 1944).

The morphology of the fixed cells has been carefully described by Pick (1926) (see figures 1 and 2). The pale, light-yellow cytoplasm is filled with a spider webb of fine fibers which form a network of irregular meshes or islets, resulting in the appearance of "crumbled tissue paper", in contrast to the foamy, "honeycomb" structure of Niemann-Pick cells. Occasionally dendritic processes are observed. Some GC, instead of a reticular structure, possess a partially or completely homogenous, acidophilic cytoplasm, and may represent young GC (Epstein 1924b), or cells which were particularly well preserved during fixing (Pick 1926). In general, mitochondria are not seen on light microscopy, but electronmicroscopic studies by Fisher and Reidbord (1962) resulted in the unequivocal demonstration of mitochondria located within round, oval or irregularly shaped cytoplasmic bodies which probably develop as a result of the metamorphosis to GC. These cytoplasmic bodies, which are surrounded by a fine membrane, contain osmiophilic, thin-walled tubuli with diameters of 250—275 A, and are, according to these authors, responsible for the cytoplasmic striations observed by PICK. Histochemical properties suggest that they contain the cerebroside-protein complex (DEMARCH and KAUTZ 1957, FISHER and REIDBORD 1962). The presence of small amounts of neutral fat is

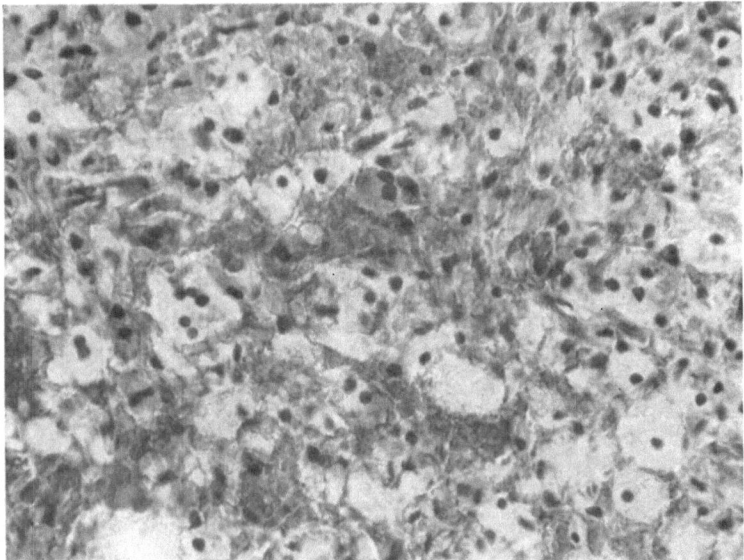

Fig. 1. Gaucher cells from bone marrow (LETTERER 1939)

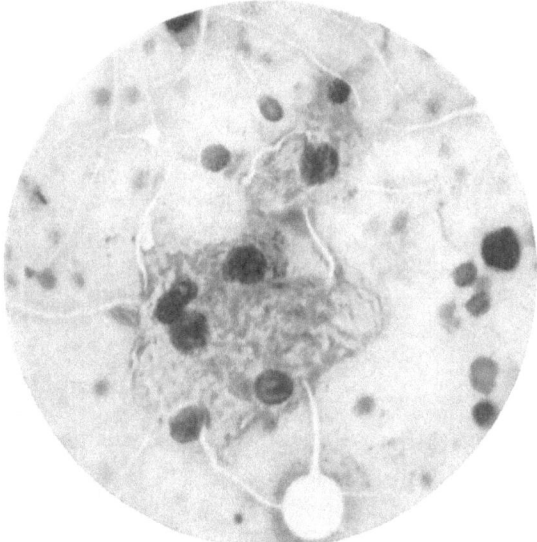

Fig. 2. So-called Pick cell in a biopsy specimen of spleen (PICK 1926)

suggested by the results of oil red-O staining. A negative peracetic acid Schiff reaction points to lack of unsaturated fatty acids which is in agreement with chemical analyses showing a predominance of lignoceric, behenic and palmitic acids among the visceral cerebroside fatty acids. A further significant histochemical finding is the high activity of an acid phosphatase (CROCKER and LANDING 1960, FISHER and

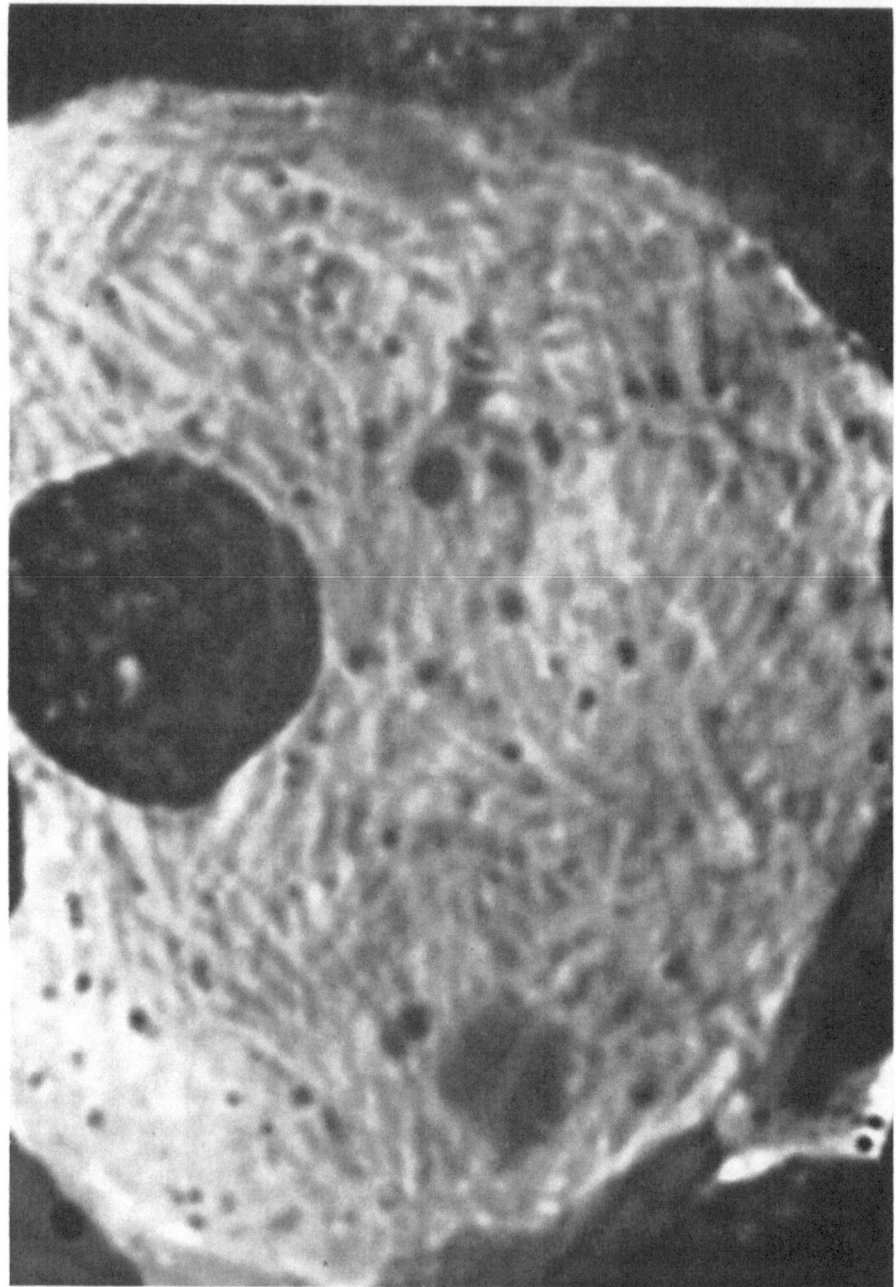

Fig. 3. "Gaucher cell" in chronic leukemia (Reproduced by courtesy of Dr. Marianne Albrecht, Berlin)

Reidbord 1962),which, according to Czitober et al. (1964), can be demonstrated in 80% of the GC. During the deposition of cerebrosides the viscosity of the cytoplasm increases (Erf 1938).

The formation of GC from reticulum cells appears to be established (Schlagen-haufer 1907, Risel 1909, Mandlebaum and Downey 1916, Kraus 1920, Bloom

1925, OBERLING 1926, PICK 1933). In addition, osteoblasts and fibroblast-like spindle cells of the bone marrow (BLOCK and JACOBSON 1948) and adventitial cells and histiocytes store cerebrosides and become GC (PICK 1926).

GÖTT and PEXA (1964), with the use of a method described by KLIMA et al. (1956), could demonstrate numerous GC in the circulating blood of an affected adult.

According to morphologic and cytochemical properties of these cells, two cell types could be differentiated: type I, representing the classical GC, with a fibrillar structure, and type II, with a granular or amorphous cytoplasm as described earlier by ALLEMANN (1941), LÜDIN (1950), ROSENSZAJN and EFRATI (1961), FÖDISCH (1962). A transformation of type I in type II may result from crystallization of the cerebroside.

Of great interest are recent reports on the occurrence of "GC" in the bone marrow of patients with chronic myelocytic leukemia, where they were found in 12 of 68 cases by ALBRECHT (1965) (see figure 3). Should this be confirmed by chemical and ultrastructural analyses, the position of the GC as pathognomonic for GD will have to be reexamined.

Spleen

Since GAUCHER's first case report, splenomegaly has been the leading clinical sign. Only about ten cases without enlargement of the spleen have been described (ERF 1938, LEVINE and SOLIS-COHEN 1943, PETIT and SCHLEICHER 1943, FIENBERG and QUIGLEY 1946, MORGANS 1947, BLOCK and JACOBSON 1948, REICH et al. 1951, SNAPPER 1957, BRINN and GLABMAN 1962).

The organ is usually larger than in Niemann-Pick disease, with an average weight of 2700 gm in (24) adults and 1800 gm in (7) children aged 5—14 years (PICK 1926). Weights of 6250 gm in a 6 year-old girl (BOVAIRD 1900) and 8100 gm ($^1/_6$ of the body weight!) in a 37 year-old patient (BRILL et al. 1905/13) have been reported. Pressure on the left kidney may result in renal atrophy (MIENZIL 1924), and compression of the ureter may produce hydronephrosis. Renal involvement has also been reported by HORSLEY et al. (1935). In spite of such enormous splenic enlargement, perisplenitis and spontaneous rupture are rare.

The surface of the spleen is smooth or slightly nodular. The capsule is tight and may show areas of thickening and adhesions in chronic cases. On cross section the organ appears greyish-red, brick-red or purple (GAUCHER 1882). A brownish coloration may result from deposition of iron pigments. Grossly, clusters of GC have a greyish pink color; they can be seen as numerous spots or may be confluent and result in the formation of a dense network. Larger foci can result from infarctions, necrosis, conglomerate tubercles or cavernous cavities which are filled with blood and may have diameters up to 4 cm (PICK 1926).

The microscopic picture is one of extensive derangement of the normal architecture by GC which had led GAUCHER to assume that the splenic tissue was completely destroyed, while PICK (1926) thought that the diminution of the normal pulp was only a relative one and resulted from the enormous enlargement of the organ. GC occur in alveolar clusters within the splenic pulp, are occasionally confluent and either surrounded by fine collagenous fibers (EVANS 1916) or by layers of flattened, endothelium-like cells. Not uncommonly small arteries are enclosed by GC clusters which infiltrate the arterial wall to the media. The absolute number of Malpighian bodies is usually not decreased (PICK 1926/33). Here, nests of GC include occasionally erythrocytes, lymphocytes and plasma cells. Whether or not GC are capable of phagocytosis is not clear. GC undergoing necrosis are replaced by nodes of a firm, fibrous tissue.

Early histologic studies have already shown the deposition of pigments, which probably result from increased breakdown of red cells and which are absent only in infants. The pigment is found in the trabecles, in endothelial cells and in GC. Hypersplenism from the disease process may contribute to anemia.

Liver

Hepatomegaly is relatively less prominent in GD than splenomegaly. The average liver weight of the adult patients collected by PICK was 3300 gm. Occasionally gross abnormalities of this organ may be absent in all age groups. In other cases a liver of normal size may show the surface changes and the histologic abnormalities of GD. Typically, the liver is firm, the margin is rounded and the surface nodular, particularly in children (HOWLAND and RICH 1926). In chronic cases signs of perihepatitis may be found.

On cross sections the color of the liver is pink to brownish-red. Small, light grey or yellow colored spots or irregular streaks form a network which in some instances resembles leukemic infiltrations. The affected areas impart a granular appearance to the cut surface and may reach diameters up to 3 cm. In spite of the similarity to morphologic findings in cirrhosis, the clinical signs of atrophic or hypertrophic cirrhosis are not observed (GAUCHER 1882). Portal hypertension does not develop (GAUCHER 1882; COLLIER 1895; EPSTEIN 1924 b; CUSHING and STOUT 1926; BÜRGER 1934; EPPINGER 1938), and portal vein thrombosis is rare (PICK 1926/33). When ascites occurred it was usually secondary to tuberculous peritonitis (MIENZIL 1924) or to extensive parenchymal infiltration of the liver by GC (MORRISON and LANE 1955).

The microscopic picture is determined by the extent to which infiltration with GC occurs. In infants, these are found mainly in the central parts of the liver lobules (PICK 1926/33), in adults they are located more peripherally. GC clusters in capillaries may cause atrophy of parenchymal cells. As a rule, bile duct proliferations are not observed (BRILL and MANDLEBAUM 1903). Although structural changes are rarely observed in the Gaucher liver (DIEZEL 1957), there may be a tendency of the GC which occur in the portal spaces to formation of a syncytium associated with connective tissue proliferation. Impairment of the lobular structure may then be seen, and parenchymal areas may become enclosed by connective tissue and GC. As in the case of the spleen, GC in the liver may be gradually replaced by callous scar tissue with central calcifications. The appearance of GC within the lumen of portal vein branches, as found frequently by MANDLEBAUM (1912), was only rarely observed by BOVAIRD (1900) and by RISEL (1909) and not et all by PICK (1926). The amount of pigment in parenchymal cells and Kupffer cells is related to the duration of the disease. In advanced cases hemosiderin is deposited in the portal spaces and around small blood vessels. Iron-free pigments are also seen, but may have no relation to the disease (PICK 1926).

In view of the morphologic changes which can be observed, there is surprisingly little impairment of liver function. Decreased clearance as evidenced by abnormalities of the bromthalein test (LEVIN 1961, GÖTT and PEXA 1964) can exist, and the bleeding tendency, although primarily on the basis of thrombocytopenia, may be enhanced through impairment of the metabolism of clotting factors.

Lymph Nodes

Involvement of lymph nodes is not obligatory in GD. Changes are more frequent in intrathoracic and intraabdominal nodes, and palpable lymph node enlargement is usually restricted to infants and small children. Nodes with a diameter greater than 2 cm are rare (PICK 1926). Since microscopic abnormalities have been observed in grossly normal lymph nodes (PICK 1926), examination of peripheral nodes does represent a valuable aid for diagnosis.

Involved nodes are smooth and soft, and the cut surface in infants and children has a pale-pink to greyish-brown color. Darker coloration is observed in adults through deposition of pigments and hemorrhage; nodes may then be brown or almost black. GC clusters form a network of light grey spots and streaks. A white color of involved nodes (RISEL 1909) has been interpreted (BARAT 1921) to result from compression of lymph and blood vessels by masses of GC.

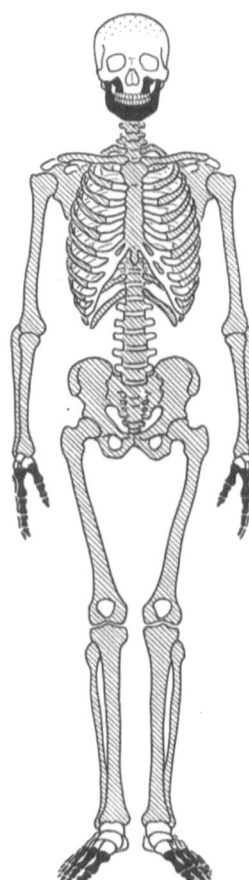

On histologic examination GC are usually found between the cells of the follicles in the medullary portions, and occasionally form long syncytia in the sinuses. The abnormalities may be limited to one segment of the node. EVANS (1916) saw GC mainly in the germinal centers, accompanied by fragmentation of lymphocytes, similar to findings in the Malpighian bodies of the spleen. In more advanced cases the supporting structure of the nodes becomes thickened, while the parenchymal cells may be almost completely replaced by accumulation of GC. When these undergo necrosis they form confluent masses with a particular hyalinous texture. The fibrous induration which is observed in spleen and liver does not take place in lymph nodes. Various stages of histologic changes may exist simultaneously. MANDLEBAUM (1912/19) has described myeloid elements (eosinophile and neutrophile myelocytes and polymorphonuclear eosinophils) in affected nodes. Occasionally the distinction is difficult between GC which contain red cells, and enlarged epithelial cells of the sinuses.

Iron-containing pigments are usually present in increased amounts, and located in reticular macrophages as well as in GC. Extracellular pigment may occur in more advanced cases.

Bones and Bone Marrow

Fig. 4. Distribution of bone lesions in GD. Black: most frequently involved. Hatched: less frequently involved. Dotted: rarely involved (SCHETTLER 1955)

The bone marrow frequently contains deposits of GC which may occur in grossly normal areas (BRILL 1905, SCHLAGENHAUFER 1907, MANDLEBAUM 1919). Most commonly affected are the phalanges of fingers and toes, vertebral bodies, ribs, sternum, pelvis, long bones of the extremities and mandibula, while the skull is usually unremarkable (see figure 4). The deposits appear as scattered light grey foci or streaks which have a firmer consistency than the red marrow. They are usually distinctly outlined in the spongiosa of the epiphyses and the sternum, where biopsy represents a valuable aid for the diagnosis (see figures 1 and 5).

The microscopic picture is characterized by the simultaneous existence of various stages of the disease process. A whole spectrum of changes, from the finding of only a few GC to almost complete replacement of the marrow, may be seen, and a relation of the changes to the duration of the disease is not apparent. The lipid-storing cells are usually located in the centers of the marrow spaces while the remaining hematopoetic tissue is restricted to the areas adjacent to the bone

spicules. The marrow which abuts upon GC nests is normal with the exception
of an increase in the plasma cell content which may be stimulated by the abnormal
marrow elements. Here, particulary, is a tendency of GC to elongation (Brill
1905, Mandlebaum 1919) and the longitudinal fibers are well seen. Occasionally
GC are found within dilated capillaries. Callous scar tissue may develop resembling
that in liver and spleen.

The deposition of pigments is less marked in the bone marrow than in other
organs, and not correlated with severity and duration of the disease.

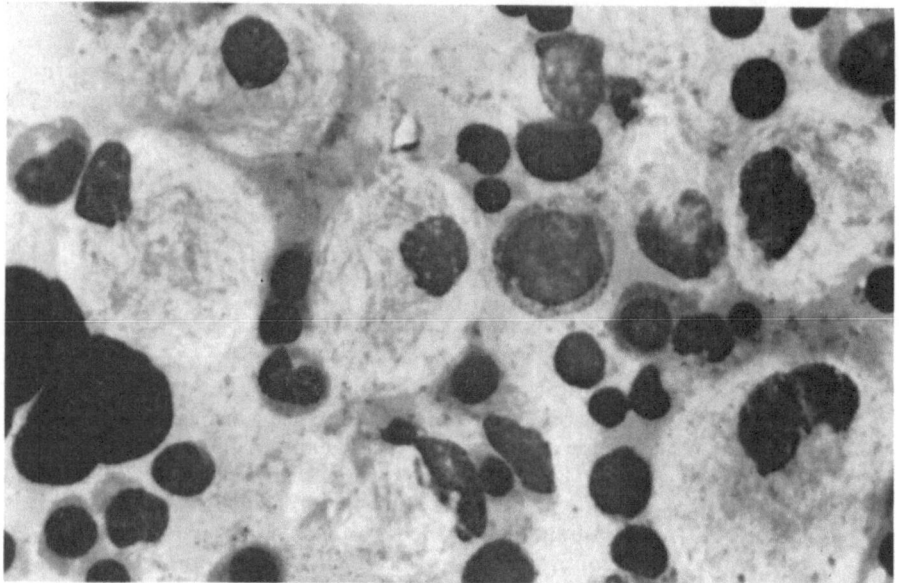

Fig. 5. GD. Bone marrow. HE-stain. Enlargement 900-fold. Reticulum cells are transformed to Gaucher
cells and store cerebrosides which impart to the cytoplasm a "crumbled tissue paper" appearance.
(Reproduced by courtesy of Prof. P. B. Diezel)

Marked bone marrow abnormalities are reflected in impairment of hematopoetic function. In addition, the mechanical stability of the skeleton will be decreased. Findings of this nature have led Pick (1926) to separate an "osseous"
type of GD from the general form. A frequent deformity of the femur is the development of an Erlenmeyer flask-like shape resulting from expansion of the cortex
in its lower portion. Spontaneous fractures occur depending on the extent of
structural abnormality and the exerted strain. Destruction of vertebrae may result
in gibbus formation. An aseptic osteomyelitis with painful swelling, redness and
bone destruction may occur (Yossipovitch et al. 1965) and GC may be found
in the drainage fluid (Gordon 1950).

A favorable effect of X-ray treatment on acute bone pain and the regression
of a large cystic area has been reported (Davies 1952). However, in the majority
of cases irradiation does not significantly affect the typical abnormalities of bone
and bone marrow (Schettler 1955).

Of particular interest is a possible relation of bone changes to splenectomy.
In patients classified as belonging to a special "juvenile" form, characterized by
a chronic course with late development of mental retardation, Herrlin and
Hillborg (1962) observed the development of visible bone changes consistently
within 3 to 3½ years after splenectomy, and independently of the time of surgery,

which was performed between 1½ and 12 years after onset of the disease. They suggest that splenectomy, eliminating the major organ of the RES, puts the load of storage to a greater degree on liver and bone marrow. Similar observations were reported by MATOTH and FRIED (1965).

Other Organs

PICK (1926) has called the "consistent limitation of abnormal findings to spleen, liver, lymph nodes and bone marrow" the most striking morphologic feature of GD. In the meantime exceptions to this rule, particularly in infants, have been described. Almost complete replacement of the thymus tissue by GC with concomitant GC deposition in the lymphatic tissue of the bowel was seen by RUSCA (1921). Since, however, deposition of lipids in reticulum cells of the thymus may also be observed in infants with nutritional problems or infections (LUBARSCH 1918), these cells may be mistaken for GC. Enlargement of the thymus in GD may occur without formation of GC.

Involvement of the lungs in adult patients has been reported on several occasions (MARKLEN et al. 1933, HERNDON and BENDER 1950), and in one case GC were found in the sputum (MARKLEN et al. 1933). HORSLEY et al. (1935) saw GC in the kidneys of an adult patient, and BANKER, MILLER and CROCKER (1962) found GC in the adrenals of several cases.

Central Nervous System

While, in general, no abnormalities can be found in the brains of affected adults (an exception is the patient described by TEILUM (1944), where pituitary gland and hypothalamus were involved) histologic and occasionally even gross changes are consistently seen in the acute, infantile cases. In these, the weight of the brain is frequently diminished (BANKER et al. 1962) due to generalized or partial cortical atrophy (mainly of the frontal and occipital cortex, LANDOLT et al. 1948). In addition, decrease in the size of thalamus and basal ganglia may occur (BANKER et al. 1961).

On microscopic examination, abnormalities of ganglion cells and the occurrence of Gaucher cells can be seen, but descriptions of such findings vary considerably. Histologic changes are rarely generalized and seem to prevail in the cerebellum, in some nuclei and in circumscribed cortical areas, while pons, diencephalon, and spinal cord are involved to a lesser degree (see figure 6).

NORMAN et al. (1956) distinguished three groups of neuropathological changes in GD: 1) nonspecific signs of degeneration without storage of lipid, 2) preponderance of nonspecific changes with scattered storage cells and 3) storage of lipid by all abnormal ganglion cells.

In three cases of BANKER et al. (1962) neuropathological changes consisted of a mild neuronal cytoplasmic accumulation of a glycolipid, nerve cell loss, and neuronophagia in the brain stem nuclei. In addition, there were foci of nerve cell loss in layers three and five of the cortex as well as infiltrates of Gaucher cells and microglia in these zones.

A detailed description of ganglion cell abnormalities in a case with involvement of the cerebellum has been given by SCHAIRER (1948). There was marked glial proliferation in place of the nucleus dentatus, where most of the ganglion cells had disappeared. The remaining ones showed a spectrum of abnormalities, from distention over loss of Nissl substance and vacuolation to shrinkage and necrosis. Many ganglion cells showed metachromasia. The myelin sheaths may be preserved (SCHAIRER 1948) or may show signs of demyelination (BANKER et al. 1961/62).

For many years GC were not found in the central nervous system, until Teilum (1944), Bird (1948) and later others (Debré et al. 1951, Barlow 1957) unequivocally demonstrated their presence. When they occur they are found either isolated within the brain tissue or in connection with the adventitia of small blood vessels, as emphasized by Barlow (1957) and by Diezel (1957), who showed in 1960 that they contained cerebrosides. GC may cause insufficient oxygenation of brain tissue by interference with vascular dilatation and with diffusion (Herrlin and Hillborg 1962), but they can hardly account for the majority of

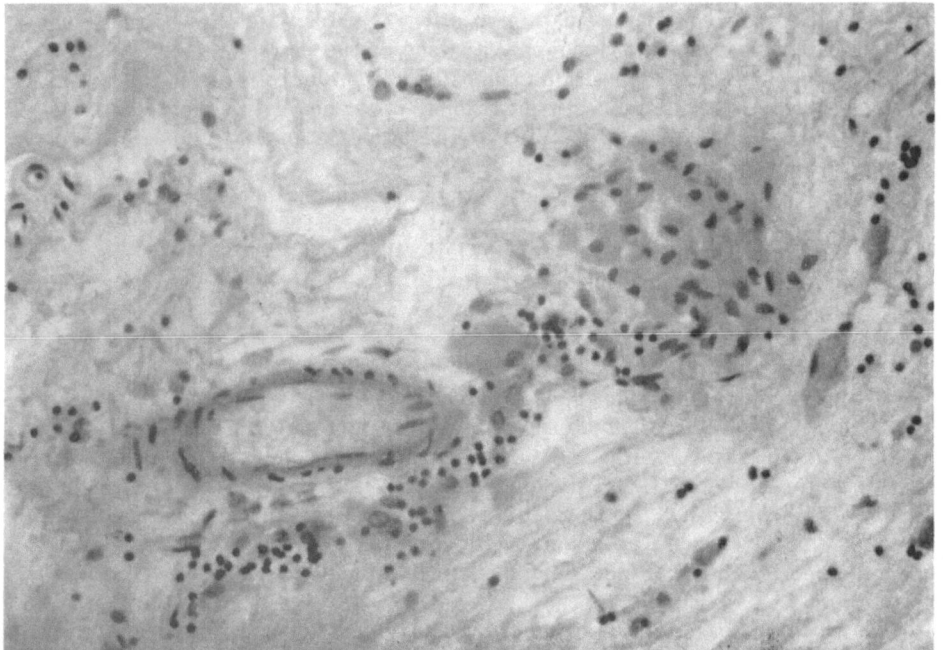

Fig. 6. GD. Cerebral white matter. HE-stain. Enlargement 300-fold. Adventitial cells store cerebrosides and are converted to Gaucher cells. (Reproduced by courtesy of Prof. P. B. Diezel)

the central nervous system symptoms which must have their basis in abnormalities of ganglion cells (Schairer 1948). Even then a considerable discrepancy frequently exists between the neurologic symptomatology on one hand and the morphologic findings on the other, which may be normal in spite of clinically severe central nervous system involvement (Woringer 1934, Rodgers and Jackson 1951).

Results of Lipid Analyses
Serum Lipids

The increased cerebroside content of many tissues has stimulated numerous attempts to measure plasma cerebroside levels, but a lack of appropriate methods has hampered such studies until recently. Thus, Jones and Thannhauser did not find differences between Gaucher patients and normals with values of 1.23 and 1.83 mg per 100 ml respectively in two subjects with GD and 1.83 mg per 100 ml in the serum of a healthy person.

In 1958 Svennerholm determined the normal serum cerebroside level with newer methods and found a value of 4.36 ± 0.18 mg per 100 ml. The average serum cerebroside level in 6 splenectomized Gaucher patients was twice normal, namely

8.1 (range 5.9 to 9.9) mg per 100 ml (HILLBORG and SVENNERHOLM 1960). Further relevant data are obviously needed. The cerebroside content of red blood cells was likewise found by these authors to be elevated, although to a lesser degree than that of the serum and with a wide variation of values.

No abnormalities of other serum lipid fractions have been found.

Brain Lipids

Most available data are not comparable due to the different origins of analyzed tissue samples and to different methods of fixation. ROUSER et al. (1965) found a 50% decrease of the cerebroside content of the brain in a chronic case without

Table 1. *Lipid composition of cerebral cortex and white matter in Gaucher's disease**

	Cortex		White matter	
	patient 7 months	normals (6 cases) 4—5 years	patient 7 months	normals (6 cases) 4—5 years
Nitrogen	9,4	9.2 — 9.9	8.5	6.0 — 6.3
Hexosamine	0.82	0.70— 0.80	0.64	0.22— 0.30
Lipid hexosamine	0.18	0.15	0.11	0.05
Total lipids	28.1	28.0 —32.4	35.6	55.6 —61.9
Cholesterol	5.5	5.0 — 7.0	7.9	12.2 —15.7
Phospholipids	22.2	21.2 —25.6	23.0	28.0 —30.6
Sphingomyelins	1.2	1.7 — 2.8	1.8	4.1 — 5.2
Cephalins	10.0	8.5 —12.2	13.6	14.4 —16.5
Lecithins	9.3	8.5 —10.2	8.8	8.5 — 9.9
Cerebrosides	0.4	0.3 — 0.7	3.7	10.3 —13.8
Sulphatides	0.1	0.4 — 0.9	1.1	1.7 — 4.1

Values expressed as per cent of dry weight.
* Source: SVENNERHOLM (1963).

neurological involvement while MALONEY and CUMINGS (1960) reported increases in brain kerasin in juvenile patients. Most analyses in cases of children with prevailing brain symptoms resulted in the finding of a normal lipid content of the gray matter. Separate analyses of morphologically affected areas might have yielded the expected abnormal chemical findings.

The white matter shows a decrease in all lipid classes which is correlated with the severity of the clinical symptoms (BANKER et al. 1962). The findings are similar to those of the immature brains of newborn infants, and appear to result from impairment of myelination rather than from defects in the maintenance of myelin, as in Tay-Sachs disease (BANKER et al. 1962). A decreased cholesterol content of the white matter is uniformly found (see table 1).

Tissue Lipids

Complete analyses of tissue lipids have rarely been performed in GD. The few cases so studied had normal values with the exception of the glycolipid content (see table 2 and 3).

Elevation of cerebrosides predominates (KLENK 1940), other glycolipids, which occur in trace amounts in normal tissues and which are probably intermediates of cerebroside synthesis, have recently received increasing attention (KLENK and RENNKAMP 1942, PARKE 1954, RAPPORT et al. 1960, MAKITA and YAMAKAWA 1962, STATTER and SHAPIRO 1963, SVENNERHOLM and SVENNERHOLM 1963). The increase in cerebroside content is more marked in the spleen than in the liver. Data from two cases examined by THANNHAUSER and REINSTEIN are as follows: Spleen cerebrosides 6.65 and 6.2 mg per 100 mg respectively (normal 0.2—0.6), and liver cerebrosides (one case only) 5.93 mg per 100 mg (normal 0.2—0.6). Cerebrosides in kidneys, lungs and heart could not be measured. Aballi and Kato (1938) found a 10- to 12-fold increase in the proportion of cerebrosides in liver and spleen lipids, and a slight elevation of total phospholipids and cholesterol. There is an increased cerebroside content of a number of tissues besides spleen, liver, bone marrow and lymph nodes in the acutely progressing infantile cases (Ottenstein et al. 1948, Thannhauser 1953/58, Banker et al. 1962).

Table 2. *Lipids of the spleen in infantile and adult patients with Gaucher's disease*

Age	Values are expressed as per cent of fresh weight		Values are expressed as per cent of dry weight			
	5 patients (pooled)* 3, 7, 8, 9 and 16 months	normal range*	patient** 7 months	patient** 18 months	patient** 40 years	normal range from 3 infants** 2 months
Total lipids	4.35	2.0—3.5	10.9	12.4	10.2	7.8 —8.8
Cholesterol	0.30	0.3—0.4	1.7	1.7	1.3	1.5 —1.8
Phospholipids	1.48	1.0—2.0	5.0	6.1	5.1	5.9 —6.6
Sphingomyelins	0.52	0.1—0.5	1.0	1.2	1.2	1.1 —1.2
Cephalins	—	—	2.2	1.7	2.3	2.2 —2.8
Lecithins	—	—	1.7	2.5	1.7	2.1 —2.7
Glycolipids	1.88	0.2—0.6	—	—	—	—
Cerebrosides	—	—	4.2	4.6	3.8	0.15—0.19
Sulphatides	—	—	0.03	0.02	0.02	0.20

Source: * Banker et al. (1962), ** Svennerholm (1963).

Apparently, the increase of glycolipid concentration, in particular that of cerebrosides, in various organs other than the brain, is dependent on the duration of the disease. While Banker et al. (1962) found 2.9 (2.6—3.5) per cent cerebrosides in the spleens and 2.0 (1.4—2.7) per cent in the livers of six children with the chronic form, the respective values for three infantile cases were 1.98 (1.58—2.35) and 1.42 (1.24—1.63). The glycolipid content of the lungs was 0.98 (0.57—1.47) per cent and thus only slightly elevated (normal 0.2—0.6). All data are as per cent of fresh weight. Philippart et al. (1965), in four cases, found the cerebrosides of the spleen to be increased 400- to 750-fold; other glycolipids were elevated to a lesser degree: hematosides (ceramide-glucose-galactose-N-acetylneuraminic acid) 8- to 15-fold, cytosides (ceramide-glucose-galactose) 1.3- and 4.2-fold (see table 3).

A very low concentration of sulfatides in Gaucher spleens was observed by Svennerholm (1963).

Chemistry of the Stored Cerebroside

The abundance of cerebrosides in the various organs of affected subjects facilitates isolation and analysis, in contrast to tissues of normals except the central nervous system. Obviously, knowledge of the nature of the stored cerebroside is of key importance for studies on the pathogenesis of GD. There are several possibilities for structural abnormalities of the cerebroside molecule, namely: 1) an abnormal sphingosine, 2) an abnormal fatty acid pattern, 3) an atypical sugar or its atypical binding to sphingosine and 4) atypical physico-chemical properties of the naturally occurring form of the molecule (as lipoprotein ?). The first three possibilities are now within the realm of available methods whereas the last one cannot yet be studied properly.

Sphingosine

Besides sphingosine, dihydrosphingosine occurs normally in varying amounts in cerebrosides and other sphingolipids. This contribution of dihydrosphingosine is probably less in GD and, for instance, ROSENBERG and CHARGAFF (1958) did not find any dihydrosphingosine in the spleen of an 8 year-old boy.

In GD, as in normals, the double bond of the sphingosine moiety is located between C-4 and C-5 in trans-configuration.

Table 3. *Chemical composition of spleen in Gaucher's disease*

Spleen	I	II	III	IV	Normal control
	(Values expressed as per cent of dry weight)				
Total lipids	32.7	47.8	11.2	24.7	12.3
Lipids-proteolipids protein	27.1	43.8	10.5	20.2	9.9
	(As per cent of lipids-proteolipids protein)*				
Cholesterol, free	8.5	6.8	8.7	7.2	24.4
Cholesterol, esterified	trace	0.7	trace	0.6	—
Total phospholipids	53.9	27.7	39.0	34.4	70.2
Sphingomyelin**	15.6	2.9	7.6	10.2	13.1
Cerebrosides***	24.4	45.7	23.4	32.4	0.06
Cytosides***	—	0.71	0.22	—	0.17
Hematosides***	—	0.24	—	—	0.3
N-acetyl-neuraminic acid	—	0.32	0.59	0.44	0.04

* All values have been expressed in terms of the weight of lipid after cleavage of proteo-lipids and removal of proteolipid protein.
** Calculated from alkali stable phosphorus x 26.2.
*** Purified.
Source: PHILIPPART et al. (1965).

While normally cerebroside sphingosine is present in the erythro-form with regard to the substituents at C-2 (N-acyl residue) and at C-3 (hydroxyl group), the sphingomyelin which is stored in Niemann-Pick disease was found in the threo-form (CUMINGS 1962). Threo-sphingosine does not occur in GD (CARTER et al. 1961).

Of interest are recent observations in a variety of mammals on an homologous sphingosine with 20 carbon atoms instead of 18 (PROSTENIK and MAJHOFER-ORESCANIN 1960, WICHA 1962, ERLAÇIN 1963). The C-20 sphingosine has now been found in minute quantities in normal human sphingolipids, but not in spleen cerebrosides of cases with GD (SUOMI and AGRANOFF 1965). The trace amounts of an unknown base with a higher number of carbon atoms which have been found in the central nervous system (RADIN and AKAHORI 1961) were possibly this homologous C-20 sphingosine.

Fatty Acid Pattern

Early studies of the cerebroside fatty acids have not shown significant differences from normal. Reevaluation of this question after the introduction of gas-liquid chromatography yielded somewhat different results. The Gaucher ceramide glucoside has a higher proportion of saturated longer-chain fatty acids and less unsaturated fatty acids than non-Gaucher ceramide glucoside, and the fatty acids consist mainly of palmitic, behenic and lignoceric acids. Most recent analyses of the cerebroside fatty acid pattern in GD are largely in agreement (see table 4).

Extensive studies of the sphingomyelin fatty acids of brain lipids by STÄLLBERG-STENHAGEN and SVENNERHOLM (1965) have shown that there is a common abnormality in all infantile cases of hereditary disorders of lipid metabolism in that the fatty acid pattern is similar to that found normally in the immature brain. This is reflected in a higher proportion of stearic acid (normally about 80 % in the newborn and 40% in adults) and a lesser proportion of the C-22 to C-26 fatty acids (normally approximately 10% in the newborn and 50% in adults). Similar studies for the brain tissue of adult Gaucher patients are lacking at present.

Table 4. *Spleen cerebroside fatty acids in Gaucher's disease*

Fatty acids	6 spleens (pooled)*	normal (average of 2 spleens)*	1 spleen (♀ 50 years)**	normal***
C_{14}	0.5	0.7	—	—
C_{16}	23.5	29.5	20	16.7
C_{17}	0.7	0.6	—	—
C_{18}	5.3	7.6	3	9.3
$C_{18:1}$	0.1	6.2	—	—
C_{19}	0.2	1.0	—	—
C_{20}	3.8	2.7	3	8.5
C_{21}	0.1	0.8	—	★
C_{22}	20.7	12.6	27	32.0
C_{23}	13.5	6.6	—	★
C_{24}	21.9	14.7	46	24.1
$C_{24:1}$	9.7	16.5	—	★

Values in mole per cent of total fatty acids recovered.
Source: * Suomi and Agranoff (1965); ** Marinetti et al. (1959); *** Wagner (1964).
★ 9.4 mole per cent of long-chain fatty acids were not identified. They were probably unsaturated fatty acids with chain lengths between C_{20} and C_{24}.

Hexose

The important question of the sugar component in the stored spleen cerebrosides has only recently been settled, whereas numerous studies before have given conflicting answers: Thus, glucose was found to be the main constituent by Halliday et al. 1940, Klenk 1940, Klenk and Rennkamp 1942, Danielson et al. 1942, Landolt et al. 1948, Sacks and Andersch 1946, Brante 1951, Halliday 1950, Devor et al. 1958, galactose by Lieb 1924, Mai 1933, Lieb 1941, and finally both sugars by Montreuil et al. 1953, Parke 1954, Uzman 1953, Woolf 1954, Schatz 1962. These have been summarized in a table by Fredrickson (1960). The confusion concerning the nature of the hexose present as the carbohydrate of Gaucher cerebrosides was increased by the report of a patient with glucose-cerebrosides, having a sibling with galacto-cerebrosides (Ottenstein et al. 1948).

Progress in methodology, in particular the use of chromatography, infrared spectroscopy and specific enzymatic methods (glucose oxidase) have now decided this controversy in favor of storage in GD of a glucocerebroside (Klenk 1955, Carter et al. 1961, Makita and Yamakawa 1962, Svennerholm and Svennerholm 1963, Suomi and Agranoff 1965, Statter and Shapiro 1965, Philippart and Menkes 1964), more specifically a D-glucose-cerebroside with beta-glycosidic binding (Neeley 1957, Rosenberg and Chargaff 1958). The conclusion that ceramide galactoside is present in Gaucher spleens, appears to be the result of analytical errors (Suomi and Agranoff 1965). In all respects the Gaucher cerebrosides are similar to glucocerebrosides which occur in traces normally.

Pathogenetic Considerations

The basic lesion in Gaucher's disease has not yet been elucidated. The storage of cerebrosides, and their identification as glucocerebrosides have stimulated intensive studies on a possible abnormality of cerebroside metabolism. These have been aided by new information regarding the normal metabolism of cerebrosides and other glycolipids which has become available during the last few years. On the other hand, the pathogenetic significance of a number of other recent findings such as the elevation of the acid serum phosphatase, is still completely unknown.

Consideration of a primary defect in cerebroside metabolism calls for answers to the following questions: 1) is there only a quantitative disturbance, i.e. a balance problem between cerebroside synthesis and breakdown, or 2) is there a qualitative abnormality of cerebroside metabolism. evidenced by a) the finding of an abnormal cerebroside and/or b) an abnormal relation between various cerebrosides which are defined by their sugar and fatty acid moieties respectively, and 3) is the presumed metabolic error limited to certain cells, i.e. cells which are to become GC, or is it a general feature of all cells with the ability to synthesize and metabolize cerebrosides.

Support for the thesis (PICK 1926) that in the lipid storage of GD uptake from circulating blood plays a part comes from the recent finding of elevated plasma cerebroside levels (SVENNERHOLM and SVENNERHOLM 1963). However, such determinations are beyond the capacity of most laboratories and have therefore been performed only in a very small number of subjects. It appears possible that all cells which synthesize cerebrosides spill any excess into the circulating blood from where it is then taken up and stored by reticulum cells, histiocytes etc. Tissues like spleen, liver, bone marrow and lymph nodes, which are those chiefly affected in GD, contain the majority of cells with the ability for storage. In addition, the capacity of the blood to keep cerebrosides in solution appears to be quite small. Further support for passive storage of cerebrosides resulting from elevated plasma levels comes from observations of HILLBORG and ESTBORN (1964), who described the development of skeletal changes in relation to splenectomy. The absence of the main storage organ may result in compensatory increase of storage by other tissues to effect the removal of excess cerebrosides.

According to information available to date a fundamental abnormality of the cerebroside molecule can be excluded as a cause for cerebroside storage (TRAMS and BRADY 1960, ROSENBERG and CHARGAFF 1958, SUOMI and AGRANOFF 1965). Glucocerebrosides, although normally present only in trace amounts in visceral organs, are nevertheless a normal constituent of the body, in addition to the prevailing galactocerebrosides in the brain.

As regards the cerebroside fatty acid pattern, deviations from the normal proportion have been described in GD (see table 4 and page 277). It is possible that in GD glycolipids accumulate as a result of an unknown primary cause. Cleavage of complex lipids leads to products which are progressively less soluble, and as tissue lipid levels increase, deposition in reticulum foam cells occurs at a rate in excess of hydrolytic degradation. This process would cause preferential deposition of less polar (saturated and long-chain fatty acids) ceramide glycosides (SUOMI and AGRANOFF 1965).

From evidence available it seems most likely that the basic disturbance in GD is located at some enzymatic step in cerebroside biosynthesis or breakdown (see figure 7). According to present knowledge, cerebrosides are normally formed from larger glycosphingolipids, the majority of which may originate in red cells. Increased formation from these precursors may result from deletion of normal feedback control; on the other hand accumulation of cerebrosides may result from a decreased rate of catabolism.

There are several studies supporting the latter possibility. BRADY's (1963) proposal that an enzymatic defect resulted in impairment of cleavage of the ceramide-glucose bond of the cerebrosides, was supported by studies on cerebrosides of affected spleens by Philippart et al. (1965) who found, in addition to large amounts of glucocerebroside, an increased content of cytoside (ceramide-glucose-galactose) which appears to be the immediate precursor of cerebrosides. Furthermore, the intermediate hematoside (ceramide-glucose-galactose-N-acetyl-neuraminic acid) was found to be increased. Earlier, Philippart and Menkes (1964) identified the increased ganglioside of GD mainly as the type A ganglioside and both, ganglioside A and hematoside, may be responsible for the increase in N-acetyl neuraminic acid (NANA) found in the Gaucher spleen.

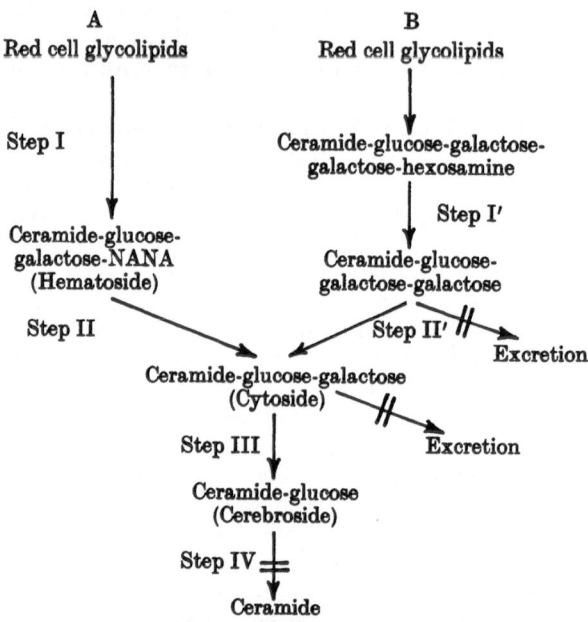

Fig. 7. Degradation of red cell glycolipids and formation of cerebrosides. Pathway A proposed by Philippart et al. (1965); pathway B proposed by Statter and Shapiro (1965). The suspected location of the lesion in Gaucher's disease is at step IV

Since NANA was not found in red cell lipids by Yamakawa and Suzuki (1953), Suomi and Agranoff (1965) suggested a different pathway for the formation of glucocerebroside. In place of the hematoside precursor of Philippart et al. (1964/65) they consider the globoside ceramide-glucose-galactose-galactose-N-acetyl-galactosamine to be the precursor of glucocerebrosides. This theory would not explain the accumulation of NANA containing compounds in GD, but synthesis of cerebrosides from red cell glycolipids could explain some aspects of the chronicity of GD; since the glycolipid content of red cells is only 2% of the stroma lipids (Yamakawa et al. 1960), lipid material derived therefrom would accumulate very slowly.

Support for a lack of a glucocerebroside-cleaving enzyme comes from studies by Brady et al. (1965) with a 1—^{14}C labeled glucocerebroside. Purified splenic extracts from Gaucher patients, and from subjects with congenital hemolytic anemia and idiopathic thrombopenic purpura were compared as regards the activities of the glucocerebroside-cleaving enzyme. Enzyme activity from Gaucher spleens was only $^1/_5$ to $^1/_{10}$ that of other splenic extracts. Similar are the findings of Patrick (1965); in addition, he found no evidence for the existence of an inhibitor of glucocerebrosidase in spleen in GD, or of an activator in control spleens.

The finding of a normal ceramide content of the Gaucher spleen may also be interpreted to result from interference in GD with cerebroside catabolism before this stage.

Among the unexplained features is the storage of glycolipid by the infantile brain in same cases of GD. Here the possiblity of an additional metabolic error exists. A case (JERVIS et al. 1962) where cytoside was the main splenic lipid instead of glucocerebroside (ROSENBERG 1962) may represent a variant of GD where the enzymetic defect is localized to the site of cleavage of cytoside to cerebroside (see figure 7).

Treatment

From the preceding discussion it is apparent that a causal therapy for GD is not available. Treatment will be symptomatic and/or directed against complications.

The possibility of dietary management is suggested by the clinical impression that "rich" food, abundant in meat and animal fat seems to hasten the development of the disease, whereas on "moderate" diets progress is slower (GROEN 1965). This possibility deserves further study. To prevent undernutrition by interference of hepatosplenomegaly with food intake, a dietary schedule with frequent small feedings should be instituted.

The question of splenectomy arises sooner or later in the course of most cases of Gaucher disease. Hematologic changes, in particular thrombocytopenia, have been the most common indication for splenectomy; occasionally the spleen was removed for alleviation of excessive pressure symptoms. While splenectomy is always followed by an immediate rise in platelet count (LOGAN 1941, THANNHAUSER 1950/58, MEDOFF and BAYRD 1954, SCHETTLER 1955, HERRLIN and HILLBORG 1962, MATOTH and FRIED 1965 and others) and cessation of the tendency to hemorrhage, there are indications that, following surgery, the liver may reach tremendous proportions (MATOTH and FRIED 1965), that frequency and severity of bone lesions may increase (HILLBORG and SVENNERHOLM 1960, HERRLIN and HILLBORG 1962, MATOTH and FRIED 1965), and that, in infants, central nervous system symptoms may be aggravated (HERRLIN and HILLBORG 1962, HILLBORG and ESTBORN 1964). On the other hand, follow-up studies by MEDOFF and BAYRD (1954) suggest some benefit of splenectomy on the survival of subjects with GD. Since in this study the decisions leading to splenectomy and the causes of death were not reported it can be of no assistance in a reevaluation of the indications for splenectomy. Awaiting further information it may be well to reserve surgery for cases with very low platelet counts and marked bleeding tendency. Anemia, as mentioned erlier, is usually moderate, and may, as in some of the 34 cases of MATOTH and FRIED (1965), improve with iron therapy or folic acid. Leukopenia, according to the same authors, seems of little importance clinically.

Decrease of splenic size and partial or complete disappearance of abdominal discomfort may result from x-ray therapy (MEDOFF and BAYRD 1954). In one case (WEINSCHENK 1964) long-term administration of B-vitamins, folic acid, methionin, choline and vitamin E was followed by decrease of hepatosplenomegaly (WEINSCHENK 1965) and this treatment is presently being evaluated in another case.

References

ABALLI, A. J., and K. KATO: Gaucher's disease in early infancy: review of literature and report of case with neurological symptoms. J. Pediat. 13, 364 (1938).

ABUL-FADL, M. A. M., and E. J. KING: Properties of the acid phosphatase of erythrocytes and of human prostate gland. Biochem. J. 45, 51 (1949).

Aghion, H.: La maladie de Gaucher dans l'enfance. Thèse, Paris 1934.

Albrecht, M.: Personal communication (1965).

— Gaucher-Zellen bei chronisch myeloischer Leukämie, in: Proceedings of the 10th Congress of the European Society of Haematology, Strasbourg, August 23—28, 1965. Basel-New York: Karger (in press).

Allemann, R.: Zur Diagnose und Therapie gleichzeitiger Milz- und Nierenerkrankungen. Z. Urol. 35, 225 (1941).

Atkinson, F. R. B.: Gaucher's disease in children. Brit. J. Child. Dis. 35, 1 (1938).

Banker, B. Q., J. Q. Miller, and A. C. Crocker: The neurological disorder in infantile Gaucher's disease. Trans. Amer. neurol. Ass. 86, 43 (1961).

— — — The cerebral pathology of infantile Gaucher's disease. In: Cerebral sphingolipidoses; S. M. Aronson, and B. W. Volk (eds.). New York: Academic Press 1962.

Barát, I.: Zur Histopathologie der großzelligen Splenomegalie Typus Gaucher. Fol. haemat. (Lpz.) 26, 303 (1921).

Barlow, C. F.: Neuropathologic findings in case of infantile Gaucher's disease. J. Neuropath. exp. Neurol. 16, 238 (1957).

Bird, A.: The lipidoses and the central nervous system. Brain 71, 434 (1948).

Block, M., and L. O. Jacobson: The histogenesis and diagnosis of the osseous type of Gaucher's disease. Acta haemat. (Basel) 1, 165 (1948).

Bloom, W.: Splenomegaly (type Gaucher) and lipoid-histiocytosis (type Niemann). Amer. J. Path. 1, 595 (1925).

Bonta, M. B.: Splenectomy in Gaucher's disease, case. Proc. Mayo Clin. 4, 262 (1929).

Bovaird jr., D.: Primary splenomegaly — endothelial hyperplasia of the spleen — two cases in children, autopsy and morphological examination in one. Amer. J. med. Sci. 120, 377 (1900).

— and F. S. Mandlebaum: cited by Marchand (1907).

Brady, R. O.: NATO Conference on the metabolism and physiological significance of lipids, R. M. C. Dawson, and D. N. Rhodes (eds.), Cambridge, England, September 1963, Jahn Wiley and Sons, Ltd., London (in press); cited by R. O. Brady, J. Kanfer, and D. Shapiro (1965).

— J. N. Kanfer, and D. Shapiro: The metabolism of glucocerebrosides. I. Purification and properties of a glucocerebroside cleaving enzyme from spleen tissue. J. biol. Chem. 240, 39 (1965).

— — — Metabolism of glucocerebrosides. II. Evidence of an enzymatic deficiency in Gaucher's disease. Biochem. Biophys. Res. Commun. 18, 221 (1965).

Brante, G.: Studies on the lipids in morbus Gaucher. I. Qualitative and quantitative determination of the hexose components in normal and Gaucher glycolipids. Acta Soc. Med. upsalien. 56, 125 (1951).

Brill, N.: Primary splenomegaly with a report of three cases occurring in one family. Amer. J. med. Sci. 121, 377 (1901).

— Large-cell splenomegaly (Gaucher's disease). Amer. J. med. Sci. 146, 863 (1903).

— F. S. Mandlebaum, and E. Libman: Primary splenomegaly — Gaucher-type. Report on one of four cases occurring in a single generation of one family. Amer. J. med. Sci. 129, 491 (1905).

— — — Primary splenomegaly of the Gaucher type. A report of the second of four cases occurring in a single generation of one family. Amer. J. med. Sci. 137, 849 (1909).

Brinn, L., and Sh. Glabman: Gaucher's disease without splenomegaly. Oldest patient on record, with review. N.Y.St. J. Med. 62, 2346 (1962).

Bürger, M.: Die Klinik der Lipoidosen. in: Neue deutsche Klinik, Bd. 12, Erg.-Bd. 2, (1934).

Carling, E. R., H. Carill, and R. J. Pulverkraft: Splenectomy in Gaucher's disease with hemoglobinuria. Proc. roy. Soc. Med. 26, 361 (1933).

Carter, H. E., J. A. Rothfus, and R. Gigg: Biochemistry of the sphingolipids: XII. Conversion of cerebrosides to ceramides and sphingosine. Structure of Gaucher cerebroside. J. Lipid Res. 2, 228 (1961).

Cazal, P.: Remarques sur la structure, l'histogenèse et la signification de la cellule de Gaucher. Sang. 16, 28 (1944).

Choisser, R. M., and R. R. Montgomery: Gaucher's disease in Negro: report of case. Amer. J. clin. Path. 19, 570 (1949).

Chung, H., K. Chin, S. Kwan, H. Weng, and C. Teng: Gaucher's disease. A report of the first case in China. China med. J. 66, 11 (1948).

Collier, W. A.: A case of enlarged spleen in a child aged six. Trans. Path. Soc. (Lond.) 46, 148 (1895).

Crefeld, S. van: The lipidoses. Advanc. Pediat. 6, 190 (1953).

Crocker, A. G., and B. H. Landing: Phosphatase studies in Gaucher's disease. Metabolism 9, 341 (1960).

CUMINGS, J. N.: Abnormalities in lipid metabolism in two members of a family with Niemann-Pick disease. in: Cerebral sphingolipidoses, S. ARONSON and B. W. VOLK (eds.), New York: Academic Press, 1962.

CUSHING, E. H., and A. P. STOUT: Gaucher's disease. Arch. Surg. 12, 539 (1926).

CZITOBER, H., E. GRÜNDIG, and B. SCHOBEL: Histochemische und biochemische Untersuchungen bei Morbus Gaucher. Klin. Wschr. 42, 1179 (1964).

DANIELSON, I. S., C. H. HALL, and M. R. EVERETT: Glucoside type of cerebroside in spleen in Gaucher's disease. Proc. Soc. exp. Biol. (N.Y.) 49, 569 (1942).

DANOPOULOS, E., and J. LOGOTHETOPOULOS: Klinische und hämatologische Beobachtungen an zwei familiären Fällen der Gaucherschen Krankheit. Dtsch. Arch. klin. Med. 201, 79 (1954).

DAVIDSOHN, L. W.: Ein Fall von Splenektomie bei der sogenannten Gaucherschen Krankheit. Langenbecks Arch. klin. Chir. 150, 537 (1928).

DAVIES, F. W. T.: Gaucher's disease in bone. J. Bone Jt Surg. 34-B, 454 (1952).

DAVIS, F. W., A. GENECIN, and E. W. SMITH: Gaucher's disease with thrombocytopenia, an instance of selective hypersplenism. Bull. Johns Hopk. Hosp. 84, 176 (1949).

DEBRÉ, R., I. BERTRAND, R. GRUMBACH and E. BARGETON: Maladie de Gaucher du nourrisson. Arch. franç. Pédiat. 8, 38 (1951).

DE MARSH, Q. B., and J. KAUTZ: The submicroscopic morphology of Gaucher cells. Blood 12, 324 (1957).

DEVOR, A. W., C. CONGER, and I. GILL: The use of resorcinol for identification and determination of monosaccharide groups: a report on a Gaucher spleen cerebroside. Arch. Biochem. 73, 20 (1958).

DIEZEL, P. B.: Die Stoffwechselstörungen der Sphingolipoide. Die Gauchersche Krankheit. Berlin-Göttingen-Heidelberg: Springer 1957.

— Lipidoses of the central nervous system. In: Modern Scientific Aspects of Neurology. J. N. CUMINGS (ed.). London: Edward Arnold Ltd. 1960.

— Die angeborenen Störungen des Lipoidstoffwechsels. In: Medizinische Grundlagenforschung, Bd. IV. Stuttgart: Thieme 1962.

EAST, T., and L. H. SAVIN: A case of Gaucher's disease with biopsy of typical pingueculae. Brit. J. Ophthal. 24, 611 (1940).

EPPINGER, H.: Die hepatolienalen Erkrankungen. Berlin: Springer 1920.

— Die Klinik der Lipoidosen. Verh. dtsch. path. Ges. 31, 51 (1938).

EPSTEIN, E.: Beitrag zur Chemie der Gaucherschen Krankheit. Biochem. Z. 145, 398 (1924a).

— Beitrag zur Pathologie der Gaucherschen Krankheit. Virchows Arch. path. Anat. 253, 157 (1924b).

— Beitrag zur Pathologie, Chemie und Systematik der Gaucherschen Krankheit. Wien. klin. Wschr. 1934c, 1179.

ERF, L. A.: Studies of Gaucher cells by supravital technique. Amer. J. med. Sci. 195, 144 (1938).

ERLAÇIN, S.: Über das Vorkommen des Sphingosins und seiner Homologen in den Sphingolipoiden des Gehirns. Dissertation, University of Cologne, 1963.

ESTBORN, B., and P.-O. HILLBORG: On the increased serum acid phosphatase in Gaucher's disease. Scand. J. clin. Lab. Invest. 12, 504 (1960).

EVANS, F. A.: Gaucher splenomegaly in a child. Proc. N.Y. path. Soc. 16, 114 (1916).

FIENBERG, R., and G. E. QUIGLEY: Osseous Gaucher's disease with macrocytic normochromic anemia. New Engl. J. Med. 234, 527 (1946).

FISHER, E. R., and H. REIDBORD: Gaucher's disease: pathogenetic considerations based on electron microscopic and histochemical observations. Amer. J. Path. 41, 679 (1962).

FÖDISCH, H. J.: Morbus Gaucher mit splenopathischer Markhemmung beim Erwachsenen. II. Pathologisch-anatomischer Teil. Wien. Z. inn. Med. 43, 334 (1962).

FREDRICKSON, D. S.: Cerebroside lipidosis: Gaucher's disease. In: The metabolic basis of inherited disease, J. B. STANBURY, J. B WYNGAARDEN, D. S. FREDRICKSON (eds.). New York-Toronto-London: McGraw-Hill 1966.

— and A. F. HOFMANN: Gaucher's disease. In: The metabolic basis of inherited disease, J. B. STANBURY, J. B. WYNGAARDEN, D. S. FREDRICKSON (eds.) New York-Toronto-London: McGraw-Hill 1960.

GÄNSSLEN, M.: Erbpathologie des Blutes und der blutbildenden Organe. In: Handb. d. Erbbiologie d. Menschen, Bd. 4, S. 411, Berlin: Springer 1940.

GAUCHER, P. C. E.: De l'epithélioma primitif de la rate. Thése, Paris 1882.

GERKEN, H., u. H.-R. WIEDEMANN: Ein Beitrag zur Genetik des Morbus Gaucher. Ann. paediat. (Basel) 203, 328 (1964).

GIAMPALMO, A.: Über die Pathologie der Gaucherschen Krankheit im frühen Kindesalter (mit besonderer Berücksichtigung der neurologischen Form). Acta paediat. (Uppsala) 37, 6 (1949).

— Über die Pathologie der Lipoidosen. II. Phosphatidosen und Cerebrosidosen. Medizinische 1953, 612.

GÖTT, E., and H. PEXA: Über andauernde Ausschwemmung von Gaucher-Zellen ins Blut. Acta haemat. (Basel) 31, 113 (1964).

GROEN, J. J.: Present status of knowledge of Gaucher's disease. Israel. J. Med. Sci. 1, 507 (1965)

GRÜNDIG, E., H. CZITOBER, and B. SCHOBEL: Vergleichende Untersuchungen von „sauren" Plasmaphosphatasen bei verschiedenen Knochenerkrankungen. Clin. Chim. Acta 12, 157 (1965).

HALLIDAY, N.: Cerebrosides from spleen and brain from an adult with Gaucher's disease. Proc. Soc. exp. Biol. (N.Y) 75, 659 (1950).

— H. J. DEUEL jr., L. J. TRAGERMAN, and W. E. WARD: On isolation of glucose containing cerebrosides of spleen in a case of Gaucher's disease. J. biol. Chem .132, 171 (1940).

HANHART, E.: Beiträge zur humangenetischen Geographie. Estratto da analecta genetica 1 (1954).

HEILMEYER, L.: Pathologische Physiologie des Eisenstoffwechsels der Leber. Verh. dtsch. Ges. Verdau.- u. Stoffwechselkr. 17, 32 (1954).

HERNDON, C. N., and J. R. BENDER: Gaucher's disease: cases in five related Negro sibships. Amer. J. hum. Genet. 2, 49 (1950).

HERRLIN, K. M., and P.-O. HILLBORG: Neurological signs in a juvenile form of Gaucher's disease. Acta paediat. (Uppsala) 51, 137 (1962).

HILLBORG, P.-O., and B. ESTBORN: Acid phosphatase activity of serum, thrombocytes and erythrocytes in a juvenile form of Gaucher's disease. Acta paediat. (Uppsala) 53, 558 (1964).

— and L. SVENNERHOLM: Blood level of cerebrosides in Gaucher's disease. Acta paediat. (Uppsala) 49, 707 (1960).

HOFFMAN, S. J., and M. I. MAKLER: Gaucher's disease. Review of the literature and case. Amer. J. Dis. Child. 38, 775 (1929).

HORSLEY, J. S., J. P. BAKER, and F. L. APPERLY: Gaucher's disease of late onset with kidney involvement and huge spleen. Amer. J. med. Sci. 190, 511 (1935).

HOWLAND, J., and A. RICH: Gaucher's disease with extensive involvement of the bones and invasion of the spinal canal. Cit. by PICK (1926).

HSIA, D. Y.-Y., J. NAYLOR, and J. A. BIGLER: Gaucher's disease. Report of two cases in father and son and review of the literature. New. Engl. J. Med. 261, 164 (1959).

HUNTER, D., and W. EVANS: Gaucher's disease 13 years after splenectomy. Proc. roy. Soc. Med. 23, 24 (1929).

JERVIS, G., R. C. HARRIS, and J. H. MENKES: Cerebral lipidosis of unclear nature. In: Cerebral Sphingolipidoses, S. M. ARONSON and B. W. VOLK (eds.). New York: Academic Press, 1962.

JONES, E., and S. J. THANNHAUSER: Cited by THANNHAUSER (1958) pg. 498.

JOSSELIN, R. DE, R. N. DE JONG, and J. S. VAN HEUKELOM: Beitrag zur Kenntnis der groß-zelligen Splenomegalie (Typus Gaucher). Beitr. path. Anat. 48, 598 (1910).

KAPLAN, M., R. GRUMBACH, A. FISCHGRUND, and J. LUNEL: Maladie de Gaucher chez un enfant de 6 ans: étude biologique du syndrome hémorragique qui l'accompagne. Bull. Soc. Méd. Paris 69, 169 (1953).

KLENK, E.: Zur Chemie der Lipoidosen: Gauchersche Krankheit. Hoppe-Seylers Z. physiol. Chem. 267, 128 (1940).

— The pathological chemistry of the developing brain. In: Biochemistry of the developing nervous system, E. WAELSCH, (ed.) New York: Academic Press, Inc. 1955.

— E. LETTERER, H. EPPINGER, and A. DETERMAN: Speicherkrankheiten. Verh. dtsch. path. Ges. 31, 6 (1938).

— and I. RENNKAMP: Nature of sugar in cerebrosides of spleen in Gaucher's disease. Hoppe-Seylers Z. physiol. Chem. 262, 280 (1942).

KLIMA, R., J. BEYREDER, and E. HERZOG: Das Leukozytenkonzentrat als einfache und ergiebige Methode für die hämatologische Diagnostik. Wien. med. Wschr. 106, 809 (1956).

KRAUS, E. J.: Zur Kenntnis der Splenomegalie Gaucher, insbesondere der Histogenese der großzelligen Wucherung. Z. angew. Anat. 7, 186 (1920).

LANDOLT, R. F., H. U. ZOLLINGER, and C. H. EUGSTER: Über die maligne, akut verlaufende Form des Morbus Gaucher. Helv. paediat. Acta 3, 319 (1948).

LANGE, C. DE: Forme maligne de la maladie de Gaucher. Acta paediat. (Uppsala) 27, 34 (1939).

LETTERER, E.: Allgemeine Pathologie und pathologische Anatomie der Lipoidosen. Zbl. Path. 71, Erg.-H., 12 (1939).

LEVIN, B.: Gaucher's disease, clinical and roentgenological manifestations. Amer. J. Roentgenol. 85, 685 (1961).

LEVINE, S., and L. SOLIS-COHEN: Gaucher's disease. Amer. J. Roentgenol. 50, 765 (1943).

LIEB, H.: Cerebrosidspeicherung bei Morbus Gaucher. Hoppe-Seylers Z. physiol. Chem. 140, 305 (1924).

— Cerebrosidspeicherung bei Splenomegalie, Typus Gaucher. Hoppe-Seylers Z. physiol. Chem. 170, 60 (1927).

— Der Zucker im Cerebrosid der Milz bei der Gaucher-Krankheit. Hoppe-Seylers Z. physiol. Chem. 271, 211 (1941).

LOGAN, V. W.: The results of splenectomy in Gaucher's disease. Surg. Gynec. Obstet. **72**, 807 (1941).

LUBARSCH, O.: Generalisierte Xanthomatose bei Diabetes. Dtsch. med. Wschr. **44**, 484 (1918).

LÜDIN, H.: Zur Cytologie des Morbus Gaucher. Schweiz, med. Wschr. **41**, 1117 (1950).

MAKITA, A., and T. YAMAKAWA: Biochemistry of organ glycolipids. I. Ceramide-oligohexosides of human, equine and bovine spleens. J. Biochem. (Tokyo) **51**, 124 (1962).

MALONEY, A. F. J., and J. N. CUMINGS: A case of juvenile Gaucher's disease with intraneuronal lipid storage. J. Neurol. Neurosurg. Psychiat. **23**, 207 (1960).

MANDELBAUM, H., L. BERGER, and M. LEDERER: Gaucher's disease. I. A case with hemolytic anemia and marked thrombopenia; improvement after removal of spleen weighing 6822 grams. Ann. intern. Med. **16**, 438 (1942).

MANDLEBAUM, F. S.: A contribution to the pathology of primary splenomegaly (Gaucher type), with the report of an autopsy on a male child four and one half year of age. J. exp. Med. **16**, 797 (1912).

— Two cases of Gaucher's disease in adults: a study of the histopathology, biology and chemical findings. Amer. J. med. Sci. **157**, 366 (1919).

— and H. DOWNEY: The histopathology and biology of Gaucher's disease (large-cell splenomegaly). Fol. haemat. (Lpz.) **20**, H. 3 (1916).

MARCHAND, F.: Über sogenannte idiopathische Splenomegalie (Typ Gaucher) Münch. med. Wschr. **1907**, 1102.

MARKLEN, P., R. WAITZ, and J. WARTER: Diagnosis of Gaucher's disease by splenic puncture. Bull. Soc. Med. Paris **49**, 36 (1933).

MASAI, H., and M. KATURADA: A case of Gaucher's disease. Ann. paediat. jap. **6**, 539 (1960).

MATOTH, Y., and K. FRIED: Chronic Gaucher's disease. Clinical observations on 34 patients. Israel J. Med. Sci. **1**, 521 (1965).

MEDOFF, A. S., and E. D. BAYRD: Gaucher's disease in 29 cases: hematologic complications and effect of splenectomy. Ann. intern. Med. **40**, 481 (1954).

MELAMED, S., and W. CHESTER: Osseous form of Gaucher's splenomegaly. Ann. Surg. **89**, 552 (1929).

— — Osseous form of Gaucher's disease, report of a case. Arch. intern. Med. **61**, 798 (1938).

MIENZIL, K.: Kasuistische Beiträge zur Kenntnis der Milzerkrankungen. Med. Klin. **1924**, 935.

MONTREUIL, J., P. BOULANGER, and E. HOUCKE: Chromatographie sur papier des constituants glucidique de cérébrosides d'une rate de Gaucher. Bull. Soc. chem. biol. **35**, 1125 (1953).

MORGANS, M. E.: Gaucher's disease without splenomegaly. Lancet **1947/II**, 576.

MORRISON, A. N., and M. LANE: Gaucher's disease with ascites: a case report with autopsy findings. Ann. intern. Med. **42**, 1321 (1955).

MOTULSKY, A. G., F. CASSERD, E. R. GIBLETT, G. O. BROUN, and C. A. FINCH: Anemia and the spleen. New Engl. J. Med. **259**, 1164 (1958).

NEELY, W. B.: Infrared spectra of carbohydrates. Advanc. Carbohyd. Chem. **12**, 13 (1957).

NORMAN, R. M., H. URICH, and O. C. LLOYD: The neuropathology of infantile Gaucher's disease. J. Path. **72**, 121 (1956).

OBERLING, C.: La maladie de Gaucher. Ann. d'Anat. Path. **3**, 353 (1926).

— and P. WORINGER: La maladie de Gaucher chez le nourrisson. Rev. franç. Pédiat. **3**, 475 (1927).

OTTENSTEIN, B., G. SCHMIDT, and S. J. THANNHAUSER: The variety of cerebrosides present in one case of infantile Gaucher's disease and 3 cases in adults. Blood **3**, 1250 (1948).

PARKE, D. V.: The occurrence of lactose in the spleen cerebrosides of a case of Gaucher's disease. Biochem. J. **56**, XV (1954).

PATRICK, A. D.: A deficiency of glucocerebrosidase in Gaucher's disease. Biochem. J. **97**, 17c (1965).

PETIT, J. V., and E. M. SCHLEICHER: "Atypical" Gaucher's disease. Amer. J. clin. Path. **13**, 260 (1943).

PHILIPPART, M., and J. H. MENKES: Isolation and characterization of the main splenic glycolipids. Biochem. biophys. Res. Commun. **15**, 551 (1964).

— B. ROSENSTEIN, and J. H. MENKES: Isolation and characterization of the main splenic glycolipids in the normal organ and in Gaucher's disease: Evidence for the site of metabolic block. J. Neuropath. exp. Neurol. **24**, 290 (1965).

PICK, L.: Zur pathologischen Anatomie des Morbus Gaucher. Med. Klin. **1922**, 1408.

— Der Morbus Gaucher und die ihm ähnlichen Krankheiten. Ergebn. inn. Med. Kinderheilk. **29**, 519 (1926).

— Classification of diseases of lipoid metabolism and Gaucher's disease (Dunham lecture). Amer. J. med. Sci. **185**, 453 (1933).

PITTALUGA, P. G., and J. GOYANES: Contribution a l'étude de la cellule de Gaucher. Arch. Mal. coeur **26**, 65 (1933).

Prostenik, M., and B. Majhofer-Orescanin: Occurrence of a new sphingolipid base C_{20}-sphingosine in horse and beef brain. Naturwissenschaften **47**, 399 (1960).

Radin, N. S., and Y. Akahori: Fatty acids of human brain and spleen cerebrosides. Fed. Proc. **20**, 269 (1961).

Rapport, M. M., L. Graf, and N. F. Alonzo: Immunochemical studies of organ and tumor lipids. VIII. Comparison of human tumor and ox spleen cytosides. J. Lipid Res. **1**, 301 (1960).

Reich, C., M. Seife, and B. J. Kessler: Gaucher's disease: A review and discussion of twenty cases. Medicine (Baltimore) **30**, 1 (1951).

Risel, W.: Über die großzellige Splenomegalie (Typ Gaucher) und über das endotheliale Sarkom der Milz. Beitr. path. Anat. **46**, 241 (1909).

Rodgers, C. L., and S. H. Jackson: Acute infantile Gaucher's disease. Pediatrics **7**, 53 (1951).

Rosenberg, A.: The sphingolipids from the spleen of a case of lipidosis. In: Cerebral sphingolipidoses, S. M. Aronson and B. W. Volk (eds.). New York: Academic Press, 1962.

— and E. Chargaff: A reinvestigation of the cerebroside deposited in Gaucher's disease. J. biol. Chem. **233**, 1323 (1958).

Rosenszajn, L., and P. Efrati: Cytochemical and phase-contrast observations on Gaucher cells. Acta haemat. (Basel) **25**, 43 (1961).

Rouser, G., C. Galli, and G. Kritchevsky: Lipid class composition of normal human brain and variations in metachromatic leucodystrophy, Tay-Sachs, Niemann-Pick, chronic Gaucher's and Alzheimer's disease. J. Amer. Oil Chemists' Soc. **42**, 404 (1965).

Rusca, C. L.: Sul morbo del Gaucher. Haematologica (Pavia) **2**, 441 (1921).

Sacks, M. S., and M. A. Andersch: Isolation of a glucose containing cerebroside from the spleen in Gaucher's disease. Amer. J. Med. Sci. **212**, 546 (1946).

Schairer, E.: Die Gehirnveränderungen bei Morbus Gaucher des Säuglings. Virchows Arch. path. Anat. **315**, 395 (1948).

Schatz, F.: Morbus Gaucher mit splenohepathischer Markhemmung beim Erwachsenen. III. Chemischer Teil. Wien. Z. inn. Med. **43**, 342 (1962).

Schettler, G.: Lipidosen. 4. Cerebrosidose. In: Handb. d. inn. Med., G. v. Bergmann, W. Frey, H. Schwiegk (eds.). Berlin-Göttingen-Heidelberg: Springer 1955.

Schlagenhaufer, F.: Über meist familiär vorkommende histologisch charakteristische Splenomegalien (Typ Gaucher). Eine Systemerkrankung des lymphatisch-hämatopoetischen Apparates. Virchows Arch. path. Anat. **187**, 125 (1907).

Sobel, A. E., and I. A. Kaye: Gaucher's disease, case with hemolytic anemia and marked thrombopenia. Ann. int. Med. **16**, 446 (1942).

Ställberg-Stenhagen, S., and L. Svennerholm: The fatty acid composition of human brain sphingomyelins: Normal variation with age and changes during myelin disorders. J. Lipid Res. **6**, 140 (1965).

Statter, M., and B. Shapiro: Metabolism of glycolipids and its relation to Gaucher's disease. Israel J. Chem. **1**, 193 (1963).

— — Studies on the etiology of Gaucher's disease. I. Catabolism of glycolipids by rat liver in vivo. Israel J. Med. Sci. **1**, 514 (1965).

Suomi, W. D., and B. W. Agranoff: Lipids of the spleen in Gaucher's disease. J. Lipid Res. **6**, 211 (1965).

Svennerholm, E., and L. Svennerholm: Quantitative estimation of cerebrosides in plasma. Scand. J. clin. Lab. Invest. **10**, 97 (1958).

— — Neutral glycolipids of human blood serum, spleen and liver. Nature (Lond.) **198**, 688 (1963).

Svennerholm, L.: Some aspects of the biochemical changes in leucodystrophy. In: Brain lipids and lipoproteins, and the leucodystrophies, J. Folch-Pi and H. Bauer (eds.). Amsterdam: Elsevier Publishing Co., 1963.

— Chromatographic separation of human brain gangliosides. J. Neurochem. **10**, 613 (1963a).

— The patterns of gangliosides in mental and neurological disorders. Biochem. J. **98**, 20 P (1966).

Teilum, G.: Gaucher's disease with changes in the pituitary and hypothalamus. Acta med. scand. **116**, 170 (1944).

Thannhauser, S. J.: Lipoidoses. New York: Oxford Press 1950.

— Diseases of the nervous system associated with disturbances of lipid metabolism. Res. Publ. Ass. nerv. ment. Dis. **32**, 238 (1953).

— Lipidoses, Diseases of the Intracellular Lipid Metabolism, 3d edition. New York: Grune and Stratton 1958.

— and H. Reinstein: Cited by Thannhauser (1958), p. 468.

Thudichum, J. L. W.: Über das Phrenosin, einem neuen stickstoffhaltigen phosphorfreien spezifischen Gehirnstoff. J. prakt. Chem **25**, 19 (1882).

— Die chemische Konstitution des Gehirns des Menschen und der Tiere. Tübingen: F. Pietzcker 1901.

TRAMS, E. G., and R. O. BRADY: Cerebroside synthesis in Gaucher's disease. J. clin. Invest. **39**, 1546 (1960).

TUCHMAN, L. R., G. GOLDSTEIN, and M. CLYMAN: Studies on the nature of the increased serum acid phosphatase in Gaucher's disease. Amer. J. Med. **27**, 959 (1959).

— H. SUNA, and J. J. CARR: Elevation of serum acid phosphatase in Gaucher's Disease. J. Mt. Sinai Hosp. **23**, 227 (1956).

— and M. SWICK: High acid phosphatase level indicating Gaucher's disease in a patient with prostatism. J. Amer. med. Ass. **164**, 2034 (1957).

TYSON, M. C., W. I. GROSSMAN, and L. R. TUCHMAN: Gaucher's disease (with elevated serum acid phosphatase level) masquerading as cirrhosis of the liver. Amer. J. Med. **37**, 156 (1964).

UZMAN, L. L.: Polycerebrosides in Gaucher's disease: isolation, composition and physical properties. Arch. Path. **55**, 181 (1953).

WECHSLER, H. F., and E. GUSTAFSON: Gaucher's disease associated with multiple teleangiectases in elderly woman. N.Y. St. J. Med. **40**, 133 (1940).

WEINSCHENK, C.: Über die Psychopathologie der juvenilen Form eines Morbus Gaucher (mit Falldemonstration). Med. Welt (Stuttg.) **1964**, 140.

— Personal communication 1965.

WICHA, H.: Dissertation, University of Cologne, 1962.

WOOLF, L. J.: The sugar containing lipids of Gaucher's disease. Biochem. J. **56**, XVI (1954).

WORINGER, P.: Cinquième enfant atteint de maladie de Gaucher dans une même famille. Méd. inf. (Paris) **41**, 190 (1934).

— S. SUZUKI: The chemistry of the lipids of post hemolytic residue or stroma of erythrocytes. IV. Distribution of lipid-hexosamine and lipid-hemat. aminic acid in the red blood corpuscles of various species of animals. J. Biochem. (Tokyo) **40**, 7 (1953).

YAMAKAWA, T., R. IRIE, and M. IWANAGA: The chemistry of lipids of posthemolytic residue or stroma of erythrocytes. IX. Silicic acid chromatography of mammalian stroma glycolipids. J. Biochem. **48**, 490 (1960).

YOSSIPOVITCH, Z. H., G. HERMAN, and M. MAKIN: Aseptic osteomyelitis in Gaucher's disease. Israel J. med. Sci. **1**, 531 (1965).

ZADEK, J.: Morbus Gaucher. Med. Klin. **1924**, 78.

ZEHNDER, M.: Klinischer und chemischer Beitrag zum Studium des M. Gaucher. Dtsch. Z. Chir. **250**, 422 (1938).

Niemann-Pick Disease

By

G. Schettler and W. Kahlke

Synonoyms: Sphingomyelin lipidosis; sphingomyelinosis.

Definition and Introduction

Niemann-Pick disease (NPD) is a rare hereditary disorder of lipid metabolism which is characterized by deposition of sphingomyelin in endothelial, mesenchymal and parenchymal cells of almost every organ and tissue. Its clinical manifestations appear in most instances during the first year of life. The symptomatology consists of hepatosplenomegaly and neurological disturbances with retardation of somatic and mental development. Affected children usually do not reach their third year of life. In exceptional cases the first symptoms appear later in life and progression of the disease is slower. The underlying error of metabolism is still not known with certainty. It appears that the metabolic lesion in the classic infantile form of NPD is attributable to a deficiency or lack of activity of the enzyme which catalyzes the cleavage of sphingomyelin (BRADY et al. 1966).

Historical Review

In 1914 the German pediatrician NIEMANN described the case of the 18 month-old daughter of Jewish parents who exhibited marked hepatosplenomegaly, enlarged lymph nodes, facial edema and pigmentation. The child appeared very ill, failed to thrive and expired before the age of two years. At autopsy yellow deposits were found in liver, spleen, lymph nodes, kidneys and adrenals. Although the large cells which were seen in these organs stained with Sudan III like the Gaucher cells which had just been described, NIEMANN differentiated his case from Gaucher's disease on the basis of the patient's age and the rapidly lethal course. Two years later KNOX et al. (1916) published as Gaucher's disease the cases of two sisters with hepatosplenomegaly and other symptoms resembling those of Niemann's case. Although their diagnosis was questioned by MANDLEBAUM and DOWNEY (1916), the relationship to the child previously described by NIEMANN (1914) was not recognized at the time. The same was true in the case of a nine month-old girl with hepatosplenomegaly whose sister had died at the age of one year with similar signs and symptoms (SIEGMUND 1921). PICK (1922, 1927) finally differentiated this new disease on the basis of careful histological studies from Gaucher's disease. His work was based on examination of the material of NIEMANN and SIEGMUND, and of two cases of his own, a 17 month-old boy published separately by SCHIFF (1926), and a 15 month-old girl. Three additional cases of NPD, two girls aged 14 and 16 months, and a boy, seven months old, were published by BLOOM in 1925 and 1928, and subsequently numerous reports of NPD appeared in the literature (DIENST and HAMPERL 1927, HAMBURGER 1927, BIELSCHOWSKY 1928, BERMAN 1928, KRAMER 1928, STRANSKY 1930, SMETANA 1930, HASSIN 1930, PONCHER 1931, WASCOWITZ 1931, GOLDSTEIN and WEXLER 1931).

Histochemical differentiation of cell lipids and the first chemical analyses of the deposited lipids were performed by WAHL and RICHARDSON (1916), SIEGMUND

(1921), BRAHN and PICK (1927), and McFATE (1928). The increased amounts of phospholipid in affected organs which were found by BLOOM and KERN (1927), SOBOTKA et al. (1930, 1933), EPSTEIN and LORENZ (1932) and BAUMANN (1935) were identified by KLENK (1934) as sphingomyelin. BAUMANN, KLENK and SCHEIDEGGER (1936) summarized in a comprehensive report clinical and post-mortem findings and biochemical data of the 25 cases of NPD which had been described up to that time.

Subsequent case reports and reviews by BAGGENSTOSS et al. (1940), MENTEN and WELTON (1946), DIDION (1949, 1950), VIDEBAEK (1949, 1952), THANNHAUSER (1950, 1953, 1958), SCHETTLER (1955), CROCKER and FARBER (1958), GARMYN (1962) and FREDRICKSON (1960, 1966) have contributed to a total of approximately 165 cases reported as NPD.

Incidence (Age, Sex, Race)

The cases of NPD which were reported during the 30 years following the first description of the disease concerned only infants who died before the age of two years, and document the strong tendency for the disease to occur in this age group. VIDEBAEK, in 1949, observed for the first time a patient who reached the age of five years. An eight year-old boy with NPD was subsequently described by THANN-HAUSER (1950), and CUMINGS (1962) studied an eight year-old girl whose affected brother had died at the age of six. The child had entered the hospital with seizures and signs of mental retardation and the diagnosis of storage disease was made by brain biopsy. Extensive chemical analyses of brain and spleen of this patient were performed. Since then a number of adults with the disease have been described. DUSENDSCHON (1946) and PFÄNDLER (1946) reported two brothers who were asymptomatic throughout their lives. One of them expired when he was 29 years old, the other reached the age of 34 and, following bronchitis, died with cor pul-monale and polycytemia. Both patients exhibited unequivocal microscopic signs of NPD, the latter with Niemann-Pick cell infiltrations in the lungs and advanced pulmonary fibrosis. A female patient (FREDRICKSON 1960), now about 25 years old, exhibited splenomegaly at the age of four and developed progressive neurological defects at the age of 12. In her the diagnosis was made by bone marrow biopsy, and at the present time she is able to live a relatively normal life. The same author (FREDRICKSON 1960) described a 42 year-old male patient who was found to have an isolated pulmonary lesion on X-ray examination. Biopsy specimens of lung, rib and liver showed histologic and clinical changes compatible with the diagnosis of NPD. TERRY et al. (1954) observed a 51 year-old male subject with NPD, in whom tissue lipid changes were very similar to those of affected infants. LYNN and TERRY (1964) described histochemical and electronmicroscopic findings in biopsy material from their 11 year-old patient.

A higher incidence of NPD in females than in males, as emphasized by GAENSS-LEN (1940), does not appear to exist, according to more recent reviews of the subject (SCHETTLER 1955, FREDRICKSON 1960, 1966).

In spite of the rarity of the disease, a number of observations on familial occur-rence have been reported. Hepatosplenomegaly in more than one family member was described by KNOX et al. (1916), SIEGMUND (1921), HAMBURGER (1927), DIENST and HAMPERL (1927), MERKSAMER and KRAMER (1939), DIDION (1949), VIDEBAEK (1949, 1952), and CROCKER and FARBER (1958). In the reviews of VIDEBAEK (1949, 1952) and CROCKER and FARBER (1958) at least 24 out of 91 cases with NPD were familial. Additional relatives with the disease might have died before it was recognized. Consanguinity was noted in six couples. For a detailed discussion on the heredity of NPD we refer to the chapter by FUHRMANN (page 497).

A relatively high incidence of NPD in Jews soon became apparent. According to SCHETTLER (1955), two thirds of the patients described up to 1955 were of Jewish ancestry. In the material compiled by VIDEBAEK (1949, 1952) and by CROCKER and FARBER (1958), 35 out of 73 patients whose racial background was known were Jewish. The majority of the remaining patients were offspring of other Caucasian families (FREDRICKSON 1960). At least one patient of CROCKER and FARBER (1958) is offspring of an American-Indian Negro and a Portuguese female. One case from Japan (TOKUJAWA 1937) and one from Turkey (FAKAÇELLI 1944) were reported by VIDEBAEK (1949).

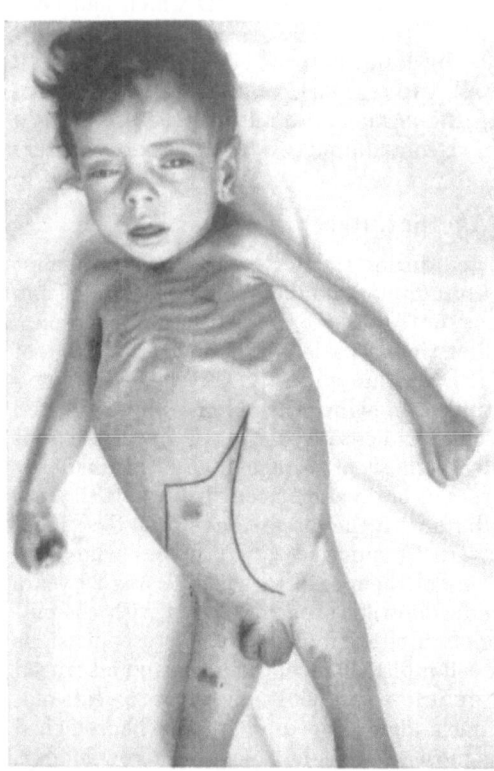

Fig. 1. Niemann-Pick disease. Case reported by BAUMANN et al. (1936)

Clinical Manifestations

In the great majority of cases the first manifestations of NPD appear during the first months of life, while affected infants are completely normal at birth. Splenomegaly in Niemann's case developed at the beginning of the second month and also occurred very early in the infant described by SIEGMUND (1921). Very soon, frequently also during the first months, feeding becomes difficult and weight loss ensues. The combination of marked hepatosplenomegaly, dehydration and loss of subcutaneous adipose tissue produces the typical appearance with protuberance of the abdomen and thin extremities as shown classically in the case of BAUMANN et al. (1936) (see figure 1 and 2). At the age of seven months the abdominal circumference in Niemann's patient was 50 cm.

In most instances enlargement of the liver is more marked than splenomegaly (SCHETTLER 1955). Due to the firm consistency of both organs, the smooth surface and the crenated margin of the spleen as well as the liver edge are easily palpated. Superficial and deep lymph nodes may be enlarged. The skin becomes pale brown or greyish-yellow and, depending on the degree of hydration, may be picked up in folds or, on the other hand, be edematous. Pigmented spots with a blueish hue resembling those of Addison's disease are occasionally found in the oral mucosa. They consist mainly of melanin and suggest infiltration of the adrenals by Niemann-Pick cells. When such infiltrations surround alveoles and blood vessels of the lungs, foci of bronchopneumonia may develop which on X-ray examination resemble silicosis. Ascites and edema of legs and eyelids may develop during the course of the disease.

A number of malformations have been reported in affected children. PICK (1927, 1933), VAN BOGAERT (1934) and VIDEBAEK (1952) found microgyria, polydactyly and cleft formations. Blueish-black moles (so-called Mongolian spots) were described by SCHIFF (1926) in the lumbosacral region and by THANNHAUSER (1958) in the oral mucosa.

Neurology

Neurological findings in NPD may vary considerably. Disturbances of mental, motor and sensory functions can occur depending on the pattern of lesions

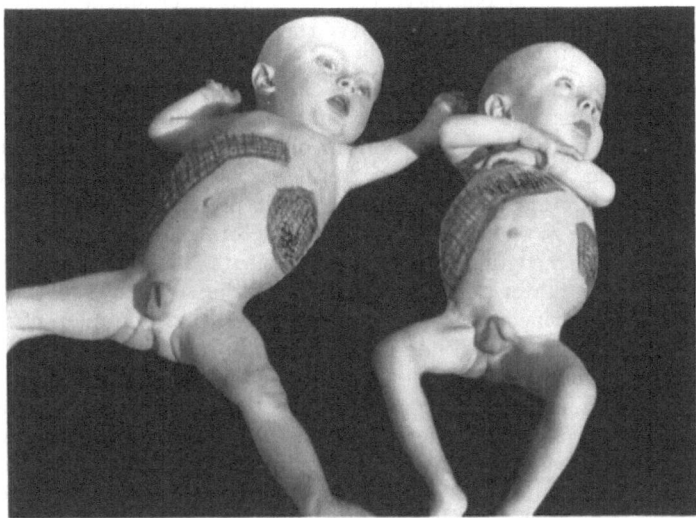

Fig. 2. Niemann-Pick disease in twins (FREUDENBERG 1937)

within the central nervous system. In most cases retardation of mental and somatic development follows the initial period of inanition. Spasticity and rigidity of the musculature are associated with involuntary contractions, incoordination, athetosis, tremors and seizures. Frequently the affected infants will be seen with their mouths open and tongues protruding. Vomiting and elevation of the basal metabolic rate with increased insensible water loss are also considered to be expressions of the central nervous system pathology (BAUMANN et al. 1936). Non-specific abnormalities may be seen in the electroencephalogram. Cranial nerves may be involved and the frequent finding of deafness may result from this cause. Progressive mental debility may result in idiotism and a vegetative state may be approached.

Hematology

Hematologic changes in NPD have been well studied by CROCKER and FARBER (1958). A mild hypochromic anemia is found in some children, even if allowance is made for the fact that hemoglobin concentration is normally lower in children than in adults. In five out of 16 patients hemoglobin levels were below 10 gm per 100 ml and in six patients they were between 10 and 12 gm per 100 ml, with red cell counts of 4—4.5 million per cubic mm. Significant abnormalities of red cells were absent even in the presence of severe bone marrow pathology. A good correlation between degree of splenomegaly and degree of anemia did not exist, but splenectomy usually resulted in improvement of anemia. Poikilocytosis, anisocytosis and polychromasia have rarely been described. The platelet count is inconsistently altered. In a number of cases, thrombocytopenia has been seen, but petechiae are rare. There is some correlation of thrombocytopenia with the degree of splenomegaly, and in cases with more severe thrombocytopenia at least a five-fold increase in the size of the spleen has been found. Prolonged thrombocytosis after splenectomy is striking; average values for thrombocytes on days 7—11 after surgery are one million, and the count may remain elevated for years without evidence of thrombotic complications.

Leukopenia (BAUMANN et al. 1936, THANNHAUSER 1950) as well as leukocytosis in the absence of infection has been described (BLOOM 1925, PICK 1927, FISHER 1932). Counts exceeding 30.000 have been recorded after splenectomy. In view of their inconsistency and non-specificity, these hematologic abnormalities are without diagnostic value.

A more specific finding is vacuolation of agranulocytes which has been described in several publications. The vacuoles have an average diameter of 1 μ and occur frequently in groups within the cytoplasm of lymphocytes and monocytes, occasionally displacing the nucleus. Upon careful search of multiple smears, CROCKER and FARBER (1958) found these cells in all their patients. There appears to be no correlation with total plasma lipids or other factors except that the vacuolated cells are more easily recognized in younger patients. It is tempting to assume the presence of lipid material, but the nature of the substance in the vacuoles has not yet been identified. Neither total white cell phospholipids nor the proportion of sphingomyelin were found to be elevated (CROCKER and FARBER 1958). The search for these cells in parents and siblings of affected children has been unsuccessful, and vacuolation of agranulocytes is therefore not a simple test for the detection of heterozygote carriers of the disease, as some workers have hoped. This is in contrast to findings in Gaucher's disease (GERKEN and WIEDEMANN 1964) where affected siblings, as well as clinically healthy ones and parents, had typical Gaucher cells in the circulating blood.

Other Laboratory Findings

There are a number of findings, the relation of which to the disease has not been established. A ten-fold elevation of serum acid phosphatase has been observed in a three year-old patient by HASTRUP and VIDEBAEK (1954). Since this enzyme differed from prostatic phosphatase by exhibiting a lower activity towards beta-glycerophosphate, it was similar to the acid phosphatase which is found elevated in Gaucher's disease and there is reason to doubt the diagnosis of NPD in this case. Elevation of serum acid phosphatase activity in NPD has not been found by other observers: for instance the relevant values were normal on 11 occasions in six patients studied by CROCKER and FARBER (1958).

Signs of a nephrotic syndrome with significant albuminuria (0.3 to 0.5%) and a low serum albumin level (46.8%) were found in a two year-old affected child with marked central nervous system involvement by ZOEPFFEL (1964); lipid chemical analyses were not performed in this case.

The results of commonly employed laboratory tests are usually normal. Even liver function tests are only occasionally altered except during episodes of jaundice. It is striking that little or no evidence of metabolic or endocrine malfunction is detectable even in cases with massive infiltration of pancreas, liver, gastrointestinal tract, heart, kidneys and adrenals with lipid-laden cells, supporting the contention of LETTERER (1939, 1947) that storage by cells is not correlated with impairment of function.

Bones

In contrast to Gaucher's disease, which occupies the first place in the differential diagnosis of NPD, typical bone abnormalities are not found in the latter. Detectable changes, consisting mainly of some enlargement of the marrow spaces and of osteoporosis, are limited to long bones, particularly the femur; they are non-specific and considerably less marked than one might expect from the bone marrow pathology. The Erlenmeyer flask deformity, typical for Gaucher's disease, has never been reported. Neither were pathologic fractures or necroses observed in spite of widespread NPC infiltration. Skeletal malformations in affected subjects have been described. Missing phalanges on one hand were reported by BLOOM (1928), and in association with anomalies of the spine by CROCKER and FARBER (1958). They were considered by these authors to represent incidental findings.

Skin

Skin changes consist of pigmentation with an ochre or yellow hue of generalized or localized occurrence, and resemble "café au lait" spots of neurofibromatosis. Blueish-black moles (the so-called Mongolian-spots) described by MERKSAMER and KRAMER (1939) and by THANNHAUSER (1958) appear to be more frequent in patients with NPD than in the general population. Xanthomas of the eruptive or infiltrative type have been seen in NPD, and it is reasonable to assume a correlation between the disturbance in lipid metabolism and the development of these lesions. MAURER (1941) and CROCKER and FARBER (1958) observed the appearance of eruptive xanthomas on face and upper extremities at the time of an increase in plasma lipids, and their disappearance during a transient remission of lipemia. Recurrence of hyperlipemia failed to reproduce xanthomatosis. Straw-colored xanthomas occurred in another subject with only slightly elevated serum cholesterol level. Tendon xanthomas have not been observed in NPD even in the presence of marked hypercholesteremia.

Eyes

A cherry-red spot in the retina has been seen by several authors. Data on its incidence vary from 20% (CROCKER and FARBER 1958) to over 50% (VIDEBAEK 1949, and others). BAUMANN et al. (1936) found it in eight out of 27 patients and considered these cases to be a combination of NPD with Tay-Sachs disease. The sign results from the red color of the fovea being visible in the middle of a greyish-white macula; it may appear at any time during the course of the disease and can occur unilaterally. Several authors (WASCOWITZ 1931, ROTHSTEIN and WELT 1941) differentiated these spots from those of amaurotic family idiocy on the basis of their color and shape. This is discussed in more detail by GOLDSTEIN and WEXLER (1931) and by RINTELEN (1935).

Course and Prognosis

Causes of death have been cachexia (KNOX and RAMSEY 1932), pneumonia (SIEGMUND 1921), heart failure (NIEMANN 1914, BLOOM 1928), pneumococcal meningitis (BLOOM 1928), enteritis (GIAMPALMO 1953) or other infections to which the debilitated infants are very susceptible. Today, prevention or treatment of complications may result in a more protracted course of the disease, and sequelae of the primary lesion may preponderate as cause of death.

A slower course is the rule when the disease begins in late childhood or in adult life, and neurologic symptoms in these patients are less marked or absent. Here the prognosis is favorable, as demonstrated by the two patients described by FREDRICKSON (1960).

Pathology

Although today's chemical methods are of greater diagnostic value than the morphologic approach, it should be kept in mind that PICK established the identity of the disease on the basis of morphologic findings. Indeed, gross and particularly microscopic changes are highly typical for NPD, and it may well be that refined morphologic studies with the aid of electronmicroscopy will eventually allow recognition of the substructural components which are responsible for abnormal biochemical findings and thus aid in tracing the metabolic defect. Most of the morbid anatomy to be described has already been recognized by Pick (1927, 1933), and little has since been added.

Niemann-Pick Cells

Since numerous tissues are involved in NPD, microscopic examination of biopsy specimens is likely to result in diagnostic findings. Niemann-Pick cells (NPC) are typical in the disease. They are lipid-storing cells which measure usually 20 to 40 μ, occasionally up to 90 μ in diameter and are thus slightly smaller than the average Gaucher cells from which they may be more reliably distinguished by their typical foamy appearance. The cytoplasm is filled rather homogenously with lipid droplets resulting in the characteristic "mulberry" or "honeycomb"-like picture (see figure 3). Although one nucleus for each cell is the rule, polynucleated NPC have been observed (Crocker and Farber 1958) with as many as 18 nuclei in one case. NPC originate mainly from cells of the reticulo-endothelial system, but parenchymal cells of liver, kidneys, adrenals, thyroid and bowel may also be transformed to lipid-storing cells. The abnormalities of glial and ganglion cells, with deposition and storage of fat, as already recognized by Pick (1927), Pick and Bielschowsky (1927) and Bloom (1928), will be discussed later.

The thesis advanced by Epstein (1932) that lipid in liver cells and kidney epithelium results from passive infiltration, while glial cells, ganglion cells, and histiocytes store lipid actively, has been convincingly repudiated by Letterer (1939, 1947).

While the typical cells in Gaucher's disease are usually limited to a few organs, NPC may be found almost everywhere in the body. However, corresponding to the distribution of the reticulo-endothelial system they will be most abundant in tissues of this system which therefore should preferably be biopsied for diagnostic purposes. As a rule, NPC cannot be recovered from circulating blood, and, according to Bloom (1928), the vascular endothelium is not a precursor for these cells.

Spleen

This organ is, in general, the seat of the most pronounced changes in NPD. The increase in weight over the age-corrected normal values may be ten-fold in some cases. In the infantile form splenic enlargement is greatest between the ages of one and three years, and less before and after this period (Crocker and Farber 1958). However, even in infants below the age of one year splenomegaly may be considerable, as in two eight and nine month-old infants with splenic weights of 235 gm (Ivemark et al. 1963), and 310 gm (Pick 1926).

The organ is usually firm and the margin rounded. On sectioning the tissue appears lighter than normal and the Malpighian bodies are seen as numerous small reddish-yellow spots. Microscopically the change of normal architecture is striking due to the deposition of NPC. These are, in milder cases, arranged mainly between the sinuses, but usually there is diffuse distribution of NPC throughout the organ with extensive involvement of the pulp, particularly around pulp arteries and trabecles and underneath the capsule. The sinuses remain distinctly outlined, and foam cells, which can be found in their lumina, may invade from the surrounding pulp (Bloom 1928). In advanced cases they may be observed

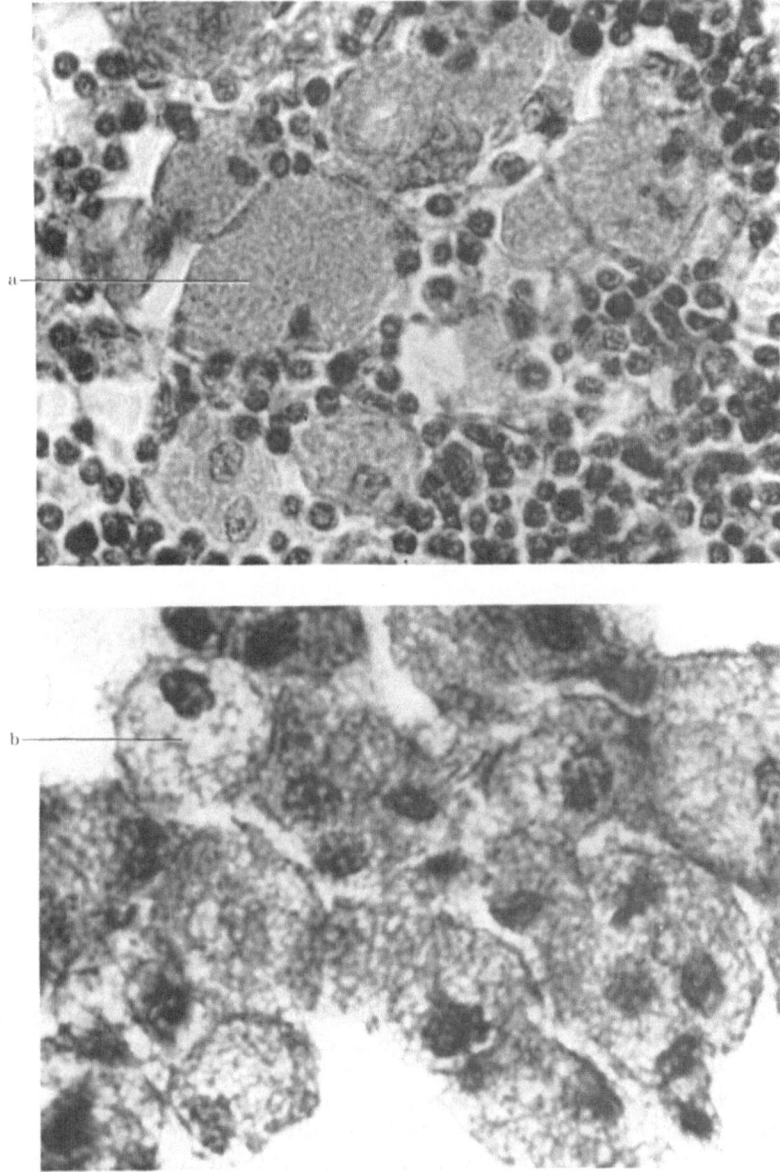

Fig. 3. Niemann-Pick disease. a) micro-vacuolated, b) macro-vacuolated foam cells.
(From LETTERER 1939)

within the Malpighian bodies, which may be decreased in number (CROCKER and
FARBER 1958). NPC may contain pigment in addition to erythrocytes and
nuclear fragments, although phagocytosis is not frequently observed. The development of these histologic changes is rapid.

Accessory spleens were described by CROCKER and FARBER (1958) in three out
of 14 cases; their detection is facilitated by an increase in size, which parallels
that of the main organ.

Liver

The liver is enlarged, although rarely as much as the spleen. The average increase in weight of ten livers was 1.5 times (range 0.8—2.7) the age-corrected normal (Crocker and Farber 1958). Hepatomegaly is less in older patients.

The organ is usually firmer than normal, although Pick (1927, 1933), in addition to very hard livers, also found organs of a doughy consistency. The cut surface is greyish-yellow, yellow or salmon colored. According to Niemann (1914) its color resembles that of the fatty liver observed in phosphorus poisoning.

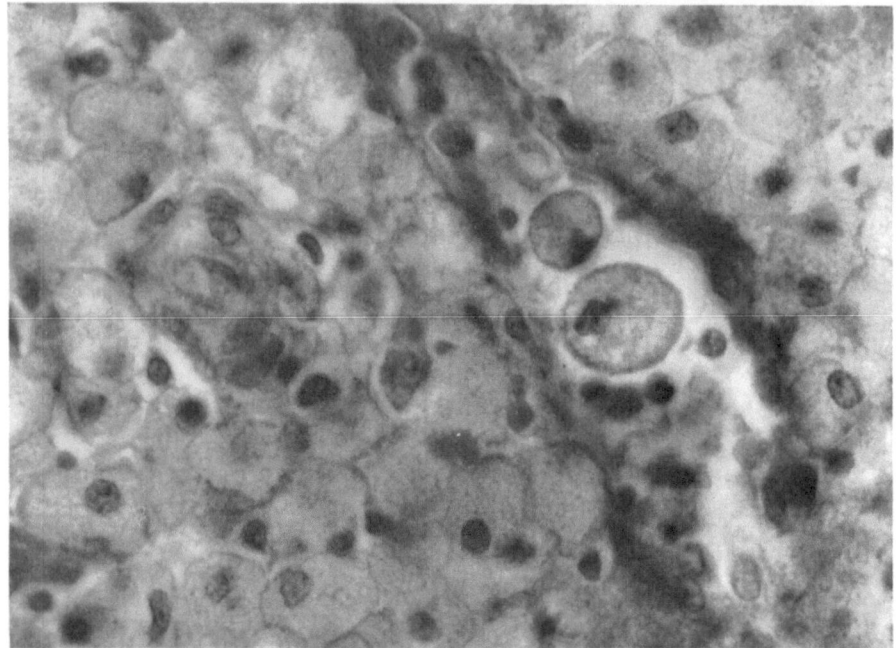

Fig. 4. Niemann-Pick disease, infantile form. Liver, PAS-reaction. Enlargement 250-fold. Liver cells and Kupffer cells (in a dilated capillary) are converted to foam cells. The depicted sphingomyelin granules are PAS-negative. (Reproduced by courtesy of Dr. P. B. Diezel)

The development of histologic abnormalities usually takes several months, and hepatomegaly may exist before histologic changes can be recognized. Liver biopsies in several affected infants during the first few months of life showed only scattered NPC or none. Later on a variety of changes develop, normal tissue being progressively replaced by foam cells which initially favor the sinuses and later extend into the portal areas. In biopsy specimens obtained during later stages of the disease the sinuses are massively infiltrated and the parenchymal cells show incipient vacuolation. Kupffer cells and parenchymal cells may be transformed into NPC (see figure 4) to such an extent that the trabecular structure is only vaguely maintained and differentiation of endothelial cells and liver cells may be difficult due to the common foamy metamorphosis. The picture may resemble that of nutritional cholesteatosis (Pick 1933). The thesis that parenchymal cells are not transformed to NPC but rather contain material resulting from cell degeneration or glycogen in place of lipid has been refuted by Diezel (1957a, b, 1960, 1962), who considered the PAS-negative granules of these cells to be sphingomyelin (see figure 4). Pick (1927, 1933) observed less staining of these modified liver cells than of NPC with the Smith-Dietrich reaction.

The lack of major connective tissue reactions is surprising. Signs of inflammation are rarely found and scarring or other cirrhotic changes are infrequent and of only minor degree. The cause for the occasional occurrence of jaundice, which begins early and lasts for several months, has not been elucidated, except for a case of CROCKER and FARBER (1958), where biliary obstruction resulted from enlarged hilar lymph nodes. In the limited number of such patients, liver function tests (flocculation tests, bromsulfalein test) reverted to normal after the icterus had subsided.

Lymph Nodes

In the full-blown disease there is generalized enlargement of lymph nodes, the degree of which varies considerably among different patients and in different areas. Lymphomegaly is particularly marked in the mesentery, in the hilus of spleen, liver and lungs, and in the head of the pancreas; thymus and tonsils are also enlarged. In contrast, swelling of peripheral nodes is often minimal.

Involved nodes are grey to yellow, their consistency varies, and conglomerates may be formed in severe cases. The fibrous structure of the nodes is usually maintained while the lymphatic parenchyma may be infiltrated or even replaced by accumulation of NPC. Strands of connective tissue separate NPC clusters and produce an alveolar picture. In other cases only scattered NPC are found without apparent diminution of lymphoid tissue. The origin of NPC in lymph nodes is controversial; according to KNOX et al. (1916) they may arise from reticular cells and from endothelial cells of blood and lymphatic vessels, while BLOOM (1928) emphasizes the sparing of the sinuses particularly in lymph nodes. As in the spleen, NPC of lymph nodes occasionally show signs of phagocytosis (inclusion of erythrocytes, leukocytes or nuclear fragments). Microscopic changes are similar in all affected lymph nodes, without apparent topographic differences.

Bone Marrow

The bone marrow, with its large reservoir of reticulum cells, is consistently involved in NPD, together with spleen and lymph nodes. Its easy availability for biopsies makes it best suited for diagnostic purposes. On gross examination the marrow appears hyperplastic; under the microscope NPC are usually numerous, occurring either singly or incorporated in the syncytium, with a maximal proportion of 3% of nucleated cells (CROCKER and FARBER 1958). NPC of the bone marrow are larger than in other organs (up to 200 μ in diameter) and polynucleated cells are more frequent. Phagocytosis of erythrocytes is rarely seen.

The blood-forming elements are, in general, morphologically normal, and, even with marked marrow involvement, peripheral smears do not reflect such changes.

It should be pointed out that NPC may not be found in the first bone marrow smear obtained from a patient with NPD, and repeated biopsies may be necessary. Furthermore, the finding of foam cells does not establish the diagnosis of NPD since atypical cells, similar to NPC, may be found in lipemia, liver tumors, during treatment with adrenocortical steroids, and occasionally in normal bone marrow. The finding of NPC should always be followed by chemical analyses of involved tissues.

Thymus

On gross examination an affected thymus resembles a lymph node in consistency and color (strikingly yellow). Microscopically, the organ is infiltrated by a great number of NPC, and some areas show almost complete replacement of normal tissue by these cells, with the exception of the Hassal bodies and residuals of surrounding lymphoid cells.

Lungs

Morbid anatomical changes as a rule include superimposed inflammatory reactions from final bronchopneumonias. These limitations have to be kept in mind in the evaluation of autopsy data. Thus the weights of 11 lungs examined by Crocker and Farber (1958) were generally increased with a maximum value of 2.4 times normal. NPC are abundant except in the lungs of very young infants on one hand and of aged subjects on the other, and are found in sections throughout the organ includ-

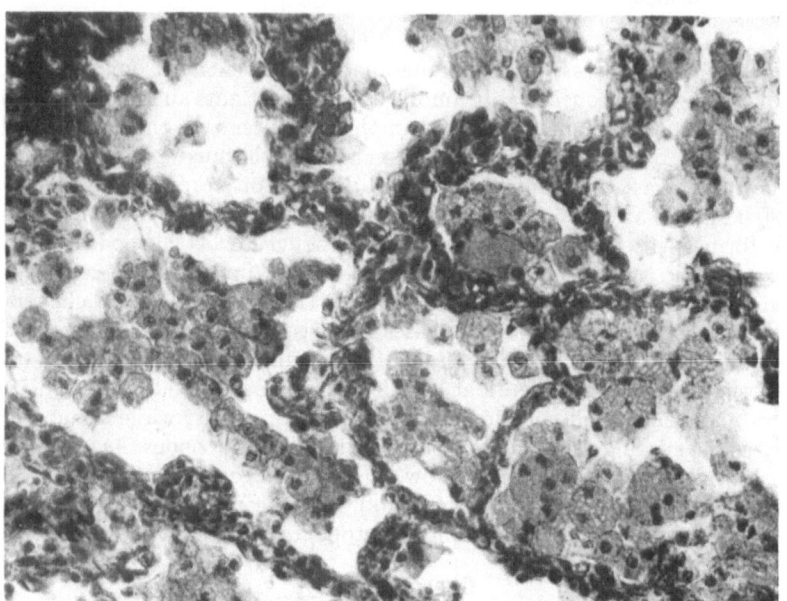

Fig. 5. Niemann-Pick disease. Foam cells in the lung. (From Letterer 1939)

ing lymphatic vessels and branches of pulmonary arteries. The occurrence of great amounts of NPC in the alveoli of severely ill patients would suggest greater impairment of gas exchange than is actually observed. An hepatic origin for NPC in pulmonary alveoli has been discussed by Bloom (1928). Occasionally deposits of NPC are limited to circumscribed areas between normal tissue (see figure 5).

On X-ray examination of such patients a diffuse and intense miliary type of mottling is observed in most cases, but normal findings are not rare. Changes from superimposed intercurrent and prefinal infections may make interpretation difficult. In general, X-ray and postmortem findings are in good agreement. Results of pulmonary function tests are scarce in the literature since most patients die during infancy; however, for at least two of the rare adult cases such data have been reported. The 19 year-old patient of Lynn and Terry (1964), for example, exhibited a 93% oxygen saturation at rest and 89% after exercise as well as other signs of early alveolar-capillary block, similar to observations in older subjects with Gaucher's disease (Thannhauser 1958).

Kidneys

In contrast to the organs which have been described so far the kidneys are usually smaller than normal, as could be shown in nine out of ten autopsies reported by Crocker and Farber (1958). On gross examination, three out of six cases examined by Pick (1928) showed a "fatty, light-yellow renal cortex". Histologic findings vary. NPC occur in only 50% of cases and may originate, according to PICK, from the tubular epithelium and from glomerular endothelial cells. They are frequently found within the capillary loops of glomeruli and occasionally in the lumen of renal arteries. Lipid casts may appear in the urine (SIEGMUND 1921).

Other non-specific abnormalities in three out of ten cases of CROCKER and FARBER (1958) included swelling and dilation of tubular cells and basal membrane thickening of glomeruli. In spite of such changes, evidence of significant functional impairment was not found. The intravenous pyelograms which were performed were normal.

Other Organs

Concomitantly with a significant enlargement of mesenteric lymph nodes, NPC frequently occur within the bowel wall and its serosal layer. Vacuolated epithelial cells have been observed by KNOX and RAMSEY (1932) in stomach and colon. In addition, lesions of the intramural plexus of the intestine have been observed. Vacuolation of epithelial cells may include salivary glands, acinus and islet cells of the pancreas and the thyroid. NPC may be found in most endocrine glands; the adrenal cortex and medulla can be severely involved. Considerable enlargement of the adrenals was a feature in the first four cases which were autopsied (PICK 1927), with weights varying from 5.5 to 8 gm. While the medulla was filled with NPC, the cortex showed only widening and marked lipid deposition in otherwise distinctly outlined cells. In spite of such pathology, no evidence for impairment of function has been reported. Finally, NPC may be found between endothelial cells and muscle cells of the heart. The heart muscle itself may show variable degrees of vacuolation by lipid droplets. Involvement of the epicardium has been seen.

Central Nervous System

Involvement of the brain in NPD is frequent. On gross examination the white matter has a leathery consistency while the grey matter is rather soft, contrary to the findings in Tay-Sachs disease. Impressive changes are seen under the microscope: the large pyramidal cells have lost their multiangular shape and are distended and ballooned, the nucleus being displaced towards the axon. The granular, pale cytoplasm may contain vacuoles in place of degenerated Nissl granules. The total number of nerve cells appears diminished, and there is a concomitant glial reaction. The changes may vary in intensity in different areas of the brain, and occasionally, particularly in very young patients, needle biopsies may yield normal tissue. No histologic abnormalities are seen in the white matter. NPC are not found within the brain parenchyma; the storage process, in analogy to Tay-Sachs disease, affects only ganglion cells.

Impairment of brain function in NPD varies considerably. It shows some correlation with the age of the patients when the disease becomes manifest. Neurologic abnormalities are most marked in infants and children up to the age of four or five years, when lipid storage coincides with myelination and general development. In this regard a resemblance to Gaucher's disease exists, where the dependence of the central nervous system involvement on age is even more apparent.

Histologic changes similar to those of the brain are found in the spinal cord and in the ganglion cells of the autonomous nervous system.

Results of Lipid Analyses

Through the work of KLENK (1934, 1935) it is known that sphingomyelin is the major component of the stored lipids in NPD. In addition, an increased cholesterol content of liver, spleen and brain has been found by SOBOTKA et al.

Table 1. Brain lipids in Niemann-Pick disease

	Cerebral cortex				Cerebral white matter			
	Patient* 15 1/2 months	Normal*	Patient** 6 years	Patient** 8 1/2 years	Patient* 15 1/2 months	Normal*	Patient** 6 years	Patient** 8 1/2 years
Total lipids	40.6	38.6			31.7	66.5		
Total cholesterol	8.0	4.3	6.0	6.8	7.7	12.0	8.8	11.9
Cholesterol ester	0.5	0.1	—	0.1	0.1	0.6	—	0.9
Total phospholipids	22.7	19.5	10.2	24.3	22.8	25.0	13.5	22.8
Sphingomyelin	5.7	1.7	2.1	5.9	5.6	2.6	5.1	5.9
Lecithin	8.3	5.2			9.8	6.0		
Cephalins	8.7	12.6			7.4	16.4		
Total hexosamine	0.550	0.695	0.29	—	0.620	0.340	0.19	0.29
Lipid hexosamine	0.180	0.182			0.148	0.052		
Neuraminic acid	0.482	0.485	0.40	0.44	0.296	0.130	—	—
Water (as per cent of fresh weight)	81.4	86.7	83.7	81.3	81.7	71.1	78.9	71.4

(Values expressed as gm/100 gm dry tissue.)
* From Norman et al. (1959); ** from Cumings (1962).

(1930, 1933), Crocker and Farber (1958), Uzman (1959), Ivemark et al. (1963), and Fredrickson (1960, 1966). An increase in brain gangliosides which is compatible with the histologic picture of the grey matter has been demonstrated by Klenk (1947, 1955, 1957), Bartsch (1957), Cumings (1957, 1962), and Jatzkewitz et al. (1965). In some more recent studies the sphingomyelin fatty acid composition was found to be altered (Thannhauser 1957, Svennerholm 1963, Ställberg-Stenhagen and Svennerholm 1965), a finding not reported in earlier studies, apparently as a result of inadequate methodology.

Differences of lipid content and composition in different organs make it desirable to discuss chemical findings for each one separately. In doing so it has to be kept in mind that comparison of reported data is limited by differences in time and methods of examination. On the other hand, variable findings may be due to the existence of subgroups of the disease, or finally, in some instances raise doubts as to the accuracy of the diagnosis.

Brain Lipids

The results of chemical analyses of brain biopsy or autopsy specimens, as reported by different laboratories, are particularly difficult to interpret. Considerable discrepancies in such data with regard to the concentrations of individual lipid fractions may to a significant degree be due to the fact that in the majority of cases analyses were performed during the period of the considerable physiologic change in brain lipid composition which accompanies myelination.

In general, the increase in sphingomyelin concentration appears to be associated with a rise in concentrations of cholesterol and gangliosides. Each of five subjects studied by Klenk (1934, 1935) had markedly increased sphingomyelins, and the total brain sphingomyelins in a case of Rouser et al. (1965)

was increased more than ten-fold if compared with normal infant brains and still 2.5-fold if compared with the adult brain. IVEMARK et al. (1963) found no increase in cerebral sphingomyelin in an infant who died at the age of eight months.

When white and grey matter were examined separately, CROCKER and FARBER (1958) found for the latter a consistently increased cholesterol content with the sphingomyelin being always at or above the upper limit of normal. In contrast, lipid values obtained from analysis of white matter, although again variable, were on the low side of normal. An interesting finding in some samples was that the lipid content of the white matter was equal to or even less than that of the grey matter, particularly with regard to total phospholipids and cholesterol. This phenomenon was interpreted by the authors to result from an overall lack of myelin, either on the basis of decreased synthesis due to insufficient amounts of precursors, of anomalies or destruction of nerve cells, or of disappearance of lipid through demyelination. CUMINGS (1962), analyzing brain tissue samples of two siblings (six and nine years old), found a normal content of total phospholipids in one and a marked decrease in the other, while sphingomyelin and cholesterol were increased in both (see table 1). On the basis of the neuraminic acid content, a small increase in ganglioside concentration to 2% of dry weight could be calculated in both cases. This finding confirms studies by KLENK (1955) who described an increase in gangliosides in three cases of NPD, and similar reports by BARTSCH (1957) and CUMINGS (1957).

It should be pointed out that histochemical methods do not allow quantitation of phospholipids and that chemical analyses of brain lipids are necessary for the determination of the content of total or individual phospholipids.

Sphingomyelin fatty acids. Normally, C-18 fatty acids prevails in the cerebral cortex and C-24 fatty acids in myelin (SVENNERHOLM 1963, PILZ and JATZKE-WITZ 1964).

Early data on the composition of brain sphingomyelin fatty acids in NPD are contradictory: KLENK (1934) reported a normal sphingomyelin fatty acid pattern, stearic acid being the most prominent component; THANNHAUSER (1957) found only traces of nervonic acid which normally makes up 12—15% of brain sphingomyelin fatty acids.

Table 2. *Fatty acid composition of brain sphingomyelin in Niemann-Pick disease*

	Patient* 10 months	Normal* 14 months	Patient** 29 months	Normal** 5 months
C 16	3.1	3.0	5.89	7.30
C 18	82.5	65.7	85.63	70.33
C 18:1	—		—	1.97
C 18:2			—	—
C 20	2.1	2.1	3.70	2.62
C 22	1.5	2.1	4.24	3.65
C 22:1	0.6	0.9	—	—
C 23	0.5	1.0	—	2.67
C 23:1	0.3	0.5		
C 24	2.1	3.9	—	4.46
C 24:1	4.2	15.9	—	8.39
C 25:0	0.7	0.5		
C 25:1	0.9	1.0		
C 26:0	trace	0.4		
C 26:1	0.9	2.5		

(Values expressed as per cent of total brain sphingomyelin fatty acids.)

 * From STÄLLBERG-STENHAGEN and SVENNERHOLM (1965).

** From ROUSER et al. (1965).

Table 3. *Lipid analyses of various organs in Niemann-Pick disease*

	Total lipids		Cholesterol		Total phospholipids		Sphingomyelin	
	Patients	Normals	Patients	Normals	Patients	Normals	Patients	Normals
Spleen (4 patients)	5.46—12.61	2.0—3.5	1.31—2.66	0.3—0.4	2.77— 7.87	1.0—2.0	1.36—4.57	0.1—0.5
Lymph nodes (3 patients)	4.04— 6.90	2.0—3.5	0.63—1.17	0.3—0.4	1.92— 5.12	1.0—2.0	0.54—2.73	0.1—0.5
Liver (5 patients)	3.48—14.8	3.0—4.0	0.34—1.07	0.3—0.4	1.49—10.1	1.5—2.5	0.26—6.58	0.1—0.25
Lung (4 patients)	2.43—16.5	2.0—3.5	0.40—0.85	0.3—0.4	1.25—12.1	1.0—2.0	0.35—6.75	0.1—0.4

(Values expressed as per cent of fresh weight.) *Source:* Crocker and Farber (1958). Data are from patients Nr. 1, 7, 8, 9, and 12.

Most recent analytical results are similar in that the proportion of stearic acid is increased while that of the longer chain fatty acids, which appear normally after the beginning of myelin function, is decreased (see table 2) (Stållberg-Stenhagen and Svennerholm 1965, Rouser et al. 1965). This change can also be deduced from absolute values (Pilz and Jatzkewitz 1964) for stearyl sphingomyelin in white and grey matter on one hand, and for lignoceric and nervonic acid-containing sphingomyelins on the other. While stearyl sphingomyelin was increased three-fold, the latter two were increased only 1.5—two-fold (Jatzkewitz 1965).

The sphingomyelin fatty acid pattern as reported for NPD is strikingly similar to that of fetal brain and thus resembles findings in other lipidoses with central nervous system involvement.

Other Organs

The results of lipid analyses of other organs are summarized in table 3. Here findings are more uniform. In nearly all affected tissues total sphingomyelin is increased as well as the proportion of sphingomyelin to total phospholipids. The sphingomyelin content may be 10—40 times normal. Equal parts of C-18 and C-24 sphingomyelin fatty acids were found by Jatzkewitz (1965) in spleens and livers of a 1½ year-old patient. Chiefly lignoceric, behenic and nervonic acids were found by Klenk (1935) in NPD and Gaucher's disease. There is a concomitant increase of free cholesterol, while ester cholesterol may be diminished (Fredrickson 1960).

The behaviour of other organ lipids is variable. A slight increase in glycerophosphatide and triglyceride content is frequent but insignificant when compared with the other fractions. It probably represents a non-specific, secondary change.

Data on individual phospholipid classes other than sphingomyelin are scarce. Klenk (1935) reported a slight increase in lecithin, Chargaff (1939) found cephalins elevated in the spleen in a case of NPD. Non-phosphorus-containing sphingolipids are not increased. The highest lipid content is found in those tissues which show the most pronounced macroscopic and histologic abnormalities, namely spleen, lymph nodes, liver and lungs. While the increase in sphingomyelin content is most marked in spleen and lymph nodes, the liver may have somewhat less sphingomyelin and a more pronounced increase in cholesterol.

Serum Lipids

Analyses of serum lipids in NPD are available in relatively few cases. From the reported data it appears that, in general, there are no specific abnormalities of serum lipids, and in particular no increase, absolute or relative, of serum sphingomyelins. Mild and often transient hyperlipidemias have been described which usually involve all lipid classes to a similar degree. In several patients of CROCKER and FARBER (1958) the degree of hyperlipidemia paralleled the increase in tissue lipids. It is likely that the mild hyperlipidemia in NPD represents a non-specific abnormality, but a definite answer to these questions has to await more precise information on the regulatory mechanisms of serum lipids.

SWEELEY (1960, 1963) examined plasma sphingomyelin fatty acids in NPD and found 18 different fatty acids with chain lengths from C-12 to C-24. As in normals, palmitic acid was the main component.

Pathogenetic Aspects

The pathogenesis of NPD, 40 years after the detection of the disease, is still largely unknown. Some possible causes of the condition are discussed below.

A genetic basis for the metabolic error is certain. An infectious etiology is as unlikely as a primary disorder of the liver, although at least two patients had liver tumors and more had jaundice of several months duration. Primary hyperplasia of reticulum cells was discussed as a cause (SCHLAGENHAUFER, see THANNHAUSER 1958) which would result in impairment of the elimination of stored lipid and thus lead to accumulation of sphingomyelin and cholesterol. When lecithin was still thought to be the prototype of stored lipids in NPD, decreased esterase activity was assumed by SOBOTKA et al. (1933) with resulting impairment of the transformation of cholesterol esters and lecithin to glycerides. This appears unlikely in view of the increased glyceride content of liver, spleen and occasionally serum of NPD-patients. EPSTEIN (1932, 1934, 1937) assumed impairment of catabolism of sphingomyelin with secondary storage of the material, similar to the pathogenesis of cystinuria. These thoughts were shared by PICK (cited from THANNHAUSER 1958) who, in addition, considered the primary lesion not to lie in the NPC themselves. THANNHAUSER (1958), in contrast, emphatically stated his belief that NPD was a disorder of "intracellular" metabolism of the enzymes concerned with sphingomyelin formation and disintegration, and postulated an imbalance of these enzymes within the cells which were to become NPC. He assumed that lignoceryl-sphingosine might be the precursor for sphingomyelins and cerebrosides and suggested similar pathogeneses for both NPD and Gaucher's disease.

If one assumes that the abnormality in NPD is basically one of sphingomyelin metabolism, two major points derserve attention, namely whether

a) there may be unchecked synthesis or impaired catabolism of normal sphingomyelin, or whether

b) there is some abnormality, either of the sphingosine moiety or its fatty acids, or of the physico-chemical state of the molecule (protein-binding, formation of aggregates) all of which may prevent entrance into degradative pathways.

Numerous chemical analyses in NPD have failed to produce evidence of an abnormal sphingomyelin molecule. As in the normal sphingosine moiety there is a double bond between carbon atoms 4 and 5. The amino group (C_2) and hydroxyl group (C_3) are in the erythro-configuration.

SRIBNEY and KENNEDY (1958) observed that for the phosphorylcholine-ceramide transferase reaction only threosphingosine could serve as substrate. They concluded that isomerisation might be a final step in normal sphingomyelin metabolism, and discussed persistence of threosphingomyelin as a possible cause for the accumulation in NPD. Since the persistence of the abnormal stereoisomer has not been established in NPD, their theory remains an interesting speculation. An argument against the presence in NPD of an altered sphingomyelin is the availability of the Niemann-Pick sphingomyelin as substrate for phospholipase-C (CROCKER and FARBER 1958).

Dihydrosphingosine and homologues with longer chain lengths are apparently present in small amounts in NPD, as is the case in normals. Whether persistence of a fetal sphingomyelin fatty acid pattern may be the cause or the result of storage, remains to be shown. There is no evidence for the occurrence in NPD of abnormal fatty acids in sphingomyelins.

The finding of poly-diaminophosphatides in Niemann-Pick organs by some authors (FRÄNKEL et al. 1933, ROSSI 1935) has been considered an artefact by KLENK (1933), and these compounds have never been found since.

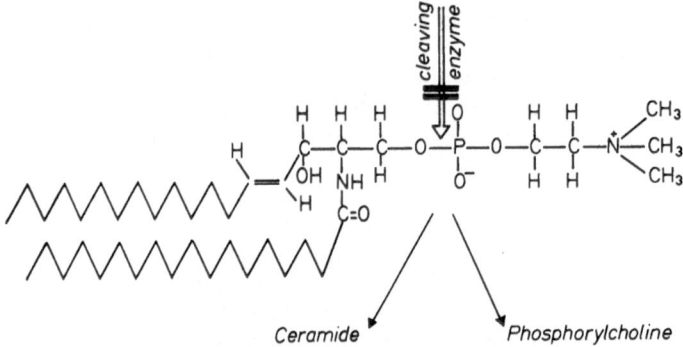

Fig. 6. Structure of sphingomyelin. The block indicates site of possible lesion in Niemann-Pick disease as suggested by findings of BRADY et al. (1966)

Abnormal intracellular protein binding as a cause for sphingomyelin storage, in analogy to findings of UZMAN (1951, 1958) in Gaucher's disease, could not be substantiated (CROCKER and FARBER 1958).

It is likely that the metabolic error in NPD consists of an enzymatic abnormality somewhere along the pathway of sphingomyelin metabolism. Whether this postulated abnormality influences synthesis or degradation of sphingomyelin has not been definitely established. The finding of a normal phospholipase C activity in tissues of Niemann-Pick patients (CROCKER and FARBER 1958), which catalyzes the hydrolytic cleavage of lecithin and sphingomyelin, does not exclude impairment of sphingomyelin degradation as the cause for NPD, since other enzymes involved in this process are still incompletely known.

Recent studies by BRADY et al. (1966) support the existence of a block of sphingomyelin catabolism. These authors presented evidence for the presence of an enzyme in normal human liver which catalyzes the hydrolysis of sphingomyelin (see figure 6), in analogy to findings in rat liver by KANFER et al. (1966). Comparison of enzyme activities in liver and kidney samples of control subjects and of six patients with NPD (FREDRICKSON 1966) showed large differences in the hydrolysis of ^{14}C-sphingomyelin. While the enzyme activity in controls ranged from 4.4 to 11.1 mμ moles of sphingomyelin cleaved per mg of protein per hour with an average of 6.6 mμ moles/mg of protein/hour, the corresponding values in tissues from NPD patients were only 0 to 0.89 mμ moles/mg protein/hour with an average value of 0.46. While inhibition of the enzyme by the accumulated sphingomyelin of Niemann-Pick tissues could be excluded, lecithin appeared to competitively inhibit the enzyme without being hydrolyzed.

If these interesting findings can be confirmed in other patients with NPD, the cause of NPD appears to be elucidated, and seems to be analogous to the lack of glucocerebroside cleaving enzyme (BRADY et al. 1965b) in Gaucher's disease.

Whether the presumed abnormality of sphingomyelin metabolism resides only in the lipid-storing histiocytes or whether it is located also in other cells capable of metabolizing sphingomyelin, has likewise not been settled. Arguments in favor of a more generalized defect include the lipid storage in cells other than reticulum cells, for instance in ganglion cells, and results of the interesting studies of HOLTZ et al. (1964). These authors studied fibroblasts of Niemann-Pick patients in tissue culture and found that their sphingomyelin contained $18.4 \pm 3.4\%$ of the total lipid phosphorus as compared to $6.8 \pm 1.7\%$ in control cultures. Even more interesting is the finding from amnion cell cultures of two children whose siblings had NPD. While in normal cultures 7.4% of the lipid phosphorus was in sphingomyelin, the respective values for the amnion culture of one infant were 7.9% and for the other 13.1% to 14.8%. While the former child was normal, the latter finally developed NPD.

Diagnosis

The diagnosis of NPD has to be considered when hepatosplenomegaly develops in an infant in association with progressive neurologic symptoms. Additional clinical evidence for the disease is a cherry-red spot in the macula similar to that seen in Tay-Sachs disease, brownish-yellow skin pigmentation, cachexia, auditory and visual disturbances and developing idiocy.

The finding of Niemann-Pick cells in biopsy specimens of spleen, bone marrow or liver supports the diagnosis which is confirmed by results of chemical analyses showing predominant elevation of sphingomyelin in various organs. While previously detailed studies of tissue lipids were rarely performed, such analyses are now facilitated by progress in methodology and ought to be performed in every case in question.

There are no significant abnormalities of serum lipids in NPD.

The differential diagnosis concerns mainly Gaucher's disease which in infants may also produce neurologic symptoms. In contrast to rigidity followed by loss of muscle tone which occurs in NPD, in Gaucher's disease general spasticity, opisthotonus and laryngospasm prevail. Furthermore, a cherry-red macular spot does not occur in Gaucher's disease. Other features of Gaucher's disease, which are not shared by NPD, are hypersplenic bone marrow inhibition, certain morphologic characteristics of the Gaucher cell, elevation of an acid serum phosphatase and storage of glucocerebrosides in reticuloendothelial tissues.

Differentiation from erythroblastoses or leukemias will be possible on the basis of hematologic findings. In the glycogenoses (v. Gierke's disease) splenomegaly is absent, the blood sugar is low and total plasma lipids are always higher than those observed in NPD although in the latter disease they may also be elevated. Essential hyperlipemia with hepatosplenomegaly does not lead to neurologic symptoms.

Finally, appropriate studies will serve to distinguish congenital syphilis, lymphogranulomatosis, Banti-syndrome and portal vein thrombosis.

Treatment

There is no way of influencing the course of the acutely progressing disease in infants. Splenectomy for mechanical reasons is rarely indicated. X-ray therapy may favorably influence local skin infiltrations (CROCKER and FARBER 1958).

Various drugs including adrenocortical steroids and vitamins have been tried without success. In contrast to Tay-Sachs disease, antibiotic treatment of intercurrent infections will postpone death only insignificantly.

References

Baggenstoss, A. H., E. F. Rosenberg, and A. E. Ostertag: Lipoid histiocytoses, report of cases with post mortem and chemical studies of the spleen. Arch. Path. **29**, 420 (1940).

Bartsch, G.: The nature of the lipids in the brain in Niemann-Pick's disease. In: Cerebral Lipidoses, p. 159. Eds.: L. van Bogaert, J. N. Cumings, and A. Lowenthal. Oxford: Blackwell 1957.

Baumann, T.: Zur Klinik und Pathogenese der Niemann-Pickschen Krankheit. Klin. Wschr. **14**, 1743 (1935).

— E. Klenk u. S. Scheidegger: Die Niemann-Picksche Krankheit, eine klinische, chemische und histopathologische Studie. Erg. allg. Path. path. Anat. **30**, 183 (1936).

Berman, S. L.: Lipoid histiocytosis (Niemann-Pick's disease). Amer. J. Dis. Child. **36**, 102 (1928).

Bielschowsky, M.: Amaurotische Idiotie und lipoidzellige Splenohepatomegalie. J. Psychiat. Neurol. (Lpz.) **26**, 103 (1928).

Bloom, W.: Splenomegaly (type Gaucher) and lipoid-histiocytosis (type Niemann). Amer. J. Path. **1**, 595 (1925).

— The histogenesis of essential lipoid histiocytosis (Niemann Pick disease). Arch. Path. **6**, 827 (1928).

— and R. Kern: Spleens from Gaucher's disease and lipoid-histiocytosis; the chemical analysis. Arch. intern. Med. **39**, 456 (1927).

Bogaert, L. van: L'idiotie amaurotique et les maladies du métabolisme lipidien. Bull. Acad. roy. Méd. Belg. **14**, 323 (1934).

Brady, R. O., J. N. Kanfer, and D. Shapiro: The metabolism of glucocerebrosides. I. Purification and properties of a glucocerebroside cleaving enzyme from spleen tissue. J. biol. Chem. **240**, 39 (1965a).

— — — Metabolism of glucocerebrosides. II. Evidence of an enzymatic deficiency in Gaucher's disease. Biochem. biophys. Res. Commun. **18**, 221 (1965b).

— — M. B. Mock, and D. S. Fredrickson: The metabolism of sphingomyelin. II. Evidence of an enzymatic deficiency in Niemann-Pick disease. Proc. nat. Acad. sci. (Wash.) **55**, 366 (1966).

Brahn, B., u. L. Pick: Zur chemischen Organanalyse bei der lipoidzelligen Splenohepatomegalie Typus Niemann-Pick. Klin. Wschr. **6**, 2367 (1927).

Chargaff, E.: A study of the spleen in a case of Niemann-Pick disease. J. biol. Chem. **130**, 503 (1939).

Crocker, A. C., and S. Farber: Niemann-Pick disease: a review of eighteen patients. Medicine (Baltimore) **37**, 1 (1958).

Cumings, J. N.: The diagnostic value of lipid estimations in the cerebral lipidoses. In: Cerebral Lipidoses, p. 112. Eds.: L. van Bogaert, J. N. Cumings, and A. Lowenthal. Oxford: Blackwell 1957.

— Abnormalities in lipid metabolism in two members of a family with Niemann-Pick disease. In: Cerebral Sphingolipidoses, p. 171. Eds.: S. M. Aronson, and B. W. Volk. New York: Academic Press 1962.

Didion, H.: Vergleichend-histopathologische Untersuchungen an einem Zwillingspaar mit Niemann-Pick'scher Krankheit. Frankfurt. Z. Path. **60**, 194 (1949).

— Die anatomischen Veränderungen des Augenhintergrundes bei Niemann-Pick'scher Krankheit. Klin. Mbl. Augenheilk. **116**, 131 (1950).

Dienst, G., u. H. Hamperl: Lipoid-Splenohepatomegalie (Typ Niemann-Pick). Wien. klin. Wschr. **40**, 1432 (1927).

Diezel, P. B.: Die Stoffwechselstörungen der Sphingolipoide. Berlin-Göttingen-Heidelberg: Springer 1957 (a).

— Histochemical study of primary lipidoses. In: Cerebral Lipidoses, p. 11. Eds.: L. van Bogaert, J. N. Cumings, and A. Lowenthal. Oxford: Blackwell 1957 (b).

— Disturbances in lipid and carbohydrate metabolism in relation to the brain. In: Mental Retardation. New York: Grune & Stratton 1960.

— Die angeborenen Störungen des Lipoidstoffwechsels. In: Medizinische Grundlagenforschg., Bd. IV, p. 239. Stuttgart: Thieme 1962.

Dusendschon, A.: Deux cas familiaux de maladie de Niemann-Pick chez adulte. Thèse, Genève 1946.

EPSTEIN, E.: Ätiologische Bedeutung der chemischen Veränderungen für die Pathologie im Gehirn bei Niemann-Pick'scher Krankheit, Beziehung zur amaurotischen Idiotie Tay-Sachs. Virchows Arch. path. Anat. **284**, 867 (1932).
— Über das gegensätzliche Verhältnis der lipoid-chemischen Beschaffenheit des Gehirns bei Niemann-Pick und infantiler amaurotischer Idiotie Tay-Sachs. Beziehung der Pathochemie zur Pathologie beider Krankheiten. Virchows Arch. path. Anat. **293**, 135 (1934).
— Beitrag zur Pathologie der generalisierten Lipoidosen. Ergebn. allg. Path. path. Anat. **33**, 280 (1937).
— and K. LORENZ: Die Phosphatidzellverfettung im Gehirn, Leber und Milz bei Niemann-Pickscher Krankheit. Z. physiol. Chem. **211**, 217 (1932).
FAKAÇELLI, N. M.: La maladie de Niemann-Pick (à propos d'un cas personnel). Ann. paediat. (Basel) **162**, 218 (1944).
FISHER, C. F.: Niemann-Pick's disease with leukemoid blood reaction. Arch. Pediat. **49**, 574 (1932).
FRÄNKEL, E., F. BIELSCHOWSKY u. S. J. THANNHAUSER: Untersuchungen über die Lipoide der Säugetierleber. III. Über ein Polydiaminophosphatid der Schweineleber. Hoppe-Seylers Z. physiol. Chem. **218**, 1 (1933).
FREDRICKSON, D. S.: Niemann-Pick disease. In: The metabolic basis of inherited disease, p. 580. Eds.: J. B. Stanbury, J. B. Wyngaarden, and D. S. Fredrickson. New York: McGraw-Hill 1960. 2nd Edition: 1966, p. 586.
GAENSSLEN, M.: Erbpathologie des Blutes und der blutbildenden Organe. In: Handbuch der Erbbiologie des Menschen, Bd. IV/2, S. 411. Berlin: Springer 1940.
GARMYN, F.: De ziekte van Niemann-Pick: Symptomatologie en evolutie. Maandschr. Kindergeneesk. **30**, 10 (1962).
GERKEN, H., u. H. R. WIEDEMANN: Ein Beitrag zur Genetik des Morbus Gaucher. Ann. paediat. (Basel) **203**, 328 (1964).
GIAMPALMO, A.: Über die Pathologie der Lipoidosen. II. Phosphatidosen und Cerebrosidosen. Medizinische **1953**, 612.
GOLDSTEIN, J., and D. WEXLER: Niemann-Pick's disease with cherry-red spots in macula, ocular pathology. Arch. Ophthal. **5**, 704 (1931).
HAMBURGER, R.: Lipoidzellige Splenohepatomegalie (Typ Niemann-Pick) in Verbindung mit amaurotischer Idiotie bei einem 14 Monate alten Mädchen. Jb. Kinderheilk. **116**, 41 (1927).
HASSIN, G. B.: Niemann-Pick's disease, pathologic studies of cases. Arch. Neurol. Psychiat. (Chic.) **24**, 61 (1930).
HASTRUP, B., and A. VIDEBAEK: Acid phosphatase in Niemann-Pick's disease and a therapeutic experiment with cortisone. Acta med. scand. **149**, 287 (1954).
HOLTZ, A. I., W. UHLENDORF, and D. S. FREDRICKSON: Persistence of a lipid defect in tissue cultures derived from patients with Niemann-Pick disease. Fed. Proc. **23**, 128 (1964).
IVEMARK, B. I., L. SVENNERHOLM, C. THORÉN, and R. TUNELL: Niemann-Pick disease in infancy: report of two siblings with clinical, histologic and chemical studies. Acta paediat. (Uppsala) **52**, 391 (1963).
JATZKEWITZ, H.: Über Sphingolipoidosen. In: 16tes Mosbacher Kolloquium. Lipoide. 1965. Berlin-Heidelberg-New York: Springer 1966.
— H. PILZ, and K. SANDHOFF: The quantitative determination of gangliosides and their derivatives in different forms of amaurotic idiocy. J. Neurochem. **12**, 135 (1965).
KANFER, J. N., O. M. YOUNG, D. SHAPIRO, and R. O. BRADY: J. biol. Chem. (in press). Cited after BRADY et al. (1966).
KLENK, E.: Über die Sphingomyeline des Herzmuskels. Hoppe-Seylers Z. physiol. Chem. **221**, 67 (1933).
— Über die Natur der Phosphatide in der Milz bei Niemann-Pickscher Krankheit. Hoppe-Seylers Z. physiol .Chem. **229**, 161 (1934).
— Über die Natur der Phosphatide und anderer Lipoide im Gehirn und Leber. Hoppe-Seylers Z. physiol. Chem. **235**, 24 (1935).
— Über die Verteilung der Neuraminsäure im Gehirn bei der familiären amaurotischen Idiotie und bei der Niemann-Pick'schen Krankheit (Beiträge zur Chemie der Lipoidosen, 6. Mitteilung). Hoppe-Seylers Z. physiol. Chem. **282**, 84 (1947).
— The pathological chemistry of the developing brain. In: Biochemistry of the developing nervous system, p. 397. Ed.: H Waelsch. New York: Academic Press 1955.
— Die Chemie der Lipoidosen und der Entmarkungskrankheiten. Wien. Z. Nervenheilk. **13**, 309 (1957).
KNOX, J. H. M., W. H. WAHL, and A. C. SCHMEISSER: Gaucher's disease in infants. Bull. Johns. Hopk. Hosp. **27**, 1 (1916).
KNOX, R. A., and G. W. RAMSEY: Niemann-Pick's disease (essential lipoid histiocytosis). Ann. intern. Med. **6**, 218 (1932).
KRAMER, B.: Lipoid-cell splenohepatomegaly, Niemann-Pick type. Med. Clin. N. Amer. **2**, 905 (1928).

Letterer, E.: Allgemeine Pathologie und pathologische Anatomie der Lipoidosen. Verh. dtsch. Ges. Verdau.- u. Stoffwechselkr. **71**, 12 (1939).
— Speicherungskrankheiten. Dtsch. med. Wschr. **73**, 147 (1947).
Lynn, K., and R. D. Terry: Lipid histochemistry and electron microscopy in adult Niemann-Pick disease. Amer. J. Med. **37**, 987 (1964).
Mandlebaum, F. S., and H. Downey: The cases of Gaucher's disease reported by Drs. Knox, Wahl, and Schmeisser. Bull. Johns. Hopk. Hosp. **27**, 104 (1916).
Maurer, L. E.: Niemann-Pick's disease, a report of four cases. Rocky Mtn. med. J. **38**, 460 (1941).
McFate, R. P.: The chemical analyses of liver and spleen from a case of lipoid histiocytosis (Niemann-Pick's disease). Arch. Path. Lab. Med. **6**, 1054 (1928).
Menten, M. L., and L. Welton: Lipid analysis in a case of Niemann-Pick's disease. Amer. J. Dis. Child. **72**, 720 (1946).
Merksamer, E., and B. Kramer: Niemann-Pick's disease. Report of three cases in one family. J. Pediat. **14**, 51 (1939).
Niemann, A.: Ein unbekanntes Krankheitsbild. Jb. Kinderheilk. **79**, 1 (1914).
Norman, R. M., H. Urich, A. H. Tingey, and R. A. Goodbody: Tay-Sachs disease with visceral involvement and its relationship to Niemann-Pick disease. J. Path. Bact. **78**, 409 (1959).
Pfändler, U.: La maladie de Niemann-Pick dans le cadre des lipoidoses. Schweiz. med. Wschr. **76**, 1128 (1946).
Pick, L.: Zur pathologischen Anatomie des Morbus Gaucher. Med. Klin. **18**, 1408 (1922).
— Der Morbus Gaucher und die ihm ähnlichen Erkrankungen. Ergebn. inn. Med. Kinderheilk. **29**, 519 (1926).
— Über die lipoidzellige Splenohepatomegalie Typus Niemann-Pick als Stoffwechselerkrankung. Med. Klin. **23**, 1483 (1927).
— Über lipoidzellige Splenohepatomegalie. Verh. dtsch. Ges. Verdau.- u. Stoffwechselkr. **5**, 8 (1928).
— II. Niemann-Pick's disease and other forms of so-called xanthomatoses. Amer. J. med. Sci. **185**, 601 (1933).
— u. M. Bielschowsky: Über lipoidzellige Splenomegalie (Typus Niemann-Pick) und amaurotische Idiotie. Klin. Wschr. **6**, 1631 (1927).
Pilz, H., u. H. Jatzkewitz: Dünnschichtchromatographische Bestimmungen von C_{18}- und C_{24}-Sphingomyelin in normalen und pathologischen Gehirnen einschließlich eines Falles von Niemann-Pickscher Erkrankung. J. Neurochem. **11**, 603 (1964).
Poncher, H. G.: Lipoidhistiocytosis (Niemann Pick's disease). Amer. J. Dis. Child. **42**, 77 (1931).
Rintelen, F.: Die Histopathologie der Augenhintergrundsveränderungen bei Niemann-Pickscher Lipoidose; zugleich ein Beitrag zur Frage der Beziehungen zwischen Tay-Sachs'scher Idiotie und Niemann-Pickscher Lipoidose. Arch. Augenheilk. **109**, 332 (1935).
Rossi, A.: Untersuchungen über die Lipoide der Säugetiere. IX. Über die enzymatische Spaltbarkeit des Leber-Polydiaminophosphatids. Hoppe-Seylers Z. physiol. Chem. **231**, 115 (1935).
Rothstein, J. L., and S. Welt: Infantile amaurotic familial idiocy of lipoid metabolism. Report of two cases of Tay-Sachs disease with necropsy. Amer. J. Dis. Child. **62**, 801 (1941).
Rouser, G., C. Galli, and G. Kritchevsky: Lipid class composition of normal human brain and variations in metachromatic leucodystrophy, Tay-Sachs, Niemann-Pick, chronic Gaucher's and Alzheimer's diseases. J. Amer. Oil Chemists' Soc. **42**, 404 (1965).
Schettler, G.: Lipidosen. 2. Sphingomyelinose. In: Handbuch der Inn. Med. Eds.: G. V. Bergmann, W. Frey and H. Schwiegk, p. 647. Berlin-Göttingen-Heidelberg: Springer 1955.
Schiff, F.: Im Leben diagnostizierte lipoidzellige Splenohepatomegalie (Typ Niemann-Pick) bei einem 17 Monate alten Knaben. Jb. Kinderheilk. **112**, 1 (1926).
Schlagenhaufer, F.: Über meist familiär vorkommende histologische charakteristische Splenomegalien (Typus Gaucher). Eine Systemerkrankung des lymphatisch-hämatopoetischen Apparates. Virchows Arch. path. Anat. **87**, 125 (1906/1907).
Siegmund, H.: Lipoidzellenhyperplasie der Milz und Splenomegalie Gaucher. Verh. dtsch. path. Ges. **18**, 59 (1921).
Smetana, H.: Ein Fall von Niemann Pickscher Erkrankung (lipoidzellige Splenohepatomegalie). Virchows Arch. path. Anat. **274**, 697 (1930).
Sobotka, H., E. Epstein, and L. Lichtenstein: The distribution of lipoid in a case of Niemann-Pick's disease associated with amaurotic family idiocy. Arch. Path. **10**, 677 (1930).
— D. Glick, M. Reiner, and L. R. Tuchman: The lipoids of spleen and liver in various types of lipoidoses. Biochem. J. **27**, 2031 (1933).
Sribney, M., and E. P. Kennedy: The enzymatic synthesis of sphingomyelin. J. biol. Chem. **233**, 1315 (1958).

STÄLLBERG-STENHAGEN, S., and L. SVENNERHOLM: The fatty acid composition of human brain sphingomyelins: Normal variation with age and changes during myelin disorders. J. Lipid Res. **6**, 140 (1965).

STRANSKY, E.: Über großzellige Splenohepatomegalie. Jb. Kinderheilk. **126**, 204 (1930).

SVENNERHOLM, L.: Some aspects of the biochemical changes in leucodystrophy. In: Brain lipids and lipoproteins, and the leucodystrophies, p. 104. Eds.: J. Folch Pi and H. J. Bauer. Amsterdam-London-New York: Elsevier Publishing Co. 1963.

SWEELEY, C. C.: Purification and partial characterization of sphingomyelin from human plasma. J. Lipid Res. **4**, 402 (1963).

— Unpublished (cit. by FREDRICKSON 1960, p. 589).

TERRY, R., W. M. SPERRY, and B. BRODOFF: Adult lipidosis resembling Niemann-Pick's disease. Amer. J. Path. **30**, 263 (1954).

THANNHAUSER, S. J.: Lipidoses: Diseases of the cellular lipid metabolism. Oxford: University Press 1950.

— Diseases of the nervous system associated with disturbances of lipide metabolism. Proc. Ass. Res. Nerv. Ment. Dis. **32**, 238 (1953).

— In: Biochemical disorders in human disease, p. 697. Eds.: R. H. S. Thompson and E. J. King. London: Churchill 1957.

— Lipidoses: Disease of the intracellular lipid metabolism. 3nd Ed., p. 524. New York: Grune & Stratton 1958.

TOKUJAWA, H.: Trans. Jap. Path. Soc. **27**, 114 (1937). Cit. by VIDEBAEK (1949).

UZMAN, L. L.: The lipoprotein of Gaucher's disease. Arch. Path. **51**, 329 (1951).

— The significance of the increase of nonspecific lipid components in primary lipoid-storage disease. Arch. Path. **65**, 331 (1958).

VIDEBAEK, A.: Niemann-Pick's disease, acute and chronic type. Acta paediat. (Uppsala) **37**, 95 (1949).

— Another case of Niemann-Pick's disease observed in Denmark. Acta paediat. (Uppsala) **41**, 355 (1952).

WAHL, H. R., and M. L. RICHARDSON: A study of lipin content of a case of Gaucher's disease in an infant. Arch. intern. Med. **17**, 238 (1916).

WASCOWITZ, B.: Niemann-Pick's disease (essential lipoid histiocytosis). Amer. J. Dis. Child. **42**, 356 (1931).

ZOEPFFEL, H.: Eine Niemann-Picksche Krankheit unter dem Bild der Lipoidnephrose. Arch. Kinderheilk. **171**, 271 (1964).

Metachromatic Leucodystrophy

By

W. Kahlke

Synonyms: Metachromatic leucoencephalopathy; degenerative diffuse cerebral sclerosis type Scholz-Bielschowsky-Henneberg; sulfatide lipidosis; sulfatidosis.

Definition and Introduction

The term "diffuse cerebral sclerosis" (leucodystrophy) is used for changes which occur in a variety of disorders and consist of demyelination in cerebrum and cerebellum, whereby reactive gliosis leads to progressive sclerosis. The axis cylinders are rather well preserved, in contrast to their condition during the demyelination which occurs following disease of ganglion cells and axons as in Tay-Sachs disease. It appears therefore that, in the leucodystrophies, there is a primary disturbance in the metabolism of myelin components. Lipid abnormalities are found in several types of congenital diffuse sclerosis or leucodystrophy, such as "globoid-cell" leucodystrophy, type Krabbe (DIEZEL 1955; LEES and MOSER 1962; AUSTIN 1963 a, b; CUMINGS and ROZDILSKY 1965; AUSTIN and LEHFELDT 1965) and Pelizaeus-Merzbacher disease (DEBUCH 1957, 1958; SEITELBERGER 1957; NORMAN and TINGEY 1963; DIEZEL et al. 1965; NISENBAUM et al. 1965).

Metachromatic leucodystrophy (ML) is a hereditary disorder of the metabolism of cerebroside-sulfuric acid esters (sulfatides) with involvement of myelin in the central nervous system and, to a lesser degree, of organs participating in excretory functions, such as the kidneys and gall-bladder. Histochemically, the accumulated sulfatides are metachromatic, whereas the material found in other leucodystrophies is not. Storage of cerebroside-sulfuric acid esters in glial and ganglion cells may result from blockage of sulfatide degradation.

Since it has not been established whether other forms of degenerative diffuse sclerosis are also due to abnormalities of lipid metabolism, the present chapter will be restricted to a discussion of ML, although analytical findings in Pelizaeus-Merzbacher disease and in diffuse sclerosis, type Krabbe, suggest that these disorders may also be lipidoses.

Historical Review

The first three juvenile cases of diffuse sclerosis were found by SCHOLZ (1925) in a family with various neurologic disorders. SCHOLZ thought that breakdown products of the myelin sheaths were not further metabolized to neutral lipids and pointed out the similarity of the stored material with the "prelipoid substances" of ALZHEIMER (1910). Since in his cases ganglion cells were not involved in the sclerotic process he proposed that the primary abnormality might reside with the glial cells. The observations of SCHOLZ were confirmed by BIELSCHOWSKY and HENNEBERG (1928) in two siblings who died at the ages of nine and 12 years, respectively. Tinctorial properties of endothelial cells within the white matter suggested to these authors a disturbance of cerebral lipid metabolism. They noted the similarities to and the differences from the amaurotic family idiocies, as SCHOLZ had done. Cases with "prelipoid degradation products" in childhood had been described earlier by HABERFELD and SPIELER (1910) and SCHILDER (1913) and a number of reports following that of BIELSCHOWSKY and HENNEBERG (1928) seems to belong to the same group on the basis of morphologic and histochemical findings (VAN BOGAERT and BERTRAND 1933; GREENFIELD 1933; BERTRAND et al. 1954; CUMINGS 1955; DIEZEL 1957 a, b; HALLERVORDEN 1957; HAIN and LA VECK 1958; PEIFFER 1959; HAGBERG et al. 1960—1962; HOLLÄNDER and PILZ 1964, and many others). A review of 65 cases in which the diagnosis of ML was confirmed neuropathologically has been prepared by HOL-LÄNDER (1964 a). Other summaries of the disease are those of POSER and VAN BOGAERT (1956), HALLERVORDEN (1957), DIEZEL (1957, 1962), PEIFFER (1959), LYON et al. (1961), POSER (1962), HAGBERG (1963), DOSS and MATIAR-VAHAR (1965), KOCH (1966), and MOSER and LEES (1966).

In 1950, BRAIN and GREENFIELD noted metachromatic deposits in cerebral white matter and in the epithelium of renal tubuli, and distention of ganglion cells and pointed out the homogeneity of reported cases. HIRSCH and PEIFFER (1955) made a systematic histochemical study of the myelin degradation products in leucodystrophy, examining the cases of SCHOLZ (1925), VAN BOGAERT and SCHOLZ (1932), SCHOLZ (1933), VAN BOGAERT and BERTRAND (1933) and WICKE (1938). Their finding of brown-metachromatic material in the ganglion cells of certain nuclei confirms earlier reports on this phenomenon (NISSL 1910; WITTE 1921; WICKE 1938; VAN BOGAERT and DEWULF 1939; CARDONA 1939; NORMAN 1947; BRAIN and GREENFIELD 1950, and LESLIE 1952). DIEZEL (1957 a, b) was able to confirm the diagnosis of ML only for the cases of VAN BOGAERT and DEWULF (1939), JACOBI (1947), and BERTRAND et al. (1954).

A similarity of leucodystrophy to some of the classic lipidoses was pointed out by EDGAR (1955, 1957) who had found increases of hexosamine-containing compounds in nine cases. On the basis of this finding ML was defined as a special type of degenerative diffuse sclerosis (HALLERVORDEN 1957).

DIEZEL (1956, 1957 a) showed that small amounts of brown-metachromatic material were actually components of the normal myelin sheaths. He contrasted cases with accumulation of brown metachromatic material and storage by ganglion cells with others exhibiting yellow myelin breakdown products with an ortho-chromatic reaction and lack of ganglion cell storage. The latter form occurs mainly in adults and does not appear to be a sulfatidosis.

In 1958, JATZKEWITZ made the important discovery that the metachromatic material in leucodystrophy consists of cerebroside-sulfuric acid esters, proving that ML was indeed a lipid storage disease. The differentiation of leucodystrophies with "prelipoid" and "metachromatic" degradation products was now abolished. Re-cent reports by AUSTIN (1957 a, b), HAGBERG et al. (1960—1962), SOURANDER and SVENNERHOLM (1962), ISLER, BISCHOFF and ESSLEN (1963), HOLLÄNDER and PILZ (1964), FULLERTON (1964), and JATZKEWITZ (1958—1965) underlined the existence of ML as a distinct cerebral sphingolipidosis.

Enzymatic studies in ML were those of WITMER and AUSTIN (1960), JATZ-KEWITZ (1963), AUSTIN et al. (1963, 1964 a, b, 1965), MEHL and JATZKEWITZ (1965) and others.

Incidence (Age, Sex, Race)

The disease may become manifest at any time between early infancy and adult life. A male infant who died at the age of six weeks was reported by FEIGIN (1954). JERVIS (1960) considered this case to be a "congenital" form of ML, and also distinguished an "infantile" form (identical with Greenfield's disease) with disease onset between the first and third year. HOLLÄNDER (1964a), who did not differentiate several forms of the disease, found that in two thirds of all cases the onset was before the age of three years. Thus, in seven out of nine cases of HAGBERG (1963) the disease began between 15 and 18 months. Some authors (BRAIN and GREENFIELD 1950; NORMAN et al. 1960; HAGBERG et al. 1960) prefer the term "late-infantile ML" for this age-group, by analogy with the late-infantile amaurotic family idiocy. The survival time of this type of ML is usually one to two years, but may be up to six years with diligent supportive care.

Subjects with the "juvenile" form were the first reported cases with degenerative diffuse sclerosis (SCHOLZ 1925; BIELSCHOWSKY and HENNEBERG 1928; NORMAN 1947). Here, manifestations appear between six and nine years of age. Although in these cases the disease may last up to eight years, its course, in general, is not much longer than in the infantile form (HOLLÄNDER and PILZ 1964).

The onset in the so-called adult form is after puberty (EINARSON and NEEL 1938; HOLLÄNDER and PILZ 1964; ETTINGER 1965). Its progression is slower than in the preceding forms and occasionally the disease may not prove fatal for several decades, but usually these patients also die after a few years (HOLLÄNDER and PILZ 1964).

For the juvenile form KOCH (1966) has found the disease to be twice as prevalent in males as in females. No such sex differences are noted in the late-infantile and adult forms. A review of 53 cases of ML, without regard to type, revealed 27 affected males and 26 affected females (HOLLÄNDER 1964a). It is likely that the various types are forms of the same disease (BARGETON 1963) and there is no evidence for biochemical differences (SVENNERHOLM 1963b). Unless otherwise noted the following discussion concerns the late-infantile form of ML.

Clinical Manifestations

Detailed reviews of the clinical picture have been given by HALLERVORDEN (1957), JEFFERSON (1958), PEIFFER (1959), JERVIS (1960), HAGBERG et al. (1960, 1962), HAGBERG (1963), and KOCH (1966). In spite of a great variability in the symptomatology, certain signs can be consistently observed, and a subdivision of the clinical course into four stages has been proposed by HAGBERG (1963) (see table 1).

Among the first signs in children is impairment of motor function with arrest of physiologic development followed by loss of acquired skills. The same applies to speech and mental development (HAGBERG 1963). Frequently, flaccid diplegic or tetraplegic paralysis develops and hypotonicity of the musculature may resemble myopathy or Werdnig-Hoffman disease (HAGBERG 1963). The further course is characterized by appearance of ataxia, coarse tremor, paralysis of ocular muscles, nystagmus and progressive impairment of speech. Muscular hypotonicity is followed by spasticity (PEIFFER 1959). Pain in the extremities is quite common, and seems to be caused by both muscular cramps and radicular involvement (HAGBERG et al. 1960) which may necessitate administration of large doses of analgesics. Tendon reflexes are diminished or absent. The peripheral nerve conduction in ML is slow (ISLER et al. 1963). While generalized seizures are rare, muscle spasms, myoclonic movements and "tonic fits" (JERVIS 1960) occur quite frequently. Complete loss of speech may be followed by the appearance of a bulbar symptomatology with feeding difficulties and impairment of respiration. Febrile periods which now occur frequently may be of cerebral origin (HAGBERG 1963). Progressive loss of mental functions results in increasing apathy and in loss of interest in and contact with the environment; it is aggravated by impairment of vision which occurs in most children following optic atrophy. Pupillary abnormalities may then occur. After this period which is characterized by a primitive, complex and marked tetraplegia with variable muscle tone, the final stage is one of decerebrate rigidity, blindness and deafness. Fever spells and hypertonic bouts become less frequent now, but bulbar symptoms progress to a point when tube feeding becomes necessary and finally intercurrent infections or cerebral hyperpyrexia terminate the disease.

A similar symptomatology is seen in juvenile cases. Here, visual and auditory disturbances may occur early, the progression of the disease may be slower and psychotic symptoms occur. In the end stage there is marked spasticity and ataxia.

The adult form is characterized by a very slowly progressing symptomatology, making the diagnosis of leucodystrophy very difficult. Clinical features simulating schizophrenia, paralysis and dementia have been described repeatedly. One case resembled in the beginning multiple sclerosis with deterioration of intellectual performance and compulsive laughter and crying (HOLLÄNDER and PILZ 1964). A correlation of the neurologic or psychiatric symptomatology with the localization of the disease process has been emphasized by PEIFFER (1959). Frontal demyelination may favor the development of a paralytic symptomatology, while lesions in the temporooccipital area may cause

Table 1. *Symptoms and signs in different clinical stages of metachromatic leucodystrophy*

	First symptoms	Stage I	Stage II	Stage III	Stage IV
Definition of stage:		Ability to walk or to stand with or without support	No ability to stand but only to sit with or without support	Bedridden without ability to stand or to sit but with some voluntary movements	Bedridden without ability to perform any voluntary movements and without contact with the surroundings
Age (years):	1—2	1¼—4½	2—5	2½—6	3—6
Duration (years):		½—2½	0—1¼	¼—3½	up to 3 (until death)
Characteristic signs:	Unsteady gait walking difficulties weak legs and feet valgus feet	Mental stagnation speech abnormalities diplegia or tetraplegia pronounced hypotonia ataxic signs CSF-protein raised weak or absent tendon reflexes (rarely)	Mental regression speech disturbances hypertonic tetraplegia pain in arms and legs absent tendon reflexes ataxia nystagmus optic atrophy (rarely)	Mental retardation violent root (?) pains no speech rigidity hypertonic fits bouts of hyperpyrexia optic atrophy bulbar signs increasing feeding and respiratory difficulties	"Burnt out stage" blindness no speech decerebrate rigidity bulbar symptoms disappearance of pains and hypertonic fits no contact with the surroundings feeding by tube

Source: HAGBERG (1963). The table is based on observations in nine cases of metachromatic leucodystrophy.

psychotic symptoms. In the absence of neurologic disturbances the differentiation from schizophrenia is not possible on clinical grounds alone.

The *electroencephalogram* is not typical in ML (THIEFFRY and LYON 1959). Frequently, focal or general delta wave activity is seen (JEFFERSON 1958; PEIFFER 1959), but the electroencephalogram may be completely normal in other cases (JERVIS 1960). PAMPIGLIONE (1961) found in six patients only mild electro-encephalographic abnormalities with a total lack of paroxysmal features. In contrast, HAGBERG et al. (1962) observed increasing preponderance of generalized delta activity with occasional spike-waves in later stages. With regard to the lack in ML of stereotyped, repeating high-amplitude complexes as commonly seen in subacute sclerosing or inclusion-body encephalitis, HAGBERG et al. (1962) consider repeated electroencephalographic studies useful for the differential diagnosis of ML.

Cerebrospinal Fluid

Elevation of cerebrospinal fluid protein is frequent. Its concentration increases during the course of the disease and may reach values of 100—200 mg/100 ml. The cell count is not elevated. In contrast to other demyelinating diseases the protein pattern in ML and in diffuse cerebral sclerosis, type Krabbe, is normal (HAGBERG and SVENNERHOLM 1960) and this finding aids in differentiation from disorders with typical deviations in the cerebrospinal fluid protein pattern such as Guillain-Barré syndrome etc. The concentration of sulfatides was very small in the material of HAGBERG (1963) and it was not possible to determine whether it was greater than in normal specimens.

Blood

There are no characteristic abnormalities of serum or of formed blood elements in ML. Non-specific hypercholesterolemia has been seen (HAGBERG 1963), but sulfatides are present in normal amounts (SVENNERHOLM and SVENNERHOLM 1962). The ratio of cerebrosides: sulfatides, which is abnormal in the central nervous system, is normal in serum (HAGBERG 1963). Some relevant serum enzymes have been studied by AUSTIN et al. (1965 a, b). According to these authors acid phosphatase activity was normal when measured with p-nitrophenylphosphate as substrate. The activity of arylsulfatase B was three to four times that of type A, and thus similar to findings in normal serum.

Urine

Urinary excretion of sulfatides in ML (AUSTIN 1957 a, b; JATZKEWITZ 1958; HAGBERG et al. 1960) was suspected as early as 1921 by WITTE who found accumulation of a metachromatic substance in the kidneys of affected subjects. Light microscopy of the stained urinary sediment shows granular and globular metachromatic bodies, but there is no complete agreement on the significance of this finding. While AUSTIN (1963) considers the presence in urine of a typical golden-brown material to be specific for ML, metachromatic substances have been found in the urine of normal subjects (HAGBERG and SVENNERHOLM 1959; HAGBERG et al. 1965) and in a number of other diseases in identical or even greater amounts than in ML (HELFANT et al. 1962; HAGBERG et al. 1965). In contrast, however, to findings in normal subjects and patients with other diseases, a substance which occurs in the "fluff" phase (interphase) of a chloroform extract from urinary sediment, shows red-pink metachromasia at pH 2 and its paper-chromatographic properties are those of brain sulfatide (AUSTIN 1960). Recent studies by HAGBERG et al. (1965) have shown that there is a typical urinary sulfatide pattern in ML, characterized by the occurrence of a second spot with a lower Rf-value in addition to the larger sulfatide spot seen in extracts of normal urine. Its chromatographic and staining properties are those of N-acylsphingosine-glucose-galactose-sulfate (SVENNERHOLM 1963a), which has been isolated from normal and ML kidneys by MARTENSSON (1963 a, b) and MÅRTENSSON et al. (1966) in addition to the prevailing sulfatide N-acylsphingosine-galactose-sulfate. According to these authors only the demonstration of this atypical sulfatide in urine is pathognomonic for ML.

Studies on sulfatases by AUSTIN et al. (1964 b) showed that in the urine of patients with ML sulfatase A activity is considerably diminished and amounts to about 2% of normal, while sulfatase B activity is not significantly altered. Although a low urinary sulfatase A activity may occasionally be found in diseases such as the nephrotic syndrome, it is now possible to detect cases of ML with a screening test of urinary sulfatase A (AUSTIN et al. 1966).

Cholecystography

Non-functioning of the gallbladder was a feature in all cases of HAGBERG's group (HAGBERG et al. 1961, 1962; HAGBERG 1963). In one patient repeated X-ray examinations showed progressive impairment of the gallbladder's ability to concentrate. The finding of a non-functioning gallbladder, which is unusual for this age-group, may be caused by deposition of sulfatides in the gallbladder wall. This was suggested by fibrous thickening and metachromasia of the wall in a case of HAGBERG (1963).

Pathology

Since sulfatides are components of the myelin sheaths the pathology of ML involves predominantly these structures.

Central Nervous System

Upon gross examination the brain appears atrophic (very markedly in the original case of SCHOLZ 1925) with narrowing of the gyri and widening of the sulci, and frequently with enlargement of the lateral ventricles. There may be slight leptomeningeal thickening. Frontal sections show symmetrical, spongy degeneration of the cerebral white matter and glial scarring. The white matter exhibits a yellowish-grey discoloration and has, in general, a leathery consistency, with particular involvement of the atrophic corpus callosum. The central grey nuclei are usually spared and U-fibers are grossly uninvolved.

Histologically, a diffuse, symmetrical, extensive *demyelination* is seen. There may be almost complete lack of myelin sheaths in the central nervous system (JERVIS 1960) with the exception, in most cases, of some U-fibers and of myelin sheaths within the central grey nuclei and the optic radiation. Demyelination is most marked in the internal capsule and pyramidal tracts; spinal roots and peripheral nerves are involved to a lesser degree (JACOBI 1947; BERTRAND et al. 1954). There may be partial loss, or in the center of involved regions, complete loss of axis cylinders. In the periphery of demyelinized areas they may be swollen and terminally distended (HOLLÄNDER and PILZ 1964). The axis cylinders of U-fibers are, in general, well preserved. Small inflammatory lymphocytic infiltrates may be seen perivascularly.

A reactive anisomorphic and fibrous *gliosis* is seen in areas of demyelination, and granule cells are numerous at the periphery of involved areas or in the neighbourhood of blood vessels. Microglial phagocytes exhibit nuclear abnormalities; proliferating astrocytes are enlarged and frequently polynuclear. Oligodendroglial elements are usually, but not always (JERVIS 1960), decreased in number and may be absent in degenerating areas or in newly formed tissue (BRANDBERG and

Sjövall 1940; Einarson and Neel 1942; Brain and Greenfield 1950). They do not seem to participate in phagocytosis. The Schwann-cells of peripheral nerves and the capsule cells of spinal ganglia may show intraplasmatic storage.

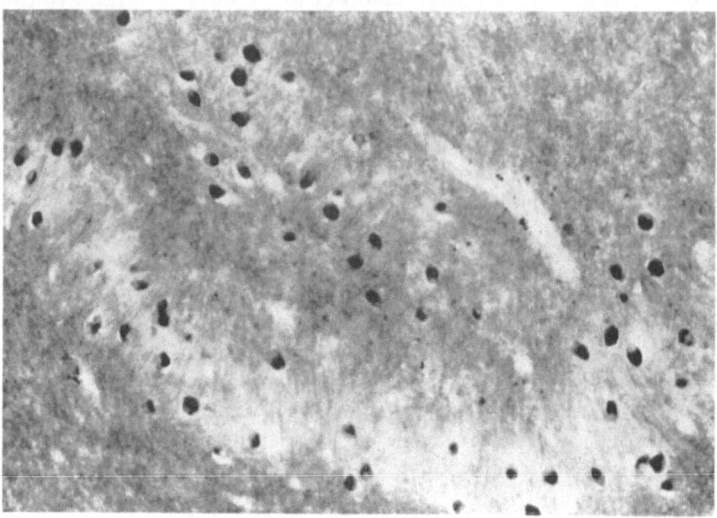

Fig. 1. Metachromatic leucoencephalopathy. Dentate nucleus of the cerebellum. Storage in ganglion cells of a brown metachromatic cerebroside sulfate. Stain: acetic acid-cresyl violet (Reproduced by courtesy of Prof. P. B. Diezel)

The occurrence of distended and ballooned *ganglion cells* is limited in most cases to certain parts of the brain, such as the dentate nucleus of the cerebellum (see fig. 1) and some nuclei of the brain stem, and to the grey matter of spinal ganglia. They are quite rare in the hypothalamus and very rare in the cerebral cortex (Norman et al. 1960). Independent of storage, rarification of ganglion cells is observed in some areas, particularly in the thalamus. A diminution of cells in the granular layer and of the Purkinje cells in the cerebellum, associated with swelling of axis cylinders and proliferation of Bergmann cells, may produce the picture of systematized atrophy (Bargeton 1963).

Extraneural Tissues

Deposition of metachromatic material in tissues other than the central nervous system was noted quite early: by Witte (1921) in the anterior lobe of the pituitary and in liver, renal tubuli and testes; by Norman (1947) in the gallbladder wall and renal tubuli, and by Einarson and Neel (1942) in the kidneys. In a case described by Kaltenbach (1922), hepatosplenomegaly was found at autopsy, but metachromasia was not looked for.

Van Bogaert and Dewulf (1939) have searched for metachromatic deposits outside the central nervous system without success, although their case, according to Holländer (1964 a), belonged to the cases verified neuropathologically as ML. Most later descriptions mention visceral involvement where this was examined (Scheidegger 1950; Brain and Greenfield 1950; Bertrand et al. 1954; Austin 1958, 1959 b; Hain and La Veck 1958; Jervis 1960; Hagberg et al. 1960, 1962; Norman et al. 1960; Hagberg 1963, and others).

Kidneys

While glomeruli are normal, the tubular cells, particularly of the loop of Henle, of the distal convoluted tubuli, and of the collecting system may be loaded with a metachromatic substance which also occurs in the tubulus lumen. It was postulated by WITTE (1921) that the stored sulfatides are formed in the kidney and do not originate in the brain. This is supported by the results of animal experiments AUSTIN (1963 a), where upon repeated subcutaneous injections of sulfatides, these remained at the site of injection and did not accumulate in kidneys, liver or lungs.

Gallbladder

The morphologic substrate for gallbladder dysfunction is cytoplasmic metachromasia of the mucosal cells. The villi are distended by accumulation of phagocytizing histiocytes, which are also filled with metachromatic lipid. This material may also be seen in small medullated nerves of deeper layers of the gallbladder wall. In addition, phagocytes contain cholesterol and other lipid which stains with Scarlet-red.

Other Organs

HAGBERG et al. (1962) found that in cases of ML the cells of pancreatic islets stained metachromatic, in contrast to normal controls. Although, according to SVENNERHOLM (1963 b), sulfatides are not stored in cells belonging to the reticulo-endothelial system, metachromatic granules have been seen by BARGETON (1963) in the cells of the splenic reticuloendothelium, and they are found in leucocytes and bone-marrow (AUSTIN 1958). Metachromatic material in the liver can occur in histiocytes of the portal fields, in Kupffer cells, in cells of the intrahepatic bile ducts and parenchymal cells (HAGBERG et al. 1962; BARGETON 1963). Macrophages and phagocytes which give a metachromatic reaction may finally be found in the bronchioles of the lungs and in the mucosa of the gastrointestinal tract. True foam cells (SCHEIDEGGER 1955) and macrophages with "foamy cytoplasm" (HAGBERG et al. 1962) were described in the lungs. A careful histologic study of the eyes in ML has been reported by COGAN et al. (1958).

Histochemical Findings

The main histochemical feature of ML is reflected in the name. Staining of frozen sections with aqueous acetic cresylviolet (HIRSCH and PEIFFER 1955) results in brown metachromasia of the myelin degradation products instead of the normal purple color of myelin. The method allows differentiation and localization of the alcohol-soluble storage material in ML, although, like most other histochemical tests, it is not completely specific for this lipid.

The first observers of degenerative diffuse sclerosis, SCHOLZ (1925) and BIELSCHOWSKY and HENNEBERG (1928) coined the term "prelipoid" for these products of myelin disintegration, on the basis of their faint orange stain with Scarlet-red, and considered this substance to be a precursor of neutral fats which stain bright red with the same dye (see fig. 2).

In addition to its typical brown metachromasia (DIEZEL 1956, 1957 a, b, 1962; DIEZEL and RICHARDSON 1957), the lipid in ML stains normally with Sudan black, is weakly PAS positive, CP*- and Bial-negative and therefore does not contain neuraminic acid. It can be selectively stained using the trypaflavin-dimethyl-aminobenzaldehyde method (HOLLÄNDER 1963, 1964 b).

Studies by HIRSCH and PEIFFER (1955), DIEZEL (1955, 1957 b), and CUMINGS (1955) of tissues from early cases (SCHOLZ 1925; VAN BOGAERT and SCHOLZ 1932; SCHOLZ 1933; VAN BOGAERT and BERTRAND 1933; WICKE 1938) where "prelipoid" material had been described resulted in the unequivocal demonstration of brown metachromasia of myelin breakdown products as well as lipid storage in ganglion

* Copper-phthalocyanin reaction.

cells of certain nuclei. Thus, the old differentiation of degenerative diffuse sclerosis into forms with simple "prelipoid" break-down products and those with meta-chromatic "prelipoid" material could not be maintained.

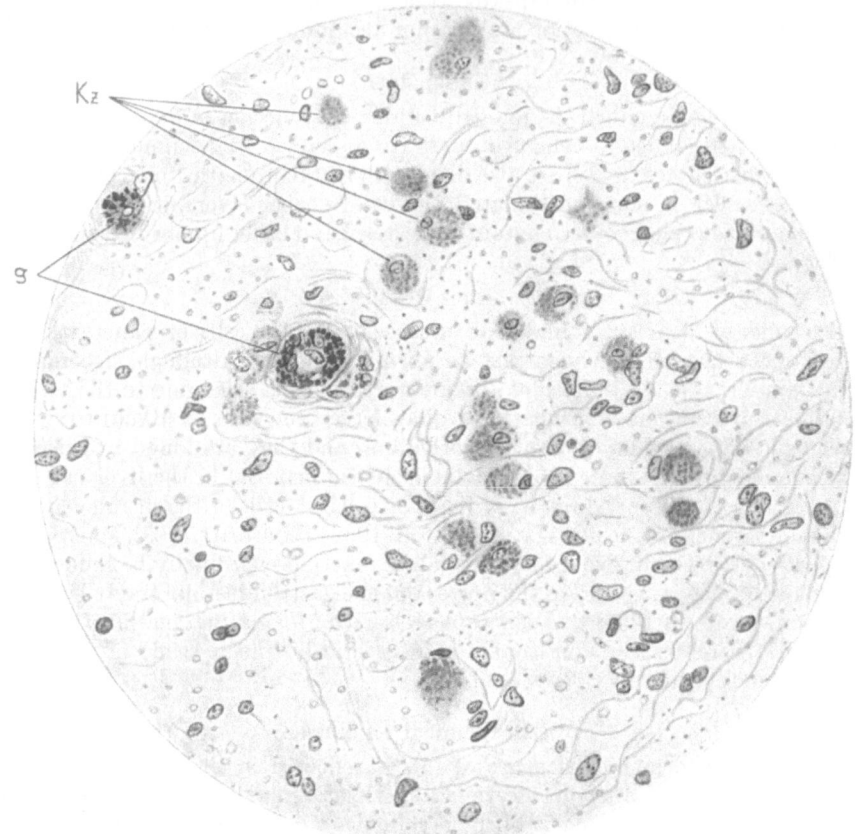

Fig. 2. Fat staining with Scarlet-red according to Herxheimer, followed by Ehrlich's haematoxylin stain. From the progressive marginal zone of a cerebellar focus. Kz = granulated glia cells with yellow red colored content; g = vessel with glowing red colored lipid break-down products. Reproduced from Scholz (1925), figure 12

There is a marked discrepancy between the great quantity of metachromatic lipids and the small amounts of sudanophilic lipids in demyelinated areas. The latter occur only in adventitial cells and perivascularly. Metachromatic lipid is found intracellularly, in phagocytic microglia or as extracellular granular material which is probably derived from necrotic granule cells. Storage is also observed in proliferating astrocytes.

Of particular interest is the finding of metachromatic material in distended ganglion cells (Nissle 1910; Witte 1921; Wicke 1938; van Bogaert and Dewulf 1939; Cardona 1939; Norman 1947; Brain and Greenfield 1950; Leslie 1952; Hirsch and Peiffer 1955; Diezel 1957 a, b, 1962). The meta-chromatic granules in nerve cells are larger than those in glial cells and are found in all cells which appear swollen and distended histologically. Therefore, meta-chromasia of the ganglion cells of the cerebral cortex, where major storage is limited to the glial cells, is either absent (Wicke 1938; Peiffer 1959; Jervis 1960) or of very minor degree.

Metachromatic bodies have been seen in ganglion cells of the retina (COGAN et al. 1958). This material apparently does not originate from myelin sheaths, since the retina does not contain myelinated nerve fibers.

A striking brown metachromasia is a frequent feature in intact myelin sheaths of white matter and peripheral nerves.

Comparative histochemical and chemical analyses have shown that the accumulated metachromatic material is identical with the sulfatide which has been isolated from brain and other organs of ML (JATZKEWITZ 1958, 1960 b; AUSTIN 1958, 1959 a, b, 1960; HAGBERG et al. 1960) (see below).

Melanin was found by DIEZEL (1957 a, b) in granule cells and storing ganglion cells, particularly of the dentate nucleus, in all six cases studied. According to this author, the finding is essential for ML.

DENGLER and DIEZEL (1958) concluded from the brown or black discoloration of involved tissues upon treatment with polyphenoloxidase to the storage of a catecholamine-lipid-complex.

Results of Lipid Analyses

Brain

Brain lipids in ML have been studied by several groups (KLENK 1955; AUSTIN 1957 a, b, 1959 b; JATZKEWITZ 1958, 1960 a—c, 1963, 1966; HAGBERG et al. 1960, 1962; JERVIS 1960; SVENNERHOLM 1963; ROUSER et al. 1965 a, b; O'BRIEN and SAMPSON 1965 a, b; SUZUKI 1966; SUZUKI et al. 1966). Discrepancies of data for grey and white matter as reported by different observers may be caused in part by difficulties in the separation of these components. Results obtained from analyses of total brain extracts show better reproducibility.

Analyses of *grey matter*, in general, show insignificant changes (see table 2a). There is a slight decrease of total lipids due to a low cholesterol and phospholipid concentration. Sphingosine phospholipids and glycerol phospholipids are diminished to a similar degree. The glycosphingolipid content is normal, and the ratio of sulfatides to cerebrosides, which together make up only about 1% of dry weight, is approximately 2:1 as in normals. Total hexosamine and lipid-hexosamine content is at the upper limit of normal.

Significant abnormalities are found in the *white matter* (see table 2b). There is a diminution of total lipids by almost one-third (HAGBERG et al. 1960, 1962) including a 50% reduction of cholesterol with a normal proportion of esterified cholesterol (1—2%), and a similar diminution of phospholipids which involves mainly cephalins and sphingomyelins and to a lesser degree lecithin (HAGBERG et al. 1960, 1962).

The most pronounced decrease is observed in the cerebroside fraction, the concentration of which is only one-third to one-fourth normal. Since sulfatides are increased to a similar degree (3—5 fold), the ratio of sulfatides to cerebrosides becomes approximately 4:1 and is thus reversed as compared with findings in normals. A similar ratio was found for the total brain by ROUSER et al. (1965 b). Comparison of absolute values for sulfatide content showed 0.3 gm for one-half brain of a normal child and 1.9 gm in a case of ML. When cerebrosides and sulfatides are measured together as "homoglycolipids" the resulting figures are normal or slightly high when related to dry weight. This small increase is more relative than absolute as can be seen if the amount is related to the nitrogen content (SVENNERHOLM 1963).

The ratio of sulfatides to cerebrosides in the spinal cord is 3:2 and in the sciatic nerve 4:1 as in brain (HAGBERG et al. 1962).

Table 2a. *Composition of cerebral cortex in metachromatic leucodystrophy*
(Analysed material from frontal lobe. All figures are expressed as per cent of dry weight)

	Normals (6 cases; 4—5 yrs.)		Sulfatidosis		
	Range	Mean value	Case A. L. 3¾ yrs.	Case R. A. 4½ yrs.	Case I. H. 29 yrs.
Nitrogen	9.2 — 9.9	9.6	10.6	10.8	
Hexosamine	0.70— 0.80	0.75	0.77		
Lipid Hexosamine		0.15	0.17	0.18	0.12
Total lipids	28.0 —32.4	30.2	26.6	22.2	31.3
Cholesterol	5.0 — 7.0	6.0	5.1	4.8	6.5
Phospholipids	21.2 —25.6	23.2	20.6	16.6	21.3
Sphingomyelin	1.7 — 2.8	2.0	1.6	1.4	2.5
Cephalins	8.5 —12.2	10.3	10.4	8.0	9.0
Lecithin	8.5 —10.2	9.8	8.6	7.6	10.0
Cerebroside	0.3 — 0.7	0.4	0.3	0.3	1.4
Sulfatide	0.4 — 0.9	0.6	0.6	0.5	2.0

Source: SVENNERHOLM (1963).

Table 2b. *Composition of cerebral white matter in metachromatic leucodystrophy*
(All figures are expressed as per cent of dry weight)

	Normals (6 cases; 4—5 yrs.)		Sulfatidosis			Normal myelin*	Case** 6 yrs.
	Range	Mean value	Case A. L. 3¾ yrs.	Case R. A. 4½ yrs.	Case I. H. 29 yrs.		
Nitrogen	6.0 — 6.3	6.1	7.9	8.0			
Hexosamine	0.22— 0.30	0.28	0.78	0.74			
Lipid Hexosamine		0.05	0.08	0.09	0.03		
Total lipids	55.6 —61.9	58.3	39.9	40.9	50.1	78—81	47.7
Cholesterol	12.2 —15.7	14.4	8.1	7.8	13.5	24.4	17.8
Phospholipids	28.0 —30.6	29.5	17.1	14.1	22.4	47.6	53.3
Sphingomyelin	4.1 — 5.2	4.6	2.5	2.2	4.7	5.6	4.0
Cephalins	14.4 —16.5	15.5	8.1	5.1	9.0	22.2***	26.8***
Lecithin	8.5 — 9.9	9.1	6.9	7.9	8.7	13.3	15.7
Cerebroside	10.3 —13.8	11.5	2.8	3.2	7.8	19.5	6.5
Sulfatide	1.7 — 4.1	2.9	12.8	15.8	6.5	5.6	20.4

Source: SVENNERHOLM (1963) and O'BRIEN and SAMPSON (1965).

  * Average of four humans aged 10 months, 6, 9 and 55 years (O'BRIEN and SAMPSON 1965 a).
 ** A boy, who expired from late infantile ML (O'BRIEN and SAMPSON 1965 b).
*** Serine glycerophosphatides = 6.0 (Normal) and 7.5 (ML).
     Ethanolamine glycerophosphatides = 16,2 (Normal) and 19,3 (ML).

The increased concentration of total hexosamine is more marked in white than in grey matter. Values three times normal have been described and are mainly due to mucoid substances such as mucopolysaccharides (HAGBERG et al. 1960) and "glycosamino-glycans" (SVENNERHOLM 1963), while lipid-hexosamine is only slightly increased.

SUZUKI (1966) found an increased concentration of total N-acetyl-neuraminic acid (NANA) in white matter (see table 3).

The sphingomyelin fatty acid pattern is characterized by a decreased proportion of long-chain fatty acids (C 22—C 26) and is similar to that of the newborn (STÄLL-BERG-STENHAGEN and SVENNERHOLM 1965; ROUSER et al. 1965a; NORTON and PODLUSO 1965). The fatty acid composition of cerebrosides and sulfatides was normal in the material of STÄLLBERG-STENHAGEN and SVENNERHOLM (1965), and NORTON and PODLUSO (1965), however, the long-chain fatty acids of cerebrosides were decreased in the study of O'BRIEN (1964) (see table 4).

Table 3. *Ganglioside patterns of grey and white matter in metachromatic leucodystrophy*

		Grey matter		White matter	
		Case	Normal control* (range)	Case	Normal control* (range)
Gangliosides		(Values expressed as per cent of NANA**)			
G_0		3.4	3.2— 4.8	5.2	2.8— 6.1
G_1	$(G_{GNT}\ IV)^{++}$	15.2	15.8—25.7	14.7	14.1—21.2
G_2	$(G_{GNT}\ III)^{++}$	22.1	14.3—19.9	22.4	12.2—18.1
G_2A^+		4.8	1.2— 4.2	7.8	1.2— 3.1
G_3	$(G_{GNT}\ II)^{++}$	30.4	29.1—43.7	21.2	30.0—38.2
G_3A^+		5.7	1.0— 2.8	11.1	1.2— 5.0
G_4	$(G_{GNT}\ I)^{++}$	14.9	13.0—15.6	12.3	14.6—21.2
G_5	$(G_{GNTr}\ II)^{++}$	2.4	1.5— 2.0	3.0	0.6— 2.0
G_6	$(G_{LACT})^{++}$	1.2	1	2.3	1
Total NANA**		(Values expressed as µg/gm wet weight)			
		790	744—918	329	80—180

Source: SUZUKI (1966).
* Average of four normal controls, aged 5 to 15 years.
** NANA = N-acetyl neuraminic acid.
+ G_2A and G_3A are two minor sialic acid-containing materials with the chromatographic mobility between G_2 and G_3 and between G_3 and G_4, respectivly (SUZUKI 1966).
++ Nomenclature of KUHN and WIEGANDT (1963, 1964) and of WIEGANDT (1965). See page 214.

Findings in adult cases (SOURANDER and SVENNERHOLM 1962; SVENNERHOLM 1963; JATZKEWITZ et al. 1964) are at variance with those in the late-infantile form of ML. In the former, the phospholipid concentration of white matter is only slightly lowered, while the concentration of cholesterol is normal. Cerebrosides are diminished by one-third to one-half; sulfatides are increased to values twice normal, their concentration being slightly below that of cerebrosides. The sulfatides of grey matter are significantly increased and amount to 2% of dry weight (normal 0.4—0.9%). Their concentration may exceed that of cerebrosides by one-third (SVENNERHOLM 1963).

Table 4. *Long-chain fatty acids of sulfatide, cerebroside and sphingomyelin of brain white matter in metachromatic leucodystrophy*

Fatty acids	Sulfatide		Cerebroside		Sphingomyelin	
	C_{14}—C_{20}	C_{21}—C_{26}	C_{14}—C_{20}	C_{21}—C_{26}	C_{14}—C_{20}	C_{21}—C_{26}
	(Values expressed as per cent of non-hydroxy fatty acids)					
Normal:	13.4	86.6	22.7	77.3	57.5	42.5
Case N. N. (9 yrs.):	25.5	74.5	84.1	15.9	72.6	27.4
Case M. T. (11 yrs.):	22.7	77.3	78.0	22.0	87.6	12.4

Source: O'BRIEN et al. (1964).

Other Organs

The accumulation of sulfatides in ML is not limited to the nervous system. Since, however, the normal sulfatide content of visceral organs is very low and measurement is difficult, data on the increase in ML vary. While AUSTIN (1959 b) found the sulfatide content of the kidneys increased nine-fold; SVENNERHOLM (1963), from comparative studies in three normal infants (aged two months) and two patients with late-infantile ML (aged $3\frac{3}{4}$ and $4\frac{1}{2}$ years respectively) found a 25—70 fold increase in kidney sulfatides (see table 5), particularly monohexosesulfatide, above normal (1.26 and 4.60% of dry weight as compared to 0.09—0.17% normally)

Table 5. *Lipid composition of kidney in metachromatic leucodystrophy*

	3 normal infants (2 months)	Case A. L. (3 ¾ yrs.)	Case R. A. (4 ½ yrs.)
	(Values expressed as per cent of dry weight)		
Total lipids	9.4 —10.5	10.8	12.5
Cholesterol	1.3 — 1.7	1.7	1.6
Phospholipids	7.4 — 8.5	6.8	5.6
Sphingomyelin	1.0 — 1.2	1.1	1.6
Cephalins	3.3 — 4.0	2.0	1.6
Lecithin	2.6 — 3.4	3.6	3.0
Cerebroside	0.41— 0.45	1.21	0.71
Sulfatide	0.09— 0.17	1.26	4.60

Source: Svennerholm (1963).

and a normal sulfatide content in the spleen (see table 6). The differences may be explained in part by the different methods employed, and by the higher normal values used by Austin (1960). A slight increase in cerebrosides may be secondary to impairment of glycolipid metabolism (Svennerholm 1963). The concentration of other organ lipids was within normal limits with the exception of that of cephalins which was lowered in kidneys and spleen. Recent analyses of renal glyco-lipids by Mårtensson et al. (1966) showed a significant increase in ML of a dihe-xose-sulfatide (ceramide-glucose-galactose-sulfate), in addition to that of ceramide-galactose-sulfate.

Table 6. *Lipid composition of spleen in metachromatic leucodystrophy*

	3 normal infants (2 months)	Case A. L. (3 ¾ yrs.)	Case R. A. (4 ½ yrs.)
	(Values expressed as per cent of dry weight)		
Total lipids	7.8 —8.8	7.3	8.8
Cholesterol	1.5 —1.8	1.8	1.9
Phospholipids	5.9 —6.6	5.5	5.9
Sphingomyelin	1.1 —1.2	1.4	1.1
Cephalins	2.2 —2.8	1.5	1.1
Lecithin	2.1 —2.7	2.7	2.1
Cerebroside	0.15—0.19	0.70	0.80
Sulfatide	0.20	0.20	0.20

Source: Svennerholm (1963).

The high sulfatide concentration in urine and bile has been mentioned. The increased concentration of kidney sulfatides may arise by formation in loco and/or transport to the organs by the blood. Although some workers (Brain and Green-field 1950; Norman et al. 1960; Mossakowski et al. 1961) consider visceral accumulation of sulfatides secondary to the central nervous system pathology, a transport from the central nervous system is unlikely since kidney sulfatides and brain sulfatides differ considerably with regard to the fatty acid pattern (Hagberg et al. 1965). In animal experiments, sulfatide turnover in visceral organs (Green and Robinson 1960) was found to be considerably more rapid than in the brain.

It is possible that sulfatides are formed in the kidney in order to yield excre-table glycolipids. Enzymic studies using renal tissues will be discussed later.

The Stored Lipid

The occurrence of sulfatides in brain was already suspected by Thudichum (1884, 1901). Koch (1910) isolated from brain a sulfur-containing lipid which, in addition, was thought to contain sugar and phosphorus. He proposed that the material was a phospholipid-cerebroside-sulfatide-complex with the sulfuric acid moiety located between phospholipid and cerebroside, but LEVENE (1912—1913) did not find phosphorus in sulfatides. A detailed study on sulfatides is that by BLIX (1933) who isolated from human brain a sulfatide which amounted to one-fifth to one-fourth of total cerebrosides and did not contain phosphorus.

The Normal Sulfatides

Until recently, therefore, the question remained unsettled whether sulfatides contained phosphorus or not. LEES et al. (1959) were able to isolate from brain white matter a "sulfatide A" in cristalline form, and a "sulfatide B" which was associated with phospholipids. Similarly BAKKE and CORNATZER (1961), and DA-VISON and GREGSON (1962) found in normal human brains sulfatides with and without phosphorus upon column chromatographic separation, and the latter authors considered the phosphorus-containing component to result from mere association of sulfatides with phospholipids. In contrast, GREEN and ROBINSON (1960), upon paper-chromatography of brain lipid extracts, observed one spot only corresponding to the authentic cerebron sulfate. Today it is generally accepted that sulfatides do not contain phosphorus.

Cerebronic acid makes up the greatest portion of brain sulfatide fatty acids according to BLIX (1933). More recent analyses showed lignoceric, nervonic and oxynervonic acids also to be present (JATZKEWITZ 1960b, 1963; SEKERIS 1964; O'BRIEN et al. 1964).

With regard to the position of the sulfuric acid moiety, NAKAYAMA (1951), on the basis of unsuccessful tritylation, suspected ester binding with the primary hydroxyl group. THANNHAUSER and BONCODDO (1953) and THANNHAUSER et al. (1955) suggested binding of the sulfuric acid moiety to the primary hydroxyl group of C_6 of galactose. More recently, it could be proved that the sulfuric acid is actually bound to C_3 (YAMAKAWA et al. 1962; HAKOMORI et al. 1962; STOFFYN and STOFFYN 1963 a, b; TAKETOMI and YAMAKAWA 1964).

According to information available to date, the sulfatide of nerve tissue is a sulfuric acid ester of cerebrosides and consists of one mole each of sphingosine, fatty acid, galactose and sulfuric acid. In addition, a dihexose sulfatide is found in the kidney (MÅRTENSSON 1963, MÅRTENSSON et al. 1966) and possibly in other tissues as well, which contains one mole glucose in addition to galactose. In this dihexose sulfatide glucose is vicinal to ceramide.

Sulfatides in Metachromatic Leucodystrophy

Sulfatides of ML have been studied by various authors. Here, too, the presence of a component containing phosphorus was suggested initially (JATZKEWITZ 1958, 1960). There are no basic differences between the sulfatide stored in ML and the normal sulfatide. The sulfatide fatty acid composition is similar to that of cerebrosides; in addition to cerebronic acid, lignoric, nervonic and oxynervonic acids are found (JATZKEWITZ 1960 b, 1963; SEKERIS 1964; O'BRIEN et al. 1964; STÄLLBERG-STENHAGEN and SVENNERHOLM 1965). While initially no significant differences of the sulfatide fatty acid composition was detected, as compared to normal brain sulfatide fatty acids (SVENNERHOLM 1963; STÄLLBERG-STENHAGEN and SVENNERHOLM 1965), more recent studies by the same group of authors show a decreased proportion of saturated C_{24} fatty acids and a small increase of the proportion of C_{22} fatty acids in sulfatides as well as cerebrosides of ML. These changes appear nonspecific, since they were found in two cases with circulatory and respiratory insufficiency as well (HAGBERG et al. 1966). Normal kidney sulfatides contain mainly

C_{22} and C_{24} fatty acids; kidney sulfatides in ML differ from those of normals by a lower content of monounsaturated fatty acids, a higher proportion of hydroxy acids and a particularly high proportion of C_{22} fatty acids, mainly in the mono-hexose-sulfatide (MÅRTENSSON et al. 1966).

Since the carbohydrate moiety of the monohexose-sulfatide is galactose, as in normals, it appears certain that the stored sulfatide in ML is identical with the normal sulfatide.

Diagnosis

The clinical picture of ML including the neurological findings is not specific. Motor involvement, rigidity and spasticity as well as mental retardation and seizures are observed in a variety of brain diseases. Sometimes, the sequence of symptoms (HAGBERG 1963) may aid in establishing the diagnosis.

A rather typical but late clinical sign in infantile ML is that of a non-functioning gallbladder. The simple finding of metachromatic material in the urine is of no diagnostic value for reasons discussed earlier. The chromatographic demonstration of two spots, one of which represents a dihexosidesulfate (N-acylsphingosine-glucose-galactose-sulfate, MÅRTENSSON 1963) appears to be pathognomonic (HAGBERG et al. 1965).

Biopsies from peripheral nerves (sciatic nerve) or from brain tissue may establish the diagnosis when a large amount of metachromatic material is found. The occurrence of small amounts is non-specific and may be seen in other demyelinating diseases (EINARSON and NEEL 1938; JERVIS 1960).

Diagnostic difficulties arise in subacute sclerosing encephalitis, although as a rule its course is more rapid and electroencephalographic changes are typical. Other virus encephalitides show unequivocally faster progression than ML.

Pathogenetic Aspects

The pathogenesis of ML is unknown. Theories proposed by various authors are difficult to substantiate, particularly since the biosynthesis of sulfatides has not been elucidated (GOLDBERG 1961; see also chapter by BURTON, page 131). The basic lesion(s) may theoretically consist of one or more of the following:

1. of a structural peculiarity of the stored sulfatide which may lead to impairment of its metabolism;

2. of overproduction, for instance from cerebrosides which are diminished in ML, or

3. of a block of degradation resulting in sulfatide accumulation.

As mentioned earlier, there is no evidence for a structural abnormality of the ML sulfatide. The sphingosine base is the D-erythro-1, 3-dihydroxy-2-amino-4-octadecene with the double-bond in trans-configuration; in addition, there are traces of the homologous C_{18}-dihydrosphingosine in human brain sulfatide (KARLSSON 1964). The galactose moiety of the monohexose-sulfatide shows beta-glycosidic binding at the C_1 position of sphingosine and is esterified at C_3 with sulfuric acid. The dihexoside, which is found in the kidney, contains glucose and galactose as in normals. The fatty acid pattern is only insignificantly altered.

A variety of pathways has been suggested for the metabolism of sulfatides, any of which could be impaired in ML. It has been proposed that galacto-cerebroside acts as a precursor for sulfatide (RADIN et al. 1957; HAUSER 1964) with phosphoadenosine-phosphosulfate (PAPS) as sulfate donor (GOLDBERG 1961) according to the following formula: Galactocerebroside + PAPS = sulfatide + PAP (McKHANN et al. 1965; BALASUBRAMANIAN and BACHHAWAT 1963, 1964).

In contrast, JATZKEWITZ (1960), on the basis of studies in normals and patients with ML, suggested that normally sulfatides are degraded to cerebrosides by removal of the sulfuric acid moiety and that the block in ML is located at this step.

Still another mechanism has been considered by HAGBERG et al. (1962) and by SVENNERHOLM (1963). These authors postulate a common precursor for the "homoglycolipids" cerebroside and sulfatide. An enzymic defect, with impairment of cerebroside anabolism would result in accumulation of the common precursor and in secondary increase of sulfatide biosynthesis, analogous to the schemes proposed in Gaucher's disease and Tay-Sachs disease (see page 280 and page 232). Since, however, a low cerebroside concentration occurs in a variety of demyelinating diseases, this finding, which correlates rather well with the morphologic extent of the demyelinating process, need not necessarily result from a specific abnormality of cerebroside synthesis.

In a more recent paper, SVENNERHOLM's group (MÅRTENSSON et al. 1966) has reviewed the subject and has interpreted the available data on the metabolic interrelationship between cerebrosides and sulfatides according to the following scheme:

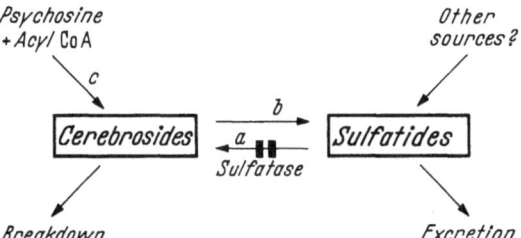

Fig. 3. Relationship between the metabolism of cerebrosides and sulfatides. From a) JATZKEWITZ (1960), b) HAUSER (1964), c) BRADY (1964). Block in lower arrow indicates the site of the possible lesion in metachromatic leucodystrophy

According to a mechanism for the pathogenesis of ML, as proposed by O'BRIEN (1964), a lack of the fatty acid chain elongation system (WAKIL 1961; FULCO and MEAD 1961; HJARA and RADIN 1963 a, b) may result in a deficiency of cerebrosides containing C_{22}—C_{26} fatty acids and a secondary increase in sulfatide content. The later finding of a normal content of long-chain fatty acids in cerebrosides (STÄLLBERG-STENHAGEN and SVENNERHOLM 1965) makes the theory unlikely. A decreased proportion of long-chain sphingomyelin fatty acids has been found by STÄLLBERG-STENHAGEN and SVENNERHOLM (1965) in ML, by ROUSER et al. (1965 a) in ML and Niemann-Pick disease, by BERRY et al. (1965), associated with a decrease of long-chain cerebroside fatty acids, in degenerating nerves, and by JATZKEWITZ and MEHL (1960) and JATZKEWITZ (1964) in demyelinating diseases of adults. It appears therefrom that sphingolipids with shorter-chain fatty acids prevail in all conditions, where the sphingolipids do not occur as components of stable myelin sheaths or membrane structures (ROUSER et al. 1965 a). It appears that such changes are the results rather than the cause of demyelination.

A number of studies examined the enzymic basis for impairment of sulfatide catabolism in ML, which is probably located at the site of the sulfate bond. The search for a cerebroside-sulfatase in normals which would catalyze the reaction cerebroside-sulfate → cerebroside + sulfuric acid (JATZKEWITZ 1958, 1960, 1963) was unsuccessful for a number of years (FUJINO and NEGISHI 1957; GREEN and ROBINSON 1960; HEALD and ROBINSON 1961; DAVISON and GREGSON 1962), but the enzyme was finally found in shellfish by FUJINO and NEGISHI (1957).

In 1963, Mehl and Jatzkewitz succeeded in isolating fractions with cerebroside-sulfatase activity from pig kidneys, and Bleszynski and Dzialoszynski (1965) purified soluble arylsulfatases from ox brain. A study by Mehl and Jatzkewitz (1965) on the significance of a lack of arylsulfatase in ML as reported by Austin (1963 a), and Austin et al. (1964 a, b), with 2-hydroxy-5-nitrophenyl-sulfate as substrate, resulted in the finding of two fractions with arylsulfatase activity in normal kidneys. While in ML the smaller of both fractions was present in normal concentration, the second component, and the predominant one in normals, was below the limits (0.005 o. d. units; Mehl and Jatzkewitz 1965) of the method in ML. It seems that diminution or lack of this heat-labile fraction, which corresponds to the arylsulfatase A of Austin, is typical for ML, and according to Mehl and Jatzkewitz (1965), supports the assumption of a block in the degradation of ML between sulfatides and cerebrosides (see fig. 3).

Recent studies in rabbit brain show a progressive physiologic increase in arylsulfatase and cerebroside-sulfatase after birth, with maximum activity upon completion of myelination. It is possible that a deficiency of the enzyme assumes significance at this time; this seems relevant to the manifestation of ML after the first year of life. An interpretation of later onset, as in adult cases (Mehl and Jatzkewitz 1965; Holländer and Pilz 1964), is more difficult. Although here a different enzymic lesion is a possibility, a quantitatively less severe enzyme defect seems more likely. In a number of adult cases sulfatide storage was less than in infantile cases (Jatzkewitz et al. 1964; Svennerholm 1963), regardless of the speed of progression of the disease.

It is not known whether glial cells become abnormal because of "glial insufficiency" (Scholz 1925) resulting from excessive myelin degradation which exceeds the metabolic capacity of glial cells (Peiffer 1959) in the presence of a normal enzymic machinery; or because they, too, harbour the enzymic lesion. It is more likely, that the enzymic lesion in ML is not limited to certain cells (Jatzkewitz 1960) but plays a role wherever sulfatides are important substrates.

References

Alzheimer, A.: Beiträge zur Kenntnis der pathologischen Neuroglia und ihrer Beziehung zu den Abbauvorgängen im Nervengewebe. Histol. Großhirnrinde 3, 521 (1910).

Austin, J. H.: Metachromatic forms of diffuse cerebral sclerosis. I. Diagnosis during life by urine sediment examination. Neurology (Minneap.) 7, 415 (1957 a).
— Metachromatic form of diffuse cerebral sclerosis. II. Diagnosis during life by isolation of metachromatic lipids from urine. Neurology (Minneap.) 7, 716 (1957 b).
— Observations in metachromatic leucoencephalopathy. Trans. Amer. neurol. Ass. 83, 149 (1958).
— Metachromatic leucoencephalopathy. Trans. Amer. neurol. Ass. 84, 203 (1959 a).
— Metachromatic sulfatides in cerebral white matter and kidney. Proc. Soc. exp. Biol. (N.Y.) 100, 361 (1959 b).
— Metachromatic form of diffuse sclerosis. III. Significance of sulfatide and other lipid abnormalities. Neurology (Minneap.) 10, 470 (1960).
— Recent studies in metachromatic and globoid body forms of diffuse sclerosis. In: Brain lipids and lipoproteins, and the leucodystrophies. Eds: J. Folch-Pi and H. J. Bauer. Amsterdam-London-New York: Elsevier Publishing Co. 1963 a, p. 120.
— Studies in globoid (Krabbe) Leucodystrophy. I. The significance of lipid abnormalities in white matter in 8 globoid and 13 control patients. Arch. Neurol. (Chic.) 9, 207 (1963 b).
— D. Armstrong, and L. Shearer: Metachromatic form of diffuse cerebral sclerosis. V. The nature and significance of low sulfatase activity: A controlled study of brain, liver and kidneys in four patients with metachromatic leukodystrophy (MLD). Arch. Neurol. (Chic.) 13, 593 (1965 a).
— — — and D. McAfee: Metachromatic form of diffuse cerebral sclerosis. VI. A rapid test for the sulfatase A deficiency in metachromatic leukodystrophy (MLD) urine. Arch. Neurol. (Chic.) 14, 259 (1966).

AUSTIN, J. H., A. S. BALASUBRAMANIAN, T. N. PATTABIRAMAN, S. SARASWATH, D. K. BASU, and B. K. BACHAWAT: Controlled study of enzyme activities in three human disorders of glycolipid metabolism. J. Neurochem. 10, 805 (1963).

— and D. LEHFELDT: Studies in globoid (Krabbe) leukodystrophy III. Significance of experimentally-produced globoid-like elements in rat white matter and spleen. J. Neuropath. exp. Neurol. 24, 265 (1965).

— D. MCAFEE, and L. SHEARER: Metachromatic form of diffuse cerebral sclerosis. Arch. Neurol. (Chic.) 12, 447 (1965 b).

— D. MCAFEE, D. ARMSTRONG, M. ROURKE, L. SHEARER, and B. K. BACHHAWAT: Low sulfatase activities in metachromatic leucodystrophy (MLD). Trans. Amer. neurol. Ass. 89, 147 (1964 a).

— — — — — Abnormal sulphatase activities in two human diseases (metachromatic leucodystrophy and gargoylism). Biochem. J. 93, 15 (1964 b).

BAKKE, J. E., and W. E. CORNATZER: Metabolism of brain and liver sulfatides. J. biol. Chem. 236, 653 (1961).

BALASUBRAMANIAN, A. S., and B. K. BACHHAWAT: Purification and properties of an arylsulphatase from human brain. J. Neurochem. 10, 201 (1963).

— — J. Neurochem. 11, 877 (1964).

BARGETON, E.: The metachromatic form of leucodystrophy and its relationship to lipidosis and demyelination in other metabolic disorders. In: Brain lipids and lipoproteins, and the leucodystrophies. Eds: J. Folch-Pi and H. J. Bauer. Amsterdam-London-New York: Elsevier Publishing Co. 1963.

BERRY, J. F., J. LOGOTHETIS, and M. BOUIS: Determination of the fatty acid composition of cerebrospinal fluid by gas-liquid chromatography. Neurology (Minneap.) 15, 1089 (1965).

BERTRAND, J., S. THIEFFRY et M. BARGETON: Leucodystrophie encéphalite et détermination splénohépatique caractérisant un trouble général du métabolisme. Rev. neurol. 91, 161 (1954).

BIELSCHOWSKY, M., u. R. HENNEBERG: Über familiäre diffuse Sklerose (Leukodystrophia cerebri progressiva hereditaria). J. Psychol. Neurol. (Lpz.) 36, 131 (1928).

BLESZYNSKI, W., and L. M. DZIALOSZYNSKI: Purification of soluble arylsulphatases from ox brain. Biochem. J. 97, 360 (1965).

BLIX, G.: Zur Kenntnis der schwefelhaltigen Lipoidstoffe des Gehirns. Hoppe-Seylers Z. physiol. Chem. 219, 82 (1933).

BOGAERT, L. VAN, et J. BERTRAND: Les leucodystrophies progressives familiales. Rev. neurol. 2, 249 (1933).

— and A. DEWULF: Diffuse progressive leucodystrophy in the adult. With production of metachromatic degenerative products (Alzheimer-Marotini). Arch. Neurol. Psychiat. (Chic.) 42, 1083 (1939).

— u. W. SCHOLZ: Klinischer und pathologisch-anatomischer Beitrag zur Kenntnis der familiären diffusen Sklerose. Z. ges. Neurol. Psychiat. 141, 510 (1932).

BRAIN, W., and J. G. GREENFIELD: Late infantile metachromatic leucoencephalopathy with primary degeneration of the interfascicular oligodendroglia. Brain 73, 291 (1950).

BRANDBERG, O., u. E. SJÖVALL: Zur Kenntnis der diffusen Hirnsklerose. (Ein Fall von familiärem spätinfantilem Typus.) Z. ges. Neurol. Psychiat. 170, 131 (1940).

CARDONA, F.: Istopatologia della malattia di Schilder familiare. Rev. Pat. Nerv. Ment. 54, 1 (1939); ref. in: Zbl. ges. Neurol. Psychiat. 96, 548 (1940).

COGAN, D. G., T. KUWABARA, E. P. RICHARDSON, and G. LYON: Histochemistry of the eye in metachromatic leucoencephalopathy. Arch. Ophthal. 60, 397 (1958).

CUMINGS, J. N.: Lipid chemistry of the brain in demyelinating diseases. Brain 78, 554 (1955).

— and B. ROZDILSKY: The cerebral lipid composition of the brain in six cases of Krabbe's disease. Neurology (Minneap.) 15, 177 (1965).

DAVISON, A. N., and N. A. GREGSON: The physiological role of cerebron sulfuric acid (sulfatide) in the brain. Biochem. J. 85, 558 (1962).

DEBUCH, H.: Nature of the linkage of the aldehyde residue in natural plasmalogens. Biochem. J. 67, 27 (1957); J. Neurochem. 2, 243 (1958).

DENGLER, H., u. P. B. DIEZEL: Speicherung eines Katecholamin-Lipoidkomplexes bei der degenerativen diffusen Sklerose vom Typus Scholz, Bielschowsky und Henneberg. Naturwissenschaften 45, 244 (1958).

DIEZEL, P. B.: Histochemische Untersuchungen an den Globoidzellen der familiären infantilen diffusen Sklerose vom Typus Krabbe. (Zugleich eine differentialdiagnostische Betrachtung der zentralnervösen Veränderungen beim Morbus Gaucher.) Virchows Arch. path. Anat. 327, 206 (1955).

— Vergleichende histochemische Untersuchungen an rein dargestellten Lipoiden des Zentralnervensystems und abgelagerten Sphingolipoiden bei den primären Lipoidosen und degenerativen diffusen Hirnsklerosen. Symposion für Histochemie Bonn 1955; ref. in: Acta histochem. (Jena) 2, 290 (1956).

Diezel, P. B.: Die Stoffwechselstörungen der Sphingolipoide. Berlin-Göttingen-Heidelberg: Springer 1957 a.
— Histochemical investigation of degenerative diffuse sclerosis (Leucodystrophy and diffuse sclerosis of the Krabbe type). Cerebral lipidoses, a symposion. Oxford: Blackwell 1957 b.
— Die angeborenen Störungen des Lipoidstoffwechsels. In: Medizinische Grundlagenforschung, Bd. IV, S. 239. Stuttgart: Thieme 1962.
— H. Fritsch u. H. Jacob: Leukodystrophie mit orthochromatischen Abbaustoffen. Ein Beitrag zur Pelizaeus-Merzbacherschen Krankheit. Virchows Arch. path. Anat. 338, 371 (1965).
— and E. P. Richardson: Histochemical and neuropathological studies in leukodystrophy (degenerative diffuse cerebral sclerosis, Scholz, Bielschowsky and Henneberg type). J. Neuropath. exp. Neurol. 16, 130 (1957).
Doss, M., u. H. Matiar-Vahar: Neurolipoidosen und angeborene Entmarkungskrankheiten. Fortschr. Neurol. Psychiat. 33, 617 (1965).
Edgar, G. W. F.: Approche biochimique des lipidoses et des leukodystrophies. Rev. neurol. 92, 277 (1955).
— Leuco-dystrophy as an "inborn metabolic error", comparable to lipidosis. In: Cerebral lipidoses. Oxford: Blackwell 1957.
Einarson, L., u. A. V. Neel: Beitrag zur Kenntnis sklerosierender Entmarkungsprozesse im Gehirn mit besonderer Berücksichtigung der diffusen Sklerose. (Strumpell-Heubner). Eine klinisch-anatomische Studie. Acta Jutlandica 10, 2 (1938); 12, 3 (1940).
— — Contribution to the study of diffuse brain sclerosis with a comprehensive review of the problem in general and a report of two cases. Acta Jutlandica 14, 2 (1942).
Erlaçın, S.: Über das Vorkommen des Sphingosins und seiner Homologen in den Sphingolipoiden des Gehirns. Dissertation Köln 1963.
Ettinger, A.: Adult form of leucodystrophy of type Scholz-Bielschowsky-Henneberg with metachromatic breakdown products in a 55-year old male (Clinical anatomic study). Psychiat. et Neurol. 149, 225 (1965).
Feigin, I.: Diffuse sclerosis in an infant (metachromatic leucoencephalopathy). J. Neuropath. exp. Neurol. 13, 393 (1954).
— Diffuse cerebral sclerosis (metachromatic leucoencephalopathy). Amer. J. Path. 30, 715 (1954).
Fujino, Y., and T. Negishi: Studies on conjugated lipids. Bull. Agr. Chem. Soc. (Japan) 21, 225 (1957).
Fulco, A. J., and J. F. Mead: The biosynthesis of lignoceric, cerebronic, and nervonic acids. J. biol. Chem. 236, 2416 (1961).
Fullerton, P. M.: Peripheral nerve conduction in metachromatic leucodystrophy (sulphatide lipidosis). J. Neurol. Neurosurg. Psychiat. 27, 106 (1964).
Goldberg, I. H.: The sulfolipids. J. Lipid Res. 2, 103 (1961).
Green, J. P., and J. D. Robinson: Cerebroside sulfate (sulfatide A) in some organs of the rat and in a mast cell tumor. J. biol. Chem. 235, 1621 (1960).
Greenfield, J. G.: A form of progressive cerebral sclerosis in infants associated with primary degeneration of the interfascicular glia. Proc. roy. Soc. Med. 26, 690 (1933).
Haberfeld, W., and F. Spieler: Zur diffusen Hirn- und Rückenmarkssklerose im Kindesalter. Dtsch. Z. Nervenheilk. 40, 436 (1910).
Hagberg, B.: Clinical symptoms, signs and tests in metachromatic leucodystrophy. In: Brain lipids and lipoproteins, and the leucodystrophies, p. 134. Eds: J. Folch-Pi and H. J. Bauer. Amsterdam-London-New York: Elsevier Publishing Co. 1963.
— P. Sourander, L. Svennerholm, and H. Voss: Late infantile metachromatic leucodystrophy of the genetic type. Acta paediat. (Uppsala) 48, 200 (1959); 49, 135 (1960).
— — — Clinical and laboratory diagnosis of metachromatic leucodystrophy. Cerebr. Palsy Bull. 3, 438 (1961).
— — — Sulfatide lipidosis in childhood. Report of a case investigated during life and at autopsy. Amer. J. Dis. Child. 104, 644 (1962).
— — and L. Svennerholm (Cited after Mårtensson et al. 1966, ref. 9).
— — and L. Thorén: Peripheral nerve changes in the diagnosis of metachromatic leucodystrophy. Acta Ped. Suppl. 135, 63 (1962).
— and L. Svennerholm: Laboratory Diagnostic Tests in Metachromatic Leucodystrophy. Acta paediat. (Uppsala) 48, 632 (1959).
— — Metachromatic leucodystrophy generalized lipidosis. Determination of sulfatides in urine, blood plasma and cerebrospinal fluid. Acta paediat. (Uppsala) 49, 690 (1960).
— — and B. Wranne: The excretion of urinary sulfatides in health and neurological disease. Acta paediat. (Uppsala) 54, 409 (1965).
Hain, F., and G. D. La Veck: Metachromatic leuco-encephalopathy review with illustrative case report. Paediatrics 22, 1064 (1958).

HAJRA, A. K., and N. S. RADIN: Isotopic studies of the biosynthesis of the cerebroside fatty acids in rats. J. Lipid Res. 4, 270 (1963a).
— — In vivo conversion of labeled fatty acids to the sphingolipid fatty acids in rat brain. J. Lipid Res. 4, 448 (1963b).
HAKOMORI, S., T. ISHIMODA, and K. NAKAMURA: Separation and characterization of two sulfatides of brain. J. Biochem. (Tokyo) 52, 468 (1962).
HALLERVORDEN, J.: Die familiäre infantile diffuse Hirnsclerose, Typus Krabbe. In: Die degenerative diffuse Sklerose (Pelizaeus-Merzbachersche Krankheit, Leukodystrophie Typus Scholz, diffuse Sklerose Typus Krabbe). In: Handbuch der spez. path. Anat., Bd. XIII/1, S. 716. Berlin-Göttingen-Heidelberg: Springer 1957.
HAUSER, G.: Labeling of cerebrosides and sulfatides in rat brain. Biochim. biophys. Acta (Amst.) 84, 212 (1964).
HEALD, P. J., and M. ROBINSON: The metabolism of sulfatides in cerebral tissues. Biochem. J. 81, 157 (1961).
HELFANT, M. H., M. BÖRJESSON, and B. HELLSTRÖM: The value of urinary sediment. Examination as a screening method in suspected cases of metachromatic leucodystrophy. Acta paediat. (Uppsala) 51, 49 (1962).
HIRSCH, T. v., u. J. PEIFFER: Über histologische Methoden in der Differentialdiagnose von Leucodystrophien und Lipoidosen. Arch. Psychiat. Nervenkr. 194, 88 (1955).
HOLLÄNDER, H.: A staining method for cerebroside-sulfuric-ester in brain tissue. J. Histochem. Cytochem. 11, 118 (1963).
— Über metachromatische Leukodystrophie. II. Relation zwischen Erkrankungsalter und Verlaufsform. Arch. Psychiat. Nervenkr. 205, 300 (1964a).
— Der histochemische Nachweis von Schwefelsäureestern mit Trypaflavin. Histochem. 3, 387 (1964b).
— u. H. PILZ: Über metachromatische Leukodystrophie. I. Kasuistische Mitteilung. Arch. Psychiat. Nervenkr. 205, 293 (1964).
ISLER, W., A. BISCHOFF u. E. ESSLEN: Die metachromatische Leukodystrophie. Diagnose durch Biopsie eines peripheren Nerven und Nachweis einer starken Verlangsamung der Nervenleitgeschwindigkeit bei einem Fall mit früh-infantiler Form. Helv. paediat. Acta 18, 107 (1963).
JACOBI, M.: Über Leukodystrophie und Pelizaeus-Merzbachersche Krankheit. Virchows Arch. path. Anat. 314, 460 (1947).
JATZKEWITZ, H.: Zwei Typen von Cerebrosid-schwefelsäureestern als sog. Prälipoide und Speichersubstanzen bei der Leukodystrophie, Typ Scholz (metachromat. Form der diffusen Sklerose). Hoppe-Seylers Z. physiol. Chem. 311, 297 (1958).
— Ergänzende Mitteilung zum Artikel Jürgen Peiffer. Über die metachromatischen Leukodystrophien (Typ Scholz). Arch. Psychiat. Nervenkr. 200, 416 (1960a).
— Die Leukodystrophie, Typ Scholz (metachromatische Form der diffusen Sklerose) als Sphingolipoidose (Cerebrosidschwefelsäureester-Speicherkrankheit). Hoppe-Seylers Z. physiol. Chem. 318, 265 (1960b).
— Cerebron- und Kerasin-schwefelsäureester als Speichersubstanzen bei der Leukodystrophie Typ Scholz (metachromatische Form der diffusen Sklerose). Hoppe-Seylers Z. physiol. Chem. 320, 134 (1960c).
— The role of cerebroside sulphuric acids in leucodystrophy. In: "Brain lipids and lipoproteins, and the leucodystrophies", p. 147. Eds: J. Folch-Pi and H. J. Bauer. Amsterdam-London-New York: Elsevier 1963.
— Eine neue Methode zur quantitativen Ultramikrobestimmung der Sphingolipoide aus Gehirn. Hoppe-Seylers Z. physiol. Chem. 336, 25 (1964).
— Über Sphingolipoidosen. In: 16. Mosbacher Kolloquium 1965. Berlin-Heidelberg-New York: Springer 1966.
— u. E. MEHL: Zur Dünnschichts-Chromatographie der Gehirnlipoide, ihrer Um- und Abbauprodukte. Hoppe-Seylers Z. physiol. Chem. 320, 251 (1960).
— H. PILZ u. H. HOLLÄNDER: Biochemische und vergleichende histochemische Untersuchungen in umschriebenen Gebieten des Gehirns bei Fällen von infantiler und adulter metachromatischer Leukodystrophie. Acta Neuropath. (Berl.) 4, 75 (1964).
JEFFERSON, M.: Late infantile metachromatic leucodystrophy. Proc. roy. Soc. Med. 51, 160 (1958).
JERVIS, G. A.: Infantile metachromatic leucodystrophy (Greenfield's disease). J. Neuropath. exp. Neurol. 19, 325 (1960).
KALTENBACH, H.: Über einen eigenartigen Markprozeß mit metachromatischen Abbauprodukten bei einem paralyseähnlichen Krankheitsbild. Z. ges. Neurol. Psychiat. 75, 138 (1922).
KARLSSON, K.-A.: Studies on sphingosines 3. C_{20}-dihydrosphingosine, a hitherto unknown sphingosine. Acta chem. scand. 18, 565 (1964).
KLENK, E.: The pathological chemistry of the developing brain. In: Biochemistry of the developing nervous system. Ed.: E. Waelsch, p. 397. New York: Academic Press 1955.

Koch, D.: Die metachromatische Leukodystrophie (Typ Scholz) mit Ganglienzellspeicherung (Cerebrosid-Schwefelsäureester-Speicherkrankheit). In: Handbuch der Humangenetik, P. E. Becker (Ed.). Bd. V. Stuttgart: Thieme 1966.

Koch, W.: Zur Kenntnis der Schwefelverbindungen des Nervensystems. II. Mitteilung. Über ein Sulfatid aus Nervensubstanz. Hoppe-Seylers Z. physiol. Chem. 70, 94 (1910).

Kuhn, R., u. H. Wiegandt: Die Konstitution der Ganglio-N-tetraose und des Gangliosids G 1. Chem. Ber. 96, 866 (1963).

— — Weitere Ganglioside aus Menschenhirn. Z. Naturforsch. 19 b, 256 (1964).

Lees, M., J. Folch, G. H. Sloane-Stanley, and S. Carr: A simple procedure for the preparation of brain sulfatides. J. Neurochem. 4, 9 (1959).

Lees, M. B., and H. W. Moser: The chemical pathology of Krabbe disease and metachromatic leukodystrophy. In: Cerebral sphingolipidoses, p. 179. Eds: S. M. Aronson and B. W. Volk. New York-London: Academic Press 1962.

Leslie, D. A.: Diffuse progressive metachromatic leucoencephalopathy. J. Path. Bact. 64, 841 (1952).

Levene, P. A.: The sulfatide of the brain. J. biol. Chem. 13, 463 (1912—1913).

Lyon, G., M. Arthuis et S. Thieffry: Leucodystrophie metachromatique infantile familiale. Etude de deux observations, dont une avec examen anatomique et chimique. Rev. neurol. 104, 508 (1961).

Mårtensson, E.: On the sulfate containing lipids of human kidney. Acta chem. scand. 17, 1174 (1963 a).

— Quantitative estimation of sulfates in lipid extracts. Biochim. biophys. Acta (Amst.) 70, 1 (1963 b).

— A. Percy, and L. Svennerholm: Kidney glycolipids in late infantile metachromatic leucodystrophy. Acta paediat. (Uppsala) 55, 1 (1966).

McKhann, G. H., R. Levy, and W. Ho: Metabolism of sulfatides. I. The effect of galactocerebrosides on the synthesis of sulfatides. Fed. Proc. 24, 361 (1965).

Mehl, E., u. H. Jatzkewitz: Über ein Cerebrosid-schwefelsäurespaltendes Enzym aus Schweineniere. Hoppe Seylers Z. physiol. Chem. 331, 292 (1963).

— and H. Jatzkewitz: Evidence for the genetic block in metachromatic leucodystrophy (ML). Biochem. biophys. Res. Commun. 19, 407 (1965).

Moser, H. W., and M. Lees: Sulfatide lipidosis: Metachromatic leukodystrophy. In: The metabolism of inherited disease, p. 539. Eds: J. B. Stanbury, J. B. Wyngaarden, and D. S. Fredrickson. New York: McGraw-Hill Book Company 1966.

Mossakowski, M., G. Mathieson, and N. Cumings: On the relationship of metachromatic leucodystrophy and amaurotic idiocy. Brain 84, 585 (1961).

Nakayama, T.: Studies on the conjugated lipids. II. On cerebron sulfuric acid. J. Biochem. (Tokyo) 38, 157 (1951).

Nisenbaum, C., U. Sandbank, and R. Kohn: Pelizaeus-Merzbacher disease "infantile acute type". Report of a family. Ann. paediat. (Basel) 204, 365 (1965).

Nissl, F.: Encyklopädie der mikroskopischen Technik. Eds.: Ehrlich, Krause, Mosse, Rosin, Weigert. 2. Aufl., Bd. II, S. 284. Berlin 1910.

Norman, R. M.: Diffuse progressive metachromatic leucoencephalopathy. A form of Schilder's disease related to the lipoidoses. Brain 70, 234 (1947).

— and A. H. Tingey: Sudanophil leucodystrophy and Pelizaeus-Merzbacher disease. In: Brain lipids and lipoproteins, and the leucodystrophies, p. 169. Eds: J. Folch-Pi and H. J. Bauer. Amsterdam-London-New York: Elsevier 1963.

— H. Urich, and A. H. Tingey: Metachromatic leucoencephalopathy. A form of lipidosis. Brain 83, 369 (1960).

Norton, W. T., and S. Podluso: Personal communication to O'Brien and Sampson (1965 b) Ref. 12.

O'Brien, J. S.: A molecular defect in metachromatic leucodystrophy (MLD). Fed. Proc. 23, 130 (1964).

— F. D. Fillerup and J. F. Mead: Quantification and fatty acid composition of cerebroside sulfate in human cerebral gray and white matter. J. Lipid Res. 5, 109 (1964).

— and E. L. Sampson: J. Lipid Res. 6, 537 (1965 a).

— — Myelin membrane: A molecular abnormality. Science 150, 1613 (1965 b).

Pampiglione, G.: EEG in inborn errors of metabolism. Excerpta med. (Amst.) (Int. Congress Ser.) 39, 2 (1961).

Peiffer, J.: Über die metachromatischen Leucodystrophien (Typ Scholz). Arch. Psychiat. Nervenkr. 199, 386 (1959).

Poser, C. M.: Concepts of Dysmyelination. In: Cerebral sphingolipidoses, p. 141. Eds: S. M. Aronson and B. W. Volk. New York: Academic Press 1962.

— and L. van Bogaert: Acta psychiat. scand. 31, 285 (1956).

RADIN, N. S., F. B. MARTIN, and J. R. BROWN: Galactolipid Metabolism. J. biol. Chem. 224, 499 (1957).

ROUSER, G., G. FELDMAN, and C. GALLI: Fatty acid compositions of human brain lecithin and sphingomyelin in normal individuals, senile cerebral cortical atrophy, Alzheimer's disease, metachromatic leucodystrophy, Tay-Sachs, Niemann-Pick diseases. J. Amer. Oil Chem. Soc. 42, 411 (1965 a).

— C. GALLI, and G. KRITCHEVSKY: Lipid class composition of normal human brain and variations in metachromatic leucodystrophy, Tay-Sachs, Niemann-Pick, chronic Gaucher's, and Alzheimer's disease. J. Amer. Oil Chem. Soc. 42, 404 (1965 b).

SCHEIDEGGER, S.: Diffuse Entmarkungs-Encephalomyelitis. Schweiz. Z. allg. Path. 13, 74 (1950).

— Diffuse Encephalopathie. Beitrag zur Frage der diffusen Sklerosen und Speicherkrankheiten. Ann. paediat. (Basel) 193, 1 (1955).

SCHILDER, P.: Zur Kenntnis der sogenannten diffusen Sklerose (über Encephalitis periaxialis diffusa). Z. ges. Neurol. Psychiat. 10, 1 (1912); 15, 359 (1913).

SCHOLZ, W.: Klinische, pathologisch-anatomische und erbbiologische Untersuchungen bei familiärer, diffuser Hirnsklerose im Kindesalter. (Ein Beitrag zur Lehre von den Heredodegcnerationen.) Z. ges. Neurol. Psychiat. 99, 651 (1925).

— Über Wesen, nosologische und pathogenetische Bedeutung der atypischen Abbauvorgänge bei den familiären Markerkrankungen. Mschr. Psychiat. Neurol. 86, 111 (1933).

SEITELBERGER, F.: Histochemie und Klassifikation der Pelizaeus-Merzbacherschen Krankheit. Wien. Z. Nervenheilk. 14, 74 (1957).

SEKERIS, K. E.: Altersbedingte Veränderungen in der Zusammensetzung der Cerebrosidfettsäuren. Dissertation Köln 1964.

SOURANDER, P., and L. SVENNERHOLM: Sulphatide lipidosis with the clinical picture of progressive organic dementia with epileptic seizures. Acta ncuropath. (Berl.) 1, 384 (1962).

STÄLLBERG-STENHAGEN, and L. SVENNERHOLM: Fatty acid composition of human brain sphingomyelins: normal variation with age and changes during myelin disorders. J. Lipid Res. 6, 146 (1965).

STOFFYN, P., and A. STOFFYN: Direct conversion of sulfatides into cerebrosides. Biochim. biophys. Acta (Amst.) 70, 107 (1963 a).

— — Structure of sulfatides. Biochim. biophys. Acta (Amst.) 70, 218 (1963 b).

SUZUKI, K.: Ganglioside patterns of normal and pathological brains. In: The 3rd international symposium on sphingolipidoses, New York 1965. Eds: S. M. Aronson and B. W. Volk. New York: Pergamon Press 1966 (in press).

— — and G. CHEN: Metachromatic leucodystrophy: Isolation and chemical analysis of metachromatic granules. Science 151, 1231 (1966).

SVENNERHOLM, E., and L. SVENNERHOLM: Isolation of blood serum glycolipids. Acta chem. scand. 16, 1282 (1962).

SVENNERHOLM, L.: Chromatographic determination of sulfatides. Acta chem. scand. 17, 1170 (1963 a).

— Some aspects of the biochemical changes in leucodystrophy. In: Brain lipids and lipoproteins, and the leucodystrophies, p. 104. Eds: J. Folch-Pi and H. J. Bauer. Amsterdam: Elsevier Publishing Co. 1963 b.

TAKETOMI, T., and T. YAMAKAWA: Further confirmation on the structure of brain cerebroside sulfuric ester. J. Biochem. 55, 87 (1964).

THANNHAUSER, S. J., and N. BONCODDO: Isolation of gangliosides and cerebrosulfatides from beef brain. Fed. Proc. 12, 280 (1953).

— J. FELLIG, and G. SCHMIDT: The structure of cerebroside sulfuric ester of beef brain. J. biol. Chem. 215, 211 (1955).

THIEFFRY, S., et G. LYON: Diagnostic d'un cas de leucodystrophie métachromatique (type Scholz) par la biopsie d'un nerf périphérique. Rev. neurol. 100, 452 (1959).

THUDICHUM, J. L. W.: The chemical constitution of the brain. London: Builliere, Tindall and Cox 1884.

— Die chemische Konstitution des Gehirns des Menschen und der Tiere. Tübingen: Franz Pietzcher 1901.

WAKIL, S. J.: Mechanism of fatty acid synthesis. J. Lipid Res. 2, 1 (1961).

WICKE, R.: Ein Beitrag zur Frage der familiären diffusen Sklerosen einschließlich der Pelizaeus-Merzbacherschen Krankheit und ihrer Beziehungen zur Amaurotischen Idiotie. Z. ges. Neurol. Psychiat. 162, 741 (1938).

WIEGANDT, H.: Ganglioside. In: Untersuchung und Bestimmung der Lipoide im Blut, S. 19. Hrsgb. N. Zöllner u. D. Eberhagen. Berlin-Heidelberg-New York: Springer 1965.

WITTE, F.: Über pathologische Abbauvorgänge im Zentralnervensystem. Münch. med. Wschr. 68, 63 (1921).

YAMAKAWA, T., N. KISO, S. HANDA, A. MAKITA, and S. YOKOYAMA: On the structure of brain cerebroside sulfuric ester and ceramide dihexoside of erythrocytes. J. Biochem. 52, 226 (1962).

Angiokeratoma Corporis Diffusum (Fabry's Disease)

By

W. Kahlke

Synonyms: Diffuse angiokeratoma; thesaurismosis hereditaria Ruiter-Pompen-Wyers; hereditary dystopic lipidosis; angiomatosis miliaris; glycolipid lipidosis.

Definition and Introduction

Angiokeratoma corporis diffusum universale (ACD) or Fabry's disease is a familial sphingolipidosis. Its first conspicuous sign is the typical skin change after which the disease is named. In addition, there is involvement of other organs, which determines the course and prognosis. The clinical picture is characterized by pains in the extremities and signs and symptoms resulting from involvement of the vasculature, kidneys and the heart. Slight corneal opacity seems to be uniformly present, but frequently goes unnoticed, since visual acuity is not impaired. The symptomatology includes vasomotor disturbances, impairment of sweat secretion, paresthesias, intolerance of high and low temperatures, fever, anemia, gastrointestinal and cerebrovascular disturbances.

While the occurrence of the full syndrome is restricted to males, an incomplete form of the disorder can be found in women.

The prognosis of ACD is determined by the extent of cardiovascular complications and kidney disease. Most affected individuals die between the ages of 30 and 60 years.

SWEELEY and KLIONSKY (1963, 1964, 1966) isolated from organs of ACD patients two glycolipids, which they identified as ceramide-dihexoside and ceramide-trihexoside. Their findings confirmed the assumption of RUITER et al. (1947) who suggested classification of ACD as a lipid storage disease. They did not confirm the postulate that the stored material was a phospholipid.

Reviews on ACD during the past 10 years have been given by FESSAS et al. (1955), LEVER (1963), DE GROOT (1964), WISE (1965), OPITZ et al. (1965), SWEELEY and KLIONSKY (1966).

Historical Review

Angiokeratoma corporis diffusum universale was first described in 1898 by the English dermatologist ANDERSON and independently by the German FABRY as purpura haemorrhagica nodularis (purpura papulosa haemorrhagica Hebrae). Fabry's patient was a 13 year-old boy who had developed peculiar skin changes when he was nine years old. The skin lesions had started in the left fossa poplitea as small, blueish-red to black indolent nodules, which consecutively involved areas of the trunk, particularly the umbilical and ileosacral region, the scrotum, the posterior aspects of thighs, the chest, and, to a lesser degree, the extensor surfaces of the lower and upper extremities. Similar lesions were observed in the oral mucosa. With the exception of slight edema of the eyelids there were no additional abnormal findings at the time. Re-examination of the patient 17 years later

(FABRY 1915) revealed an increase of skin lesions and of the edema. In addition, signs of asthma and albuminuria had appeared. On the basis of histologic examination, the skin changes were initially interpreted to result from hemorrhage. There was also aneurismal dilatation of small vessels of the cutis and subcutis and partial hypertrophy of the stratum corneum. The patient expired at the age of 35 years from lung disease. His disease was named angiokeratoma corporis diffusum (universale) in Fabry's second report (1915, 1916).

In the "angiokeratoma" case of ANDERSON (1898), there was again proteinuria in addition to skin lesions. ANDERSON suggested that the lesions which he observed in the skin might also occur in a generalized form and pointed out the differences between these changes and those which had been described earlier as angiokeratoma by COTTLE (1878) and MIBELLI (1889). The possibility of a systemic disorder was also ventilated by STEINER and VOERNER (1909) and by GÜNTHER (1913).

In subsequent reports on ACD additional symptoms were described such as temperature intolerance, anhidrosis, cramplike pains in the extremities (STÜMPKE 1916, SIBLEY 1918), cardiac enlargement (WEICKSEL 1925), accentuation of the second aortic sound, and "fat cells" in the urine (SIBLEY 1918). Varicosis of conjunctival veins, corneal opacity and caliber changes of retinal vessels were described by WEICKSEL (1925). A close relationship between external and internal involvement was pointed out by RUITER and POMPEN (1939) who, in addition to the typical skin changes, found evidence of cardiac, vascular and renal lesions in three affected brothers. One of these three patients and an additional patient who died from uremia were the first cases of ACD in which autopsies were performed. There was thickening of the media of blood vessels resulting from deposition of hyaline material, particularly in renal arteries of medium and large size, and also in blood vessels of other organs (RUITER et al. 1947, POMPEN et al. 1947). On the basis of these findings the authors suspected an inborn error in the metabolism of muscle cells of the heart and blood vessels.

Subsequently HORNBOSTEL et al. (1950, 1951) reported two more cases of ACD and published detailed descriptions of pathologic changes. Studies by SCRIBA (1950) resulted in the demonstration of vacuolation of muscle cells which was caused by a material appearing birefringent with polarized light. A similar material was found in other organs and in ganglion cells of the central and peripheral nervous system. Chemical analyses of the heart musculature showed storage of a substance which was considered a phosphatide at a level which was ten times normal (KÜHNAU 1950, 1958). However, the stored lipid was not further identified in this case. On the basis of these findings the authors concluded that they were dealing with an unknown lipid storage disease.

All patients reported up to that time were males, many of them brothers (STÜMPKE 1916, SIBLEY 1918, WEICKSEL 1925, RUITER and POMPEN 1939). In 1952, BROWN and MILNE made the observation, that each of two half-brothers, from different fathers but one mother, suffered from ACD. In 1958, COLLEY's group studied tissues of the mother of an affected subject, whose nephew also had ACD. There was a typical "honeycomb" like vacuolation of the glomerulus epithelium (COLLEY et al. 1958, WALLACE 1958), but it appears that this female patient, who had died at the age of 47 years, never had the skin lesions of ACD, and it is not known whether other signs and symptoms of ACD were present. The authors suggest from their findings that the metabolic error of ACD can also occur in female subjects, with or without the typical skin manifestations. Shortly thereafter WISE (1960) and WISE et al. (1962) reported skin lesions and corneal opacity in a female subject, thus confirming that the occurrence of ACD is not restricted to the male sex. From the finding of lipid storage in females DE GROOT (1964) concluded that

in female patients skin changes may be lacking and clinical symptoms may appear
only at an advanced age. According to DE GROOT the disease may be transmitted
by females as well as by males. Extensive investigations on the mode of inheritance
are those by OPITZ et al. (1965).

In 1963, SWEELEY and KLIONSKY succeeded in chemical identification of the
stored material in ACD. They isolated from the kidney of a patient (KLIONSKY
et al. 1966) large amounts of a glycolipid incorporating three hexose units and
another component with two hexose units and sulfur and thus established that
ACD was not a phospholipid storage disease.

Incidence (Age, Sex, Race)

Angiokeratomas are the first sign of ACD in almost all cases. In a few patients
they were observed before the tenth year of life (FABRY 1898, 1916, 1930, BROWN
and MILNE 1952), but in most they appeared with the onset of puberty, and only
rarely after the 18th year (STEINER and VOERNER 1909, LAPIÈRE 1957). According
to the review of DE GROOT (1964) which includes 47 patients, the onset of skin
changes occurred during childhood in 14 subjects, and between the age of six and
14 years in 17 subjects. At the time of the skin eruption, or a little later, episodes
of pain in hands and feet make their appearance, while disturbances of other
organs, particularly the heart, vasculature and kidneys generally become manifest
later.

As mentioned above, ACD is not restricted to the male sex. On the basis of
the reported cases (GÜNTHER 1913, SIGUIER et al. 1956, WISE 1960, CURRY and
FLEISHER 1961, RAHMAN et al. 1961, CROSS 1962, WISE et al. 1962, DE GROOT
1964) it appears that in females the disease produces less symptoms than it does
in males. Typical skin changes may be missing or are considerably less marked
than in males (WISE 1960, DE GROOT 1964).

Occurrence of ACD in several generations seems frequent. Relevant reports
have been given by PRICE (1955), with ACD in a male and his maternal aunt,
by WISE (1960), who identified the cousins described by COLLEY et al. (1958)
as grandchildren of the subject described by ANDERSON (1898), by CROSS (1962),
by DE GROOT (1964) whose seven cases come from three generations (three females
and four male patients), including the cases of POMPEN et al. (1947), and by OPITZ
et al. (1965) whose detailed review on the heredity of ACD contains the pedigrees
mentioned. Consanguinity of parents has not been described. For details on the
genetics of ACD see the chapter by FUHRMANN.

With the exception of a 15 year-old Chinese patient (YU 1956) all reported
cases occurred in the white race.

Clinical Manifestations

First complaints in over half of the juvenile patients are pains in the extremities,
usually localized to the joints and initially attributed to a rheumatic disorder. Some
patients state that the pain increases with physical activity. Attacks of pain can
be triggered by high or low temperatures. This was shown by DE GROOT (1964)
in one of his patients: immersion of the hands in water below 22—23°C consistently initiated the painful episodes, which became intolerable when the temperature was lowered to 13—14°C. This sensory disturbance is most probably
due to morphologic changes in the nervous system (see page 343).

In addition to the symptoms described, there may be paresthesias of hands
and feet, and vasomotor and vegetative disturbances such as impaired sweat

secretion, which is usually manifested as hypo- or anhidrosis, or occasionally as hyperhidrosis (NETHERTON 1934, DUPERRAT and PLUVINAGE 1956, FONE and KING 1964). In a case described by DE GROOT (1964) sweat secretion was normal up to the age of 20 years, but thereafter a period of excessive sweating occurred with a final loss of sweating ability.

Difficulties in temperature adaption are suggested by the occurrence of episodes of blueish or white discoloration of the hands or the sign of digitus mortuus.

Skin Lesions

The angiokeratomas, which have been observed in all male patients, consist of numerous small spots or papules, the color of which ranges from purple through dark-blue to black. They are diffusely distributed over large parts of the body with predilection for certain areas, such as the lower parts of the trunk, particularly the lumbosacral area, umbilical area, genital area, inguinal folds and buttocks (see fig. 1). They are also found in great numbers on the posterior aspects of the thighs, while other portions of the extremities and the thorax are involved to a lesser degree. Skin lesions are rarely observed on the face and on hands and feet. The papules are minimally hyperkeratotic, and show incomplete blanching with pressure. The diameter of the lesions is rarely more than a few millimeters, and many are found only by diligent searching. The angiokeratomas show no tendency to spontaneous bleeding, and there is little hemorrhage after puncture of the lesions, apparently due to the fact that circulation through them is very limited (BROWN and MILNE 1952).

This description does not apply to females suffering from ACD.

In about one-third of cases mucosal changes were reported, while in about

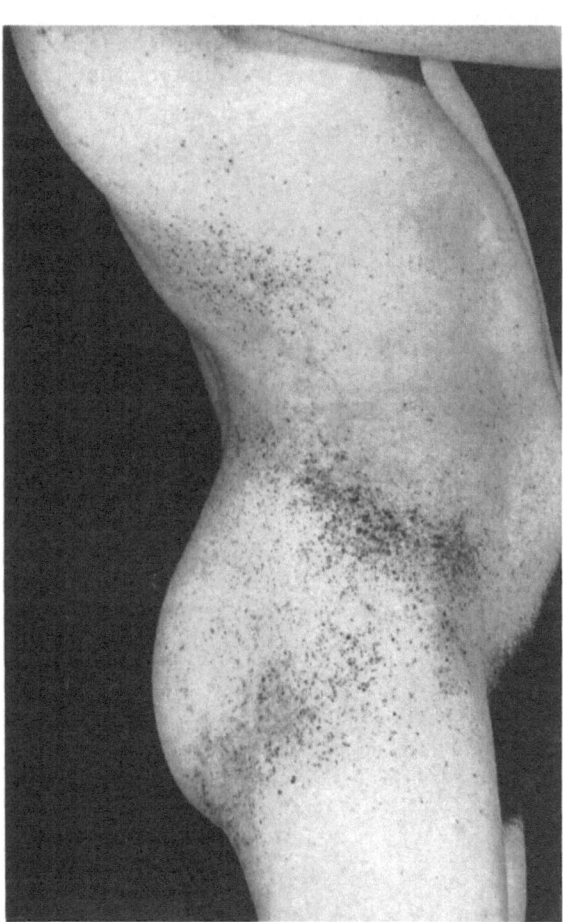

Fig. 1. Typical skin lesions of the trunk in ACD. (Reproduced by courtesy of Prof. K. W. KALKOFF)

50 per cent of cases their presence or absence has not been documented. The oral mucosa may show blueish papules; conjunctival veins may be dilated and have the appearance of a sausage or of a string of pearls.

Kidneys

Changes in the kidneys usually determine the prognosis. Most frequent signs of renal involvement are proteinuria, hypo- or isosthenuria, microhematuria, and cylindruria. The lack of concentrating ability might indicate that the distal tubule and collecting duct epithelium has become relatively insensitive to antidiuretic hormone (Henry and Rally 1963). A striking finding, although rarely described in early cases, is lipid excretion with the urine (Sibley 1918, Pittelkow et al. 1955, Fessas et al. 1955, Bethune et al. 1961, Kalkoff 1966). The renal disease usually becomes manifest during the fourth decade, although its onset is probably many years earlier. It results in a progressive rise of blood urea nitrogen and finally uremia. Occasionally uremia appears before age 40.

Cardiac Disturbances

Involvement of the heart is less frequent than that of the kidneys, and results in less impairment of function. In a number of reported cases, particularly those of younger patients, there is no information on the cardiac status. According to

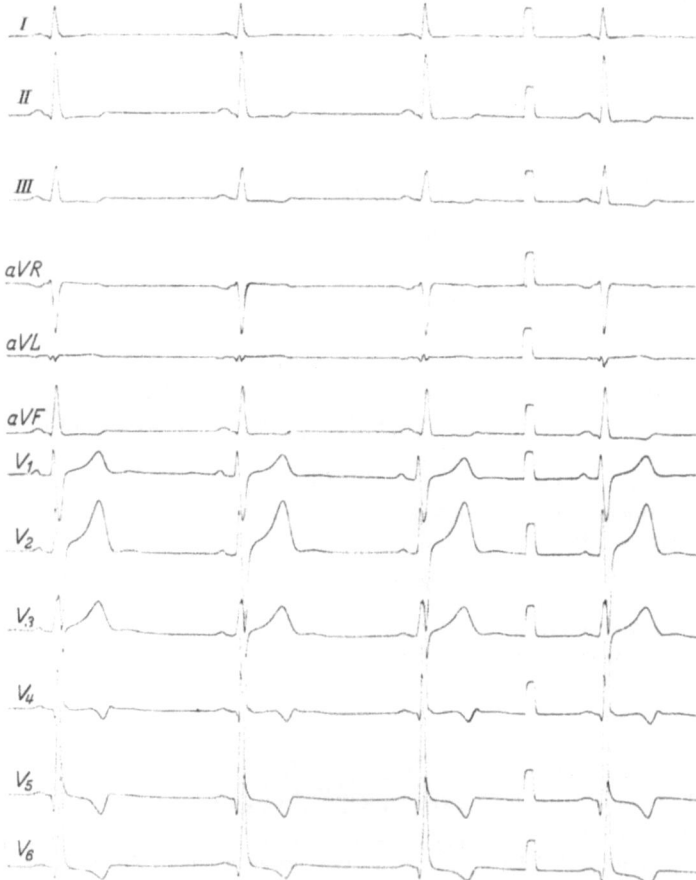

Fig. 2. ECG in a 39 year-old male patient with ACD. (Reproduced by courtesy of Prof. E. Zeh). Sinus bradycardia, heart rate 48/min. Intermediate heart position. P: 0.01, PQ: 0.13, QRS: 0.10 and QT 0.42 sec. Lowering of ST in lead *II* and *III*. T—*I* flattened, T—*II* and T—*III* biphasic. Lowering of ST and biphasic T-wave in lead *aVF*. High amplitudes in the chest leads. Left-ventricular Sokolow-index positive. Transition at V_3. Slight lowering of ST-segments in V_4—V_6; preterminal negativity of T. Interpretation: Left ventricular hypertrophy and left heart strain. Additional right ventricular hypertrophy is suggested by the heart position which is relatively far to the right ((Dr. R. Thorspecken)

DE GROOT (1964) heart symptoms appear during the third decade. Left ventricular hypertrophy and/or electrocardiographic changes (see fig. 2) compatible with diffuse myocardial lesions are found in over 30 per cent of affected subjects. Heart failure seems rare (HORNBOSTEL 1952, both cases).

Mild hypertension is found in almost 25 per cent of cases. Very high blood pressure values or fixed hypertension are not a feature of ACD. Involvement of heart valves, such as the lesion of the aortic valve in the case of KUSKE and BAUMGARTNER (1962) are exceptions and seem to be unrelated findings.

Edema

Edema of the extremities is one of the most frequent symptoms of ACD and has been reported in about 50 per cent of cases. In some patients there is simultaneous swelling of the eyelids, or periorbital edema only (CURRY and FLEISHER 1961). Rarely, the edema becomes quite severe as in the case of HOFMANN and HAUSER (1962) and VORSTER (1964). Here elephantiasis of the left lower leg developed in addition to bilateral ankle edema and swelling of the hands (see fig. 3 and 4). In some cases it is restricted

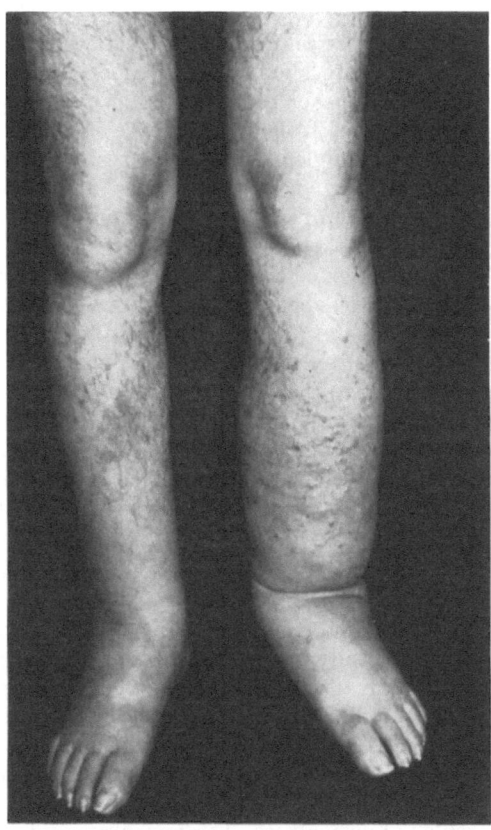

Fig. 3. Edema and elephantiasis of the left lower leg and sclerodermatitis in ACD. Picture taken after bed rest for ten days. (Reproduced by courtesy of Dr. K. VORSTER)

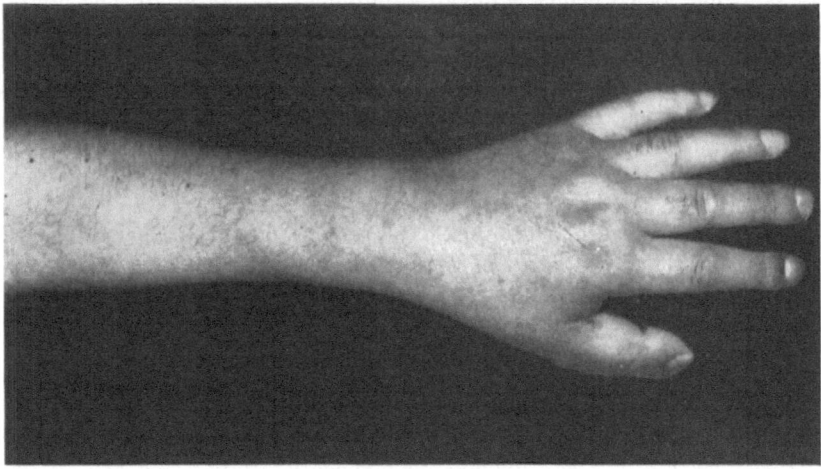

Fig. 4. Edema and clubbing of fingers with scaly lesions of the lower arm in ACD. (Reproduced by courtesy of Dr. K. VORSTER)

to the summer months or increases during this time (FESSAS et al. 1955, DE GROOT 1964).

Neurologic Disturbances

About 30 per cent of patients with ACD complain of symptoms referable to the nervous system. The neurologic symptomatology may be quite complex, and it is not possible in each case to decide whether symptoms result from cerebrovascular involvement or from lipid storage in nerve cells. Acute hemiparesthesia, hemiparesis or hemiplegia in some cases is suggestive of a vascular cause, and may be fatal (DUPERRAT and PLUVINAGE 1956, BASS 1958).

Frequent complaints are headache, dizziness, nausea and vomiting. Epileptic seizures are rarely observed (BETHUNE et al. 1961). Involvement of cranial nerves such as pareses of the oculomotorius and/or trigeminus nerves and impairment of the senses of smell and taste have been described (HOFMANN and HAUSER 1962, CURRY and FLEISHER 1961). Occasionally symptoms of cerebrovascular insufficiency (HORNBOSTEL 1952) appear which are undistinguishable from those resulting from atherosclerotic vascular lesions (HOFMANN and HAUSER 1962). In a case of STOUGHTON and CLENDENNING (1959) there was deafness and evidence of hydrops of the labyrinth. DE GROOT (1964) described a Menière syndrome in one of his cases and excessive need for sleep in three of his seven patients. Ataxia and nystagmus (BASS 1958) are suggestive of cerebellar involvement.

Eyes

Various eye lesions are manifestations of the vascular process. These include aneurysmal dilatation and varicosis of the conjunctival vessels. Since there is no systematic study on these symptoms their prevalence is not known. Angiectasias of conjunctival vessels were observed in four of the seven patients described by DE GROOT (1964). In a patient described by PITTELKOW et al. (1955) involvement of the conjunctiva was observed at the age of 26, but upon re-examination of this patient 20 years later, the conjunctivas were completely normal. Lid edema has been mentioned; it is not known whether it is related to the renal disease or to local vascular abnormalities. The appearance of corneal opacities is a sign which was rarely noticed in earlier cases, but which is apparently closely related to lipid storage. The lesion can be recognized with the aid of a slitlamp as a slight fogginess. As a rule, visual acuity is impaired minimally or not at all. The symptom is found in the majority of patients upon careful search and was present in six out of seven patients of DE GROOT (1964) and in all twelve cases of SPAETH and FROST (1965). This dystrophy of the corneal epithelium (WEICKSEL 1925, RAHMAN 1963, WISE et al. 1962) is considered characteristic for ACD by OPITZ et al. (1965). Examination of the cornea is utilized for the detection of carriers. Other findings include anisocoria and cataract of the right eye (HOFMANN and HAUSER 1962).

Upon fundoscopy vascular changes have been seen in a number of cases. As a rule, they consist of tortuosity of the arteries, which show an uneven caliber or aneurysmal dilatation. In addition, localized venous dilatation has been described. In some cases there was papilledema (BASS 1958, HOFMANN and HAUSER 1962, DE GROOT 1964).

Other Signs and Symptoms

A number of other symptoms which have been described cannot be related to ACD with certainty. These include splenomegaly (BROWN and MILNE 1952), and hepatosplenomegaly and thrombopenia (WÖHNLICH 1949). The classification of the latter author's case is not certain. Hepatomegaly may result from cardiac involvement (FESSAS et al. 1955). Emphysema was present in both cases of HORNBOSTEL (1952) and in the patients of FESSAS et al. (1955). PITTELKOW et al. (1955) described necrosis of the femoral epiphysis, and related it to a vascular lesion. Abnormalities of nails were observed by FESSAS et al. (1955), KARR (1959), HOFMANN and HAUSER (1962) and DE GROOT (1964). One patient died from a severe form of gastroenteritis (RUITER 1957, case 4). OPITZ et al. (1965) emphasize that puberty is delayed in patients with ACD, and fertility seems to be impaired. Impairment of development of secondary sex characteristics has been described, such as decreased growth of the beard (PRICE 1955), while in two patients of DE GROOT (1964) the opposite was observed. A large ulcer of the lower leg was present in a 35 year-old patient reported by COLLEY et al. (1958).

Serum

Abnormal chemical findings in blood are usually restricted to those which result from decreased renal function, such as progressive rise of blood urea nitrogen and uremia. When isosthenuria is established, abnormalities of serum electrolytes may develop. Total serum protein is normal.

The creatinine clearance in two cases was 48 ml/min. and 94.5 ml/min. respectively (COLLEY et al. 1958).

Hematology

Hematologic findings include mild to moderate anemia, anisocytosis and poikilocytosis. In two out of six cases (FESSAS et al. 1955) in which white blood cells were differentiated, eosinophilia was observed.

Thrombocyte count and function is normal with the exception of the case of WÖHNLICH (1949), in which the diagnosis of ACD is not certain. A bleeding tendency or specific abnormalities of the blood clotting mechanism have not been reported. Findings from bone marrow biopsies will be reported in the section on pathology (see page 344).

Urine

Urinary abnormalities consist of proteinuria, cylindruria (hyaline and granular) microhematuria and pyuria. Inability to concentrate may occur simultaneously or may follow such findings after years.

Urinary lipid excretion occurs mainly in the form of vacuolated cells (SIBLEY 1918, FESSAS et al. 1955, PITTELKOW 1955, YU 1956, DEMPSEY et al. 1965) which resemble macrophages; some free lipid droplets are also found (FESSAS et al. 1955, WACHTEL and MATTEI 1964, KALKOFF 1966). According to RUITER (1958) the lipid-laden cells are desquamated epithelial cells of the loop of Henle.

Pathology

The description of pathologic changes in ACD is based on autopsies by RUITER et al. (1947), SCRIBA (1950), HORNBOSTEL (1952), FALCK (1955), FALCK and WEICKSEL (1957), WALLACE (1958), RAHMAN and LINDENBERG (1963). In addition, reports on histologic findings in skin lesions and in biopsies of kidney, liver, muscle, bowel, lymph nodes and bone marrow have been given (FESSAS et al. 1955, RAHMAN and LINDENBERG 1963, LEDER and BOSWORTH 1965, VON GEMMINGEN et al. 1965, WALLACE and COOPER 1965, DUBACH and GLOOR 1966). The main morphologic changes in ACD consist of thickening of the walls of blood vessels, occurrence of foam- or storage cells in reticulo-endothelial tissues and generalized ganglion cell storage.

22*

Vasculature

Vascular abnormalities may be grossly visible. Ectasia of blood vessels was observed by SCRIBA (1950) in the mucosa of numerous organs such as the trachea, esophagus, stomach and appendix and in the renal pelvis. Similar ectasias were found in the same patient in the perichondrium of the ribs. In a patient who had

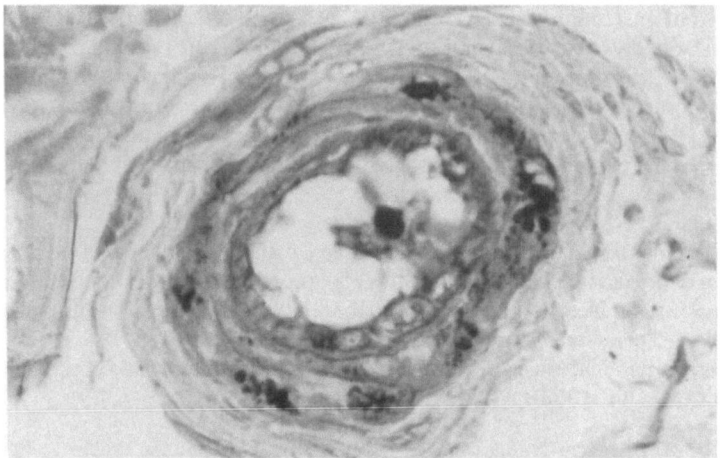

Fig. 5. Skin biopsy in ACD. Arteriole of the corium containing aggregates of black lipid granules in smooth muscle fibers of the vessel wall (Fig. 3 from RUITER 1958)

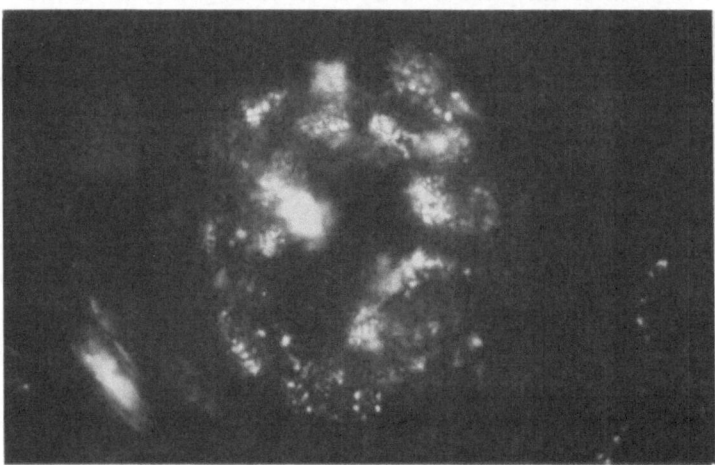

Fig. 6. Skin biopsy in ACD. Appearance of an unstained frozen section with polarized light. Birefringent material in the vessel wall and endothelial cells (Fig. 2 from RUITER 1958)

died from gastrointestinal hemorrhage (RUITER 1957), there were blueish-red papules distributed over the entire intestinal mucosa. The most prominent finding upon histologic examination is marked thickening of the media of arteries in almost every tissue. Intimal swelling may or may not be present (RUITER et al. 1947). In spite of thickening of the vessel wall, encroachment on the vessel lumen is rare (HORNBOSTEL 1952). The thickening of the media is caused by deposition of a light, hyaline material, which is found mainly between muscle fibers (see fig. 5). Intracellular storage of this material results in vacuolation of the cytoplasm. There may be deformities of the nuclei of the smooth muscle cells (SCRIBA 1950). Changes are most marked in the aorta and in renal arteries of medium and large size; qualitatively similar changes, however, are observed in the blood vessels of other organs as well. The absence of thickening of renal blood vessels is an exception (LEDER and BOSWORTH 1965). Involvement of the musculature of veins was described by SCRIBA (1950).

Examination of the material contained in vacuolated muscle cells, even in those which appear only minimally involved, shows birefringence with polarized light (SCRIBA 1950) (see fig. 6). Histochemically, this material stains faint yellowish-red with hematoxylin-scarlet red, which, according to SCRIBA, is suggestive of the presence of lipid. Staining with Sudan III is negative (POMPEN et al. 1947). According to RUITER (1954, 1958), the stored material is stainable with Sudan black or scarlet red after chromate fixation. Comparative studies by DE GROOT (1964), who examined material from 25 patients with various diseases, including angiokeratoma scroti, angioma senile, Letterer-Siwe's disease etc. with the same methods, suggest that this behaviour is specific for ACD. DUBACH and GLOOR (1966) deduce the presence of phospholipids from a positive Luxol-blue-reaction. These phospholipids are rather unsoluble and possibly bound to carbohydrate or protein.

Kidneys

Grossly, the kidneys appear decreased in size and atrophic (RUITER et al. 1947, SCRIBA 1950, HORNBOSTEL 1952, FALCK and WEICKSEL 1957, COLLEY et al. 1958, WALLACE 1958). The weight of both kidneys in case 3 of COLLEY et al. (1958)

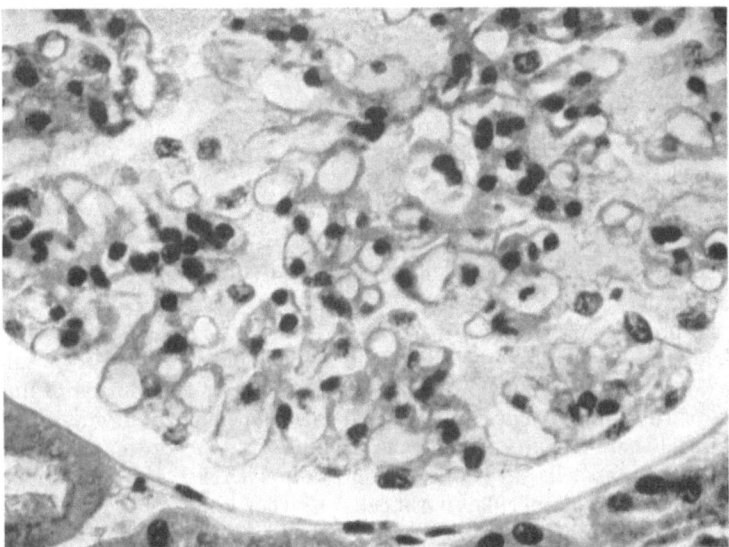

Fig. 7. Renal biopsy in ACD; section of glomerulus. Glomerulus epithelium with foamy metamorphosis (Fig. 2 from DUBACH and GLOOR 1966. Reproduced with permission of Georg Thieme Verlag, Stuttgart)

was 240 gm, the surface showed large depressed scars, and there were irregularities of the cortex on cross sections. In a 47 year-old affected subject (SCRIBA 1950) each kidney weighed 125 gm, there were scars secondary to vascular occlusions and small, spotty, yellowish-grey deposits resembling those seen in chronic nephrosis, as well as fibrosis of the renal medulla.

Microscopic changes were similar in all reported cases when whole organs were studied. In contrast, findings in samples from small areas, such as these obtained by needle biopsy, were variable (WACHTEL and MATTEI 1964). Typical changes resulting from lipid deposition concern the glomeruli (see fig. 7), the Bowman capsule and distal parts of the tubuli. The involvement of the loop of Henle (see fig. 8) and the interstitium is less marked and proximal tubuli are not involved. Visceral and parietal cells of the Bowman capsule are dilated and contain numerous small vacuoles, which impart to them the appearance of foam cells (see fig. 7). When the Bowman capsule is filled with such vacuolated foam cells, a typical honeycomb appearance results. There may be thickening of the basal membrane

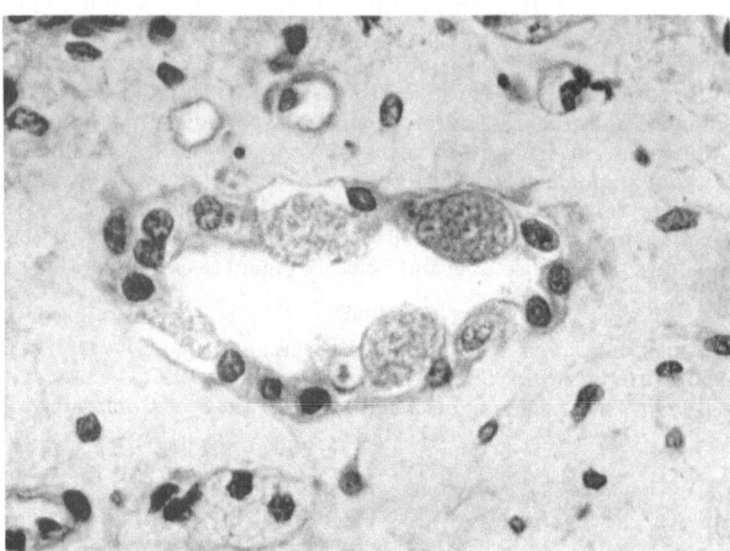

Fig. 8. Renal biopsy in ACD. Foam cells in the loop of Henle. Marked swelling of the tubulus epithelium. Foamy metamorphosis of the cytoplasm. Droplets stain with Luxol fast-blue and are PAS-positive. Paraffin section, enlargement 570-fold. (Fig. 4 from Dubach and Gloor 1966. Reproduced with permission of Georg Thieme Verlag, Stuttgart)

at the vascular pole of the glomerulus. Numerous glomeruli are obliterated and appear amorphous. Frequently, cells of the distal tubuli and of Henle's loop are also converted to foam cells (see fig. 8) (Colley et al. 1958, Dubach and Gloor 1966). With progression of the disease (case 1 of Colley et al. 1958), and in the final stages (Hartley and Miller 1963) foam cells may decrease in number, and extensive degeneration of the epithelium with flattening, dissolution of nuclei and distention of the tubuli ensues. In addition to replacement of glomeruli by amorphous material there is connective tissue proliferation. According to Dubach and Gloor (1966), foam cells of Henle's loop stain with Luxol-blue and PAS (see fig. 8), in contrast to glomerular foam cells. Neither kind of foam cell stains with fat-red, Sudan-black, Nile-blue sulfate and Astra-blue. Electronmicroscopic studies of renal tissue by these authors showed various osmiophilic inclusions. There was evidence for uptake of stored material by mitochondria. Electronmicroscopic findings by Hartley and Miller (1963) were similar. Dempsey et al. (1965) observed well-organized onion skin figures in the intercapillary areas of the glomerulus on electron microscopy.

Heart and Skeletal Muscle

The heart was found to be enlarged in all autopsied cases. Its weight in the 47 year-old patient of Scriba (1950) was 550 gm, in the 47 year-old patient (case 3) of Colley et al. (1958) 630 gm and in the 38 year-old patient reported by Falck and Weicksel (1957) 620 gm. Although both ventricles are hypertrophied, the musculature of the right heart may be thicker than that of the left (Scriba 1950).

Microscopic examination shows widening and hypertrophy of muscle fibers. Numerous muscle cells are vacuolated. Vacuoles are particularly numerous in the center of muscle fibers and displace the muscle fibrils peripherally (SCRIBA 1950). In a patient described by LEDER and BOSWORTH (1965) who, in addition to ACD, suffered from mitral stenosis, there was edematous, fibrous thickening of the endocardium of the left auricular appendix, which extended into the interstitium. The nuclei of involved cells are usually large, rarely pyknotic; they frequently appear irregularly outlined, lobulated and hyperchromatic (RUITER et al. 1947, SCRIBA 1950, HORNBOSTEL 1952, LEDER and BOSWORTH 1965).

The material which is stored in the heart muscle is birefringent (SCRIBA 1950) and stains faintly yellowish-red with hematoxylin-scarlet red.

Involvement of the skeletal musculature is qualitatively similar to that of the heart muscle, although storage is less marked and a predilection of vacuoles for the center of muscle fibers is not apparent.

Skin

Skin lesions are multiple. Their size is that of a pin head or greater and they appear grossly as angiectasias with focal hyperkeratosis of the surface, which is particularly marked in older lesions. Detailed histopathological reports have been given by RUITER (1952, 1954), FESSAS et al. (1955), PITTELKOW et al. (1957), LEVER (1963), DE GROOT (1964), VON GEMMINGEN et al. (1965), HASHIMOTO et al. (1965) and others. The prevailing change consists of thickening of the walls of capillaries, arterioles and venules, which is caused by deposition of birefringent material (see fig. 5 and 6). This was not found in a patient described as suffering from ACD by VINEYARD and KAMIN (1960). In addition to blood vessels, there are large spaces with and without endothelium located intraepidermally and filled with blood. In the upper layers of the corium are nests of dilated tubuli which contain red cells and are frequently surrounded by lymphocytes and histiocytes. Upon rupture, ectatic vessel leave accumulations of red blood cells and a conglomerated amorphous material which forms intraepidermal nests. There is no evidence of new blood vessel formation as in angiomatosis (WERTHEIM 1932) and the changes described appear to result from dilation of pre-existing blood vessels (RUITER 1958), as illustrated by the ampullary dilations of conjunctival vessels. Smooth muscle cells of the media of small arteries in the corium and subcutis show the typical vacuolation and deposition of birefringent material. The nucleus seems suspended in an apparently empty space (HORNBOSTEL and SCRIBA 1953, RUITER 1954). Other elements of the skin such as the arrector pilorum muscles, may show similar changes.

Histochemical properties of skin vessels are similar to those of the vasculature of other tissues. The diagnosis of ACD is therefore established most easily by means of a skin biopsy. RUITER (1954), PITTELKOW et al. (1957), DE GROOT (1961, 1964), VON GEMMINGEN (1965) have described specific staining methods for the stored lipid. Although its histochemical behaviour resembles that of phospholipids, LAPIÈRE (1957) could not find increased phosphatides upon chemical analyses. In most other cases chemical analyses were not performed.

Nervous System

Due to the limitation of nervous system changes to certain groups of neurons, which belong mainly to the autonomous nervous system, RAHMAN et al. (1961) coined the term "hereditary dystopic lipidosis". Whether this restriction of changes to certain groups of neurons is a general feature of the disease is not yet known since complete neuropathological studies in ACD are rare. A detailed review of neuropathologic findings is that by RAHMAN and LINDENBERG (1963).

Grossly, Scriba (1950) found moderate bilateral atrophy of the anterior poles of the frontal lobes of the brain. Crawford (1958) reported enormous dilation of the vessels of the brain base, particularly of vertebral, left carotid and basilar arteries, the diameter of the latter vessel being 12,5 mm. Moderate generalized edema of cerebrum and cerebellum was described by Falck and Weicksel (1957). Areas of ischemic degeneration have been seen in cross sections (Scriba 1950, Wallace 1958).

On microscopy, Scriba (1950) observed groups of markedly distended ganglion cells in the dorsal autonomic nuclei of the vagus and in the hippocampus. The cells showed honeycombing and the nuclei were displaced. Scattered ganglion cells exhibiting similar changes were found in the reticular formation of the pons, in the medulla oblongata and in the nuclei of Goll and Burdach. Ganglion cells in other areas of the brain, and in particular the Purkinje cells of the cerebellum, were not involved. Rahman and Lindenberg (1963) found corresponding ganglion cell changes in the amygdaloid nucleus, the supraoptic nuclei, the paraventricular nuclei, the anterior thalamus and the substancia nigra. There was also involvement of cells of the intermedio-lateral column of the thoracic section of the spinal cord. Findings similar to those reported by Rahman and Lindenberg were reported by Carter and Clark (1963). In contrast, Wallace (1958) observed storage in vessels of the basal ganglia only.

Nerve cells showing changes similar to those in the central nervous system are found in the myenteric plexus of the gastrointestinal tract, in the membranous portion of the trachea (Scriba 1951, Falck and Weicksel 1957, Ruiter 1957, Rahman and Lindenberg 1963), in the autonomous ganglion cells of the thoracolumbar sympathicus, and in the pancreas, thyroid, rectum and tongue (Rahman and Lindenberg 1963, Dubach and Gloor 1966). Birefringence of stored material in these neurons was first shown by Scriba (1950) and confirmed by others. Smith-Dietrich or myelin stains are negative, and there is no metachromasia with the inclusion staining technique of Feyrter (Scriba 1950). In frozen sections, staining for lipids was positive for all storing nerve cells (Rahman and Lindenberg 1963).

Reticuloendothelial Tissues

There may be lipid storage in bone marrow, spleen, lymph nodes and Kupffer cells of the liver. Foam cells in bone marrow were demonstrated first by Fessas et al. (1955). In addition, von Gemmingen et al. (1965) described a second cell type measuring about 16 μ in diameter and exhibiting pyknosis of the nucleus and degeneration of the cell wall while the cytoplasm encloses the nucleus like a parcel. Histochemically, the cytoplasm is PAS-positive and staines with Sudan black B. Upon enzymatic treatment with amylase, there were decreased amounts of the PAS-positive cytoplasmic material. Marti (1966), examining the bone marrow of case 1 of Dubach and Gloor, found scattered, large storage cells with a small round nucleus and a basophilic fragmented material in the cytoplasm Other reports on storing cells in bone marrow have been given by Hofmann and Hauser (1962) and Wallace and Cooper (1965).

Splenic enlargement was found in only one proved case of ACD (Brown and Milne 1952). Grossly, the architecture of the organ appeared normal. Upon histologic examination foam cells were found in the white as well as in the red pulp occurring singly or in groups and containing birefringent material (Scriba 1950, Hornbostel 1952, Fessas et al. 1955, Falck and Weicksel 1957). Findings from lymph node biopsies were similar (Fessas et al. 1955, Falck and Weicksel 1957). On the basis of histochemical studies, Wallace and Cooper (1965) suggest that the macrophages of lymph nodes contain a glycolipid. Moderate lipid storage in Kupffer cells of the liver was described by SCRIBA (1950).

Other Organs

Cells exhibiting storage of birefringent material were found in the parenchyma of liver and spleen, in the adrenals (SCRIBA 1950), in ganglion cells of the submucous

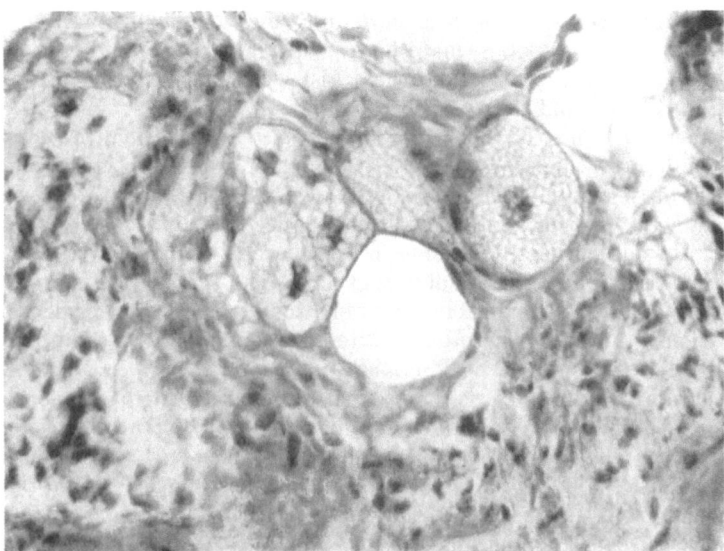

Fig. 9. Rectum biopsy in ACD. Ganglion cells of the submucous plexus are converted to foam cells. Paraffin section, van-Gieson stain, enlargement 400-fold. (Fig. 7 from DUBACH and GLOOR 1966. Reproduced with permission of Georg Thieme Verlag, Stuttgart)

plexus (see fig. 9) (DUBACH and GLOOR 1966) and in muscle cells of the gastrointestinal tract (RUITER 1957), while liver biopsies gave completely normal results in the cases of FESSAS et al. (1955), and WALLACE and COOPER (1965). Apparently, lipid storage in ACD is not restricted to vessel walls, ganglion cells and reticuloendothelial cells, although forthcoming reports may modify the impression resulting from the few ones that have been published.

Results of Lipid Analyses

From the time of reports of KÜHNAU (1950, 1958), ACD has been considered a phospholipid storage disease by most authors, although complete chemical analyses and structural identification of the stored material were not performed at the time. In 1963, SWEELEY and KLIONSKY isolated from the kidney of a 28 year-old patient two lipid fractions which together amounted to 20 mg/gm of wet weight. The larger fraction was a trihexoside (ceramide-glucose-galactose-galactose). The second and smaller fraction was also a glycolipid, the sole carbohydrate of which was galactose. Therefore, the two fractions are different in that the hexose bound directly to the sphingosine is glucose in one and galactose in the other. The composition of the dihexoside was determined by SWEELEY and KLIONSKY (1963, 1966) who found that it contained sulfur in contrast to the trihexoside and had a fatty acid composition similar to sphingolipids.

The fatty acids of the trihexoside consist to 75% of C_{22}—C_{24} fatty acids while palmitic and stearic acids together amount to only about 10%.

It is probable that the stored lipid of ACD occurs normally in small amounts. Svennerholm and Svennerholm (1963) found a trihexoside with a proportion of ceramide : glucose : galactose of 1 : 1 : 2 in plasma and Mårtensson et al. (1966) found a trihexoside in kidney lipids of normals in addition to dihexoside.

Pathogenetic Aspects

An hereditary occurrence, histologic findings by Ruiter et al. (1947) and the discovery of birefringent storage material by Scriba (1950) constitute the basis for consideration of the disease as a lipid-thesaurismosis. Various signs and symptoms probably result from lipid storage.

Pathogenetic interpretation is difficult for vascular abnormalities in skin and mucous membranes, which far exceed those which might be expected from storage alone, and which partly resemble angiomatous tumors. Some authors interpret vascular changes to result from the loss of muscle tone, particularly of small arteries and arterioles, whereby storage in vessel walls would impair active regulation of the vessel lumen. The involvement of various parts of the nervous system by lipid storage may be responsible for vasomotor disturbances, episodes of fever, pain sensations, and other symptoms. Extensive foam cell formation in the kidneys results in progressive loss of function.

A further unsolved problem is the predisposition of the media of blood vessels, ganglion cells, renal epithelium and reticuloendothelial system for accumulation of the lipid. This may be related to the function of the stored material or of some material associated with it or else may result from its physical properties, particularly its solubility. In the case of the kidney, impaired excretion of these glycolipids may be the cause of storage.

A significant structural difference of the oligosaccharide in glycolipids of neural as compared to extraneural tissues has been pointed out by Sweeley and Klionsky (1966): While glycolipids of neural tissues contain N-acetyl-galactosamine as the third carbohydrate component (counting from the ceramide moiety), glycolipids of extraneural tissues, such as the globoside of red cells (Yamakawa et al. 1960, 1963) contain non-substituted galactose. Since the ceramide-trihexoside which was isolated by Sweeley and Klionsky from kidneys of affected subjects corresponds to glycolipids of extraneural origin with regard to its third carbohydrate moiety, predominant involvement of extraneural tissues in ACD may be explained that way. However, arguments against the thesis of specificity of glycolipids as regards extraneural and neural tissues are on the one hand the findings of visceral involvement in neurovisceral gangliosidosis and late-infantile amaurotic idiocy with storage of the major monosialoganglioside ($G_{GNT}I$) and on the other the involvement of ganglion cells of the central nervous system in ACD and in infantile Gaucher's disease.

The origin of the stored ceramide-trihexoside in ACD has not been clarified. The structural similarity with the globoside of red cells suggests a relationship of the two glycolipids. This assumption is supported by similarities of their fatty acid patterns (Sweeley and Klionsky 1963, 1966). While mammalian sphingolipids usually contain considerable amounts of palmitic and stearic acids, these two fatty acids are found in very small concentrations in the trihexoside of ACD (Sweeley and Klionsky 1963) and of normals (Mårtensson 1963) and in the globoside (Yamakawa et al. 1963). Here, C_{16} and C_{18} fatty acids make up only about 10% of total fatty acids. It is possible that the ceramide trihexoside is an intermediate of the degradative pathway of red cell glycolipids and that ACD is in a way similar to Gaucher's disease. While the block in ACD may be located between globoside and trihexoside (see figure 10) that of Gaucher's disease appears to reside between the monohexoside (cerebroside) on the one hand and ceramide and glucose on the other (see figure 7 page 280). However, the degradation of globoside to trihexoside has not been demonstrated in the normal organism, and neither has a defect at this step been demonstrated in ACD. If the theory as outlined can be

Glycolipids
(red cells, other nonneural cells)
↓
Ceramide-glucose-galactose-
galactose-hexosamine
↓ Step I
Ceramide-glucose-galactose-galactose
↓ Step II
Ceramide-glucose-galactose
(Cytoside)
↓ Step III
Ceramide-glucose
(Cerebroside)
↓ Step IV
Ceramide

Fig. 10. Hypothetical scheme of degradation of glycolipids. A block at step II would lead to accumulation of ceramide-trihexoside and might represent the lesion in ACD. Blockage of step III is a possibility in the case of JERVIS et al. (1962), and of step IV in Gaucher's disease

confirmed, a case of JERVIS et al. (1962) with storage of the dihexoside "cytoside" (ROSENBERG 1962) becomes particularly interesting as a possible link between ACD and Gaucher's disease.

Diagnosis

The leading sign in ACD is the appearance of skin lesions with a typical color, size and distribution, which permit experienced dermatologists to make an unequivocal diagnosis. Somewhat similar skin lesions are seen in the angiokeratoma of Mibelli; however, here the localization is different in that primarily the dorsal surfaces of hands and fingers are involved, the lesions are larger and warty, and appear after exposure to cold. The lesions of angioma serpiginosum of Hutchinson are not palpable, in contrast to ACD. Angiokeratoma naeviforme (circumscriptum) can be differentiated by its sharp border and the unilateral appearance of the lesions. The angiokeratoma of Fordyce is characterized by its localization on the scrotum of old men, and is usually found along larger scrotal veins, while in ACD skin lesions are distributed over the entire scrotum and frequently overlying small veins (WISE 1966).

Difficulties may be encountered in differentiation of ACD from purpura or from hereditary teleangiectasia (Osler's disease). In this situation the localization of lesions to the umbilical area and the centripetal distribution in ACD may be of help. In contrast to purpura, the lesions of ACD are permanent; in contrast to those of hereditary teleangiectasia, they are darker.

When skin lesions suggest the diagnosis of ACD, it is supported by complaints of attacks of pain in the extremities, of paresthesias and of oversensitivity towards hot and cold temperatures, at a time when involvement of kidneys, heart and vessels is not yet manifest. Strong evidence for the diagnosis is the slight corneal opacity, which can be demonstrated upon slit lamp examination. This finding had already been emphasized by RUITER (1958) and was seen by WISE (1966) in all of 40 examined cases, which contained eight women and children in whom angiokeratomas of the skin were missing. In patients with typical skin lesions the corneal abnormality was always present.

When, in younger patients, skin manifestations are as yet absent, the complaints are frequently misinterpreted to result from rheumatic fever, polyarteritis nodosa, erythromelalgia or even psychoneurosis. The diagnosis may be particularly difficult in women, in whom ACD is more rare and in whom skin lesions are usually absent; it may be established only on the basis of the familial nature of the disease.

The diagnosis is confirmed by histologic and histochemical studies with demonstration of lipid storage and its typical distribution in the angiokeratomas. Renal biopsy is usually not necessary. Chemical analyses with the finding of the typical glycolipid are desirable in each case.

Treatment

There is no causal treatment for ACD, as there is none in other hereditary storage diseases. Therapy is restricted to symptomatic measures and the alleviation of disability resulting from chronic progressive kidney- and/or vessel disease.

References

ANDERSON, W.: A case of "angeio-keratoma". Brit. J. Derm. **10**, 113 (1898).

BASS, B. H.: Angiokeratoma corporis diffusum. Brit. med. J. **1958/I**, 1418.

BETHUNE, J. E., P. L. LANDRIGAN, and C. D. CHIPMAN: Angiokeratoma corporis diffusum universale (Fabry's disease) in two brothers. New Engl. J. Med. **264**, 1280 (1961).

BROWN, A., and J. A. MILNE: Diffuse angiokeratoma: Report of two cases with diffuse skin changes, one with neurological symptoms and splenomegaly. Glasg. med. J. **33**, 361 (1952).

CARTER, H. W., and D. CLARK: Unpublished data. Cited after RAHMAN and LINDENBERG (1963) ref. [5].

COLLEY, J. R., D. L. MILLER, M. S. R. HUTT, H. J. WALLACE, and H. E. DE WARDENER: The renal lesion in angiokeratoma corporis diffusum. Brit. med. J. **1958/I**, 1266.

COTTLE, W.: Warty growths. St. George's Hosp. Rep. **9**, 758 (1878); cited after WISE (1966).

CRAWFORD: Refer to COLLEY et al. (1958) and WALLACE (1958).

CROSS, E. G.: The familial occurrence of erythromelalgia and nephritis. Canad. med. Ass. J. **87**. 1 (1962).

CURRY, H. B., and T. L. FLEISHER: Angiokeratoma corporis diffusum. A case report. J. Amer. med. Ass. **175**, 864 (1961).

DEMPSEY, H., M. W. HARTLEY, J. CARROLL, J. BALINT, R. E. MILLER, and W. B. FROMMEYER: Fabry's disease (Angiokeratoma corporis diffusum). Case report on a rare disease. Ann. intern. Med. **63**, 1059 (1965).

DUBACH, U. C., u. F. GLOOR: Fabry-Krankheit (Angiokeratoma corporis diffusum universale). Phosphatidspeicherkrankheit bei zwei Familien. Dtsch. Med. Wschr. **91**, 241 (1966).

DUPERRAT, B., et G. PLUVINAGE: Angiokératose diffuse de Fabry avec hémiplégie. Bull. Soc. Méd. Hôp. Paris **72**, 748 (1956).

FABRY, J.: Ein Beitrag zur Purpura haemorrhagica nodularis (Purpura papulosa haemorrhagica Hebrae). Arch. Derm. Suppl. **43**, 187 (1898).

— Über einen Fall von Angiokeratoma circumscriptum am linken Oberschenkel. Derm. Z. **22**, 1 (1915).

— Zur Klinik und Ätiologie des Angiokeratoma. Arch. Derm. Suppl. **123**, 294 (1916).

— Weiterer Beitrag. Zur Klinik des Angiokeratoma naeviforme (Naevus angiokeratosus). Derm. Wschr. **90**, 339 (1930).

FALCK, I.: Angiokeratoma corporis diffusum Fabry mit vasorenalem Symptomenkomplex. Samml. selt. klin. Fälle **9**, 20 (1955).

— u. A. WEICKSEL: Angiokeratoma corporis diffusum Fabry mit vasorenalem Symptomenkomplex. Samml. selt. klin. Fälle **13**, 20 (1957).

FESSAS, PH., M. M. WINTROBE, and G. E. CARTWRIGHT: Angiokeratoma corporis diffusum universale (Fabry). First American report of a rare disorder. Arch. intern. Med. **95**, 469 (1955).

FONE, D. J., and W. E. KING: Angiokeratoma corporis diffusum (Fabry's syndrome). Aust. Ann. Med. 13, 339 (1964).

GEMMINGEN, G. V., R. R. KIERLAND, and J. M. OPITZ: Angiokeratoma corporis diffusum (Fabry's disease). Arch. Derm. Syph. (Berl.) 91, 206 (1965).

GROOT, W. P., DE: Thesaurismosis hereditaria Ruiter-Pompen-Wyers (Angiokeratoma corporis diffusum Fabry). Thesis, Amsterdam 1961.

— Angiokeratoma corporis diffusum Fabry (Thesaurismosis hereditaria Ruiter-Pompen-Wyers). Dermatologica (Basel) 128, 321 (1964).

GÜNTHER, H.: Anhidrosis und Diabetes insipidus. Z. klin. Med. 78, 53 (1913).

HARTLEY, M. W., and R. E. MILLER: Renal and vascular changes in Fabry's disease, a dysphospholipidosis. J. Cell. Biol. 19, 31 A (1963).

HASHIMOTO, K., B. G. GROSS, and W. F. LEVER: Angiokeratoma corporis diffusum (Fabry). Histochemical and electron microscopic studies of the skin. J. invest. Derm. 44, 119 (1965).

HENRY, E. W., and C. R. RALLY: The renal lesion in angiokeratoma corporis diffusum (Fabry's disease). Canad. med. Ass. J. 89, 206 (1963).

HOFMANN, A., u. W. HAUSER: Angiokeratoma corporis diffusum Fabry mit cerebralen Manifestationen. Dtsch. Z. Nervenhlk. 183, 351 (1962).

HORNBOSTEL, H.: Das Angiokeratoma corporis diffusum universale mit Cardio-vaso-renalem Symptomenkomplex als neuartige Thesaurismoseform. Helv. med. Acta 19, 388 (1952).

— u. K. SCRIBA: Zur Diagnostik des Angiokeratoma Fabry mit kardio-vasorenalem Symptomenkomplex als Phosphatidspeicherungskrankheit durch Probeexcision der Haut. Klin. Wschr. 31, 68 (1953).

— W. SPIER u. H. KOCH: Angiokeratoma corporis diffusum universale (Fabry) mit kardiovaso-renalem Symptomenkomplex als Allgemeinerkrankung. Ärztl. Wschr. 6, 49 (1951).

— — — u. K. SCRIBA: Angiokeratoma corporis diffusum Fabry mit cardio-vaso-renalem Symptomenkomplex als Allgemeinerkrankung auf dem Boden einer Thesaurismose. Hautarzt 1, 183 (1950).

JERVIS, G., R. C. HARRIS, and J. H. MENKES: Cerebral lipidosis of unclear nature. In: Cerebral Sphingolipidoses, p. 101. Eds.: S. M. Aronson and B. W. Volk. New York: Academic Press 1962.

KALKOFF, K. W.: Personal communication 1966.

KARR, W. J.: Fabry's disease (angiokeratoma corporis diffusum universale). Amer. J. Med. 27, 829 (1959).

KLIONSKY, B., C. C. SWEELEY, F. D. BEYER, and R. FONT: Fabry's disease — glycolipid lipidosis: morphologic, chemical and histochemical observations from an autopsy. In preparation. Cited after SWEELEY and KLIONSKY (1966) [ref. 40].

KÜHNAU, J.: Personal communication to SCRIBA 1950, and RUITER 1958.

KUSKE, H., u. P. BAUMGARTNER: Demonstration. Dermatologica (Basel) 124, 298 (1962).

LAPIÈRE, S.: Angiokeratoma corporis diffusum (Fabry). (Syndrome cardio-vaso-rénale de Ruiter-Pompen.) Dermatologica (Basel) 115, 572 (1957).

LEDER, A. A., and W. C. BOSWORTH: Angiokeratoma corporis diffusum universale (Fabry's disease) with mitral stenosis. Amer. J. Med. 38, 814 (1965).

LEVER, W. F.: Angiokeratoma corporis diffusum. In: Handb. d. Haut- u. Geschlechtskrkh., Bd. III/1, p. 133. Ed.: H. A. Gottron. Berlin-Göttingen-Heidelberg: Springer 1963.

MARTI, H. R.: Refer to DUBACH and GLOOR 1966.

MÅRTENSSON, E.: On the neutral glycolipids of human kidney. Acta chim. scand. 17, 2356 (1963).

— A. PERCY, and L. SVENNERHOLM: Kidney glycolipids in late infantile metachromatic leucodystrophy. Acta paediat. scand. 55, 1 (1966).

MIBELLI, V.: Di una nuova forma di cheratosi „Angiocheratoma". G. ital. Mal. vener. 30, 285 (1889), cited after WISE et al. (1962).

NETHERTON, E. W.: A case for diagnosis (demonstration). Arch. Derm. (Chicago) 29, 965 (1934).

OPITZ, J. M., F. C. STILES, D. WISE, R. R. RACE, R. SANGER, G. R. V. GEMMINGEN, R. R. KIERLAND, E. G. CROSS, and W. P. DE GROOT: The genetics of angiokeratoma corporis diffusum (Fabry's disease) and its linkage relations with the Xg locus. Amer. J. hum. Genet. 17, 325 (1965).

PARKINSON, J. E., and A. SUNSHINE: Angiokeratoma corporis diffusum universale (Fabry). Presenting as suspected myocardial infarction and pulmonary infarcts. Am. J. Med. 31, 951 (1961).

PITTELKOW, R. B., R. R. KIERLAND, and H. MONTGOMERY: Angiokeratoma corporis diffusum. Arch. Derm. 72, 556 (1955).

— — — Polariscopic and histochemical studies in angiokeratoma corporis diffusum. Arch. Derm. 76, 59 (1957).

Pompen, A. W. M., M. Ruiter, and H. J. G. Wyers: Angiokeratoma corporis diffusum (universale) Fabry, as a sign of an unknown internal disease; two autopsy reports. Acta med. scand. 128, 234 (1947).
Price, J. H.: Angiokeratoma corporis diffusum. Brit. J. Derm. 64, 105 (1955).
Rahman, A. N.: The ocular manifestations of hereditary dystopic lipidosis. Arch. Ophthal. 69, 708 (1963).
— and R. Lindenberg: The neuropathology of hereditary dystopic lipidosis. Arch. Neurol. (Chic.) 9, 373 (1963).
— F. A. Simeone, D. B. Hackel, P. W. Hall III, E. Z. Hirsch, and J. W. Harris: Angiokeratoma corporis diffusum universale (hereditary dystopic lipidosis). Trans. Ass. Amer. Phycns 74, 366 (1961).
Rosenberg, A.: The sphingolipids from the spleen of a case of lipidosis. In: Cerebral Sphingolipidoses, p. 119. Eds.: S. M. Aronson and B. W. Volk. New York: Academic Press 1962.
Ruiter, M.: Angiokeratoma corporis diffusum (universale) Fabry als Symptom einer Phosphatidspeicherungskrankheit. Hautarzt 3, 557 (1952).
— Histological investigation of the skin in angiokeratoma corporis diffusum in particular with regard to the associated disturbance of phosphatide metabolism. Dermatologica (Basel) 109, 273 (1954).
— Some further observations on angiokeratoma corporis diffusum. Brit. J. Derm. 69, 137 (1957).
— Das Angiokeratoma corporis diffusum — Syndrom und seine Hauterscheinungen. Übersicht und eigene Erfahrungen der letzten zehn Jahre. Hautarzt 9, 15 (1958).
— u. A. W. M. Pompen: Angiokeratoma corporis diffusum universale mit cardio-vaso-renalem Symptomenkomplex bei drei Brüdern. Arch. Derm. Suppl. 179, 165 (1939).
— — u. H. J. G. Wyers: Über interne und pathologisch-anatomische Befunde bei Angiokeratoma corporis diffusum (Fabry). Dermatologica (Basel) 94, 1 (1947).
Scriba, K.: Zur Pathogenese des Angiokeratoma corporis diffusum Fabry mit cardio-vaso-renalem Symptomenkomplex. Verh. dtsch. Ges. Path. 34, 221 (1950).
Sibley, W. K.: Case for diagnosis. Proc. roy. Soc. Med. 2, 70 (1918).
— Case for diagnosis (demonstration). Brit. J. Derm. 30, 109 (1918).
Siguer, F., B. Duperrat, C. Bétourné et A. Hanaut: Angiokératose de Fabry, expression cutaneé d'une maladie générale nouvellement individualisée. Bull. Soc. méd. Hôp. Paris 72, 291 (1956).
Spaeth, G. L., and P. Frost: Fabry's disease. Its ocular manifestations. Arch. Ophthalm. 74, 760 (1965).
Steiner, L., u. H. Voerner: Angiomatosis miliaris, eine idiopathische Gefäßerkrankung. Dtsch. Arch. klin. Med. 96, 105 (1909).
Stoughton, R. B., and W. E. Clendenning: Angiokeratoma corporis diffusum (Fabry). Arch. Derm. 79, 601 (1959).
Stümpke, G.: Ein Fall von Angiokeratoma corporis diffusum. Arch. Derm. Syph. (Berl.) Suppl. 121, 291 (1916).
Svennerholm, E., and L. Svennerholm: Neutral glycolipids of human blood serum, spleen and liver. Nature (Lond.) 198, 688 (1963).
Sweeley, C. C., and B. Klionsky: Fabry's disease: Classification as a sphingolipidosis and partial characterization of a novel glycolipid. J. biol. Chem. 238, 3148 (1963).
— — Fabry's disease; the isolation and characterization of a ceramide trihexoside from kidney. Abstracts 6th Internat. Congr. Biochem. New York 1964.
— — Glycolipid lipidosis: Fabry's disease. In: The metabolic basis of inherited disease, p. 618. Eds.: J. B. Stanbury, J. B. Wyngaarden, and D. S. Fredrickson. New York: McGraw-Hill Book Co. 1966.
Vineyard, W. R., and E. J. Kamin: Angiokeratoma corporis diffusum. Arch. Derm. 82, 817 (1960).
Vorster, K.: Fabry-Syndrom. Münch. med. Wschr. 106, 1402 (1964).
Wachtel, H. L., and I. R. Mattei: Angiokeratoma corporis diffusum universale. Arch. intern. Med. 114, 805 (1964).
Wallace, H. J.: Angiokeratoma corporis diffusum. Bull. Soc. franç. Derm. Syph. Suppl. 65, 348 (1958).
— Angiokeratoma corporis diffusum. Brit. J. Derm. 70, 354 (1958).
Wallace, R. D., and W. J. Cooper: Angiokeratoma corporis diffusum universale (Fabry). Amer. J. Med. 39, 656 (1965).
Weicksel, J.: Angiomatosis, bzw. Angiokeratosis universalis (eine sehr seltene Haut- und Gefäßkrankheit). Dtsch. med. Wschr. 51, 898 (1925).
Wertheim, L.: Hämangiome. In: Handb. d. Haut- und Geschlechtskrankheiten, Bd. 12/2, S. 423. Herausgeber: J. Jadassohn. Berlin: Springer 1932.

WISE, D.: Diffuse angiokeratoma. Thesis. University of Cambridge, 1960.
— Diffuse Angiokeratoma (J. Fabry). In: Jadassohn's Hdb. d. Haut- und Geschlechtskrankh., Bd. 7, S. 743. Berlin: Springer 1966.
— H. J. WALLACE, and E. H. JELLINEK: Angiokeratoma corporis diffusum. A clinical study of eight affected families. Quart. J. Med. 31, 177 (1962).
WÖHNLICH, H.: Zur Symptomatologie multipler Angiome. Arch. Derm. Syph. (Berl.) 187, 528 (1949).
YAMAKAWA, T., R. IRIE, and M. IWANGA: The chemistry of lipid of posthemolytic residue or stroma of erythrocytes. IX. Silicic acid chromatography of mammalian stroma glycolipids. J. Biochem. (Tokyo) 48, 490 (1960).
— S. YOKOYAMA, and N. HANDA: Chemistry of lipids of posthemolytic residue or stroma of erythrocytes. XI. Structure of globoside, the main mucolipid of human erythrocytes. J. Biochem. (Tokyo) 53, 28 (1963).
YU, K.-Y.: Angiokeratoma corporis diffusum universale (Fabry). Report of a case with lipoiduria. Chin. med. J. 74, 478 (1956).

Heredopathia Atactica Polyneuritiformis (Refsum's Disease)

By

W. Kahlke*

Definition and Introduction

The first description of heredopathia atactica polyneuritiformis (HAP) was given 20 years ago by the Norwegian neurologist SIGVALD REFSUM. Main clinical features of this hereditary disorder are symptoms and signs of chronic polyneuropathy with progressive pareses of the distal parts of the extremities and distal muscular atrophy, and cerebellar involvement with ataxia and nystagmus. Deep tendon reflexes are absent. The cerebrospinal fluid protein is always considerably increased while the cell count is normal (albuminocytologic dissociation). Other clinical signs include atypical or (less frequently) typical pigmentary retinitis with night blindness and concentric narrowing of the visual fields, skeletal malformations which are usually symmetrical in approximately 75% of cases, and cardiac involvement which may give rise to various electrocardiographic abnormalities. Further facultative symptoms consist of impairment of hearing and sense of smell, skin changes resembling ichthyosis and other non-characteristic changes.

The typical laboratory findings in HAP concern the occurrence in plasma and organ lipids of large amounts of an atypical fatty acid, namely 3,7,11,15-tetramethylhexadecanoic acid (phytanic acid) which may amount to 20% of total plasma fatty acids.

On the basis of neurological findings HAP was considered to belong to the group of heredoataxic disorders; and there are similarities to progressive neural amyotrophy. The finding of lipid storage, which seems to be related to the causal defect, forms the basis for consideration of the disorder as a lipidosis.

Historical Review

First studies of the disease were performed between 1937 and 1943 by REFSUM among the members of two Norwegian kindreds (REFSUM 1944, 1945, 1946a, b). The almost simultaneous manifestations of the disease in five subjects between the ages of 25 and 41 years permitted recognition of the typical symptomatology which is described by the term "heredoataxia hemeralopica polyneuritiformis" (REFSUM 1945, 1946a) and less concisely by the later version "heredopathia atactica polyneuritiformis" (1946b).

In 1939, THIÉBAUT et al. had already described a case with a similar symptomatology. In a later report (1961) they suggested the diagnosis of HAP which was subsequently confirmed by chemical analyses (KAHLKE 1964a).

In 1944, DEREUX observed the case of a 41 year-old patient with "affection familiale caractérisée par une rétinite pigmentaire avec héméralopie associée à des accidents de type polynévritique avec ataxie évoluant par poussées" thus recog-

* Supported in parts by funds from Deutsche Forschungsgemeinschaft.

nizing the typical features of the syndrome which he later (1961) classified as HAP. This case, too, was confirmed biochemically (KAHLKE 1964 a).

Soon after Refsum's reports several authors published cases which were diagnosed clinically as HAP. SALOMONSEN and SKATVEDT (1949) described four children from three Norwegian families, including twins, all of whom manifested the disease between the fourth and seventh year of life. At the time of examination, deafness was present in all four. One of the patients died at the age of nine years and findings at autopsy (CAMMERMEYER 1946, CAMMERMEYER et al. 1954) were in agreement with those in the first patient with HAP and his sister (REFSUM 1946). In another of the four children acutely progressing ataxia led to almost complete paralysis, which was later followed by a remission, as also seen in other patients.

The tenth case has been described by REESE and BARETA (1950) in the U.S.A. Their 25 year-old patient was described under the heading of HAP, but was placed clinically into the group of progressive interstitial polyneuropathies. It was differentiated from the heredoataxias.

Already in 1946, CAMMERMEYER had pointed out lipid deposition in swollen nerve cells and areas of demyelination with the formation of fatty macrophages. These findings were subsequently confirmed (CAMMERMEYER 1956). There were also significant amounts of fat in liver and kidneys of Refsum's first case (CAMMERMEYER et al. 1954). On the basis of CAMMERMEYER's findings, SALOMONSEN and SKATVEDT (1949) considered HAP a lipidosis and discussed its relation to amaurotic family idiocy and to Niemann-Pick disease. In contrast to the former, Schaffer's ganglion cell process which according to GLOBUS (1923, 1942) is typical for amaurotic family idiocy (REESE and BARETA 1950) is absent in HAP.

The next case reports came from England (CLARK 1951) and from Sweden (KJELLSON 1953, two patients). Although autopsy findings in one of the latter (GELLERSTEDT 1953) were in agreement with those of the earlier cases, the disorder was not considered a lipidosis but was classified as heredofamilial ataxia.

GELLERSTEDT proposed, as did REFSUM in a later publication (1957), that the original designation "heredoataxia hemeralopica polyneuritiformis" would best fit the symptomatology.

Subsequent reports include cases which differ slightly from the typical description of HAP or which show additional complications. OLESEN (1957) did not find night blindness or retinitis in his 40 year-old patient, but saw paralysis of conjugate eye movements and chorioiditis-like changes. There was little evidence of polyneuritis or of a disturbance of cerebellar function. In the subject described by HEYCOCK and WILSON (1958) there were diabetes mellitus and slightly different ophthalmologic findings as compared to those seen typically in HAP. FLEMING (1957) described subjects in some affected families who did not have the disease, but showed psychiatric abnormalities and mental retardation. One of four unaffected siblings of a HAP-family (DEREUX 1961) had impairment of vision and hearing, another one was mongoloid and died at the age of ten years. Night blindness was found in two out of five siblings of the mother and in a number of their children.

Three siblings with HAP were described by ASHENHURST et al. (1958) and three by EDSTRÖM et al. (1959); two affected siblings and an additional patient were reported by GORDON and HUDSON (1959). TOUSSAINT et al. (1959) reviewed 20 cases of HAP and performed a nerve biopsy in one patient. They suggested a possible relationship of the disease with the neural heredodegenerative amyotrophies. Further case reports were those of VELTEMA and VERJAAL (1961), RAVIN and SCHWARTZ (1962), PECKER et al. (1963), BLANC et al. (1963) and NORDHAGEN and GRÖNDAHL (1964).

Support for the assumption of a disturbance of lipid metabolism (CAMMER-MEYER 1946, 1956, SALOMONSEN and SKATVEDT 1949) came from studies in an affected child of seven years, who had a fatty liver proved by biopsy in addition to lipuria (RICHTERICH et al. 1963, 1965). Studies on urinary and liver lipids of this patient, with the use of gas-liquid chromatography, showed the occurrence in both lipid extracts of an unusual fatty acid which made up a major portion of the total fatty acids. This finding was confirmed by analyses of liver-, muscle-, kidney- and brain lipids of the same case. Isolation and identification of the fatty acid showed it to be a branched chain fatty acid with 20 carbon atoms (3,7,11,15-tetra-methylhexadecanoic acid, phytanic acid, KLENK and KAHLKE 1963). At this time the first cases (two siblings) of HAP were diagnosed in Germany (HARDERS and DIECKMANN 1964) and phytanic acid was found in significant quantities in the serum (KAHLKE 1963). As can be seen in table 1, phytanic acid could subsequently be demonstrated in six serum samples from patients who had been described earlier (KAHLKE 1964) and was also repeatedly found in plasma and tissues of one of Refsum's original cases (T. E.), (KAHLKE 1964a, KAHLKE and RICHTERICH 1965).

Recently the finding of phytanic acid in HAP was confirmed by TRY et al. (1965) in two additional patients.

The similarity between HAP and more common neurologic disorders (Friedreich's ataxia, Déjérine-Sottas disease etc., GREENFIELD 1958) suggest that among such patients a number of unrecognized cases of HAP may be found. On the other hand, atypical cases have been reported as HAP (OLESEN 1957, RAVIN and SCHWARTZ 1962) which could be classified with certainty only by chemical analyses.

Incidence (Age, Sex, Race)

The disease may become manifest at any time from childhood to adult life. The youngest patients with the complete symptomatology were four years old (REFSUM et al. 1949, SALOMONSEN and SKATVEDT 1949, RICHTERICH et al. 1963), the oldest ones over 40 (REFSUM 1946, GORDON and HUDSON 1959, DEREUX 1961, 1963). When less typical symptoms are looked for, such as progressive loss of vision, the disease onset may be noticed several years earlier than might otherwise be the case. Sometimes the progression of symptoms may be noted by the sufferer, as in the case of GORDON and HUDSON (1959), where the patient, a mariner, registered his own progressive concentric narrowing of visual fields.

Course and severity of the disease do not seem to depend on the time of its clinical onset. Remissions and deaths have been described for each age group (see table 2).

Of the 44 cases of HAP 24 are males and 20 are females. A sexual prevalence cannot be derived therefrom, particularly since the numbers become equal when two male patients with a somewhat confusing clinical picture are omitted from the series. On the other hand, a systematic study on sex distribution would have to include subjects who remain asymptomatic for many years and possibly throughout their lives, as was the case in the mother of the patients described by THIÉBAUT (1961). Clinical manifestations were the same in male and female patients.

As in any inborn error of metabolism the prevalence among different races is of interest. Of the 41 known patients with HAP four were Jews (REESE and BARETA 1950, GORDON and HUDSON 1959, case III, THIÉBAUT 1939, 1961, RAVIN and SCHWARTZ 1962), and possibly all originate in Scandinavia (RICHTERICH et al. 1965). In 13 affected families consanguinity of the parents, and in 4 kindreds consanguinity

of grandparents was noted. In one kindred there was consanguinity in two generations (for details see chapter on genetics by FUHRMANN).

In some kindreds with HAP, siblings of patients with the full-blown disease
show only a few of the typical symptoms (FLEMING 1957, GORDON and HUDSON
1959, DEREUX 1961, 1963, VELTEMA and VERJAAL 1961). Mentally abnormal
siblings were found in other kindreds (FLEMING 1957, OLESEN 1957). Finally,
siblings of affected subjects may show signs and symptoms at the first examination, which are only suggestive of the disease, and later also develop the complete
symptomatology of HAP. Some maternal cousins of such subjects were found to
have night blindness (DEREUX 1963, 1965).

The literature contains a number of cases where the symptomatology did not completely fit the picture of HAP. Some of these have been presented as HAP, others
have not. Such case reports will be discussed briefly in the chapter on diagnosis.

Clinical Manifestations

When the patient goes to see the physician for the first time, his complaints are
usually compatible with those of polyneuritis. There may be an unstable gait with
weakness of the lower extremities and with consecutive involvement of other parts
of the body. Sensory disturbances include paresthesias which may be initially
associated with severe pain in the knees, the legs or the whole body. Within a few
weeks pareses of all four extremities may develop, resulting in almost complete
inability to move.

Upon questioning, the patient may complain of night blindness dating back
for many years, and of symptoms compatible with constriction of the visual fields.
Frequently a "cold" or "flu" is reported to have preceded the appearance of the
specific symptomatology (HEYCOCK and WILSON 1958, ASHENHURST et al. 1958,
EDSTRÖM et al. 1959), or recurrences of the disease. It is not known whether this
represents a chance observation, whether stress may trigger the development of
clinical polyneuritis, or whether the infection is secondary to HAP on the basis
of an increased susceptibility as observed in other heredodegenerative disorders
(REFSUM 1946). In a patient of DEREUX (1963) first symptoms of HAP appeared
immediately following a gynecologic operation.

Occasionally, non-characteristic symptoms such as loss of appetite, nausea,
vomiting or diffuse abdominal pain may appear initially (SALOMONSEN and
SKATVEDT 1949, PECKER et al. 1963).

A typical feature of HAP is the consistency of its symptomatology. In over
40 cases (see table 2) signs and symptoms were very similar to those in the first
five patients of REFSUM (1946).

Neurologic Disturbances

Involvement of the *motor system* leads to pareses, predominantly of the lower
extremities and usually symmetrical; the distal distribution is indicative of a
polyneuritic type of lesion. As a result, the musculature of calves, feet, lower arms
and hands shows hypotonicity and/or atrophy, which, if not apparent initially,
develops during the course of the disease. Its morphologic substrate can be
demonstrated in biopsy specimens. Occasionally, muscular fasciculations are seen
or felt, involving for instance the small muscles of the hands. Motor involvement
may be so severe as to result in tetraplegia.

Sensory disturbances are frequent, but their pattern is less uniform. Superficial sensation may be unimpaired or may show a variety of alterations, ranging from slight
differences in the sensation of touch and temperature to painful paresthesias.

Table 1. *Clinical data of*

No.	Author(s)	Case	Year born	Sex (m = male, f = female)	Cousanguinity	Ataxia	Superficial sensory disturbance	Impairment or loss of tendon reflexes	Muscle atrophy	Increased cerebrospinal fluid protein	Retinitis pigmentosa	Night blindness	Constriction of visual fields	Cataract	Nystagmus
1	REFSUM (1945/46)	H.B.	1896	m	+	+	+	+	+	+		+	+		+
2	REFSUM (1945/46) sibs	G.B.	1908	f	+	+	(+)	+	+			+	+		+
3	REFSUM (1945/46)	T.A.	1920	m		+	—	+	+	+	+	+	+		+
4	REFSUM (1945/46) sibs	G.N.	1903	f		+	+	+	+	+	+	+	+		+
5	REFSUM (1945/46)	R.K.	1906	f		+		+	+		+	+	+		
6	REFSUM et al. (1949) twins	I	1938	f	+	(+)	—	+	+		+	(+)	—		
7	REFSUM et al. (1949)	II	1938	m	+	(+)	—	+	+		+	(+)	—		
8	REFSUM et al. (1949)	III	1939	m	—	(+)	—	+	+		+	(+)	—		
9	REFSUM et al. (1949)	IV	1939	f	+	+	—	+	+		+	—			
10	REESE and BARETA (1950)	B.A.	1910*	m	+	+	—	+	+	+	+	+	+		(+)
11	CLARK (1951); FLEMING (1957) sibs	N.C.	1924*	m	+	+	+	+	+	+	+	+	+		(+)
12	FLEMING (1957)	M.P.	1928*	f	+	+	+	+	+	+		+	+		
13	KJELLSON (1953) sibs	I	1922*	m	+	+	+	+	+	+	+	+	+		
14	KJELLSON (1953)	II	1921*	f	+	+	(+)	+	+		+	+	+		
15	OLESEN (1957)		1916*	m	—	—	—	—		+	—	—	—		(+)
16	BILLINGS et al. (1957)		1935	m		+	+	+	+	+	+	+	+	+	
17	HEYCOCK and WILSON (1958)		1948	f	—	+	(+)	+	+	+	+	(+)			(+)
18	ASHENHURST et al. (1958)	I	1932*	m	—	(+)	(+)		+	(+)	+	+	+		+
19	ASHENHURST et al. (1958) sibs	II	1934*	f	—	—	+	+	(+)	+	—	+	+		
20	ASHENHURST et al. (1958)	III	1937*	f	—	—	—	(+)	—	+		+			
21	TOUSSAINT et al. (1959)	L.D.	1925*	f	—		+	+	(+)	+	+	+		+	
22	EDSTRÖM et al. (1959)	i.M.S.	1919	f	—	+	—	+	+	+		+	+		
23	EDSTRÖM et al. (1959) sibs	A.E.B.	1909	m	—	+	—	+	(+)	+	+	+	+		
27	EDSTRÖM et al. (1959)	A.L.B.	1916	f	—	+	(+)	+	+	+		+	+		
25	GORDON and HUDSON (1959) sibs	G.O.	1912*	m	—	(+)	+	+	+	+		+	+		
26	GORDON and HUDSON (1959)	F.O.	1921*	m	—	(+)	+	+	+	+					
27	GORDON and HUDSON (1959)	H.S.	1907*	m	+	+	+	+	+	+		+			
28	THIÉBAUT et al. (1939/61)	E.H.	1911	m	+		+	+	+	+	+	+	+	+	
29	DEREUX (1961) sibs	E.L.		m	+						+	+			
30	DEREUX (1961)	S.G.		f	+						+				
31	VELTEMA and VERJAAL (1961)	H.v.d.K.	1923	m	+	+	+	+	+	+	+		+	+	—
32	RAVIN and SCHWARTZ (1962)			m	—	+	—	(+)		+	+	—		+	+
33	PECKER et al. (1963); PETIT (1963)	M.C.	1930	f	+	+		+	+	+	+	+			
34	RICHTERICH et al. (1963)	R.B.	1954	f	—	+		+	+	+	+	+		+	
35	BLANC et al. (1963)			m	+	(+)	+	+	+	+					
36	HARDERS and DIECKMANN (1964) sibs	W.M.	1942	m	—	+	(+)	(+)	—	+	+	+	+		
37	HARDERS and DIECKMANN (1964)	E.H.	1938	f	—		—	(+)		+	+	+	+	+	
38	REFSUM (1965/66)	T.E.	1920	f	+	(+)	(+)	+	+	+	+	+	+	—	—
39	NORDHAGEN and GRØNDAHL (1964)	N.B.	1952*	m	+	+		+	+	+	+	+			
40	ALEXANDER (1966)	E.M.W.	1929*	m		+	+	+	+						+
41	PRIOR and BERGIN (1966)	J.M.	1912	f	—	+	+	+	+	+		—		+	—	+
42	DEREUX (1965)	G.L.		m											
43	SABOURAUD (1965/66)	J.M.	1948*	m	—		+	+							
44	KEHLER (1966)	I.V.	1924	f	—	+	+	+	+	+		+	+	+	+

* The occurrence of phytanic acid could be demonstrated in cases 21, 28, 29, 30, 33, 34, 36, 37, 38, 42, 43 and 44 (KAHLKE 1963—1966).

• Estimated from age of subject at time of report.

Anosmia	Deafness	Skin changes	Skeletal deformities	Cardiac involvement	Mental retardation	Remissions	Symptoms in family members	Initial signs or symptoms	Additional signs or symptoms	Kind or cause of death	Autopsy (A.), Nerve biopsy (N. B.), Muscle biopsy (M. B.)
	+		+	+				Auditory disturbance, instability of gait		Respiratory paralysis	A. (Brain)
+		+	+	+						Respiratory paralysis	A. (Brain)
			+	(+)				Impairment of vision	Psychosis symptomatica		A.
+	+	+		+						Sudden death	
	+	+			—			Loss of appetite, instability of gait		Cachexia	A.
(+)	+				—	+		Dry skin			
(+)	+				—	+		Impairment of hearing			
	+	+			(+)	+		Deafness since age 5			
+	+	—	+	—	—			Night blindness		Dyspnoe, cardiovascular collaps	M. B., A. N. B.
(+)		+	—					Pain in knees			
	+	+		+	—		+	Instability of gait	Psychosis, appendectomy		A.
	+										
+	+	—	+	(+)	—			Instability of gait (first noticed during pregnancy)	Mild hypertension, slight urinary incontinence	Cardiovascular collaps	
	(+)		—		+			Limitation of ocular movements	Congenital ptosis		
	+	+	+	+	—			Impairment of vision			
	+	—	—	+			—	Anorexia, ptosis (Diabetes)	Diabetes; weakness of external rectus movement		
+	(+)	+	—				+	"Flu"-like infection Influenca, severe			
	+	+	(+)					root pain	Aminoaciduria	Collaps, sudden death	
		+	+								
—	+	+	+	+				Instability of gait, severe pains			M. B.
+	+	+	(+)	+	—	+	—	Pain and weakness in the legs			N. B.
+	+	+		+			—	Respiratory tract infection	Congenital polycystic kidney	Respiratory failure	A.
+	+	+	+			—		Common cold			
					+		+	+	Impairment of vision	Absence of spermatozoa, atrophy of testes	Sudden death in spite of adequate pulmonary ventilation	N. B., M. B., A.
	+	—	+	+	(—)		+	Weakness of eye muscles	Blindness, atrophy of testes		
	+	+	+				+	Night blindness, impairment of vision	Difficulties in swallowing	Sudden death (tracheotomy)	
	+		+		—			Imbalance, night blindness	Glaucoma (operated)		
			+	—			+		Gynecological operation		
—	+		—		+	+		Imbalance			N. B.
	+			+					Ptosis, ophthalmoplegia externa, tinnitus		
—	+	+		—	+	—		Vomiting, anorexia diffuse abdominal pains			N. B., M. B.
—	+		+	+	+			Paresis of all extremities	Hepatomegaly, lipiduria	Sudden death	A.
+									Loss of hair		N. B.
—	—	+	+					Night blindness since childhood, muscle weakness	Polycytemia		M. B.
—	+	—	—					Night blindness since childhood			
(+)	+	+	+	+	(+)	+		Night blindness	Paranoid psychosis		M. B.
	+	+	+		(+)		(+)	Instability of gait			
+	+				+						A.
+	+	+	—	(+)	—	—		Weakness in lower limbs	Opacity of both corneae		N. B.
+	+	+	—		+	—	—	Polyneuritis in lower limbs			

** We would like to thank Dr. I. PRIOR, Wellington, New Zealand, for information regarding the clinical data of his patient.

Deep sensation is impaired in most cases, particularly the position and vibratory sense of the distal parts of the extremities. Sometimes muscle pain appears with motion.

Of the signs referable to the *cerebellum*, ataxia is consistently found in HAP. Although initially it may be mild, it is always progressive and much more marked than that observed in polyneuritis from other causes. In some cases the gait is so markedly ataxic as to significantly impair balance. In association with pareses, ataxia contributes to loss of ability to move about without assistance. Other cerebellar signs such as adiadochokinesis, tremor, abnormal finger-to-nose test, positive Romberg sign and nystagmus occur singly or together, mainly in later stages of the disease.

Involvement of *cranial nerves* consistently includes the optic nerve (see page 365), and in most cases the cochlear and olfactory nerves. Progressive loss of hearing is heralded by loss of perception of high sounds and may be an initial symptom as mentioned earlier. Although involvement is bilateral, the lesion may be more marked on one side. Even in children it may lead to complete deafness rather rapidly. Vestibular nerve function is unimpaired. Olfactory involvement is less frequent and occurs in about 75% of cases (RICHTERICH et al. 1965 a).

Progressive diminution and finally absence of deep *tendon reflexes* is an obligatory sign; reflexes do not disappear simultaneously and some may still be present while others are lost. Subsequently, abdominal reflexes may be found decreased or absent, although the loss of other superficial reflexes is rare. In some cases superficial nerves appear thickened on palpation, in agreement with findings at biopsy or autopsy.

In general, there are no other signs of involvement of either the pyramidal or extrapyramidal system. Seizures as well as mental retardation have not been reported and the electroencephalogram is normal.

Ophthalmologic Disturbances

There are obligatory and facultative ophthalmologic symptoms in HAP. Night blindness develops in all patients, although its recognition in children may be difficult. Its absence in patients reported by OLESEN (1957) and by RAVIN and SCHWARTZ (1962) argues against the correctness of the diagnosis in these cases.

Another consistent symptom in adults is progressive, concentric narrowing of the visual fields. In children, it may not be found initially, but develops during the course of the disorder. Finally, a telescopic field of vision remains (REFSUM 1946) with central vision being only slightly impaired or not at all.

Involvement of the retina is a classic finding in HAP (FRANCESCHETTI et al. 1963). Although it may not be seen in children, and may be of only minor degree, even in some older patients pigmentary retinitis, usually of the atypical kind, always develops eventually. In some cases the presence of cataracts prevented proper examination. Differences reported by different authors are partly due to the lack of a standardized nomenclature. The appearance of the vasculature and macula and the electroretinogram fit the generally accepted criteria for retinitis pigmentosa (see figure 1).

In addition to cataracts, miosis and asymmetric pupils with abnormal reaction to light have been described. Nystagmus may be present, as mentioned earlier. Ptosis and/or ophthalmoplegia externa were described only in questionable cases of HAP (OLESEN 1957, HEYCOCK et al. 1958, RAVIN and SCHWARTZ 1962) and do not seem to be typical features of the disease.

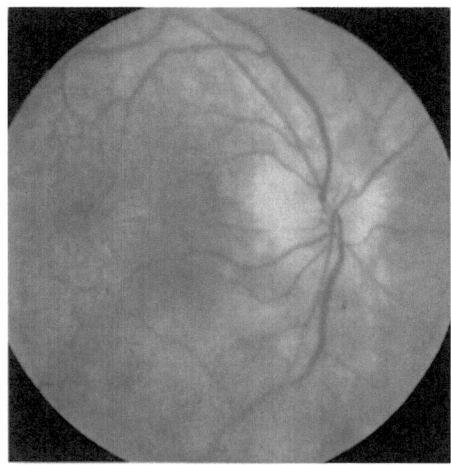 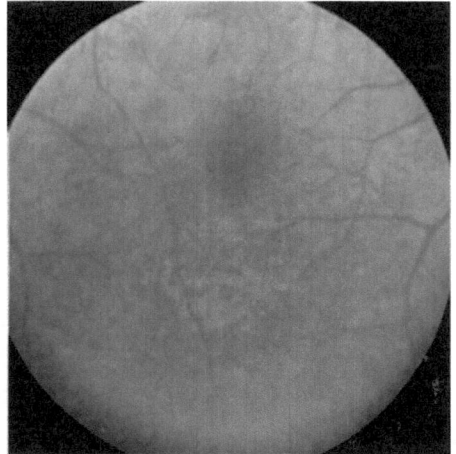

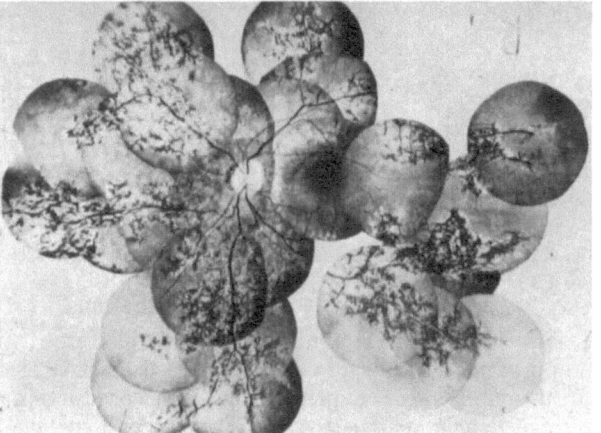

Fig. 1a—c. Fundus photographs in HAP. Fine-granular depigmentation of the macular area. The optic disc is pale and its margin blurred. The retinal vessels are narrowed. (Reproduced by courtesy of Dr. H. Dieckmann, Hamburg)

Cardiac Disturbances

Cardiac involvement was present in most patients and is certainly related to the underlying disease. Although the signs and symptoms referable to the heart vary in different subjects, angina pectoris and congestive failure occur rarely, while tachycardias and arrhythmias are frequent. Enlargement of the heart and non-specific systolic murmurs have been described.

Electrocardiographic changes occur consistently and consist of conduction disturbances and signs compatible with lesions of the myocardium. Sudden deaths have been reported repeatedly and may have been of cardiac origin, even though significant morphologic findings were absent.

Skin Changes

Skin changes occur in all patients with HAP and usually resemble ichthyosis (see figure 2). The findings may vary in degree from dry skin to severe scaling. In general, the skin of infants which reacts more intensely, shows the most marked changes, while skin involvement in adults is usually less severe, and shows regression during the course of remissions.

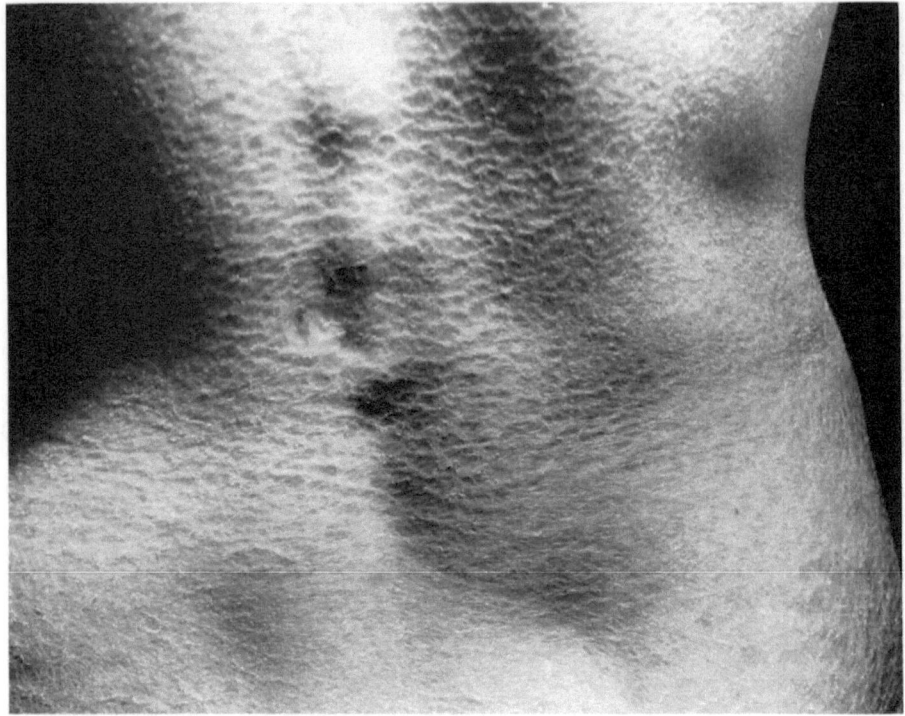

Fig. 2. Ichthyosis-like skin changes in HAP. (Reproduced by courtesy of Dr. H. DIECKMANN, Hamburg)

Malformations

Associated skeletal abnormalities are bilateral in most cases and were found in approximately 75% of all reported cases of HAP. Shortening of the fourth metatarsal bone is most frequent, usually in conjunction with malformations of toes or fingers, such as hypertrophy of the second toe, claw hand formation, and elongation or shortening of other metatarsal bones.

In addition, postural abnormalities are observed resulting from spondylitis deformans of the thoracic or cervical spine, with kyphosis and kyphoscoliosis. Other patients exhibit pes cavus deformities, hallux valgus, or hammer toes.

X-ray examination in one of Refsum's families showed symmetrical epiphyseal dyplasias of various joints; similar findings were described in other patients with HAP. Bone erosion and degenerative changes of the cartilages may also occur symmetrically. Deformities of the articular surfaces of femur and tibia, flattening of the condyles and reactive bone changes were described by HARDERS and DIECKMANN (1964) in a male patient (see figure 3).

Other Findings

In addition to obligatory and facultative signs and symptoms, occasionally other findings were reported, the relationship of which to the underlying disease remains to be clarified. These include hepatosplenomegaly, testicular atrophy (with azoospermia in one case) and irregularities of the menstrual cycle. Since affected females as well as affected males had children, impairment of fertility is not a consistent feature of HAP. Unrelated findings may be aminoaciduria (ASHENHURST et al. 1958) and polycystic kidneys (EDSTRÖM et al. 1959), while lipuria (RICHTERICH et al. 1963) may be explained by damage to the renal tubular epithelium from storage of lipids. Polycythemia was described by HARDERS and DIECKMANN (1964) in the male of their siblings. There does not seem to be an increased incidence of diabetes mellitus in HAP.

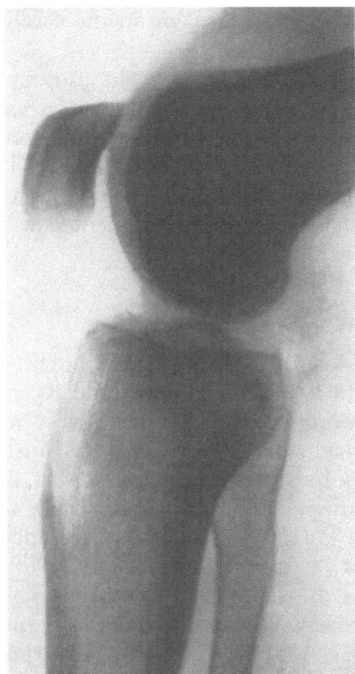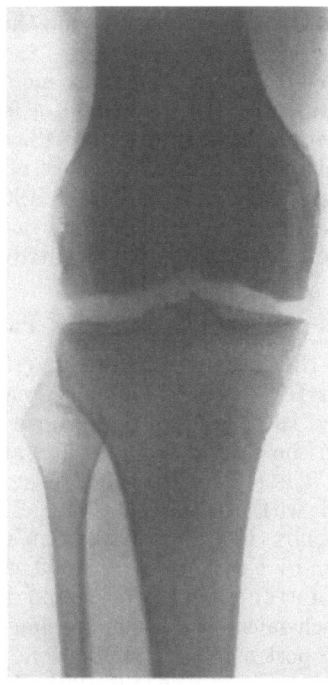

a   b

Fig. 3 a and b. Involvement of the knee joints in HAP. Deformities of the articular surfaces of femur and tibia and flattening of the condyles with reactive bone formation at their margins. (Reproduced with permission of Georg Thieme Verlag, Stuttgart)

Laboratory Findings

Serum

With the exception of the occurrence of phytanic acid there are no typical serum findings in HAP. Total serum lipids and total serum cholesterol may be low, but are usually normal. Lipoprotein electrophoresis, performed in a few cases, gave normal results. In contrast to a-beta-lipoproteinemia, with which HAP has many common symptoms, beta-lipoproteins are present.

A questionable and inconsistent increase of alpha-2 macroglobulins in one patient was found by HARDERS and DIECKMANN (1964) by immunoelectrophoresis. A recent ultracentrifugal study by ELDJARN et al. (1965 a) also revealed an abnormal serum protein pattern in three patients with HAP, consisting of a slight increase of the total protein and elevated levels of the M ("19 S") component. In addition, there was diminution of the G ("7 S") component in one subject.

Serum enzyme studies by RICHTERICH et al. (1963) showed elevation of glutamic-oxalacetic transaminase, glutamic-pyruvic transaminase and creatine-phosphokinase, while HARDERS and DIECKMANN (1964) reported normal values for these enzymes. Phosphatases, flocculation tests, serum bilirubin, albumin/globulin ratio, non-protein nitrogen and protein electrophoresis were normal. An elevated plasma copper level and increased concentration of ceruloplasmin support the diagnosis of a lipidosis, according to RICHTERICH et al. (1965 b).

Cerebrospinal Fluid

The cerebrospinal fluid protein is elevated in all cases of HAP, while the cell count is normal. Protein levels usually range from 100 to 700 mg per 100 ml, but may be higher in some cases. Frequently there is some correlation between the severity of the clinical picture and the protein concentration in the cerebrospinal fluid.

An elevated N-acetyl-neuraminic acid content relative to the protein content was described by RICHTERICH in a female patient, and is found in a variety of central nervous system disorders (SAIFER and GERSTENFIELD 1962). Spinal fluid protein electrophoresis in the case of HARDERS and DIECKMANN (1964) showed a normal pattern. ELDJARN et al. (1966) also found a normal protein distribution of the spinal fluid upon electrophoresis; 94% of the protein sedimented with the A ("4 S") component in the ultracentrifuge.

Pathology

At the time of REFSUM's reports (1944—1946) two of his original cases (brother and sister H. B. and G. B.) had already died at the age of 41 and 32 years, respectively. In both cases the brain was examined. The next autopsies were performed in the case of SALOMONSEN and SKATVEDT (1949) and in a third case of REFSUM. These were thoroughly reviewed by CAMMERMEYER et al. (1954) and compared with the histopathological findings of REESE and BARETA (1950), GELLERSTEDT (1953) and KJELLSON's case T. (1953). Other autopsy reports have been given by EDSTRÖM et al. (1959, case II), GORDON and HUDSON (1959, cases 1 and 3), RICHTERICH et al. (1963), and ALEXANDER (1966). In several cases histologic and histochemical studies on specimens from nerve- and/or muscle biopsies preceded the post mortem examinations (REESE and BARETA 1950, EDSTRÖM et al. 1959, VELTEMA and VERJAAL 1961, PECKER et al. 1963, PETIT 1963, DEREUX and GRUNER 1963a, b, DEREUX 1963, BLANC et al. 1963, HARDERS and DIECKMANN 1964).

Peripheral Nerves

Peripheral nerves, in particular those of the brachial and lumbosacral plexus, show the major neuropathologic changes observed in HAP (GORDON and HUDSON 1959). A striking finding upon gross examination is thickening of the entire nerve (CAMMERMEYER 1956, EDSTRÖM et al. 1959, ALEXANDER 1966). The thickness of the sciatic nerve at the level of the proximal thigh was 1.8×1 cm instead of 1.0×0.45 cm normally, and the vagus nerve was about twice as thick as normal in patients of GORDON and HUDSON (1959). Thickening of peripheral nerves was less in other cases (REESE and BARETA 1950). There is whitish discoloration and occasionally local gelatinous swelling. In cross-sections the nerve tissue appears prominent, as if under pressure; it has a viscous consistency and a greyish-red color (CAMMERMEYER 1956).

Under the microscope perineurium and endoneurium are thickened. Typically (DEREUX 1963) but not always (VELTEMA and VERJAAL 1961) the appearance resembles that of hypertrophic polyneuritis, type Déjérine-Sottas (EDSTRÖM et al. 1959). Microscopic lesions vary in intensity in different sections, and are most marked where the tissue appears edematous on gross examination. Here, the axis cylinders are diminished in number and are separated by an amorphous material which stains metachromatic with cresyl violet, toluidin blue and PAS (CAMMERMEYER 1956). The accumulation of serous fluid which apparently is responsible for the swelling (GORDON and HUDSON 1959, ALEXANDER 1966) may be limited to peripheral bundles, and the metachromatic material may become less or may even disappear upon treatment with hyaluronidase. In some fibers axis cylinders may be completely missing, in other areas they are swollen (see figure 4); only a few uninvolved ones remain (REESE and BARETA 1950, CAMMERMEYER 1956). When axons are concentrically surrounded by connective tissue fibers, a characteristic onion bulb structure appears in cross sections (REESE and BARETA 1950,

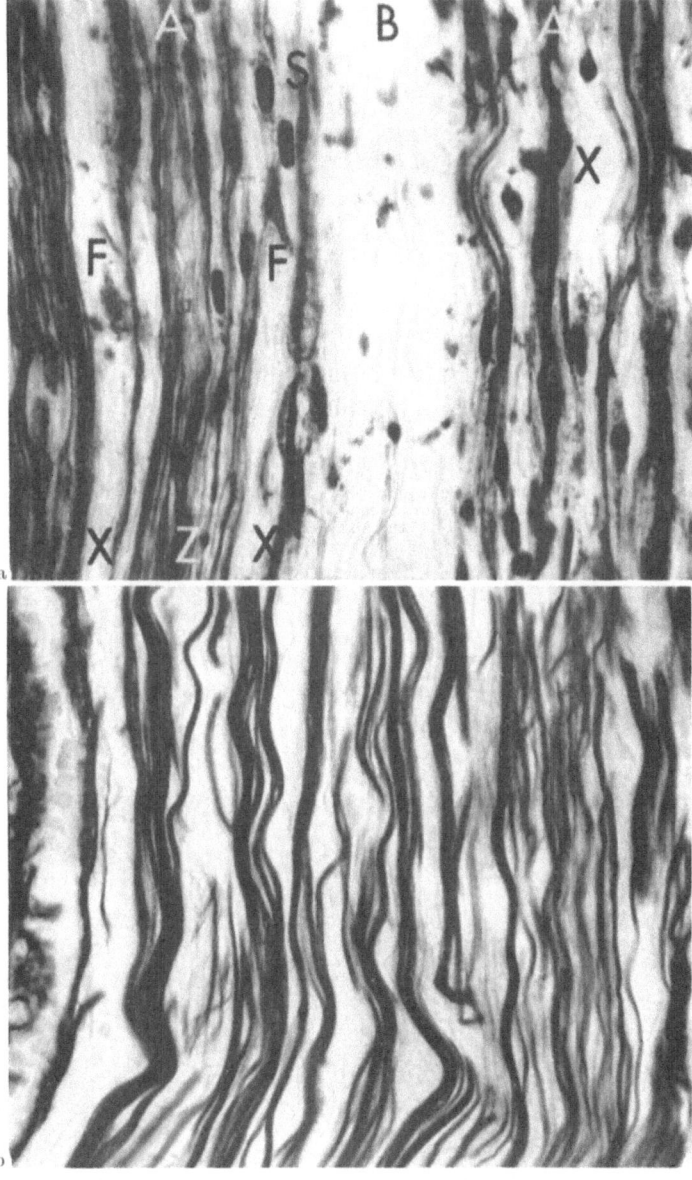

Fig. 4a and b. a Irregular damage of nerve with areas of diffuse (A) and complete (B) loss of axons. Some axons are irregularly thickened (X), others beaded (Z). Intermingled are some delicate axons, Schwann cell nuclei (S) and hypertrophied stellate fibroblasts (F). Paraffin embedded, longitudinal section, Bodian silver method; ×600. b Irregular spacing of longitudinal argentophilic collagenous fibers corresponding to varied disappearance of nerve fibers. Same block as in a. Wilder silver reticulum modification; ×600. — Norwegian case T.A. Source: CAMMERMEYER (1956). (Reproduced with kind permission of *Journal of Neuropathology and Experimental Neurology* and the author)

CAMMERMEYER 1956, EDSTRÖM et al. 1959) (see figures 5, 6 and 7 b, c). Occasionally these onion shells may be formed by polynucleated cells, and sometimes they

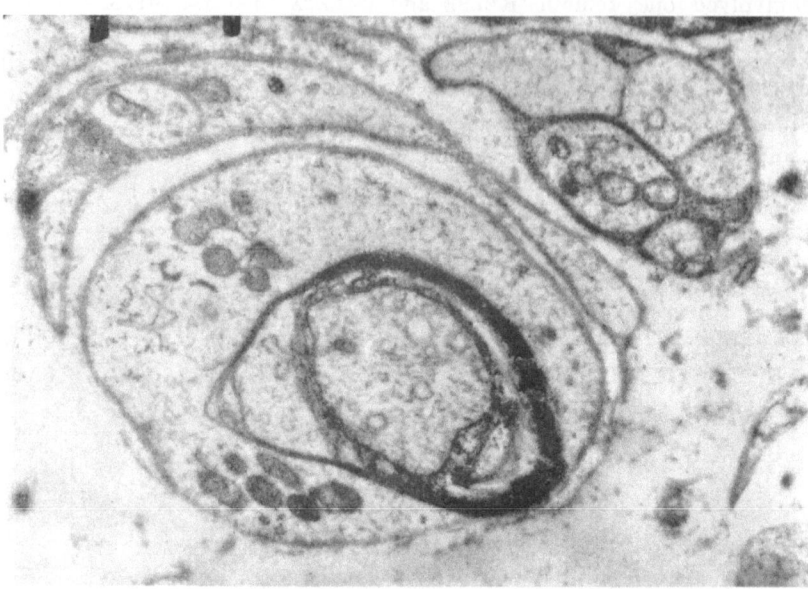

Fig. 5. Initial stage of hypertrophy of Schwann cells. Unfolding of myelin. The onion bulb structure is apparent. Source: DEREUX (1963). (Reproduced with kind permission of *Revue neurologique* and the author)

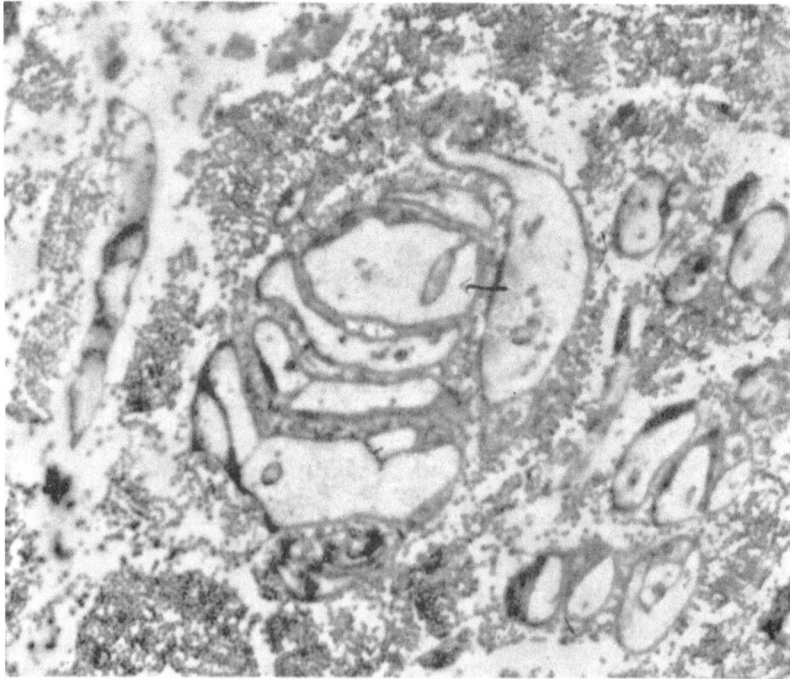

Fig. 6. Onion bulb with alternating layers of Schwann cells and collagen fibers which surround a demyelinated nerve fiber (axon at top of arrow). Source: DEREUX (1963). (Reproduced with kind permission of *Revue neurologique* and the author)

have a hyaline appearance. The case of BLANC et al. (1963) was an exception: in the presence of interstitial hypertrophic neuritis, proliferation of Schwann cells and onion shell formation were missing.

The myelin sheaths which surround thickened nerve fibers are thin and atrophic. They may appear granular and fragmentated or may disappear completely. Granular myelin material stains well with Sudan-red; portions of the myelin which are close to the axis cylinders give a pale color with Baker's phospholipid stain and in some bundles the myelin does not stain at all (CAMMERMEYER 1956). In longitudinal sections the Schwann cell nuclei appear to be increased in number (GORDON and HUDSON 1959). Hyperplasia of Schwann cells and myelinoclasis have been observed (CAMMERMEYER 1956). There are no signs of an inflammatory reaction.

The blood vessels of nerves appear moderately sclerotic. The subcapsular space is frequently widened by an exudate containing protein and fat. In summary, nerve changes are similar to those occurring with Wallerian degeneration, associated with variable degrees of connective tissue hyperplasia. Histochemical studies show that there is lipid deposition as droplets or in the form of phagocytized material (CAMMERMEYER 1956, ALEXANDER 1966) along the whole course of peripheral nerves.

Spinal Cord

The firmness of the spinal cord is usually increased (REESE and BARETA 1950, EDSTRÖM et al. 1959). In contrast to the components of the cauda equina, which may be thickened, the spinal cord tends to be atrophic (GORDON and HUDSON 1959).

The anterior horns show yellow discoloration and appear increased in size, the roots leaving the anterior and posterior horns may be thinner than normal. Spinal ganglia are enlarged, and the roots are swollen distally (GORDON and HUDSON 1959, case III). There are large amounts of fat in the leptomeninges, which appear in the form of sudanophilic granules in endothelial cells, histiocytes and macrophages of pia and arachnoidea, with particular involvement of the outer layer of the latter (KJELLSON 1953, CAMMERMEYER 1956).

Histologic findings consist of localized and moderate degeneration of myelin and ganglion cells. Anterior horn cells are reduced in number and show pyknosis, swelling, chromatolysis, hyalination, rarefication or only slight shrinkage (REFSUM et al. 1949, REESE and BARETA 1950, GORDON and HUDSON 1959). EDSTRÖM points out the lack of gliosis with these changes. A frequent finding is atrophy of the posterior tracts with reduction in the number of nerve fibers; the changes may be restricted to the fasciculi graciles (KJELLSON 1953, CAMMERMEYER 1956), where EDSTRÖM et al. (1959) observed marked myelin degeneration. Numerous amyloid bodies were seen by REESE and BARETA (1950) in the white matter of the spinal cord.

The appearance of nerve roots is similar to that of peripheral nerves. In addition to partial demyelination there is extensive connective tissue proliferation. Blood vessels of the spinal cord may appear hyaline and the vessel wall shows increased eosinophilia (REESE and BARETA 1950).

The overall picture in the spinal cord consists of degenerative changes of motor neurons; involvement is less intensive than that of peripheral nerves.

Sympathetic ganglia (CAMMERMEYER 1956) may be slightly fibrotic with rare lymphocytic nodules. There were conspicuous reactive changes and loss of ganglion cells in one of this author's case (T. A.). Sympathetic nerve fibers traversing the ganglia were not involved.

Brain

The brains of the cases H. B., G. B. and T. A. (REFSUM 1946b) and of case I (REFSUM et al. 1949, SALOMONSEN and SKATVEDT 1949) have been thoroughly studied by CAMMERMEYER (1946, 1956) and by CAMMERMEYER et al. (1954). To date autopsy data on about ten brains of patients with HAP are available (REESE and BARETA 1950, GELLERSTEDT 1953, EDSTRÖM et al. 1959, GORDON and HUDSON 1959, ALEXANDER 1966).

On gross examination the leptomeninges show moderate patchy or diffuse thickening. Pacchionian granulations may be more prominent than usual (REESE

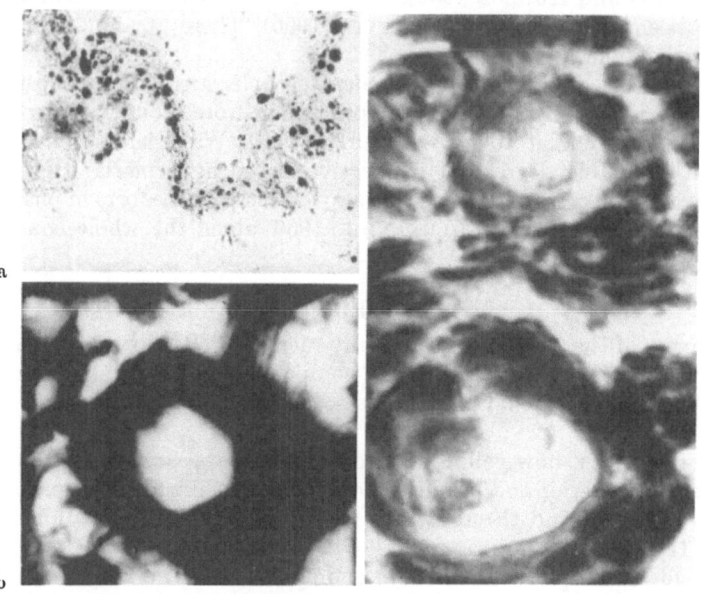

Fig. 7a—c. a Fat droplets deposited in macrophages of leptomeninges of cauda equina. Norwegian case G. B. Gelatin embedded; frozen section, sudan red stain; ×150. b Argentophil connective tissue fibers condensed around unstained nerve fibers. Thick section, Bielschowsky silver method; ×2000. c Darkly stained longitudinal collagenous fibers aggregated around preserved nerve fibers seen in cross section. Separation of "onion bulb"-like structures in retroperitoneal nerve. Same block as in b. Paraffin embedded, Heidenhain trichrome method; ×2000. — Norwegian case G. B. Source: CAMMERMEYER (1956). (Reproduced with kind permission of *Journal of Neuropathology and Experimental Neurology* and the author)

and BARETA 1950). In the 37 year-old patient of the latter authors the brain weighed 1360 gm and exhibited thickening of the optic nerves and the optic chiasm. In cross sections a relative increase of the white matter was apparent. Brain weight in a 27 year-old patient of EDSTRÖM et al. (1959) was 1250 gm. Here, yellowish liquid was found below the thickened pia.

Histochemical studies of the meninges reveal the presence of a considerable amount of lipid (see figure 7a), which is partly phagocytized by macrophages. Lipid can also be found in the epithelium of the chorioideal plexus and the ependymal granulations of the ventricular walls (CAMMERMEYER 1946). Intimal thickening of the smaller meningeal arteries was observed by REESE and BARETA (1950).

Histologic findings in the various brains are not uniform, which may be due in part to different durations of the disease (REFSUM 1960). Changes are most frequent and most marked in the brain stem, but there is usually involvement of other areas as well. Signs of cell degeneration such as pyknosis or loss of ganglion cells prevail in the posterior olivary nuclei and in the dorsal nuclei of the vestibular and acustic nerves. Involvement of nuclei of the vagus, of the dentate nucleus and the red nucleus is less frequent. Pyknosis and cytoplasmic shrinkage of Purkinje cells were described by REESE and BARETA (1950) and by EDSTRÖM et al. (1959). The trigeminus nerve may atrophy (GELLERSTEDT 1953). A yellowish cytoplasmic pigment and eccentric nuclei were found by REESE and BARETA (1950) in numerous nerve cells of the dentate nucleus. These authors also observed numerous amyloid bodies in the outer molecular layers of the hemispheres, in

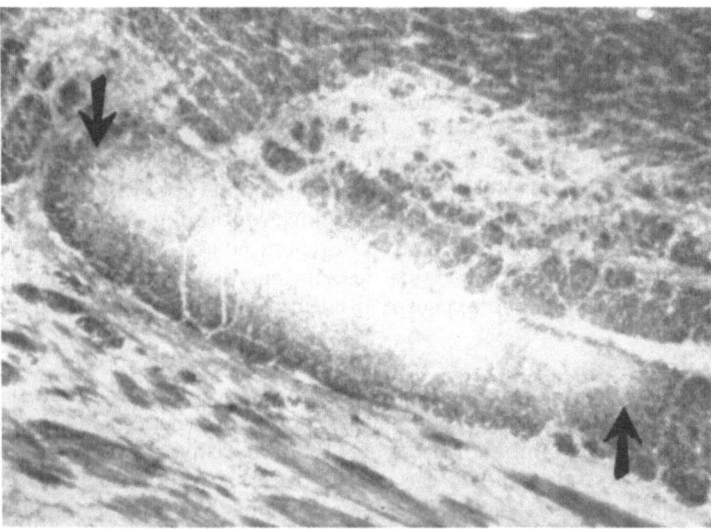

Fig. 8. Loss of myelinated fibers in center of medial lemniscus in pons. Norwegian case H. B. Frozen section, Spielmeyer method; × 50. Source: CAMMERMEYER (1956). (Reproduced with kind permission of *Journal of Neuropathology and Experimental Neurology* and the author)

thalamus, cerebellum, pons, medulla oblongata and in the olfactory and optic nerves. In contrast to other workers CAMMERMEYER (1946, 1956) found marked swelling and lipid storage in nerve cells of all areas. Lipid deposition in nerve cells was also observed in KJELLSON's (1953) case I. There was no alteration in the cerebellum of ALEXANDER's (1966) case.

Abnormalities of the white matter consist of localized, mild to moderate loss of myelin, particularly in the lemniscus medialis, in the Monakow bundle, in the olivocerebellar tract, in the anterior and posterior cerebellar peduncles and in the area surrounding the dentate nucleus (see figure 8). The defect of myelin is frequently most marked in the center of some bundles or in the neighbourhood of blood vessels (EDSTRÖM et al. 1959). Axis cylinders seem to be involved to a minor degree. In the white matter, lipid storing macrophages are found in involved areas (CAMMERMEYER 1956, EDSTRÖM et al. 1959, REFSUM 1960). The finding of deposition of fat droplets in the pallidum of all four adult cases of CAMMER-MEYER (1956) is of interest. Here, free lipid was present in the tissue which otherwise appeared normal, and there was no cellular reaction.

In addition to lipid storage, signs of focal gliosis are found in involved areas. Frequently astrocytes hypertrophy (CAMMERMEYER 1956) and oligodendroglial cells increase in number (REESE and BARETA 1950).

Eyes

In all cases, in which the optic system was thoroughly examined, there were significant changes corresponding to the clinical manifestations with the exception of the case of ALEXANDER (1966). Involvement of the optic nerve is qualitatively similar but quantitatively more marked than that of peripheral nerves. The edematous or myxomatous inner portion is completely replaced by fibrous tissue (EDSTRÖM et al. 1959). In one case (REESE and BARETA 1950) there was infiltration of the optic nerve and of most of the brain with numerous amyloid bodies and thickening and hyaline metamorphosis of the leptomeninges surrounding the optic nerve.

The pathological findings in the eye itself are those of pigmentary retinitis (REESE and BARETA 1950, EDSTRÖM et al. 1959, GORDON and HUDSON 1959, ALEXANDER 1966). All layers of the retina are atrophic, and the ganglion cell layer as well as inner and outer molecular layers show a diminished number of cells (REESE and BARETA 1950, GORDON and HUDSON 1959). Rods and cones showed vacuolation, fragmentation and partial replacement by spheroid bodies in the case of ALEXANDER (1966) or had disappeared in that of REESE and BARETA (1950), and the pigmented layer was atrophic, containing only small remnants of pigment. Bruch's membrane appeared degenerated and could not be recognized in places. Although the few available descriptions do not allow generalizations, changes as described may be expected in all cases with pigmentary retinitis.

Musculature

Biopsy specimens (KJELLSON 1953, TOUSSAINT et al. 1959, PECKER et al. 1963, HARDERS and DIECKMANN 1964) and autopsy specimens (REESE and BARETA 1950, CAMMERMEYER 1956, GORDON and HUDSON 1959, EDSTRÖM et al. 1959, RICHTERICH et al. 1963, ALEXANDER 1966) of the musculature show muscular atrophy as the predominant finding. Localized proliferation of connective tissue and small amounts of fat may be seen between muscle fiber bundles (REESE and BARETA 1950).

The histologic picture is compatible with atrophy, which in case III B of REFSUM was most marked in intercostal muscles, and less severe in the diaphragm, psoas, pectoralis, gastrocnemius and levator ani muscles (CAMMERMEYER 1956). Changes in ALEXANDER's (1966) case involved mainly the peroneus muscles, while the pectoralis muscles were hardly altered. Some parts of the atrophic musculature appear as filaments only (CAMMERMEYER 1956). Muscle striation is nevertheless maintained; the nuclei are frequently increased in number (REESE and BARETA 1950, CAMMERMEYER 1956, HARDERS and DIECKMANN 1964). The degree of atrophy may vary considerably within involved bundles. Very large (CAMMERMEYER 1956) and hypertrophic (HARDERS and DIECKMANN 1964) fibers can be found between atrophic ones. In addition to reactive fibrosis in atrophic areas, CAMMERMEYER (1956) found significant amounts of lipid surrounded by fibrous tissue in portions where loss of muscle fibers was most marked. Scattered portions of the muscle showed signs of necrosis and accumulations of hypertrophic histiocytes. Signs of inflammation are not observed.

Neuromuscular changes were described in detail by TOUSSAINT et al. (1959). Degeneration of the neural elements occurs rarely and is suggestive of a chronic process. The sum of pathologic changes in muscle corresponds to the clinical finding of neurogenic muscular atrophy.

Heart

The high incidence of sudden deaths and of signs and symptoms referable to the heart prompted thorough studies of the myocardium. REESE and BARETA (1950) found basophilic degeneration and moderate vacuolation of muscle fibers. EDSTRÖM et al. (1959) saw signs of diffuse atrophy without evidence of fibrosis or cellular infiltration, in contrast to ALEXANDER (1966) who described markedly fibrotic areas of the myocardium which were surrounded by swollen muscle fibers with hyperchromatic and irregularly shaped nuclei. Extensive histologic and histochemical studies of the myocardium and of the conducting system have been performed by GORDON and HUDSON (1959). There was no evidence of inflammation, amyloid infiltration or glycogen storage, and stains for iron and lipid were negative. In large areas muscle fibers had lost much of their identity and appeared empty and somewhat atrophic. The sinus node was enlarged; autonomous fibers and ganglia were unusually prominent. Swollen and partially vacuolated cells were situated beneath the ventricular endocardium including the Purkinje cells, the terminal elements of the conducting system (GORDON and HUDSON 1959).

Other Organs

Detailed studies on changes of visceral organs and of blood vessels are not yet available. In case I of the B-family (REFSUM 1946 b) there was significant lipid deposition in liver and kidneys (CAMMERMEYER et al. 1954). Other cases of this series were not examined in this regard. In the cases of REESE and BARETA (1950) and ALEXANDER (1966) there was extensive fatty degeneration of the liver and numerous fat globules were found in the renal tubular epithelium. Marked fatty infiltration of liver and kidneys was also a finding in the case of RICHTERICH et al. (1963); here extensive histologic and electronmicroscopic studies were performed (ROOS and RICHTERICH 1965). The testes were diminished in size in case I of GORDON and HUDSON (1959) and the tissue appeared orange in cross sections. In another case (REESE and BARETA 1950) there was evidence of impaired spermiogenesis. In the same patient small yellow plaques were found in the intima of the aorta adjacent to the origin of the coronary arteries; in addition there was intimal thickening of leptomeningeal arteries and spinal cord vessels.

Results of Lipid Analyses

Serum Lipids

The pathognomonic and consistent finding in serum is the occurrence of 3,7,11,15-tetramethylhexadecanoic acid (phytanic acid), as demonstrated by

3,7,11,15–Tetramethylhexadecanoic acid

gas-liquid chromatography of total serum fatty acids (see figure 9). While phytanic acid occurs only in traces or not at all in normal controls, in patients with other diseases and in the parents of the patients with HAP, in affected subjects it is usually present to the extent of 10—20% (in some cases only 3%) of total plasma fatty acids (see table 2). Studies on the distribution of phytanic acid among the various serum lipid fractions show that it may make up over 30% of triglyceride fatty acids, and 5—10% of phospholipid fatty acids. An intermediate proportion of phytanic acid is found in the free fatty acid, diglyceride and monoglyceride fatty acid fractions. It is of interest that plasma cholesterol ester fatty acids contain only traces of phytanic acid; its concentration is always below 1% and frequently cannot be measured. The proportions of plasma lipid fatty acids other than phytanic acid are normal (KAHLKE 1963, 1964 b).

The concentration of phytanic acid in different lipoprotein classes as separated by precipitation with dextran sulfate (SAKAGAMY and ZILVERSMIT 1962) is twice as high in the beta-lipoprotein fraction as in the alpha-lipoprotein fraction (KAHLKE and WAGENER 1966 a) due to the higher triglyceride content of beta-lipoproteins. The concentration of phytanic acid in triglycerides and phospholipids is similar in each lipoprotein fraction (see table 3).

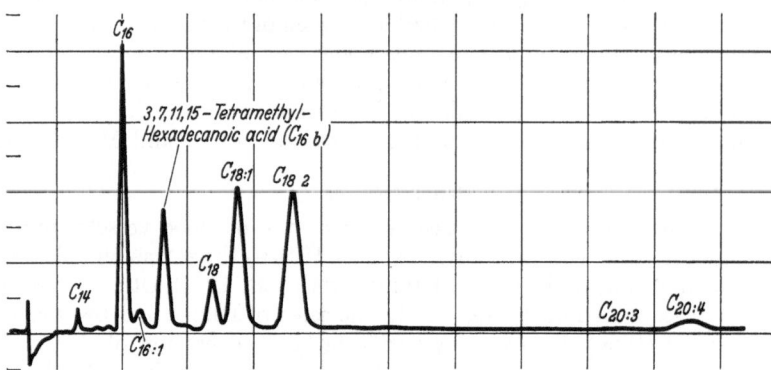

Fig. 9. Gas chromatographic separation of plasma fatty acids in a patient with HAP. Model 872 Packard Instruments; DEGS-column 4 × 180 mm, 160°C., 65 ml argon/minute, 500 volts, sensitivity 1 × 10⁻⁸ amperes, 5 minutes/inch

Red Cells

Phytanic acid of total red cell lipids may amount to 12% of total red cell fatty acids. Its concentration in the various lipid fractions of washed red cells varies; the main portion is found in red cell phospholipids, although here cholesterol esters also contain phytanic acid.

Organ Lipids

Analyses of tissue lipids from biopsy and autopsy material (case of RICHTERICH et al. 1963) were performed by KLENK and KAHLKE (1963); the organs of a male patient, who had died at the age of 33 years (ALEXANDER 1966) were studied by HANSEN (1965 b), (see table 4). Phytanic acid was found in variable but considerable amounts in total tissue lipids. The phytanic acid fraction in the liver of both cases amounted to over 50% of total fatty acids and the concentration of phytanic acid in kidneys, heart and skeletal muscle was almost as high. In contrast, depot fat contained only about 1% phytanic acid. Urinary findings vary. The high urinary lipid excretion in the patient of RICHTERICH et al. (1963) was partly the result of sequestration of renal cells since a portion of the lipid was seen intracellularly. The proportion of phytanic acid in total urinary fatty acids of this case was 41% and similar to that found in other cases (KAHLKE 1965).

Brain lipid fatty acids contained less than 10% of total fatty acids as phytanic acid. The corresponding figure for the sciatic nerve was about 14% (HANSEN 1965 b).

Study of *lipid fractions* from liver, kidney and brain showed liver cholesterol ester fatty acids to contain the highest proportion of phytanic acid with over 60%; significant amounts of the acid were also found in liver and kidney triglycerides. Phytanic acid in brain was present only in the aceton soluble fraction, and, in small concentration, in fatty acids of glycerophosphatides (see table 5).

The Atypical Fatty Acid

Isolation and identification of the unknown fatty acid was first performed using liver lipids of the case of RICHTERICH et al. (1963), (KLENK and KAHLKE

Table 2. Fatty acid patterns of plasma lipids of 12 patients with HAP.
(Fatty acid values calculated from gaschromatograms by triangulation, expressed as per cent of total fatty acids)

Patient	Sex m = male, f = female	Author(s) of original case report	Fraction	14:0	16:0	16:1	16b*	18:0	18:1	18:2	20:3	20:4
T. E.	f	REFSUM (1965, 1966)	Total lipids	4	23	8	14	3	25	21	0.5	1.5
			Triglycerides	5	24	7	16	5	28	10		2
			Cholesterol esters	2	8	8	—	1	22	53		3
			Lecithin*	—	38		7	47	20:0 = 8	8	22:0 = 21	
			Sphingomyelin*	2	45		7	17	20:0 = 9,	9,		
J. M.	m	SABOURAUD (1965, 1966)	Total lipids	2	25	1	23	5	18	20	Trace	5
			Triglycerides	3	23	0,5	51	1.5	17	4	—	
			Cholesterol esters	4	13	2	1	1	23	49	Trace	6.5
			Phosphatides	2	29	0.5	17	11	14	15	Trace	10
W. M.	m	HARDERS and DIECKMANN (1964)	Total lipids	4	37	2	11	5	18	21	0.5	2
			Triglycerides	2	25	5	34	3	24	7	—	
			Cholesterol esters	3	13	3	1	1	18	58	—	
			Phosphatides	2	28	1	11	14	16	21	Trace	7
E. H.	f	HARDERS and DIECKMANN (1964)	Total lipids	1	21	6	20	4	23	21	—	5
L. D.	f	TOUSSAINT et al. (1959)		1	21	5	21	5	21	20	—	5
M. C.	f	PECKER et al. (1963)		1	21	3	7	7	24	31	—	5
E. H.	m	THIÉBAUT et al. (1939, 1961)		1	22	7	16	4	27	23	**	**
N. H.	f	(Mother from E. H. m, not yet reported)		1	28	6	18	4	24	19	**	**
G. S.	f	DEREUX (1961, 1963)		1	27	6	14	4	23	24	**	**
E. L.	m	DEREUX (1963, 1965)		4.5	24	3	4.5	5	24	29	1	4.5
G. L.	m	DEREUX (1963, 1965)		2.5	26	5	2.5	6	28	25	0.5	4
K. M.	m	REFSUM et al. (1949)		2	31	1	11	7	25	20	—	2

* = Tetramethylhexadecanoic acid.

* Fatty acid pattern calculated from gaschromatograms after hydrogenation of fatty acid methyl esters.

** Only acetone soluble lipids were available.

Table 3. *Fatty acid distribution between plasma lipoproteins in HAP. (Fatty acid values calculated from gaschromatograms by triangulation, expressed as per cent of total fatty acids)*

Patient	Lipoprotein-fraction	14:0	16:0	16:1	16b*	18:0	18:1	18:2	20:3	20:4
K. M.	α	5	33.5	1.5	7	4.5	18.5	26.5	—	2.5
	β	3	32	1.5	13	3.5	22.5	22	—	2
T. E.	α	3.5	31	3	3.5	6.5	26.5	22	0.5	3
	β	2.5	29.5	3.5	6.5	4	29.5	23	—	1
E. L.	α	3	31	3	4	5.5	20.5	27	0.5	5.5
	β	2	26.5	3.5	5.5	3.5	26.5	29.5	0.5	3
G. L.	α	1.5	35	5	1.5	5.5	26	21.5	0.5	3.5
	β	2	28	6.5	4	4	28	24	0.5	3
L. D.	α	1.5	29	1.5	4	7	23.5	28	—	5
	β	5.5	23	1.5	7.5	4	19	35.5	—	4
L. D.	Triglycerides α	3.5	30.5	2.5	12	2.5	39	8	—	9,5
	Triglycerides β	6.5	28.5	3.5	13.5	2	35	8	—	—
L. D.	Phosphatides α	2	38	1.5	3	11.5	21.5	16.5	0.5	6
	Phosphatides β	3.5	33	0.5	4	12.5	13	23.5	1	9

Source: Kahlke and Wagener (1966a)

* = Tetramethylhexadecanoic acid.

Table 4. *Fatty acid composition of several organs in 2 cases with HAP. (Values expressed as per cent of total fatty acids after gaschromatography)*

	Liver			Heart muscle			Adipose tissue			Kidney			Urine
	EMW	RB	Control	EMW	RB	Control	TE	RB	Control	EMW	RB	Control	RB
$C_{12:0}$		—	Trace	0.4	0.5	Trace	1	1	1	0.7	—	Trace	3
$C_{14:0}$	1	2	3.5	3.2	4	1.5	5	9	5	4.5	—	2	4
$C_{16:0}$	20.1	20	35	23.6	29	29.5	19	34	27	24	26	25	25
$C_{16:I}$		1	4		5	5	14	4	8		3	2	5
C_{16b}*	53.6	56	Trace	42.2	20.5	—	1	1	—	44.1	47	Trace	41
$C_{18:0}$	5.1	6	7.5	9.5	5	11	2	7	5	8.4	10	12.5	6
$C_{18:I}$	18.1	14	37	18.4	34	27.5	44	44	44	18.3	14	22	8
$C_{18:II}$	1.5	1	9	0.7	2	12	8	—	7	Trace		14	—
C_{20} (and above)		—	4	1.1	—	14	—	—	1			19.5	—

Sources: Case EMW from Hansen (1965). All samples from EMW had been preserved in formalin for about 2 years.
Cases RB and TE from Klenk and Kahlke (1963), and Kahlke (1964).
Controls from Kahlke (1965a, b; 1966).

* = Tetramethylhexadecanoic acid.

1963, Kahlke and Richterich 1965) and plasma lipids of Refsum's (1946) case T. E. (Kahlke 1964a)*. Methods and results were identical in both instances although a nuclear resonance spectrum was obtained only in the first case and a complete mass spectrometric analysis only in the second case. Phytanic acid was isolated by preparative gas-liquid chromatography from a mixture of fatty acid methyl esters. Traces of stearic acid were removed as the urea inclusion compound by treatment with a saturated methanolic solution of urea (Cason et al. 1953). After repeated crystallization from acetone at minus 70—80°C and drying under vacuum at minus 10°C, phytanic acid was obtained as a white crystalline powder with a melting point of minus 7—6°C. At room temperature phytanic acid is a colorless, odorless oil. The lack of hydrogen uptake with exhaustive

* For repeated shipments of samples I want to thank Dr. Jens Christian Arbo, Bodø, Rønvik Sykehus Norway and Dr. S. Refsum, Rikshospital/Oslo, Norway.

Table 5. *Fatty acid composition of nervous tissue in 2 cases with HAP.*
(Values expressed as per cent of total fatty acids after gaschromatography)

| | Sciatic nerve | | Brain | | | | |
| | Total lipids | | Total lipids | | Neutral lipids | Glycero-phospha-tides | Sphingo-lipids |
	EMW	Control	EMW	Control	RB	RB	RB
$C_{12:0}$	0.8	0.5			—	—	—
$C_{14:0}$	5.9	5.3	0.7	0.4	1	—	—
$C_{16:0}$	38.2	33.2	31.6	22.9	27	11	20
$C_{16:I}$		6.7			—	—	—
$C_{16b}*$	13.8		8.5		10	3	—
$C_{18:0}$	7.9	4.2	26.5	25.9	45	74	58
$C_{18:I}$	24.7	44.9	28.0	43.5	18	10	16
$C_{18:II}$	0.7	0.4	0.4	0.2	—	—	—
C_{20} (and above)	3.7	0.7	3.2	4.8	3	2	6

Sources: Case EMW and Controls from HANSEN (1965). All samples from EMW and from
controls had been preserved in formalin, those from EMW for about 2 years.
Case RB from KLENK and KAHLKE (1963).
* = Tetramethylhexadecanoic acid.

hydrogenation over platinum oxide and the lack of bromine uptake indicate its
fully saturated nature. The retention time of phytanic acid methyl ester during
gas-liquid chromatography on columns of reoplex, apiezon, EGS, etc. suggests
that the molecule contains between 16.9 and 17.2 carbon atoms, and separation
from the C-17 (margaric) acid is not always possible. The equivalent weight obtained by titration of the free acid corresponded to an acid containing 20 carbon
atoms. Elementary analysis in addition to infrared spectroscopy, mass spectroscopy (see fig. 10) and nuclear resonance finally suggested that the material examined was the 3,7,11,15-tetramethylhexadecanoic acid. A standard compound
prepared from phytol by hydrogenation over platinum oxide and followed by
chromic acid oxidation, showed essentially identical behaviour.

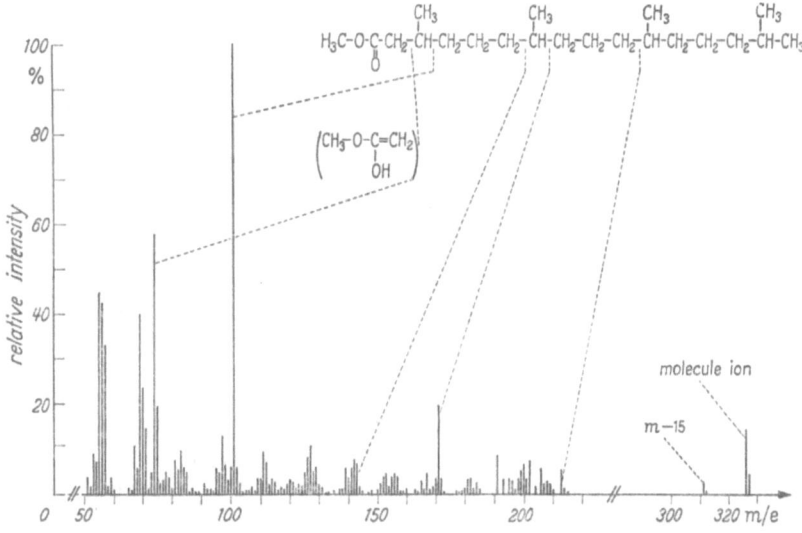

Fig. 10. Mass spectroscopic analysis of 3, 7, 11, 15-tetramethylhexadecanoic acid isolated from plasma
of a patient with HAP

Phytanic acid had been isolated earlier from butter fat by HANSEN and SHOR-
LAND (1951, 1953), BJURSTAM et al. (1961), SONNEVELD et al. (1962) and HAN-
SEN and MORRISON (1965). It is also present in ox plasma (DUNCAN and GARTON
1963, LOUGH 1963, 1964) and in ox and sheep fat (HANSEN 1965 a and c). After
complete hydrogenation of beef plasma fatty acids we found a fraction amounting
to about 3% which corresponded to the phytanic acid peak on gas-chromatography. BILLETER et al. (1964) could show in pigeons that the side chain of
phyllochinone which is split off by the action of intestinal bacteria, is converted

Phytol

to phytanic acid or a derivative of it. The similarity of the acid with the alcohol
phytol which makes up the side chain of the chlorophyll molecule, and the demonstration of its synthesis from this alcohol (STOFFEL and KAHLKE 1965) suggest
that at least traces of phytanic acid occur in all animals which consume large
amounts of chlorophyll.

Diagnosis

HAP should be suspected in a patient with polyneuritic symptoms, which occur
in association with changes of the skeletal musculature, night blindness and abnormal retinal pigmentation. In younger patients eye changes may not yet be fully
developed. In almost all cases ataxia exceeds that which occurs in polyneuritis
from other causes. Cerebrospinal fluid protein is increased while the cell count is
normal. The diagnosis is supported in most cases of HAP by findings such as
partial or complete nerve deafness, anosmia, miosis, and concentric narrowing of
the visual fields. Diagnostic difficulties result from the fact that many of these
symptoms are found in other diseases (CLAUSS 1924, JEQUIER and STREIFF 1947,
ROTH 1947, DUREUX 1957). It is the particular merit of REFSUM that he recognized
the disease as a separate entity solely on the basis of clinical findings and compiled
(1946) the criteria for a complete neurologic differential diagnosis from other
heredofamilial degenerative disorders such as Friedreich's ataxia and cerebellar
ataxias, in which nerve deafness and pigmentary retinitis are rare. Other diseases
to be considered are peroneal muscular atrophy (Charcot-Marie-Tooth) and hypertrophic neuritis (Déjérine-Sottas).

Today, demonstration of phytanic acid in plasma and organ lipids of patients
with HAP by gas-liquid chromatography has eliminated differential diagnostic
difficulties and is pathognomonic for the disease.

The literature contains a number of cases which are very similar to HAP and
which have been published in part under this heading. Some of these show external
ophthalmoplegia in addition to pigmentary degeneration of the retina (BARNARD
and SCHOLZ 1944, WALSH 1947, CHAMLIN and BILLET 1950, ALFANO and BERGER
1957, ERDBRINK 1957). In addition, deafness and/or heart block — frequent signs
of HAP — were described in such cases (KEARNS and SAYRE 1958, JAGER et al.
1960). Disorders without pigmentary retinitis such as the Landry-Guillain-Barré
syndrome where the cerebrospinal fluid protein concentration is also elevated and
which may occur in families (SAUNDERS and RAKE 1965), or the so-called Fisher
syndrome (FISHER 1956, SMITH and WALSH 1957, GOODWIN and POSER 1963)
where motor weakness of the extremities is absent, can usually be differentiated
from HAP on the basis of their clinical course. Of the cases described but not

confirmed as HAP, ophthalmoplegia externa was present only in that of RAVIN and SCHWARTZ (1962), limitation of ocular movements in that of OLESEN (1957), and weakness of the ocular muscles in that of GORDON and HUDSON (1959).

In the former two cases some of the classic findings of HAP are missing, such as night blindness, which was absent in both and ataxia, which was missing in one. Both patients, however, had bilateral ptosis. Lack of night blindness and ptosis was also reported in the younger patient of BAUM et al. (1965); there was only minimal narrowing of the visual fields and normal pupils, but evidence of corneal involvement. With the exception of the ankle jerks, deep tendon reflexes were present bilaterally. Further findings were dysarthria and diabetes. Diabetes, dysarthria and bilateral ptosis were also found in a patient of HEYCOCK and WILSON (1958); in addition, there was weakness of the rectus externus muscles of the eyes. In another case, which was diagnosed as Refsum's disease (SAUER 1964), diabetes, paresis of ocular muscles and dysarthria existed in conjunction with the typical symptomatology of HAP. Only in the youngest of the cases mentioned in this paragraph (BAUM et al. 1965) were fatty acids analyzed. Since in this patient plasma, urinary and liver lipids did not contain phytanic acid, he certainly does not belong to the category which is now designated as HAP. The same applies to the last mentioned unpublished case, where serum, liver, spleen and muscle lipids were examined (KAHLKE 1964a). The case of OLESON (1957) which has already been reported as an atypical one and those of HEYCOCK and WILSON (1958), and RAVIN and SCHWARTZ (1962) cannot be classified correctly without the results of lipid analyses. Accumulation of phytanic acid should be considered the only pathognomonic finding for HAP.

Treatment

As yet, there are no reports of any successful therapy for HAP. Generally employed methods for treatment of neuritis, such as the administration of adrenocortical steroids and B-vitamins have not resulted in significant improvement. Based on the assumption that phytanic acid is the harmful agent and that it is synthesized mainly from exogenous phytol, it appears reasonable to restrict the intake of dietary phytol. Such trials employing chlorophyll-free diets are presently in progress. It remains to be seen whether this procedure results in significant lowering of the plasma and total body phytanic acid content, and whether elimination of phytanic acid will prevent progression of the disease or result in clinical improvement (ELDJARN et al. 1966 b).

Pathogenetic Aspects

The cause of the disease is not known. By analogy with other storage diseases, it is suspected that accumulation of phytanic acid is closely related to the basic cause of HAP. Since lipids are important for the structure and function of the nervous system, it is likely that the morphologic changes observed are related to the appearance of the atypical lipid. However, the abnormalities are not specific; similar polyneuritic changes are seen in disorders where phytanic acid does not play any role.

No information is available on the pathogenesis of the cardiac disturbances which are frequent in HAP, although large amounts of phytanic acid can be found in the heart. Cardiac disturbances occur frequently in heredoataxic diseases, particularly in Friedreich's disease and Pierre-Marie's disease (BERGMANN 1921, HALLERVORDEN 1936, SJÖGREN 1943, REFSUM 1946 b); they are not found in neurospinal amyotrophy and other disorders which should be considered in differential diagnosis.

The mechanism by which accumulation of phytanic acid may produce the features of the disease is not known. The possibility of competitive depression of another, essential fatty acid is not supported by available data; low concentrations of acids, such as linoleic or other polyenoic acids are relative rather than absolute when the increase in total lipid content of involved organs is considered. It is possible that certain effects result from the particular molecular structure of phytanic acid, since it possesses four methyl groups and is considerably less polar than acids of similar chain length (palmitic) on one hand and the straight chain fatty acids with the same number of carbon atoms (C-20, eicosanoic acid) on the other. The methyl groups rather than the carboxyl group may determine the behaviour of the acid and its interactions, for instance, with membrane lipids of nerves or with the conducting system.

From this point of view the retinal changes are of particular interest. While phytanic acid could well play an (unfavorable) role in the rhodopsine cycle (WALD 1960, BAUM et al. 1965), in the majority of patients with pigmentary retinitis this change develops in the absence of phytanic acid storage, either as a disease of its own or during the course of other disorders such as a-beta-lipoproteinemia (see page 382).

While practically no information is available on the effect of an accumulation of phytanic acid in the production of tissue lesions, information is beginning to come forth on the cause of its accumulation.

Theories on the in vivo synthesis of phytanic acid concentrate mainly on two possibilities. One of them deals with the possible formation of phytanic acid from isopren units or four molecules of mevalonic acid (or mevalonate), (KAHLKE 1964a, KAHLKE and RICHTERICH 1965). Instead of an end-to-end condensation of two molecules of farnesyl pyrophosphate which results in the formation of squalene and finally cholesterol, a fourth active isoprenoid unit might be attached to farnesyl pyrophosphate. From this intermediate several steps of hydrogenation and oxidation would be required for the formation of phytanic acid. This hypothesis now appears unlikely since STEINBERG (1965) was unable to detect any activity in the phytanic acid fraction after administration of labeled mevalonate to a patient with HAP (case T.E. of REFSUM).

The other possible pathway for the formation of phytanic acid is its synthesis from phytol which is the corresponding alpha-beta-monounsaturated alcohol. STOFFEL and KAHLKE (1965), administering tritium labeled phytol orally to a patient with HAP (case W. M., HARDERS and DIECKMANN 1964), found significant amounts of label in the phytanic acid fraction of the plasma, while other fatty acids did not contain any radioactivity, proving that phytanic acid can be formed from exogenous phytol in HAP (see figure 11). Their findings were confirmed shortly thereafter by STEINBERG et al. (1965a and b) in animal experiments, and in patients with HAP. Further studies (KAHLKE et al. 1965, KAHLKE and WAGENER 1966) showed that labeled phytanic acid could be recovered in each plasma lipid fraction.

The natural source of exogenous phytol is mainly dietary chlorophyll which contains about 30% of phytol. The extent to which the alcohol is split from the chlorophyll molecule, and its absorption characteristics are not yet known.

It is not certain whether phytol is transformed to phytanic acid via the alpha-beta-unsaturated (phytenic) acid, or wether phytanic acid is formed by hydration of phytol to dihydrophytol and consecutive oxidation. The latter possibility seems to be more likely. While a small amount of phytenic acid was found in beta-lipoprotein triglycerides (KAHLKE 1965, KAHLKE and WAGENER 1966a), and in urinary and bile lipids of some cases of HAP by gas liquid chromatography no labeled phytenic acid, as shown upon oxidative ozonolysis of the phytanic acid fraction was found in plasma lipids of a case of HAP after labeled phytol had been administered orally (STOFFEL and KAHLKE 1965).

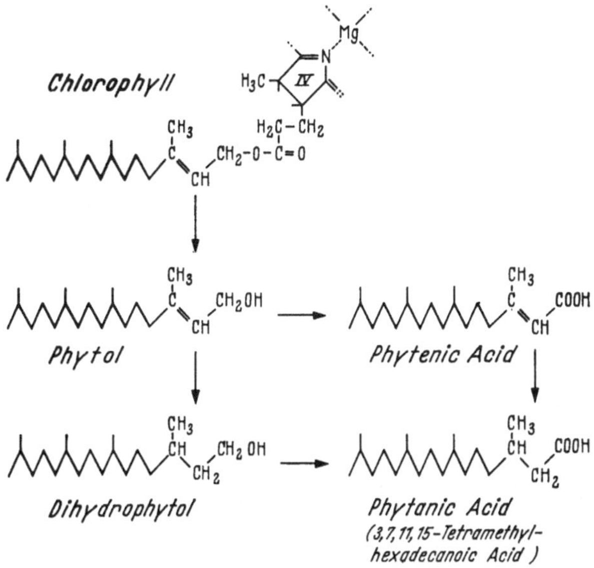

Chlorophyll

Phytol

Phytenic Acid

Dihydrophytol

Phytanic Acid
(3,7,11,15-Tetramethyl-hexadecanoic Acid)

Fig. 11. Hypothetical scheme of formation of phytanic acid from phytol. Exogenous sources of phytol may be chlorophyll or other compounds containing the isoprenoid or phytyl-side chain, such as phyllochinone

Elucidation of a possible defect in the degradation of phytanic acid requires information on the catabolic pathway. Oxidation of phytanic acid in HAP is apparently very slow (STEINBERG 1965). Only 10% of the [14]CO$_2$ which is formed from ^{14}C-labeled phytanic acid in normal subjects appeared in the expired air of patients with HAP during the first 12 hours (STEINBERG et al. 1965b). According to a suggestion of ELDJARN (1965a, ELDJARN et al. 1965b) phytanic acid accumulates as a result of impaired omega-oxidation. When three patients with HAP were given 25 gm tricaprin by mouth, less than 50 mg sebacic acid was excreted in the urine over 24 hours in each case, while the corresponding amounts of sebacic acid excreted in 18 normal subjects lay between 190 and 1180 mg (with one exception where excretion was 16 mg). However, other substances such as geraniol and 2,2-dimethyloctadecanoic acid, which cannot be oxidized at the beta-carbon atom because of the presence of a methyl group at this position, and which (like cholesterol and alpha-tocopherol) are oxidized only at the terminal carbon atom, are degraded normally by patients with HAP (ELDJARN et al. 1966a). Therefore, the authors suggest, there may be an alternative mode of degrading branched-chain fatty acids, which possibly includes a CO$_2$-fixation step, in addition to beta-oxidation, omega-oxidation and the breakdown mechanism of isovaleric acid. This pathway may be impaired in HAP.

Information on the pathogenesis of HAP can be summarized as follows: It could be shown that phytanic acid can be formed in the body. Very probably, impaired catabolism results in the accumulation of this material. The localization of this defect is not known. It remains to be shown whether the accumulation of phytanic acid is directly responsible for neurologic and neuro-ophthalmologic symptoms, or whether the defect which leads to the accumulation of phytanic acid, involves other metabolic processes, the impairment of which may in turn produce the symptoms of HAP.

References

ALEXANDER, W. S.: Phytanic acid in Refsum's syndrome. J. Neurol. Neurosurg. Psychiat. (1966) **29**, 412. Personal communication.

ALFANO, J. E., and J. P. BERGER: Retinitis pigmentosa, ophthalmoplegia, and spastic quadriplegia. Amer. J. Ophthal. **43**, 231 (1957).

ASHENHURST, E., J. MILLAR, and T. MILLIKEN: Refsum's syndrome affecting a brother and two sisters. Brit. Med. J. **1958/II**, 415.

BARNARD. R. I., and R. O. SCHOLZ: Ophthalmoplegia and retinal degeneration. Amer. J. Ophthal. **27**, 621 (1944).

BAUM, J. L., M. TANNENBAUM, and E. H. KOLODNY: Refsum's syndrome with corneal involvement. Amer. J. Ophthal. **60**, 699 (1965).

BERGMANN, E.: Studies in Heredo ataxia. Uppsala Läk.-Fören. Förh. **26**, 1 (1921).

BILLETER, M., W. BOLLIGER u. C. MARTIUS: Untersuchungen über die Umwandlung von verfütterten K-Vitaminen durch Austausch der Seitenkette und die Rolle der Darmbakterien hierbei. Biochem. Z. **340**, 290 (1964).

BILLINGS, J. J., J. O'CALLAGHAN, and K. O'DAY: Refsum's syndrome: Heredopathia atactica polyneuritiformis. Trans. ophthal. Soc. Aust. **17**, 131 (1957).

BJURSTAM, N., B. HALLGREN, R. RYHAGE u. S. STÄLLBERG-STENHAGEN: Cit. by STENHAGEN: Massenspectrometrie als Hilfsmittel bei der Strukturbestimmung organischer Verbindungen, besonders bei Lipiden und Peptiden. Z. analyt. Chem. **181**, 462 (1961).

BLANC, M., A. SEILHCAN, J. JULIEN et BOURGEOIS: Maladie de Refsum: Limites du syndrome de Guillain-Barré. Ann. méd.-psychol. **1**, 732 (1963).

CAMMERMEYER, J.: Om de anatomiske Gunn i to tilfelle av dr. Refsum's materiale av "et tidligere ikke beskrevet (?) familiaert syndrom". Nord. Med. **29**, 617 (1946).

— Neuropathological changes in hereditary neuropathies: manifestation of the syndrome heredopathia atactica polyneuritiformis in the presence of interstitial hypertrophic polyneuropathy. J. Neuropath. exp. Neurol. **15**, 340 (1956).

— W. HAYMAKER, and S. REFSUM: Heredopathia atactica polyneuritiformis: The neuropathologic changes in three adults and one child. Amer. J. Path. **30**, 643 (1954).

CASON, J., G. SUMRELL, C. F. ALLEN, G. A. GILLIES and S. ELBERG: Certain characteristics of the fatty acids from the lipides of the tubercle bacillus. J. biol. Chem. **205**, 435 (1953).

CHAMLIN, M., and E. BILLET: Ophthalmoplegia and pigmentary degeneration of the retina. Arch. Ophthal. **43**, 217 (1950).

CLARK, D. B.: Heredopathia atactica polyneuritiformis. J. Neuropath. exp. Neurol. **9**, 385 (1951).

CLAUSS, O.: Über hereditäre cerebellare Ataxie in Verbindung mit Pigmentdegeneration und Degeneration des N. cochlearis. Z. ges. Neurol. Psychiat. **23**, 294 (1924).

DEREUX, J.: Maladie de Refsum. VII. Int. Congres Neurol., Roma. Excerpta med. (Amst.). Int. Congr. Series **38**, 103 (1961).

— La maladie de Refsum. Rev. Neurol. **109**, 599 (1963).

— Personal communication (1965).

— and J. E. GRUNER: Maladie de Refsum. Étude d'une biopsie nerveuse au microscope électronique. Rev. neurol. **109**, 564 (1963a).

— — Maladie de Refsum. Étude biopsique d'un nerf au microscope électronique. Soc. Franç. de Neurologie, Séance du novembre 1963b.

DUNCAN, W. R. H., and G. A. GARTON: Blood lipids. 3. Plasma lipids of the cow during pregnancy and lactation. Biochem. J. **89**, 414 (1963).

DUREUX, J. B.: Les génopathies et embryopathies neuro-ophtalmiques. Encéphale **3**, 253 (1957).

EDSTRÖM, R., O. GRÖNTOFT, and H. SANDRING: Refsum's disease. Three siblings, one autopsy. Acta psychiat. scand. **34**, 40 (1959).

ELDJARN, L.: Heredopathia atactica polyneuritiformis (Refsum's disease) — A defect in the omega-oxidation mechanism of fatty acids. Scand. J. clin. Lab. Invest. **17**, 178 (1965a).

— Biokjemiske synspunkter pa phytansyrens opprinelse. Nord. Med. **73**, 571 (1965b).

— K. TRY, and O. STOKKE: Abnormal serum protein pattern in Refsum's disease. Scand. J. clin. Lab. Invest. **17**, Suppl. 86, 137 (1965a).

— — — Studies on the defect in the degradation of branched-chain fatty acid structures in Refsum's disease. Scand. J. clin. Lab. Invest. **17**, Suppl. 86, 138 (1965b).

— — — The existence of an alternative pathway for the degradation of branched-chain fatty acids, and its failure in heredopathia atactica polyneuritiformis (Refsum's disease). Biochim. biophys. Acta (Amst.) **116**, 395 (1966a).

ELDJARN, L., K. TRY, O. STOKKE, A. M. MUNTHE-KAAS, S. REFSUM, D. STEINBERG, J. AVIGAN, and C. MIZE: Dietary effects on serum-phytanic acid levels and on clinical manifestations in heredopathia atactica polyneuritiformis. Lancet 1966 b/I, 691.

ERDBRINK, W. L.: Ocular myopathy associated with retinitis pigmentosa. Arch. Ophthal. 57, 335 (1957).

FISHER, M.: Unusual variant of acute idiopathic polyneuritis syndrome of ophthalmoplegia, ataxia and areflexia. New. Engl. J. Med. 255, 57 (1956).

FLEMING, R.: Refsum's syndrome. An unusual hereditary neuropathy. Neurology (Minneap.) 7, 476 (1957).

FRANCESCHETTI, A., J. FRANÇOIS et J. BABEL: Les hérédo-dégénérescenses chorio-rétiniennes (dégénérescenses tapéto-rétiniennes), p. 851 et 1085. Paris: Masson 1963.

FREYCON, F.: Revue critique. Le syndrome de Refsum. Pédiatrie 16, 411 (1961).

GELLERSTEDT, in: KJELLSON (1953).

GLOBUS, J. H.: Ein Beitrag zur Histopathologie der amaurotischen Idiotie (mit besonderer Berücksichtigung der Beziehungen zu den hereditären Kleinhirnerkrankungen und zur Merzbacher-Pelizaeusschen Krankheit). Z. ges. Neurol. Psychiat. 85, 424 (1923).

— Amaurotic family idiocy. J. Mt Sinai Hosp. 9, 451 (1942); cited after REESE and BARETA, 1950.

GOODWIN, R. F., and C. M. POSER: Ophthalmoplegia, ataxia and areflexia. J. Amer. med. Ass. 186, 258 (1963).

GORDON, N., and R. E. B. HUDSON: Refsum's Syndrome. Heredopathia atactica polyneuritiformis. A report of three cases, including a study of the cardiac pathology. Brain 82, 41 (1959).

GREENFIELD, J. G.: Diseases of the lower motor and sensory neurones (peripheral neuritis and neuropathy) in hypertrophic interstitial neuropathy of Déjérine and Sottas (heredopathia atactica polyneuritiformis Refsum). In: Neuropathology. Ed.: Arnold, p. 607. London 1958.

HALLERVORDEN, J.: Die hereditäre Ataxie. In: Bumke, O., and O. Foerster (Herausgeb.): Handbuch der Neurologie, Bd. 16, S. 657. Berlin: Springer 1936.

HANSEN, R. P.: 3, 7, 11, 15-tetramethylhexadecanoic acid: its occurrence in sheep fat. N. Z. J. Sci. 8, 158 (1965a).

— 3, 7, 11, 15-tetramethylhexadecanoic acid: its occurrence in the tissues of humans afflicted with Refsum's syndrome. Biochem. biophys. Acta (Amst.) 106, 304 (1965b).

— Occurrence of 3, 7, 11, 15-tetramethylhexadecanoic acid in ox perinephric fat. Chem. Industry 1965c, 303.

— and F. B. SHORLAND: The branched chain fatty acids of butter fat. II. The isolation of a multibranched C_{20} saturated fatty acid fraction. Biochem. J. 50, 358 (1951).

— — Biochem. J. 55, 662 (1953); cited after HANSEN (1965 b).

— — and J. D. MORRISON: Identification of a C_{20} multibranched fatty acid from butterfat as 3, 7, 11, 15-tetramethylhexadecanoic acid. J. Dairy Res. 32, 21 (1965).

HARDERS, H., u. H. DIECKMANN: Heredopathia atactica polyneuritiformis. Klinik und Diagnostik des Refsum-Syndroms. Dtsch. med. Wschr. 89, 248 (1964).

HEYCOCK, J. B., and J. WILSON: Diabetes mellitus in a child showing features of Refsum's syndrome. Arch. Dis. Childh. 33, 320 (1958).

JAGER, B. V., H. L. FRED, R. B. BUTLER, and W. H. CARNES: Occurrence of retinal pigmentation, ophthalmoplegia, ataxia, deafness and heart block. Report of a case with findings at autopsy. Amer. J. Med. 29, 888 (1960).

JÉQUIER, M., et E. B. STREIFF: Paraplégie, dystrophie scelettique et dégénérescense tapéto-rétinienne familiale. Arch. Klaus-Stift. Vererb.-Forsch. 22, 129 (1947).

KAHLKE, W.: Über das Vorkommen von 3, 7, 11, 15-Tetramethylhexadecansäure im Blutserum bei Refsum-Syndrom. Klin. Wschr. 41, 783 (1963).

— Refsum-Syndrom. — Lipoidchemische Untersuchungen bei 9 Fällen. Klin. Wschr. 42, 1011 (1964a).

— Unpublished results (1964b).

— Lipoide (Lipide). Fortschr. Med. 83, 517, 552 u. 634 (1965).

— and R. RICHTERICH: Refsums disease (heredopathia atactica polyneuritiformis): An inborn error of lipid metabolism with storage of 3, 7, 11, 15-tetramethylhexadecanoic acid. II. Isolation and identification of the storage product. Amer. J. Med. 39, 237 (1965).

— and H. WAGENER: Destribution of 3, 7, 11, 15-tetramethylhexadecanoic acid between plasma lipoproteins in Refsum's syndrome. In: Protides of the biological fluids, XIII. Colloquium Brugge 1965, p. 351. Ed.: H. Peeters. Amsterdam: Elsevier 1966a.

— — Conversion of ³H-phytol to phytanic acid and its incorporation into plasma fractions in heredopathia atactica polyneuritiformis. Metabolism 15, 687 (1966b).

— u. H. DIECKMANN: Untersuchungen über den Phytolstoffwechsel bei der Lipidose Heredopathia atactica polyneuritiformis (Refsum-Syndrom): Umwandlung von ³H-Phytol in die 3. 7. 11. 15-Tetramethylhexadecansäure (Phytansäure) der Plasmalipoidfraktionen. Klin. Wschr. 43, 1345 (1965).

KEARNS, T. P., and G. P. SAYRE: Retinitis pigmentosa, external ophthalmoplegia and complete heart block. Arch. Ophthal. **60**, 280 (1958).

KJELLSON, L.: Refsum sjuledom. Refsum's disease. Nord. Med. **49**, 460 (1953).

KLENK, E., u. W. KAHLKE: Über das Vorkommen der 3, 7, 11, 15-Tetramethylhexadecansäure (Phytansäure) in den Cholesterinestern und anderen Lipoidfraktionen der Organe bei einem Krankheitsfall unbekannter Genese. Verdacht auf Heredopathia atactica polyneuritiformis (Refsum-Syndrom). Hoppe Seylers Z. physiol. Chem. **333**, 133 (1963).

LOUGH, A. K.: Isolation of 3, 7, 11, 15-tetramethylhexadecanoic acid from ox plasma. Biochem. J. **86**, 14 (1963).

— Blood lipids. 4. The isolation of 3, 7, 11, 15-tetramethylhexadecanoic acid (phytanic acid) from ox-plasma lipids. Biochem. J. **91**, 584 (1964).

NORDHAGEN, E., and J. GRÖNDAHL: Heredopathia atactica polyneuritiformis (Refsum's disease). Acta ophthal. (Kbh.) **42**, 629 (1964).

OLESEN, TH. B.: A case of heredopathia atactica polyneuritiformis (Morbus Refsum). Acta psychiat. scand. **32**, 83 (1957).

PECKER, J., Y. M. FEUVRIER et Y. LEHUEROU: Maladie de Refsum. Diagnostic avec certaines polyradiculonévrites à rechutes. Rev. neurol. **109**, 1 (1963).

PETIT, J. F.: Le syndrome de Refsum. Les manifestations ophthalmologiques à propos d'une observation. Thèse, Rennes, No. 354 (1963).

PRIOR, I.: Personal communication (1966).

RAVIN, B., and H. SCHWARTZ: Case report: Refsum's disease. Anesthesiology **23**, 269 (1962).

REESE, H., and J. BARETA: Heredopathia atactica polyneuritiformis. J. Neuropath. exp. Neurol. **9**, 385 (1950).

REFSUM, S.: Staff meeting Rikshospitalet, Oslo, June 1944.

— Heredoataxia hemeralopica polyneuritiformis — et tidligere ikke beskrevet familiaert syndrom? En foreløbig meddelelse. Nord. Med. **28**, 2682 (1945).

— Et tidligere ikke beskrevet (?) familiaert syndrom: "Heredoataxia hemeralopica polyneuritiformis". Nord. Med. **29**, 617 (1946a).

— Heredopathia atactica polyneuritiformis. A familial syndrome not hitherto described. Acta psychiat. scand. Suppl. **38** (1946b).

— Heredopathia atactica polyneuritiformis. J. nerv. ment. Dis. **116**, 1046 (1952).

— Heredopathia atactica polyneuritiformis. Acta genet. (Basel) **7**, 344 (1957).

— Heredopathia atactica polyneuritiformis. Wld Neurol. **1**, 334 (1960).

— Heredopathia atactica polyneuritiformis, en metabolisk betinget nervesykdom. Nord. Med. **73**, 570 (1965).

— Personal communication (1966).

— L. SALOMONSEN, and M. SKATVEDT: Heredopathia atactica polyneuritiformis in children; a preliminary communication. J. Pediat. **35**, 335 (1949).

RICHTERICH, R., W. KAHLKE, P. VAN MECHELEN u. E. ROSSI: Refsum's Syndrom (Heredopathia atactica polyneuritiformis): Ein angeborener Defekt im Lipoidstoffwechsel mit Speicherung von 3, 7, 11, 15-Tetramethylhexadecansäure. Klin. Wschr. **41**, 800 (1963).

— H. MOSER, and E. ROSSI: Refsum's disease (heredopathia atactica polyneuritiformis). An inborn error of lipid metabolism with storage of 3, 7, 11, 15-tetramethylhexadecanoic acid. A review of the clinical findings. Humangenetik **1**, 322 (1965a).

ROOS, B., P. VAN MECHELEN and E. ROSSI: Refsum's disease (heredopathia atactica polyneuritiformis): An inborn error of lipid metabolism with storage of 3, 7, 11, 15-tetramethylhexadecanoic acid. I. Report of a case. Amer. J. Med. **39**, 230 (1965b).

— and R. RICHTERICH: Refsum's disease (heredopathia atactica polyneuritiformis): An inborn error of lipid metabolism with storage of 3, 7, 11, 15-tetramethylhexadecanoic acid. V. Biochemical, histological and electron microscopical studies on biopsy material from the liver and the kidney. (In preparation.) Cited by RICHTERICH et al. (1965a).

ROTH, M.: On a possible relationship between hereditary ataxia and peroneal muscular atrophy; with a critical review of the problems of "intermediate forms" in the degenerative disorders of the central nervous system. Brain **71**, 416 (1948).

SABOURAUD, O.: Personal communication (1965/1966).

SAIFER, A., and S. GERSTENFIELD: Photometric determination of sialic acid in serum and in cerebrospinal fluid with the thiobarbituric acid method. Clin. chim. Acta **7**, 467 (1962).

SAKAGAMY, T., and D. B. ZILVERSMITH: Separation of dog serum lipoproteins by ultracentrifugation, dextran sulfate precipitation, and paper electrophoresis. J. Lipid Res. **3**, 111 (1962).

SALOMONSEN, L., and M. SKATVEDT: Four cases of heredopathia atactica polyneuritiformis (Refsum) in children. Acta paediat. (Uppsala) Suppl. **77**, 44 (1949).

SAUER: Personal communication (unpublished data) 1964.

SAUNDERS, M., and M. RAKE: Familial Guillain-Barré Syndrome. Lancet **1965/II**, 1106.

SJÖGREN, T.: Klinische und erbbiologische Untersuchungen über die Heredoataxien. Acta psychiat. scand. Suppl. **27**, 1 (1943).

Smith, J. L., and F. B. Walsh: Syndrome of external ophthalmoplegia, ataxia, and areflexia (Fisher). Arch. Ophthal. **58**, 109 (1957).

Sonneveld, Z. W., P. Haverkamp-Begeman, G. J. van Beers, R. Keuning, and J. C. M. Schogt: 3.7.11.15-tetramethylhexadecanoic acid: a constituent of butter-fat. J. Lipid. Res. **3**, 351 (1962).

Steinberg, D.: Remarks on the biochemical basis of Refsum's disease. Nord. Med. **73**, 571 (1965).

— J. Avigan, C. Mize, and J. Baxter: Phytanic acid formation and accumulation in phytol-fed rats. Biochem. biophys. Res. Commun. **19**, 412 (1965a).

— — — L. Eldjarn, K. Try, and S. Refsum: Conversion of U-C^{14}-phytol to phytanic acid and its oxydation in heredopathia atactica polyneuritiformis. Biochem. biophys. Res. Commun. **19**, 783 (1965b).

Stoffel, W., and W. Kahlke: The transformation of phytol into 3, 7, 11, 15-tetramethyl-hexadecanoic (phytanic) acid in heredopathia atactica polyneuritiformis (Refsum's syndrome). Biochem. biophys. Res. Commun. **19**, 1 (1965).

Thiébaut, J., J. Lemoyne et L. Guillaumat: Deux syndromes oto-neuro-oculistiques d'origene congenitale. Leurs rapports avec les placomatoses de van der Stolve et autres dysplasies neuro-ectodermiques. Rev. neurol. **72**, 71 (1939).

— — — Maladie de Refsum. Rev. neurol. **104**, 152 (1961).

Toussaint, D., C. Coers et N. Toppet: Heredopathia atactica polyneuritiformis (syndrome de Refsum). Constatation cliniques et biopsiques. Bull. Soc. belge Ophtal. **122**, 383 (1959).

Try, K., O. Stokke, and L. Eldjarn: Two new cases of heredopathia atactica polyneuritiformis (Refsums syndrome). Demonstrated phytanic acid accumulation. Scand. J. clin. Lab. Invest. **17**, Suppl. **86**, 195 (1965).

Veltema, A. N., et A. Verjaal: Sur un cas d'hérédopathie ataxique polyneuritique. Maladie de Refsum. Rev. neurol. **104**, 15 (1961).

Wald, G.: The visual function of the vitamins A. Vitam. and Horm. **18**, 417 (1960).

Walsh, F. B.: Clinical Neuro-Ophthalmology. Baltimore: Williams & Wilkins 1947.

A-ß-Lipoproteinemia

By

W. Kahlke

Synonyms: Bassen-Kornzweig syndrome, familial low density lipoprotein deficiency, acanthocytosis.

Definition and Introduction

A-β-lipoproteinemia has been known for 15 years. It is characterized by neuromuscular disturbances, mainly progressive ataxic neuropathy, by retinal changes consisting of atypical pigmentary retinitis with involvement of the macula, by deficiency or lack of serum β-lipoproteins, by morphologic abnormalities of red cells (acanthocytosis) and by steatorrhea. Lack of β-lipoproteins and acanthocytosis are found in all cases. They are specific symptoms and exist from birth, while other symptoms may occur in other disorders as well. Ataxic neuropathy and retinitis pigmentosa may or may not develop during the course of the disease, and steatorrhea or a celiac syndrome are early symptoms in most cases, but may not be found in others.

As long as incomplete knowledge of the pathogenesis of the disease prevents the use of a more specific term, the name Bassen-Kornzweig syndrome or a-β-lipoproteinemia should be used.

Historical Review

BASSEN and KORNZWEIG, in 1950, described the case of an 18 year-old Jewish girl with atypical retinitis pigmentosa and degenerative central nervous system disease affecting the cerebellum, the long tracts of the spinal cord and the peripheral nerves. The red cells showed irregular pseudopodia giving them a crenated appearance, and there was impaired rouleaux formation. The course of the disease in the 11 year-old brother of the patient was described by the same authors in 1957, and results of detailed metabolic studies and laboratory data were reported by EDER (1962) and SCHWARTZ et al. (1963) who also noted the lack of β-lipoproteins which had been found by SALT et al. (1960), LAMY et al. (1960), and MABRY et al. (1960) in their respective patients.

In 1952 SINGER et al. described the red cell changes and progressive ataxic neuropathy in a 13½ year-old boy, and coined the term "acanthrocytosis" for the former abnormality, which they thought was due to an hereditary disturbance of a control system for normal red cell architecture. Later, DRUEZ (1959) and others used the etymologically correct form "acanthocytosis" (acanthos = thorn or sharp point). A reexamination of the case of SINGER et al. (1952) by JAMPEL and FALLS (1958) now revealed the presence of retinopathy and steatorrhea. The ataxic neuropathy had become more marked, and the serum cholesterol level was 37 mg/100 ml. The fourth case of a-β-lipoproteinemia was studied by DRUEZ (1959) and by DRUEZ et al. (1961). Their 30 year-old patient exhibited non-pigmentary retinitis, a serum cholesterol level of 60 mg/100 ml, steatorrhea and ataxia since childhood. In addition, hyperglycemia and diabetic acidosis developed in this patient; she had three miscarriages and one hypotrophic infant, who died from pneumonia at the age of two months. The authors (1961) described "acanthocytosis" as a disease with congenital lack of β-lipoproteins.

This lack of serum β-lipoproteins had been found one year earlier by SALT et al. (1960) in a 17 months-old girl, who had episodes of diarrhea and vomiting since the age of five weeks and who later developed anemia and acanthocytosis. SALT et al. discussed the pathogenetic significance of a very low serum concentration of vitamin A for the development of ataxia and retinopathy, and attempted replacement therapy. The sixth and seventh patients with Bassen-Kornzweig syndrome were described during the same year (1960) by LAMY et al. and by MABRY et al. respectively; neither of their patients had retinopathy but in both serum β-lipoproteins were absent. The next case of the syndrome is probably that of a 36 year-old man (FRIEDMAN et al. 1960) with hypocholesterolemia (25—45 mg/100 ml), signs of sprue, neurologic symptoms and polydactyly. β-lipoproteins were not determined but acanthocytosis was found. Other cases described during 1960 and later were those of MIER et al. (1960), WOLFF and BAUMAN (1961), WAYS et al. (1962) and KUO and BASSETT (1962). Results of metabolic studies, nerve biopsies and muscle biopsies were published by SCHWARTZ et al. (1963) for a case of their own and for a patient of KORNZWEIG and BASSEN (1957). In the latter case demyelination of peripheral nerves was noted.

The first patient with a-β-lipoproteinemia who came to autopsy had died from heart-failure at the age of 37 years (SOBREVILLA et al. 1964). In her bilateral pes cavus deformities had necessitated orthopedic measures at age 15; the initial diagnosis of Friedreich ataxia was later dropped in favor of the diagnosis "spinocerebellar degeneration", type Roussy-Levy. Post-mortem findings included demyelination of anterior columns and spino-cerebellar tracts.

The 15th case of a-β-lipoproteinemia is that of a 7 year-old boy (FORSYTH et al. 1965), who exhibited, in addition to all symptoms described, congenital abnormalities of the toes and signs of mental retardation. The latter feature had already been described for the cases of SINGER et al. (1952), LAMY et al. (1960), and DRUEZ et al. (1961).

A-β-lipoproteinemia in a Maori child, who died at the age of 18 months, was described by BECROFT et al. (1965). In addition to the typical symptoms of the disease, disturbances of renal function with aminoaciduria and recurrent pulmonary infections were noted in this child.

The most recent reports of a-β-lipoproteinemia are those by AHRENS et al. (1966) and FREDRICKSON et al. (1966). Clinical data in 20 cases of a-β-lipoproteinemia are summarized in table 1.

Incidence (Age, Sex, Race, Family)

Although the cardinal symptom, namely a-β-lipoproteinemia exists from birth, the disease may not become manifest before adolescence or adult life. Frequently, however, diarrhea starts immediately after birth or during the first weeks and months. The youngest patients were 17 months old at the time of diagnosis (SALT et al. 1960; BECROFT et al. 1965), the oldest 36 years (FRIEDMAN et al. 1960). Of the 20 reported cases 14 are males and six are females. Familial occurrence has been observed by BASSEN and KORNZWEIG (1950/1957) and KUO and BASSETT (1962), who described acanthocytosis in the three siblings of their 41 year-old patient. Neuromuscular disability was an additional feature in one of them. Serum α-lipoproteins and S_f 0—12 β-lipoproteins were slightly increased in the mother,

Table 1. *Clinical data in 20 cases of α-β-lipoproteinemia**

Case No.	References (first description of case)	Case**	Ethnic origin	Year born**	Sex (m = males, f = females)	Consanguinity	β-lipoprotein deficiency	Decreased α-lipoproteins	Hypocholesterolemia	Acanthocytosis	Anemia (permanent or transitory)	Steatorrhea	Neurological signs, particularly ataxia	Retinal involvement	Mental retardation	Cardiac manifestations	Skeletal deformities	Lipid storage by small bowel mucosa	Muscle biopsy (M.B.), nerve biopsy (N.B.), or autopsy (A.)
1	BASSEN and KORNZWEIG (1950)	R.K.	Jewish	1932	f		+		+	+	+	+	+	+	–	+			M.B.
2	KORNZWEIG and BASSEN (1957)	L.Z.	Jewish	1938	m	+	+		+	+		+	+	+	–	+			N.B.
3	SINGER et al. (1952)	R.C.	Jewish	1938	m	+			+	+	+	+	++	+	++		++	+	
4	DRUEZ (1959)	C.S.	French	1927	f	–			+	+	+	+	+	–	++			+	
5	SALT et al. (1960)	G.F.	English	1958	f		+	+	+	+	+	+	(±)	–	+				
6	LAMY et al. (1960)	C.R.	French	1953	m				+	+		+	+	–					
7	MABRY et al. (1960)	M.R.	Negro	1947	f		+		+	+		+	+	–					
8	DiGEORGE et al. (1966)	N.S.	Negro	1950	m		+		+	+		+	+	+					
9	FRIEDMAN et al. (1960)	A.C.	Jewish	1923	m	–	+		+	+	(±)	+	++	+			++	+	
10	MIER et al. (1960)	R.B.	Jewish	1943	m		+	+	+	+		+	++	–	–				
11	WOLF and BAUMAN (1961)	M.S.	Jewish	1956	m		+	+	+	+		+	+	+|					
12	WAYS et al. (1961)		Jewish	1954	m		+		+	+		+	+	–					
13	KUO and BASSETT (1962)***	R.I.	Jewish	1953	m		+		+	+	+	+	+(±)	+	+		+	+	
14	SCHWARTZ et al. (1963)	A.E.	Italian	1926(?)	f	+	+		+	+	+	+	++	+	–		+		M.B.
15	SOBREVILLA et al. (1964)	J.M.	Maori	1962	m	++		+	+	+			++	+|	–	–	+++		N.B.
16	BECROFT et al. (1965)	A.L.	Scottish	1956	m	++	++		+++	+++	+		+	–	–				A.
17	FORSYTH et al. (1965)	J.G.	Old Amer.	1957	m		++		+++	+++			+(±)			++	+++		
18	WAYS (1966)												+	+	+	+			
19	FARQUHAR et al. (1966)	J.V.	Italian	1953	m		++		++	++		++			–				
20	FARQUHAR et al. (1966)	A.V.	Italian	1957	f		++		++	++		++		+	+				

* In a number of cases some of the symptoms were diagnosed during a later reexamination by the same or by another author.

** Names and dates of birth are from SIMON and WAYS (1964), unless mentioned in the original case reports.

*** Abstract without detailed description of case (41 year old white male).

HDL$_3$ and S$_f$ 0—400 lipoproteins decreased in the patient and his three siblings. In seven of the reported cases there was consanguinity of the parents (BASSEN and KORNZWEIG 1950; SINGER et al. 1952; KORNZWEIG and BASSEN 1957; DRUEZ 1959; LAMY et al. 1961; BECROFT et al. 1965; FORSYTH et al. 1965). The incidence of mental retardation was increased in the offspring of these marriages (FORSYTH et al. 1965).

Heterozygotes, in general, are asymptomatic and do not exhibit acanthocytosis. Exceptions may be the case of a maternal uncle of the patient of MIER et al. (1960), who at the age of 19 developed ataxic neuropathy and deterioration of vision, and who expired at the age of 27 years. A paternal cousin of the same patient had instability of gait and impairment of vision at the age of 6 years (cit. after SCHWARTZ et al. 1963). SALT et al. (1960) examined all four grandparents, the parents and two maternal uncles of their patient. Serum lipids were abnormal in both parents and in the paternal grandfather, the level of β-lipoproteins being one half of normal. Total lipids, cholesterol and phospholipids were decreased accordingly. Chylomicrons were observed in both parents after a fatty meal.

Normal β-lipoprotein levels were found in other heterozygotes (WAYS et al. 1963). FORSYTH et al. (1965) even reported elevation of S$_f$ 3—9 β-lipoproteins, of total lipids and cholesterol in both parents, in the maternal grandmother, and in two siblings of the mother of his case. α-lipoproteins tended to be low. One sibling of the mother and a sister of the father had normal serum lipid levels.

In this disease, too, there is a predilection for the Jewish race. Five of the reported cases were of Jewish ancestry (BASSEN and KORNZWEIG 1950; SINGER et al. 1952; KORNZWEIG and BASSEN 1957; MIER et al. 1960; WAYS et al. 1961). The remaining patients came from English, French and Italo-American families; one case each was of Negro and Maori origin. The mode of transmission appears to be autosomal recessive (see chapter on genetics).

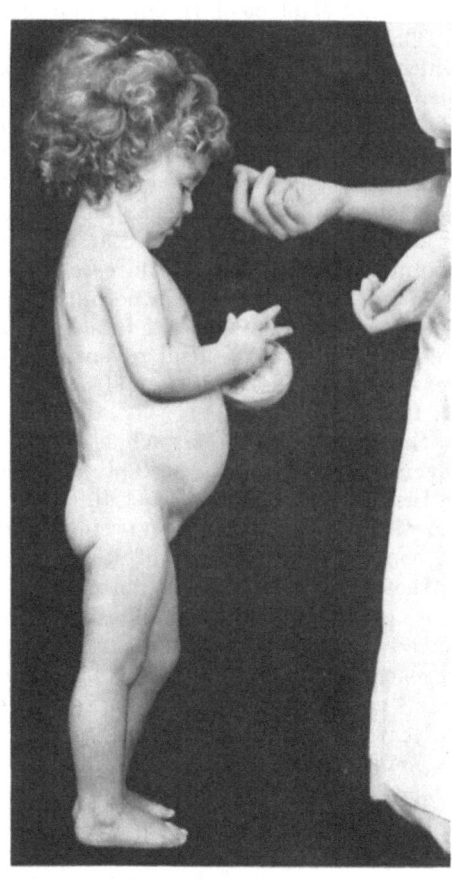

Fig. 1. The patient of SALT et al. (1960), aged 17 months, showing distended abdomen and wasted buttocks (WOLFF 1965)

Clinical Manifestations

Upon inspection of patients with a-β-lipoproteinemia a disproportioned habitus may be noted. The extremities are thin, shoulders and buttocks may appear flattened, there may be kyphoscoliosis and, particularly in children, abdominal distension (see fig. 1). Atrophy of the skin may exist. Impairment of growth leads to underweight and small stature. An adult female patient of SOBREVILLA et al. (1964) measured 147 cm in length and weighed 46 kg. The bone age in the 7 year-old patient of FORSYTH et al. (1965) was 4 years.

In spite of an increased susceptibility to infections, the majority of affected children will survive into adulthood. We know of the death of only three patients, one of whom was the above mentioned patient of SOBREVILLA et al. (1964) who died from an acute cardiac disturbance at the age of 37 years. The second is probably the patient of FRIEDMAN et al. (1960), according to a personal communication from GOLDNER to SCHWARTZ et al. (1963). The third fatal case was that of an 18 month-old child (BECROFT et al. 1965) who died from cardiac failure with pulmonary edema during an episode of bronchitis and asthma.

Neurologic Disturbances

Neurologic disturbances have never been observed before the second year of life. They develop during the course of the disease, producing its most prominent signs and symptoms. The earliest signs of neuropathy were found by BECROFT et al. (1965) in their 17 month-old patient, while another affected infant had no neurologic symptoms at the same age, and did not show any such disturbance before he was 5 years old (WOLFF et al. 1965). The appearance of neurological signs at the age of 2 years has been reported by DRUEZ (1959) and by DRUEZ et al. (1961). Deep tendon reflexes of the lower extremities were absent in the $3\frac{1}{2}$ year-old child observed by WAYS et al. (1963). Neurological disturbances in the case of MIER et al. (1960) did not develop before the age of 17.

The first sign consists of a loss of deep tendon reflexes of the lower extremities, which is found in almost all patients. Subsequently, cerebellar signs become prominent, with development of an ataxic gait, or ataxic signs of the trunk and of the upper extremities. Similarly frequent is a marked proprioceptive deficiency. Since kyphoscoliosis and a positive Babinski sign may also be present, the neurological status may resemble Friedreich's ataxia, which was a preliminary diagnosis in a number of cases (BASSEN and KORNZWEIG 1950; SINGER et al. 1952; MIER et al. 1960; SOBREVILLA et al. 1964). Muscular weakness may suggest the diagnosis of muscular dystrophy, as in cases of KORNZWEIG and BASSEN (1957) and of FRIEDMAN (1960), although no muscular atrophy was found in the sister of the patient of KORNZWEIG and BASSEN (1957). The neural origin of the muscular weakness may be difficult to substantiate, but is supported by findings from nerve biopsies (SCHWARTZ et al. 1963) and by autopsy findings (SOBREVILLA et al. 1964).

Sensory disturbances, such as loss of vibratory sense, have been observed in several cases, vibratory perception being absent up to the level of the clavicles in the patient of FRIEDMAN et al. (1960). This patient also exhibited ophthalmoparesis. Atypical signs of spino-cerebellar degeneration led SOBREVILLA et al. (1964) to consider the diagnosis of Roussy-Levy syndrome in their case. There was apallesthesia in both lower limbs below the knee, which gradually improved as more proximal portions were tested, approaching a normal response at the level of the costal margins (MIER et al. 1960). The sum of neurological signs suggest degeneration of posterior and lateral tracts of the spinal cord, the pyramidal tracts and cerebellar pathways. Sensory disturbances in some cases point to involvement of peripheral nerves.

Mental retardation was a feature in five cases (SINGER et al. 1952; LAMY et al. 1960; DRUEZ et al. 1961; BECROFT et al. 1965; FORSYTH et al. 1965). The latter authors emphasize that in all these cases consanguinity of the parents was noted. There was no consanguinity in the families of the patients with normal intelligence with the exception of the patient of SCHWARTZ et al. (1963), whose parents were 4th degree cousins. For the parents of the first case of a-β-lipoproteinemia consanguinity was reported initially (BASSEN and KORNZWEIG 1950), but this could not be confirmed subsequently (SCHWARTZ et al. 1963). A patient described by MIER et al. (1960) developed aggressive behaviour towards other children when he reached school age and had to be enrolled in a special school for this reason.

Skeletal Abnormalities

Deformities of the feet were seen by MIER et al. (1960), SCHWARTZ et al. (1963), SOBREVILLA (1964), FORSYTH et al. (1965), usually as unilateral or bilateral pes cavus. Congenital deformities of the toes (FORSYTH et al. 1965) and polydactyly (FRIEDMAN et al. 1960) have been described.

Ophthalmologic Disturbances

The retinopathy has been described as typical retinitis (KORNZWEIG and BASSEN 1957; SINGER et al. 1952; DRUEZ et al. 1961), as atypical retinitis (BASSEN and KORNZWEIG 1950; WOLFF 1965) or as retinitis punctata albescens with retinal pigmentary degeneration (MIER et al. 1960). Retinal changes, too, develop during the course of the disease and are not found in the beginning. This is illustrated by a number of cases: by that described by SINGER et al. (1952) and JAMPEL and FALLS (1958), by the patient of SALT et al. (1960) who had a normal fundus at the age of 17 months and developed retinal changes at the age 5 years in spite of continuous vitamin A administration, and by WOLFF et al. (1965) who observed the appearance of blueish pigment in the macular area of the left eye when their patient was 5 years old. In this subject evidence for slight impairment of rod function was detectable at the age of 6, the finding being typical for the initial stages of retinitis pigmentosa. REY (1961) found an abnormal *electro-retinogram* with no visible fundus changes in a child who was almost 6 years old. This was followed with advancing age by impairment of vision and night blindness.

Retinitis is not limited to the periphery but involves also the macula. Pigmentary degeneration and proliferation of the typical bone corpuscle and clumped type are characteristic of the advanced lesion (BASSEN and KORNZWEIG 1950; MIER et al. 1960). It remains to be seen whether the subjects with normal retinas at the ages of 9 and 13 years respectively (SCHWARTZ et al. 1963; DI GEORGE et al. 1961) will eventually develop retinopathy.

Eye findings other than retinal changes include bilateral lenticular opacities and myopic chorioiditis (FRIEDMAN 1960), macular degeneration with ocular hemorrhage (SOBREVILLA et al. 1964), signs of incipient ophthalmoparesis with bilateral ptosis (SCHWARTZ et al. 1963), strabismus divergens alternans and nystagmus bilateralis horizontalis (FRIEDMAN et al. 1960) and ptosis and strabismus (WAYS et al. 1963).

Hematologic Abnormalities

The main hematologic change is acanthocytosis, a red cell abnormality (see figure 2) which has been used by some authors as a name for the disease. It is uniformly present in a-β-lipoproteinemia and can be seen upon inspection of a wet blood smear. In cases where anisocytosis is suspected initially rather than acanthocytosis, other findings such as the low serum cholesterol level aid in differentiation. Over 50 per cent (WOLFF 1965) and up to 80 per cent (SOBREVILLA et al. 1964) of red cells show the typical changes: they resemble "thorn-apples" with spinelike processes of various sizes that impart a crenated appearance. Bone-marrow examinations show the reticulocytes to be normal. The lack of rouleaux formation may contribute to the low red cell sedimentation rate (about 1 mm in the first hour) or else may result from a common cause.

The acanthocytes are of normal size. Osmotic resistance is usually decreased, while mechanical resistance is increased. Hemoglobin concentration is normal or slightly decreased; an atypical hemoglobin has not been found. Mild anemia was seen in some patients. Upon incubation at 37° and 4°C for 48 hours hemolysis is increased in the presence of acanthocytosis (WAYS and SIMON 1964).

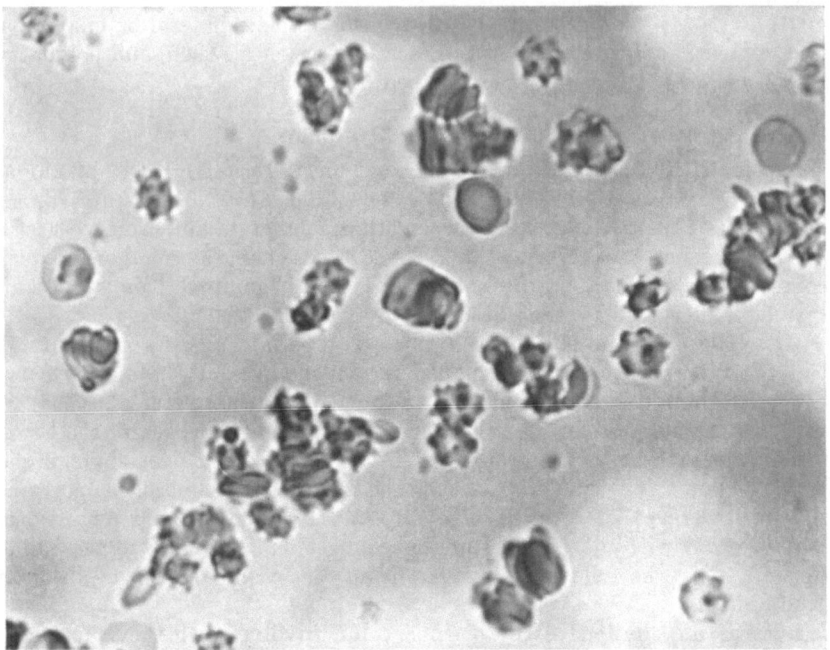

Fig. 2. Wet preparation of blood showing acanthocytes and absence of rouleaux formation (WOLFF 1965)

Other findings suggestive of increased hemolysis are an elevated stercobilinogen content of the stool, reticulocytosis, lack or deficiency of serum haptoglobin, and erythroid hyperplasia of the bone marrow (SOBREVILLA et al. 1964; WOLFF et al. 1965). In contrast to the latter finding, MIER et al. (1960) saw significant reduction of erythropoesis, suggestive of hypoplastic anemia. Red cell survival, as measured with ^{51}Cr, was found to be shortened in three cases so studied (MIER et al. 1960; DRUEZ 1959; WAYS et al. 1963). In the case of WAYS et al. (1963) the half-life of red cells was approximately 22 days (normal 26—27 days).

Gastrointestinal Disturbances

Failure to thrive was caused in a number of children by the early onset (in some immediately after birth) of a celiac syndrome. The prominent symptom is diarrhea. The bulky stools are loose or liquid and may be associated with vomiting. Such stools can appear before any gluten-containing food is fed, and, in contrast to true celiac disease, there is no improvement on a gluten-free diet. In other cases signs of chronic enteritis appear. Grossly bloody stools were occasionally seen by MIER et al. (1960) during bouts of diarrhea. Steatorrhea may improve with increasing age or, as was the case in some patients, on a variety of self-chosen diets, but chemical evidence for impaired fat absorption will be found in most patients. Lack of steatorrhea in a-β-lipoproteinemia is a rare exception (SOBREVILLA et al. 1964).

X-ray examination of the gastrointestinal tract shows distention of the small bowel similar to that found in celiac disease. Segmental puddling of the small intestine and hypotony of the colon were described (FRIEDMAN et al. 1960). A marked exaggeration of the mucosal folds may exist in the upper jejunum (MIER et al. 1960).

Examination of intestinal secretions yields normal values (FRIEDMAN et al. 1960; LAMY et al. 1961; SCHWARTZ et al. 1963). In duodenal contents pancreatic enzyme activity and concentrations of bile acids were found to be normal (WOLFF 1965).

Small Bowel Biopsy

Small bowel biopsies were performed in a number of cases (SALT et al. 1960; MABRY et al. 1960; LAMY et al. 1961; SCHWARTZ et al. 1963; WAYS et al. 1963; AHRENS et al. 1966). In all reports the histology of the jejunal mucosa is similar, and unlike that found in celiac disease (SALT et al. 1960). While the lamina propria is normal with regard to thickness and cellularity and has the normal complement of plasma cells, the columnar cells covering the villi exhibit an unusually clear cytoplasm (see figure 3), which is PAS negative. Staining of the frozen sections with Oil-red 0 or Sudan black suggests the presence of lipid (SALT et al. 1960; MABRY et al. 1960) which is distributed in droplets throughout the cell. Qualitative and quantitative analyses of the stored lipid as well as fat absorption studies have been performed by a number of authors and will be discussed below.

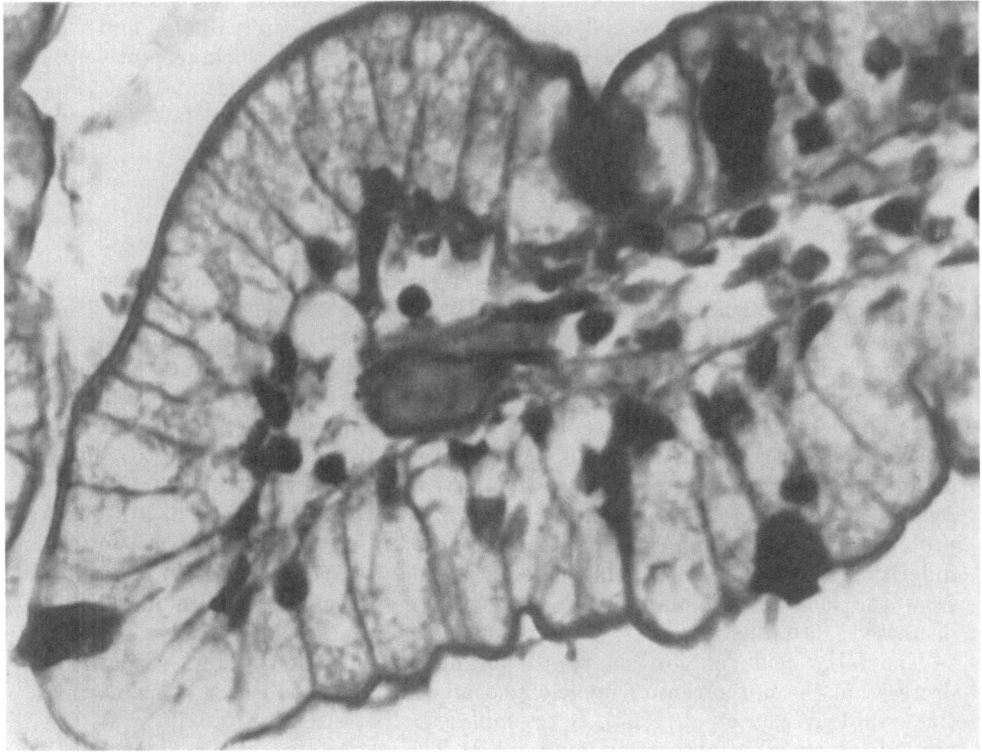

Fig. 3. Jejunal biopsy, high power (PAS), showing columnar cells covering surface of villi with unusually clear cytoplasm which does not stain with PAS (WOLFF 1965)

Pathology

The time which has elapsed since the description of the first case of a-β-lipoproteinemia is too short for detailed information on the morbid anatomy of the disease. Of the three affected subjects who have died, an autopsy was performed in only one (SOBREVILLA et al.). The following describes the findings in this case.

Central Nervous System

Gross examination of the brain in this 37 year old patient showed an organ with normal weight (1340 g) which was symmetrically shaped, and appeared normal with the exception of a brown discoloration of the lumbosacral area of the anterior horns bilaterally.

Microscopic examination confirmed the clinical diagnosis of involvement of the posterior, lateral and anterior columns, and of the pyramidal and cerebellar tracts. There was demyelination of the anterior columns, of the spino-cerebellar tracts and of the cerebellum, with loss of anterior horn cells and cerebellar nuclei. Sections of peripheral nerves, too, showed foci of demyelination. Histochemical studies were not performed in this case.

Other Organs

The visceral organs appeared normal, the weight of the liver was 1500 gm, that of the spleen 250 gm and that of the kidneys 120 gm and 110 gm respectively. There were no gross or microscopic abnormalities of the gastrointestinal tract of this subject, in whom steatorrhea was never observed. The heart weighed 300 gm, the coronary arteries were normal, the ventricles were moderately dilated and the musculature of the left and right ventricles was 1.2 and 0.4 cm thick, respectively. There was some pulmonary congestion and the weight of both lungs was 1150 gm. The pathological findings did not explain the clinical picture with its fatal cardiac disturbance.

Results of Lipid Analyses

Serum Lipids

Total serum lipid levels in a-β-lipoproteinemia are lower than in other malabsorption syndromes, with a range of reported values from 80—285 mg/100 ml. The decrease involves all lipid fractions (see table 2), but the most striking finding is a serum cholesterol level which is always below 100 mg/100 ml (19—86 mg/100 ml). Serum triglycerides are usually less than 20 mg/100 ml (3—15 mg/100 ml). Of total phospholipids, the concentration of which ranges from 23 to 97/100 ml, lecithin is decreased more than sphingomyelin, and the ratio of lecithin to sphingomyelin in the patients of WAYS et al. (1963) was 5:4 (normal about 3:1). This finding is difficult to explain, since α-lipoprotein, which is present in a-β-lipoproteinemia, contains more lecithin than β-lipoprotein, so that the relative decrease in lecithin and increase in sphingomyelin (WOLFF 1965) does not seem to result from the lack of β-lipoproteins (WOLFF 1965). Cephalins are also markedly decreased (PHILLIPS 1962).

The fatty acid composition of all plasma lipid fractions shows a marked decrease in the proportion of linoleic acid and an increase in that of oleic acid (REY 1961; WAYS et al. 1963). It resembles the pattern observed in sprue or other disorders of fat absorption (see table 3). The fasting free fatty acid level has been found to be within normal limits by SALT et al. (1960); the composition of free fatty acids has not been determined.

Table 2. *Serum lipids in a-β-lipoproteinemia*

Units: Cholesterol, Triglycerides, Lipid-phosphorus for the first group are (in mM/L); Total Lipids, Cholesterol, Triglycerides, Total Phospholipids, Lecithin for the second group are (in mg/100 ml); Lecithin, Lyso-lecithin, Sphingomyelin, Cephalins are (in per cent of total phospholipids); Carotenoids in μg/100 ml; Vitamin A in I.U.

Reference	Subjects*	Total Lipids	Cholesterol	Triglycerides	Lipid-phosphorus	Total Phospholipids	Lecithin	Lyso-lecithin	Sphingomyelin	Cephalins	Carotenoids	Vitamin A
	Normals		4.62	0.74	3.22		68.2	7.7	19.1	5.0		
PHILLIPS (1962)	R.K.		0.97	0.15	0.69		58.1	7.0	33.0	1.9		
PHILLIPS (1962)	R.B.		0.75	0.13	0.49		57.6	7.5	32.0	3.0		
PHILLIPS (1962)	L.Z.		2.20	0.19	1.24		64.5	5.1	29.8	0.6	0	62
SCHWARTZ et al. (1963)	R.I.		1.22	0.19	0.74		50.4	12.7	35.2	1.7	0	136
FRIEDMAN et al. (1960)	Normals	400—750	145—285	20—225		150—250	100—175	4—8	30—50	8—14	60—260**	80—180**
SALT et al. (1960)	N.S.	108—110	25—47			58—67						
	C.S.	80	22			45					0	19
WAYS et al. (1963)	M.S.		34		1.8							
WAYS et al. (1963)	C.R.	180	59				55		29			
WAYS et al. (1963)	A.C.	96	26				49		47			
BECROFT et al. (1965)	J.M.		23			58	42.5		35.5		12.5	
FORSYTH et al. (1965)	A.L.	110	29								0	
FREDRICKSON (1966)	A.C.		46	<10		73	27	8	31		0	55

* For author of original case report see table 1.
** From SALT et al. (1960).

Table 3. *Fatty acid composition of serum lipids in a-β-lipoproteinemia and sprue*

Fatty acid	Total Lipids		Triglycerides			Cholesterolesters			Phospholipids		
	Normal[1]	Sprue[2]	Normal	A-β-lipoproteinemia[3]	Sprue	Normal	A-β-lipoproteinemia[4]	Sprue	Normal	A-β-lipoproteinemia[4]	Sprue
$C_{12:0}$	0.5			8.2							
$C_{14:0}$	1.5	2.2	2.5	5.5	3.0	1	1.6	4.4	0.5	1.7	1.1
$C_{14:1}$	trace	—		1.4			1.7	2.7			
$C_{16:0}$	28	33.9	29	26.0	34.1	12.5	19.6	15.3	31	23.3	46.8
$C_{16:1}$	5.5	13.0	8	6.8	15.3	7	14.4	30.2	3	6.8	5.8
X_1		0.7			0.4			1.2			
X_2		0.5			0.4			1.7			
$C_{18:0}$	7	3.8	5	13.7	1.7	2	7.6	0.5	12	10.5	5.4
$C_{18:1}$	24.5	42.3	36.5	34.3	44.3	19	44.2	37.8	15	30.9	34.5
$C_{18:2}$	23.5	1.6	11	1.9	0.6	50	4.2	6.0	22	2.1	2.2
$C_{20:3}$	1	—	<1		—	1	5.0	—	1	13.1	4.1
$C_{20:4}$	5	—	3		—	4.5	1.6	—	9	5.0	trace

Source: [1,2] KAHLKE (1965, 1966); [3] FRÉZAL et al. (1966); [4] AHRENS jr. (1966).

Lipoproteins

The typical finding is a marked decrease or lack of β-lipoproteins (d = 1.019 — 1.063) which can be demonstrated with paper-electrophoresis (see figure 4), ultracentrifugation and immunoelectrophoresis (see table 4). It is not known with certainty whether or not there are traces of β-lipoproteins, as suggested by SALT et al. (1960) from studies with a sensitive immunochemical technique (GELL 1957) using rabbit antiserum against human β-lipoproteins. Upon paper-electrophoresis, there was a marked reduction, but not a complete lack of β-lipoproteins (SCHWARTZ et al. 1963) in some cases. Studies with a turbidimetric method (WALTON and SCOTT 1964) resulted in the finding of 10—20 mg β-lipoproteins per 100 ml plasma instead of 130—500 mg normally, but these small amounts may be due to precipitated globulin (BECROFT et al. 1965). A further possibility is the presence of an abnormal β-lipoprotein.

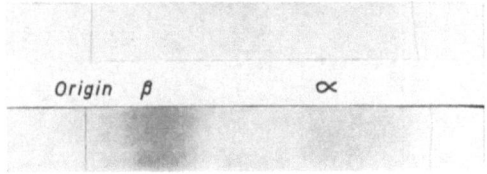

Origin β ∝

Fig. 4. Electrophoretic strip stained for lipid, showing absence of beta-lipoprotein and depletion of α-lipoprotein (WOLFF 1965)

Table 4. *Serum lipoproteins in a-β-lipoproteinemia*

	α-lipoproteins	β-lipoproteins		β/α ratio
		(mg/100 ml serum)		
	as lipid by paper electrophoresis		by dextran sulfate precipitation	
patients:				
SALT et al. (1960)	80	0	20*	0
BECROFT et al. (1965)			15	
FORSYTH et al. (1965)	110	0		0
normals:				
SALT et al. (1960)	150—280	300—580		1.5—3.0
BECROFT et al. (1965)			0—10 yrs.: 120—570 30—40 yrs.: 250—780	

* Determination performed by BECROFT et al. (1965).

Chylomicrons are not found in a-β-lipoproteinemia after fatty meals or with fat loading (see figure 5).

In most cases the concentration of α-lipoprotein (HDLP) was also found to be low (SALT et al. 1960; WOLFF and BAUMANN 1961). This seems to be a non-specific abnormality since it also occurs in steatorrhea resulting from other causes. The lipid pattern of α-lipoproteins (phospholipid/cholesterol ratio 53:26) is reflected in that of total plasma lipids (FORSYTH et al. 1965). The lipid phosphorus and cholesterol content of the fraction with d > 1.063 is about ½ normal (WAYS et al. 1963). The cause for the lowered α-lipoprotein concentration is not known. A possibility is decreased formation from lipoproteins of lower density (chylomicrons and β-lipoproteins), due to the decreased concentration or absence of the latter.

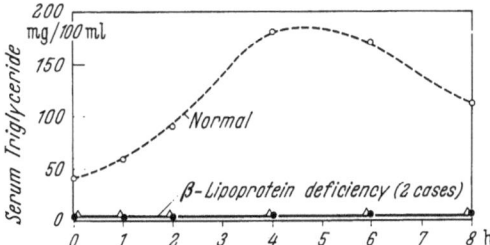

Fig. 5. Serum triglycerides following the ingestion of 30 ml corn oil in normal subjects and in two cases with beta-lipoprotein deficiency. In normal subjects the peak level occurs at 4 hours. In cases 1 and 2 fasting triglycerides were 3 and 6 mg/100 ml serum and no detectable increase occurred for 8 hours (ISSELBACHER et al. 1964). (With kind permission of Dr. KURT J. ISSELBACHER)

A further finding in a-β-lipoproteinema is a low postheparin lipoprotein lipase activity (0.16 μ Eq/min/ml; normal 0.28—0.41 μEq/min/ml, KUO and BASSETT 1962), which is also found after low fat feeding in normals.

Serum vitamin A levels were low in all cases so studied, and this finding is the rule for disorders where the absorption of fat is interfered with (SALT et al. 1960). Serum carotenoids which are normally transported with β-lipoproteins may be missing (SALT et al. 1960) or be markedly lowered (12.5 μg as compared to the normal range of 60—260 μg/100 ml, BECROFT et al. 1965).

Red Cells

Morphologic abnormalities of erythrocytes stimulated studies on red cell lipids (WAYS et al. 1963; SIMON and WAYS 1964; FREDRICKSON 1966) (see table 5). A normal total lipid content (PHILLIPS and ROOME 1959; REED et al. 1960;

Table 5. *Red-cell phospholipids in a-β-lipoproteinemia*

Subjects*	Lipid-phosphorus	Le-cithin	Sphin-go-myelin	Ethanol-amine-cephalin	Serin-cepha-lin	Lyso-lecithin	Total recovery
	mM/L			*per cent of total phospholipids*			
PHILLIPS (1962)							
13 normal adults	4.50	32.7	23.1	42.4		1.8	97
R. K.	3.87	24.2	28.7	45.0		2.1	90
R. B.		27.9	26.5	44.3		1.3	100
L. Z.	3.46	31.2	21.4	45.6		1.8	101
	mg/cell						
WAYS et al. (1963)							
normal	1.16×10^{-11}	29.5	23.8	25.7	15.0	5.9**	95
M. S.	1.15×10^{-11}	19.9	31.4	22.9	15.0	9.0	93
C. R.	0.97×10^{-11}	18.4	36.2	19.5	15.9	9.3	101
A. C.	1.20×10^{-11}	15.0	28.5	24.0	17.0	15.0	96
	$\mu M/10^{12}$						
FREDRICKSON (1966)	A. C.	446	18	36	30	—	—	—

* For author of original case report see table 1.
** Lysolecithin and other unidentified lipids.

HANAHAN et al. 1960; DEGIER and VAN DEENEN 1961; FARQUHAR 1962) was found in three cases studied by MABRY et al. (1960), MIER et al. (1960) and WAYS et al. (1963), respectively. Lipid phosphorus was slightly low in one of the cases. As in plasma, red cell lecithin was absolutely and relatively decreased, while the sphingo-myelin concentration was increased. Plasmalogens were low. The concentrations of cephalin and of cholesterol were normal (WAYS et al. 1963; FREDRICKSON 1966).

Red cell phospholipid fatty acids show a low concentration of linoleic acid. Of the lecithin fatty acids, stearic acid is also decreased, and the proportion of palmitic and oleic acids is increased; these changes appear to result from pre-vailing endogenous lipogenesis (KUO and BASSETT 1962). Surprisingly, the arachidonic acid concentration was normal in red cell lecithin and only slightly decreased in total red cell phospholipids (WAYS et al. 1963). The lowering of linoleic acid concentration and the reversal of the lecithin to sphingomyelin ratio in red cells as found in a-β-lipoproteinemia is more marked than in other disorders where fat absorption is impaired.

Findings in red cell ghosts which contain all the red cell cholesterol and phos-pholipids (DODGE et al. 1963; WEED et al. 1963), were similar to those in total erythrocytes (WAYS et al. 1963).

Small Intestine

A greatly increased lipid content of the small bowel epithelium can already be recognized histochemically. Values up to 3 times normal are observed even in the postabsorptive state (WAYS and PARMENTIER 1963), although ingestion of fat-free diets for 10 days or longer restores the mucosal fat content almost to normal (AHRENS et al. 1966). The stored intracellular lipid is mainly triglyceride (WAYS and PARMENTIER 1963; ISSELBACHER 1965); as regards the phospholipids, the ratio of lecithin to sphingomyelins appears to be normal (WAYS and PARMENTIER 1963). Impairment of fat absorption by distended mucosal cells leads to increased fecal fat excretion, the quantity and quality of the excreted fat being dependent on the fed fat.

Pathogenetic Aspects

A discussion on the pathogenesis of a-β-lipoproteinemia should include an attempt to correlate the various symptoms. The red cell lesion seems to be related to, or even caused by, the abnormal lipid composition of the acanthocyte mem-brane. Retinitis pigmentosa and cerebellar ataxia also seem related to a disturb-ance of lipid metabolism; they are non-specific and can also occur in the Refsum-syndrome and in the syndrome described by HOOFT (1962).

The mechanism of impaired fat absorption has not been elucidated, but is probably related to the lack of β-lipoproteins, which seems to be important for the trans-port of fat including carotenoids. Intracellular functions of β-lipoproteins, for in-stance for intracellular membrane formation, have not been sufficiently studied.

In favor of the hypothesis that development of acanthocytosis is secondary to abnormal serum lipids, is the occurrence of normal red cell precursors in the bone-marrow, and the fact that red cell changes become more marked in aging cells (SIMON and WAYS 1964). Interference with the exchange of lipid between red cell membranes and serum due to the absence of low density lipoproteins and the low levels of high density lipoproteins might result in the abnormal lecithin/ sphingomyelin ratio and the low concentration of linoleic acid (PHILLIPS 1962; WAYS et al. 1963, 1964). In addition, WAYS et al. (1963) consider a primary abnormality of the red cell membrane to be the cause of acanthocytosis. Acantho-cytosis persists when washed red cells of patients are suspended in normal homologous serum (SALT et al. 1960). Another possibility cannot be excluded, namely that the low levels of plasma lipids and low density lipoproteins are not responsible as such for the red cell abnormality, but rather some substances which are normally transported by them. Of interest are findings by DI GEORGE et al. (1961) who observed almost complete disappearance of acanthocytes after intravenous infusions of a cottonseed oil emulsion for 39 days. The acanthocytes reappeared upon discontinuation of the infusion and the effect of lipomul was probably due to the detergent (tween 80) contained in the emulsion. Similarly SWITZER and EDER (1962) were able to convert acanthocytes to normal red cells by the addition of small amounts of tween 80 or other oleyl ethers or esters of nonionic detergents. It is not known whether the membrane lipid pattern became normal as a result of this procedure.

The retinopathy may be related to vitamin A or carotenoid deficiency (SALT et al. 1960, and others), and low serum levels of vitamin A were found by CAMP-BELL and TONKS (1963) in other patients with retinitis pigmentosa. However, in the patient of SALT et al., normal serum levels of this vitamin were maintained from the age of 22 months by the administration of water-soluble vitamin A preparations and he nevertheless showed the first signs of retinitis pigmentosa at the age of 5 years (WOLFF et al. 1966). Similarly FORSYTH et al. (1965) administered vitamin A to their patients in daily doses of 20,000 to 40,000 IU, and achieved serum levels of 55 IU/100 ml (normal 72 IU/100 ml) but were unable to prevent the development of retinitis and the appearance of neurological signs at the age of 7. Even with normal serum levels of vitamin A, its transport to important sites may not be secured, and coupling with β-lipoproteins may be necessary for its action. In addition, some cells may need carotenoids which are almost completely absent in the serum of a-β-lipoproteinemic patients.

The cause of the neurologic symptomatology is obscure. The co-occurrence of ataxia and atypical pigmentary retinitis is a feature in several other hereditary syndromes, so that a common pathogenesis is likely for both symptoms. GAI-TONDE (1963) has emphasized the importance of lipoproteins for the metabolism of the nervous system, but the causal relation of a-β-lipoproteinemia and ataxic disturbance has not yet been elucidated. It is possible that there is a common factor essential for the normal structure and function of the nerve cell on one hand, and the production of β-lipoproteins on the other (SALT et al. 1960), but it appears more likely that the lack of β-lipoprotein formation actually represents the central lesion.

Numerous studies have dealt with the epithelium of the small intestine. Entry of fat from the bowel lumen into the mucosal cells appears to proceed as evidenced by the extreme degree of fat accumulation in these cells. Steatorrhea may result when the maximal absorptive capacity of these cells is exceeded. There is no evidence of selective absorption of certain fats, as could be shown by analysis of mucosal lipids and feces. In particular, the lowering of plasma linoleic acid concentration in a-β-lipoproteinemia and other forms of malabsorption does not appear to be due to impairment of absorption of „essential" fatty acids. After administration of diets rich in polyenoic acids WAYS and PARMENTIER (1963) found more linoleic acid in mucosal phospholipids and triglycerides than was found with the normal diet. There was a simultaneous increase in the proportion of linoleate in plasma cholesterol esters. Linoleic acid, given for a period of three years, was absorbed to about 97 per cent (FRÉZAL et al. 1966). Its administration resulted in a significant increase of the proportion of linoleic acid in the plasma lipid fatty acids. Normal values were reached in the triglyceride and phospholipid fractions (see table 6).

Table 6. *Plasma lipid fatty acid patterns in a-β-lipoproteinemia after dietary treatment**

Fatty acids	Triglycerides					Cholesterol esters				Phospholipids			
	Normal**	Before	After 6 mths.	After 2 yrs.	After 3 yrs.	Normal**	Before	After 2 yrs.	After 3 yrs.	Normal**	Before	After 6 mths.	After 2 yrs.
$C_{12:0}$	1	8,2	1,5	0,3	6,2	1	6,6	Trace	0,8	—	11,7	Trace	0 7
$C_{14:0}$	2,5	5,5	5,5	0,7	6,6	1	7	2,3	1,7	0,5	7,6	0,8	1,2
$C_{14:1}$		1,4	1,0		Trace		3	Trace	Trace		1,5	Trace	0,2
$C_{16:0}$	29	26	27,5	11,4	29,7	12,5	25,9	14,3	20,6	31	28	35,4	17
$C_{16:1}$	8	6,8	4,2	1,1	5,5	7	10,6	1,6	6,7	3	6,3	2	4,4
$C_{18:0}$	5	13,7	11,9	9,6	5,8	2	5	5,4	10,3	12	9,7	26,7	14,9
$C_{18:1}$	36,5	34,3	42,2	64,3	34,4	19	31,9	54,5	44,7	15	27,9	27,8	43,8
$C_{18:2}$	11	1,9	2,8	12,6	9,6	50	5,3	18,6	14,9	22	3,1	4,5	15,1

* Source: FRÉZAL et al. (1966). Patient G. F., treated over a period of three years with 10 g per day of grape stone oil containing 70 per cent of linoleic acid.
** Source: KAHLKE (1965).

Triglyceride synthesis from absorbed fatty acids and monoglycerides by the mucosal cells also seems to be intact, since the major portion of the intracellular lipid is triglyceride (see chapter by SHAPIRO page 40). Esterification of fatty acids by mucosa from patients with a-β-lipoproteinemia proceeds normally in vivo and in vitro (SABESIN et al. 1964).

SHEARER (1965), administering β-carotenes orally to an affected subject, was able to show that it appeared in the blood in the form of vitamin A, as in normals. It seems therefore that the intestinal epithelium in a-β-lipoproteinemia, as in normals, is capable of cleaving carotene (THOMPSON et al. 1949, 1950).

Normally, absorbed lipids leave the mucosal cells in the form of chylomicrons which are discharged into the lymphatic system. Only short and medium chain fatty acids (up to C_{10}) are carried by portal vein blood (ISSELBACHER 1964). In a-β-lipoproteinemia no fat is seen in the lymphatic spaces of the small bowel (ISSELBACHER 1965), and no chylomicrons appear in the plasma after fat loading (see figure 5). It appears that the defect in a-β-lipoproteinemia concerns the lipid transport from the mucosal cells into the lymphatic system. For the formation of chylomicrons, β-lipoproteins (ISSELBACHER 1965), but not α-lipoproteins (FREDRICKSON 1966) seem to be necessary. The fat absorption defect is not improved with transfusion of normal β-lipoproteins (FRÉZAL et al. 1961).

ISSELBACHER (1965) was able to show that the absorption of short and medium chain fatty acids is not impaired in a-β-lipoproteinemia, and that, on a diet rich in such fatty acids, there is a significant decrease of the mucosal fat content.

As regards the disturbance of fat transport and the lack of β-lipoproteins there are two important questions:
1. Does the defect of β-lipoprotein formation lie in the mechanism for coupling of lipid to protein, or
2. Is there a deficiency of a specific protein moiety which is necessary for the formation of β-lipoproteins and/or chylomicrons (see fig. 6).

A model for the first possibility might be the specific depression of lipoprotein synthesis, particularly of very low density lipoproteins (d < 1.019) (ROHEIM et al. 1965) which is observed after administration of orotic acid to rats. Since orotic acid does not affect the protein moiety of the lipoprotein, the authors deduce the presence of one or more steps after the synthesis of the protein which would be necessary for the formation and release of lipoproteins. Any of these steps could be blocked in a-β-lipoproteinemia.

Another possibility is an alteration of the protein moiety resulting in deficient lipid binding, in spite of maintenance of its antigen specificity. However, SCHWARTZ et al. (1963) examining sera of patients with a-β-lipoproteinemia by means of immunoelectrophoresis using rabbit antisera against normal human β- and α_2 lipoproteins, could not identify the arc for β- and α_2 lipoproteins. These findings support the thesis that a specific protein moiety (of β-lipoproteins) is diminished or absent in the serum of patients with a-β-lipoproteinemia, in analogy to findings

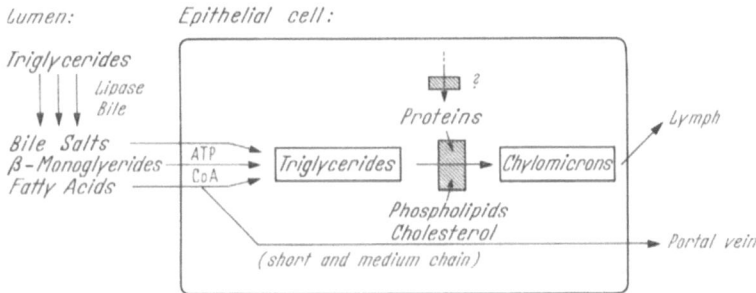

Fig. 6. Scheme of triglyceride absorption. Hatched blocks indicate site(s) of possible lesion in a-β-lipoproteinemia

in Wilson's disease, congenital a-γ-globulinemia, analbuminemia and Tangier disease (hypo-α-lipoproteinemia) (SCHWARTZ et al. 1963). The sites affected by this specific defect in protein synthesis are probably liver and intestinal mucosa.

Results of animal experiments by ISSELBACHER et al. (1964) and by SABESIN et al. (1964) favor deficient synthesis of the protein moiety as a pathogenetic mechanism in a-β-lipoproteinemia. When protein synthesis was inhibited in the rat by administration of puromycin, acetoxycycloheximide or ethionin, these authors found biochemical and morphological abnormalities which were very similar to those observed in a-β-lipoproteinemia. The mucosal cells accumulated fat, serum triglycerides were low, and did not rise after fat loading, and the serum β-lipoprotein level decreased precipitously. In these studies the dose of inhibitors was such that visible cell damage and a decrease in activation and esterification of fatty acids was not observed (ISSELBACHER 1965).

An interesting observation is that by BLUMBERG (1963) who found precipitins in the serum of two subjects with a-β-lipoproteinemia which reacted with β-lipoproteins from normal subjects. It is not known whether these precipitins were naturally occurring antibodies or whether they occurred as the result of an immunologic phenomenon (cit. after BECROFT et al. 1965).

Obviously further studies are necessary to determine the location of the lesion in a-β-lipoproteinemia, as well as the correlation between the lack of this lipoprotein and the various symptoms.

Diagnosis

If the disease is thought of, diagnosis should not be difficult. The appearance of steatorrhea at a time when the diet does not yet contain gluten, and its persistence in spite of a gluten-free diet both aid in excluding sprue. Correspondingly, biopsies of the intestinal mucosa show a picture which is quite different from that of sprue. The very low sedimentation rate of the red cells may lead to the specific finding of acanthocytes in a fresh blood smear. In contrast, retinitis pigmentosa and neuroataxic symptoms occurring during the course of the disease or representing the first symptoms in older patients, are not restricted to a-β-lipoproteinemia. The finding of extremely low levels of serum cholesterol and total lipid levels makes the diagnosis very likely; it can be confirmed by demonstration of the lack of β-lipoproteins through chromatography, electrophoresis, or ultracentrifugation.

A special case of a-β-lipoproteinemia seems to be that described by Anderson et al. (1961). This patient had steatorrhea which could be controlled with a fat-free diet and findings on jejunal biopsy were identical with those in a-β-lipoproteinemia. Accordingly, total serum lipids and total serum cholesterol were 200 mg and 58 mg per 100 ml, respectively, and serum carotenoids were absent. There were, however, no acanthocytes and β-lipoproteins were not absent, but only reduced to $\frac{1}{2}$ the normal concentration; furthermore, chylomicrons were found after fat loading. Further observation of this patient will be of interest and detailed lipid analyses including those of red cell membranes are desirable.

Treatment

Although there is no causal treatment for a-β-lipoproteinemia, improvement can be achieved by symptomatic measures.

Steatorrhea improves with limitation of fat intake, preferably after a brief fat-free period. Thus in the patient of Salt et al. (1960) steatorrhea subsided on a diet containing less than 20 gm fat per day, the weight of the patient increased and the general condition improved considerably. Good results have been reported with the use of medium chain triglycerides (Isselbacher 1965), the intake of which does not have to be restricted, while histologic findings in the intestinal mucosa become normal (Ahrens et al. 1966). Kuo and Bassett (1962) saw clinical improvement with omission of dairy and meat fat and the administration of a diet rich in polyunsaturated fatty acids (60 g corn oil per day emulsified with tween 80).

Although DiGeorge et al. (1961), while administering cottonseed oil emulsions intravenously to patients with a-β-lipoproteinemia did not observe any changes of serum lipids or β-lipoproteins, there was significant improvement of the clinical picture and disappearance of acanthocytes. As mentioned earlier, this latter effect might have resulted from the emulsifying agent. When, after 39 days, treatment had to be discontinued because of the development of a typical fat-overloading syndrome, recurrence of acanthocytosis was associated with clinical deterioration.

Whether long-term administrations of water-soluble vitamin A preparations, which are customarily given in each case of retinitis pigmentosa, are of any benefit remains to be seen. As mentioned earlier, ingestion of vitamin A over years by some patients (Wolff et al. 1965/1966) with a-β-lipoproteinemia, failed to prevent the development of retinitis pigmentosa and ataxia, in spite of satisfactory serum levels. Nevertheless, the fat soluble vitamins A, D and E, and possibly vitamin K in the presence of hypoprothrombinemia, should be substituted. The lack of plasma carotenoids persists in spite of these measures.

Hypochromic anemia was successfully treated with intramuscular iron by Salt et al. (1961) and the hemoglobin rose with this therapy from 9.7 to 13.1 gm/ 100 ml.

The usefulness of repeated infusions of fresh β-lipoproteins remains to be proved. In the patient of Frézal et al. (1961) there was no improvement of fat absorption.

The improvement of autohemolysis has been proposed (Ways and Simon 1964) as an indication of the effectiveness of therapeutic measures, since procedures that reduce abnormal autohemolysis might also benefit the membranes of the central nervous system.

References

Ahrens jr., E. H.: Personal communication (1966).
— A. Novikoff, and N. Spritz: Fat transport from the intestine in a-betalipoproteinaemia. (In preparation.)

ANDERSON, C. M., R. R. W. TOWNLEY, M. FREEMAN, and P. JOHANSEN: Unusual causes of steatorrhoea in infancy and childhood. Med. J. Aust. 2, 617 (1961).

BASSEN, F. A., and A. L. KORNZWEIG: Malformation of the erythrocytes in a case of atypical retinitis pigmentosa. Blood 5, 381 (1950).

BECROFT, D. M. O., J. M. CASTELLO, and P. J. SCOTT: A-β-lipoproteinaemia (Bassen-Kornzweig-Syndrom). Report of a case. Arch. Dis. Childh. 40, 40 (1965).

BLUMBERG, B. S.: Multiple inherited antigenic differences in serum beta-lipoproteins. Clin. Res. 11, 202 (1963).

CAMPBELL, D. A., and E. L. TONKS: Biochemical findings in human retinitis pigmentosa with particular relation to vitamin A deficiency. Brit. J. Ophthal. 46, 151 (1962).

DE GIER, J., and L. L. M. VAN DEENEN: Some lipoid characteristics of red cell membranes of various animal species. Biochim. biophys. Acta (Amst.) 49, 286 (1961).

DIGEORGE, A. M., C. C. MABRY, and V. H. AUERBACH: A specific disorder of lipid transport (acanthrocytosis): treatment with intravenous lipids. Amer. J. Dis. Child. 102, 580 (1961).

— — — Personal communication to FARQUHAR and WAYS (1966); ref. [37].

DODGE, J. T., C. MITCHELL, and D. J. HANAHAN: The preparation and chemical characteristics of hemoglobin-free ghosts of human erythrocytes. Arch. Biochem. 100, 119 (1963).

DRUEZ, G.: Un nouveau cas d'acanthocytose: dysmorphie érythrocytaire congénitale avec rétinite, troubles nerveux et stigmates dégénératifs. Rev. Hémat. 14, 3 (1959).

— M. LAMY, J. FRÉZAL, J. POLONOVSKI et J. REY: L'acanthocytose: ses rapports avec l'absence congénitale de bêta-lipoprotéines. Presse méd. 69, 1546 (1961).

EDER, H., Acanthocytosis, case 525 from the medical grand rounds. Amer. Practit. 13, 225 (1962).

FARQUHAR, J. W.: Human erythrocyte phosphoglycerides. I. Quantification of plasmalogens, fatty acids and fatty aldehydes. Biochim. biophys. Acta (Amst.) 60, 80 (1962).

— J. HORNE, and M. ERLANDSEN: (In preparation). Cit. after FARQUHAR and WAYS (1966) ref. [11].

— and P. WAYS: Abetalipoproteinemia. In: The metabolic basis of inherited disease. Eds.: J. B. Stanbury, J. B. Wyngaarden, and D. S. Fredrickson. New York: McGraw-Hill Book Co. 1966, p. 509.

FORSYTH, C. C., J. K. LLOYD, and A. S. FOSBROOKE: A-β-lipoproteinaemia. Arch. Dis. Childh. 40, 47 (1965).

FREDRICKSON, D. S.: Symposium on pathophysiological and clinical aspects of lipid metabolism, Heidelberg 1965. Ed.: G. Schettler. Stuttgart: Thieme 1966 (in press).

— Familial high-density lipoprotein deficiency: Tangier disease. In: The metabolic basis of inherited disease. Eds.: J. B. Stanbury, J. B. Wyngaarden, and D. S. Fredrickson. New York: McGraw-Hill Book Co. 1966, p. 486.

FRÉZAL, J., et M. LAMY: Influence d'une huile riche en acide linoléique sur la composition en acides gras des lipides plasmatiques dans l'absence congénitale de β-lipoprotéines. Rev. franç. Étud. clin. biol. 11, 69 (1966).

— J. REY, J. POLONOVSKI, G. LÉVY et M. LAMY: L'absence congénitale de β-lipoprotéines: étude de l'absorption intestinale près exsanguinotransfusion: mesure de la demiviede, lipoprotéines injéctees. Rev. franç. Étud. clin. biol. 6, 677 (1961).

FRIEDMAN, J. S.: Personal communication to MIER et al. (1960); ref. [15].

— H. COHN, M. ZYMARIS, and M. G. GOLDNER: Hypocholesterolemia in idiopathic steatorrhea. Arch. intern. Med. 105, 136 (1960).

GAITONDE, M. K.: The turnover of proteolipids and phosphatidopeptides in the brain; in "Brain lipids and lipoproteins, and the leucodystrophies". p. 42. Ed.: J. Folch Pi and H. Bauer. Amsterdam-London-New York: Elsevier 1963.

GELL, P. G. H.: The estimation of the individual human serum proteins by an immunological method. J. clin. Path. 10, 67 (1957).

GOLDNER, M. G.: Personal communication to SCHWARTZ et al. Arch. Neurol. (Chic.) 8, 438 (1963).

HANAHAN, D. J., R. M. WATTS, and D. PAPPAJOHN: Some chemical characteristics of the lipids of human and bovine erythrocytes and plasma. J. Lipid Res. 1, 421 (1960).

HOOFT, C., P. DE LAEY, J. HERPOL, F. DE LOORE, and J. VERBEECK: Familial hypolipidaemia and retarded development without steatorrhoea. Helv. paediat. Acta 17, 1 (1962).

ISSELBACHER, K. J.: Metabolism and transport of lipid by intestinal mucosa. Fed. Proc. 24, 16 (1965).

— R. SCHEIG, G. R. PLOTKIN, and J. B. CAULIFIELD: Congenital β-lipoprotein deficiency: an hereditary disorder involving a defect in the absorption and transport of lipids. Medicine (Baltimore) 43, 347 (1964).

JAMPEL, R. S., and H. F. FALLS: Atypical retinitis pigmentosa, acanthrocytosis, and heredodegenerative neuromuscular disease. Arch. Ophthal. 59, 818 (1958).

KAHLKE, W.: Lipoide I. Fortschr. Med. 83, 517 (1965).

— Unpublished results (1966).

KORNZWEIG, A. L., and F. A. BASSEN: Retinitis pigmentosa, acanthrocytosis and heredodegenerative neuromuscular disease. Arch. Ophthal. 58, 183 (1957).

KUO, P. T., and D. R. BASSETT: Blood and tissue lipids in a family with hypo-beta-lipo-proteinemia. Circulation **26**, 660 (1962).

LAMY, M. J., J. FRÉZAL, J. POLONOVSKI et J. REY: L'absence congénitale de β-lipoprotéines. C. R. Soc. Biol. (Paris) **154**, 1974 (1960).

— — — et G. DRUEZ: L'absence congénitale de beta-lipoprotéines. Presse méd. **69**, 1511 (1961).

MABRY, C. C., A. M. DIGEORGE, and V. H. AUERBACH: Studies concerning the defect in a patient with acanthocytosis. Clin. Res. **8**, 371 (1960).

MIER, M., S. O. SCHWARTZ, and B. BOSHES: Acanthocytosis, pigmentary degeneration of the retina and ataxic neuropathy: a genetically determined syndrome with associated metabolic disorder. Blood **16**, 1586 (1960).

PHILLIPS, G. B.: Quantitative chromatographic analysis of plasma and red blood cell lipids in patients with acanthocytosis. J. Lab. clin. Med. **59**, 357 (1962).

— and N. S. ROOME: Phospholipids of human red blood cells. Proc. Soc. exp. Biol. (N. Y.) **100**, 489 (1959).

REED, G. F., S. N. SWISHER, G. V. MARINETTI, and E. G. EDEN: Studies of the lipids of the erythrocyte. I. Quantitative analysis of the lipids of normal human red blood cells. J. Lab. clin. Med. **56**, 281 (1960).

REY, J.: L'absence congénitale de bêta-lipoprotéines. Paris: Foulon et Cie. 1961.

ROHEIM, P. S., S. SWITZER, A. GIRARD, and H. A. EDER: The mechanism of inhibition of lipoprotein synthesis by orotic acid. Biochem. biophys. Res. Comm. **20**, 416 (1965).

SABESIN, S. M., G. D. DRUMMEY, D. M. BUDZ, and K. J. ISSELBACHER: Inhibition of protein synthesis: a mechanism for the production of impaired fat absorption. J. clin. Invest. **43**, 1281 (1964).

SALT, H. B., O. H. WOLFF, J. K. LLOYD, A. S. FOSBROOKE, A. H. CAMERON, and D. V. HUBBLE: On having no beta-lipoprotein – a syndrome comprising a-beta-lipoproteinaemia, acantho-cytosis, and steatorrhoea. Lancet **1960/II**, 325 (1960).

SCHWARTZ, J. F., L. P. ROWLAND, H. A. EDER, P. M. MARKS, E. OSSERMANN, H. ANDERSON, and E. HIRSCHBERG: Bassen-Kornzweig Syndrome; neuromuscular disorder resembling Friedreich's ataxia associated with retinitis pigmentosa, acanthocytosis, steatorrhea, and an abnormality of lipid metabolism. Trans. Amer. Neurol. Ass. **86**, 49 (1961).

— — — — — É. HIRSCHBERG, and H. ANDERSON: Bassen-Kornzweig Syndrome; deficiency of serum beta-lipoprotein. Arch. Neurol. (Chic.) **8**, 438 (1963).

SHEARER, J. A.: Absorption and conversion of beta-carotene. Exp. Eye Res. (in press).

SIMON, E. R., and P. WAYS: Incubation hemolysis and red cell metabolism in acanthocytosis. J. clin. Invest. **43**, 1311 (1964).

SINGER, K., B. FISHER, and M. A. PERLSTEIN: Acanthocytosis. A genetic erythrocyte mal-formation. Blood **7**, 577 (1952).

SOBREVILLA, L. A., M. L. GOODMAN, and CH. KANE: Demyelinating central nervous system disease, macular atrophy and acanthocytosis (Bassen-Kornzweig-Syndrome). Amer. J. Med. **37**, 821 (1964).

SWITZER, S., and H. A. EDER: Interconversion of acanthocytes and normal erythrocytes with detergents. J. clin. Invest. **41**, 1404 (1962).

THOMPSON, S. Y., R. BRAUDE, M. E. COATES, A. T. COWIE, J. GANGULY, and S. K. KON: Further studies of the conversion of β-carotene to vitamin A in the intestine. Brit. J. Nutr. **4**, 398 (1950).

— J. GANGULY, and S. K. KON: The conversion of β-carotene to vitamin A in the intestine. Brit. J. Nutr. **3**, 50 (1949).

WALTON, K. W., and D. J. SCOTT: Estimations of the low-density (beta) lipoproteins of serum in health and disease using large molecular weigh dextran sulphate. J. clin. Path. **17**, 627 (1964).

WAYS, P.: Unpublished data. Cited after FARQUHAR and WAYS (1966); ref. [21].

— and C. PARMENTIER: Mucosal lipids in acanthocytosis. Clin. Res. **11**, 77 (1963).

— C. F. REED, and D. J. HANAHAN: Abnormalities of erythrocyte and plasma lipids in acanthocytosis. J. clin. Invest. **40**, 1088 (1961).

— — — Red cell and plasma lipids in acanthocytosis. J. clin. Invest. **42**, 1248 (1963).

— and E. R. SIMON: The role of serum in acanthocyte autohemolysis and membrane lipid composition. J. clin. Invest. **43**, 1322 (1964).

WEED, R. J., C. F. REED, and G. BERG: Is hemoglobin an essential structural component of human erythrocyte membranes. J. clin. Invest. **42**, 581 (1963).

WOLFF, J. A., and W. A. BAUMAN: Studies concerning acanthocytosis: a new genetic syndrome with absent beta-lipoprotein. Amer. J. Dis. Child. **102**, 478 (1961).

WOLFF, O. H.: A-beta-lipoproteinaemia. In: Erbliche Stoffwechsel-Krankheiten. Ed.: F. Linne-weh, p. 603. Berlin: Urban & Schwarzenberg 1962.

— A-β-Lipoproteinaemia. Ergebn. inn. Med. Kinderheilk. **23**, 190 (1965).

— K. J. LLOYD, and E. L. TONKS: A-β-Lipoproteinaemia; with special reference to the visual defect. Exp. Eye Res. (1965); cited after WOLFF (1965).

Tangier Disease

By

W. Kahlke

Synonyms: Familial high density lipoprotein deficiency; hypo-α-lipoproteinemia.

Definition and Introduction

Tangier disease (TD) is a very rare disorder which is named after the island of Tangier in the Chesapeake Bay where the first cases have been found. It is characterized by very low concentrations in plasma of high density lipoproteins (HDL) and by storage of cholesterol esters in various organs, particularly in those belonging to the reticuloendothelial system.

At first glance affected subjects do not present with remarkable features. Closer examination reveals striking discoloration and enlargement of the tonsils; in addition, spleen, lymph nodes and liver may be enlarged. Organomegaly is caused by storage of lipids, particularly of cholesterol esters. Changes compatible with lipid deposition have also been described in the cornea and in the intestinal mucosa.

Detailed descriptions of the few known cases have been given by FREDRICKSON et al. (1961), FREDRICKSON and ALTROCCHI (1962), FREDRICKSON (1964), HOFFMAN and FREDRICKSON (1965) and FREDRICKSON (1966). The present report is mainly based on the recent review of the disease by FREDRICKSON (1966).

Historical Remarks

In 1961/1962 the first case of the disease was described by FREDRICKSON's group. Their patient was a five year-old boy who had undergone tonsillectomy for marked tonsillar enlargement. Because of the particular color of the tonsils a lipid storage disease was considered. Further clinical findings in this otherwise healthy and intelligent child included enlargement of spleen, liver and lymph nodes. The lipid content of a lymph node which was removed was approximately 100 times normal with cholesterol esters predominating (FREDRICKSON et al. 1961).

The second case of TD, the only sibling of the first patient, was a girl in whom at the age of six enlargement and orange discoloration of the tonsils were found. Here, too, the concentration of cholesterol esters in the tonsils was extremely high. In both children plasma total cholesterol levels were below 100 mg per 100 ml. and plasma HDL were absent (FREDRICKSON et al. 1961; FREDRICKSON and ALTROCCHI 1962).

The third and fourth patients with TD were detected in 1962 (FREDRICKSON et al.). They were sisters from Missouri, aged 8 and 12 years respectively, in whom tonsillar changes had again given the clue to the diagnosis, and in whom plasma HDL were absent.

The last two patients, again siblings, were found in Kentucky. One of them was 45 years old and exhibited splenomegaly and signs of hypersplenism. His plasma total cholesterol level was below 50 mg per 100 ml. His brother, 3 years older, died suddenly, presumably from myocardial infarction. Plasma HDL could not be found in either subject.

Incidence (Age, Sex, Race, Family)

Obviously more than six cases are necessary to make any generalizations with regard to the incidence of TD. In the patients reported the disease was discovered accidentally on the basis of peculiar tonsillar enlargement; splenomegaly or palpable lymph nodes may also be the first findings of note. HDL deficiency which very probably exists at birth, does not produce symptoms; its discovery rests upon laboratory findings. The reported cases include both males and females, whites and Negroes.

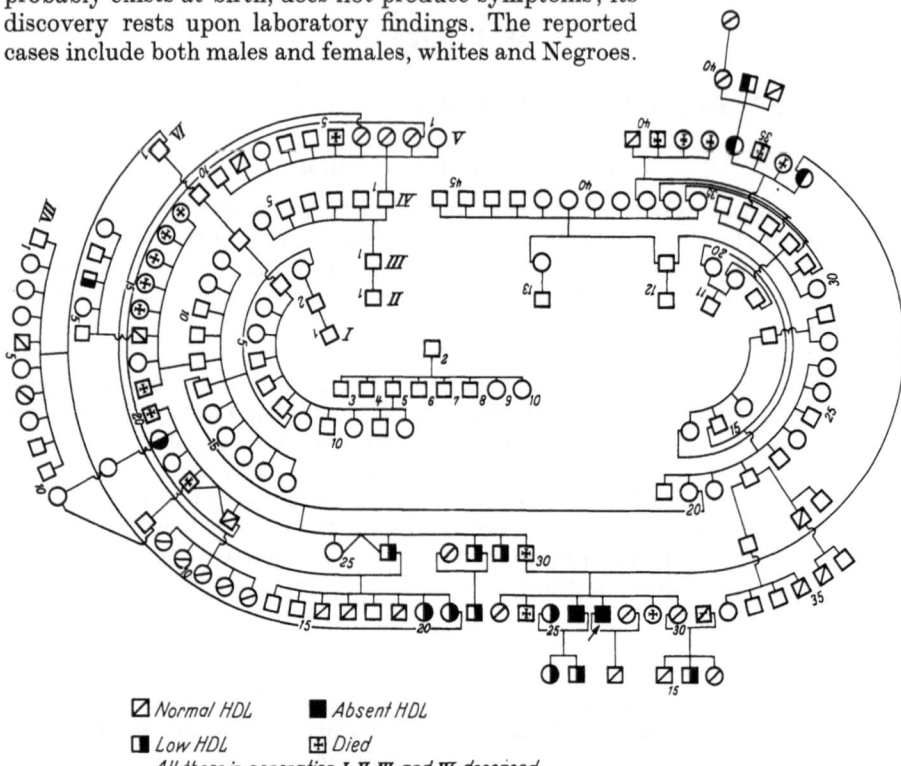

Fig. 1. Pedigree of Kentucky propositi, showing distribution of high density lipoprotein concentrations among forty-eight relatives. Source: Hoffman and Fredrickson (1965). (Reproduced with kind permission of *The American Journal of Medicine* and the authors)

The parents and a large number of close relatives of the first two patients had low plasma HDL levels as compared with normal controls. Out of 45 close relatives plasma HDL were abnormally low in 70% of the males and in over 50% of the females as determined by the cholesterol content of the ultracentrifugal lipoprotein fraction of $d > 1.063$. Abnormal HDL concentrations were less frequently found in distant relatives (see figure 1).

Consanguinity could not be established for any of the parents and certainly does not exist in the kindred from Missouri.

Clinical Manifestations

The clinical findings common for all six cases of TD is enlargement and typical discoloration of the tonsils. The latter appears as an orange or yellowish-white coating of the reddish tissue (see figure 2). Upon inspection of the tonsillar area following tonsillectomy follicles of similar color may be seen. Some mucosal tags show a translucent orange ring which is not found in any other tonsillar condition

(FREDRICKSON 1966). Therefore, inspection of the pharynx may already give some clue to the diagnosis.

Splenomegaly was found in three cases, while in the youngest patient hepatomegaly and recurrent swelling of lymph nodes were additional features (see table 1).

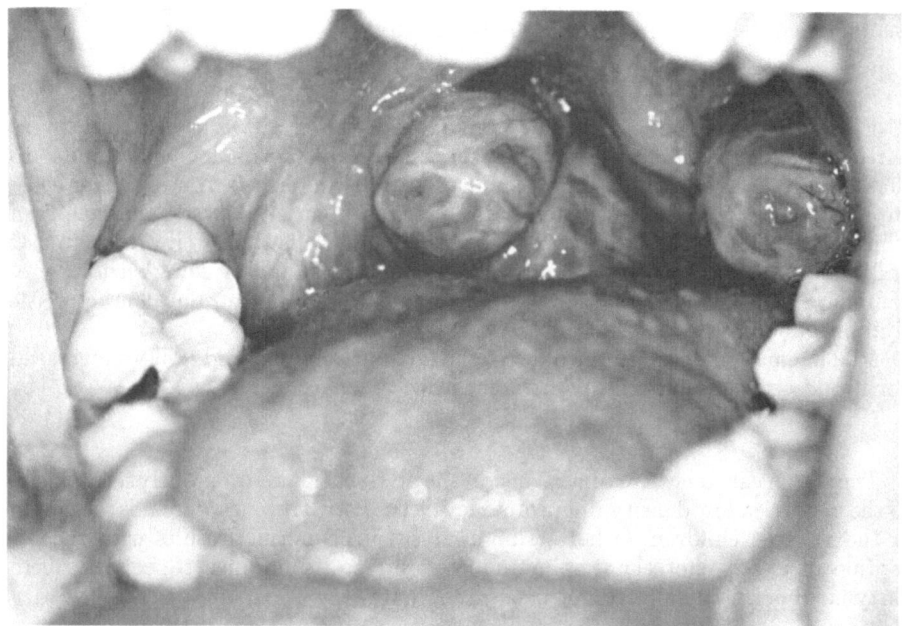

Fig. 2. Tonsils in Tangier disease. Patient E. L., age 6. The lighter bands on the tonsils appear orange in situ, yellow-white after removal. Source: FREDRICKSON et al. (1961). (Reproduced with kind permission of *Annals of Internal Medicine* and the authors)

In one case splenomegaly was associated with thrombocytopenia and leukopenia which were both reversible with splenectomy.

A hazily flocculent infiltration of the cornea may develop with advancing age. This was a finding in one subject, in whom visual acuity was not impaired.

A heart murmur and findings compatible with pulmonary stenosis were present in the 8 year-old child of the Missouri family. Electrocardiographic evidence for

Table 1. *Clinical features in Tangier disease*

Patient	Sex	Age at detection years	Abnormal tonsils	Spleno-megaly	Hepato-megaly	Enlarged lymph nodes	Corneal infiltration	Abnormal rectal mucosa	Neurologic abnormality	Foam cells in bone marrow
Tangier:										
T. L.	M	5	+*	+	+	+	0	?	0	+
E. L.	F	6	+*	0	0	0	0	?	0	+
Missouri:										
Pe. Lo.	F	8	+*	0	0	0	0	?	0	0
Pa. Lo.	F	12	+	+	0	0	0	?	0	0
Kentucky:										
C. N.	M	45	+	+	0	+	+	+	0	+
L. N.	M	48	+	0	0	0	+	+	0	+

* Tonsils shown to have increased content of cholesterol esters; remainder judged abnormal by history and presence of persistent tags or follicles having distinctive orange or yellow-white color. Source: FREDRICKSON (1966).

coronary heart disease was found in the patient from Kentucky who died suddenly. Both abnormalities cannot yet be related to TD (FREDRICKSON 1966).

Neurological symptoms have never been noted and mental and somatic development was unimpaired in every case. There is no evidence of progression of the disease during the course of four years in the two young patients from Tangier island, one of whom appears completely healthy.

Hematology

Foam cells were found in the bone marrow of the first two patients and were particularly numerous in the third sibship. They are morphologically similar to those found in other storage diseases, but can be distinguished from Gaucher cells. Birefringence can be demonstrated with polarized light, and crystals may be seen which are similar to those found in the tonsils. Foam cells stain well with oil red-O and Sudan dyes. A positive Schultz reaction is suggestive of a high cholesterol content. Smith-Dietrich reaction, Nile blue and PAS stains are not characteristic (FREDRICKSON 1966).

Mild anemia is present in the older of the Missouri siblings, and signs of increased hematopoesis were found in his bone marrow.

Serum

The serum carotenes are diminished in the adult patients, apparently secondarily to the decreased low density lipoprotein levels (LDL). Carotenes were not measured in the affected children. Other serum analyses yield normal results with the exception of electrophoretic and immunoelectrophoretic findings to be described. Enzyme abnormalities have not been observed.

Histology
Spleen

Histologic examination of a spleen following removal (weight 1116 gm) showed the reticuloendothelial cells of the pulp to be filled with intracytoplasmic fat droplets. There were scattered nests of cells containing cholesterol crystals (see figure 3).

Liver Biopsy

Liver biopsy specimens from the two adult patients of HOFFMAN and FREDRICKSON (1965) showed mild intralobular accumulation of foam cells. Histochemically, the foam cells as well as a granular material within parenchymal cells stained well with oil-red and were weakly PAS-positive. The Schultz reaction for cholesterol revealed small foci of blue-green coloration in the parenchymal cells and brillant blue-green staining of the foam cells.

Bowel Biopsy

While the jejunal mucosa of the adult cases was normal, the mucosa of the rectum showed the histological picture of lipid deposition in foam cells, and there was an orange-yellow tinge and tiny, flat, red-brown spots (HOFFMAN and FREDRICKSON 1965, FREDRICKSON 1966).

Other Organs

Lymph node biopsy showed marked fatty degeneration. Other organs were not examined in TD. There was no autopsy in the only fatal case.

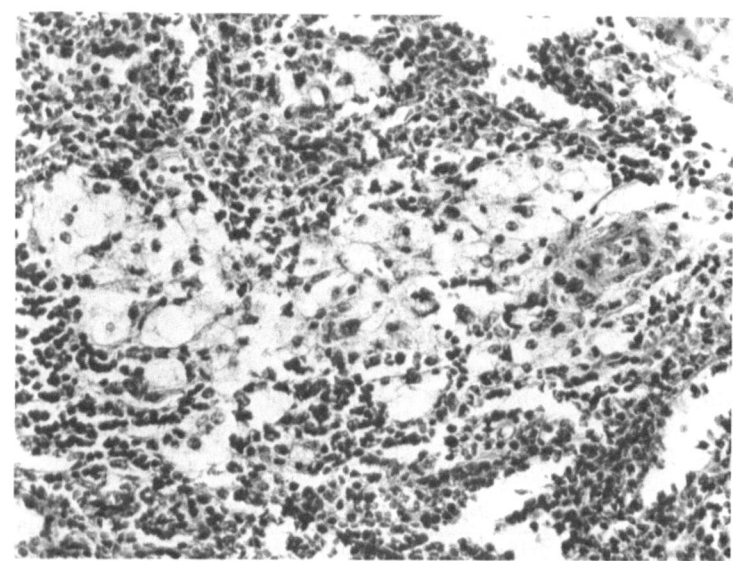

Fig. 3. Spleen showing lipid-filled reticulo-endothelial cells of pulp. Hematoxylin and eosin stain, original magnification × 250. Case 1 from HOFFMAN and FREDRICKSON (1965). (Reproduced with kind permission of *The American Journal of Medicine* and the authors)

Results of Lipid Analyses

Exhaustive plasma lipid analyses of all six cases were performed by FRED-RICKSON's group at the National Institutes of Health, and in addition, tonsillar lipids were studied in three cases and lipids of spleen and lymph nodes in one case.

Plasma Lipids

The most significant plasma lipid abnormality is a decreased cholesterol level. The lowest values are below 50 mg per 100 ml; similarly low levels are found

Table 2. *Plasma lipids in Tangier disease*

Patient	Sex	Age, years	Mean and range, mg/100 ml			
			Total cholesterol	Free cholesterol	Phospholipids	Triglycerides
Normal subjects	M, F	1—19	180 (115—240)		215 (155—265)	70 (20—120)
T. L.	M	5	101 (54—126)	31	144 (124—175)	225 (118—269)
E. L.	F	6	77 (50—96)	24	101 (82—148)	205 (191—237)
Pe. Lo.	F	8	112 (107—117)	33	137 (136—137)	224
Pa. Lo.	F	12	72 (67—76)	20	104 (96—111)	151
C. N.	M	45	38 (30—45)	14	86 (68—104)	142 (136—152)
L. N.	M	48	69 (50—88)	21	114 (104—124)	213 (195—238)
Normal subjects	M	40—49	250 (176—324)		280 (205—355)	70 (20—120)

Source: FREDRICKSON (1966).

only in a-β-lipoproteinemia (Bassen-Kornzweig syndrome). The highest values measured in TD lay between 100 and 130 mg per 100 ml and thus approached low normal levels. The free cholesterol levels are between 14 and 33 mg per 100 ml, the ratio of esterified to free cholesterol being normal in all cases.

Phospholipids are also decreased to about one half to two third of control values (see table 2). Again, some determinations in TD patients fell within the lower limit of normal. Although lecithin seems to be decreased to a greater degree than sphingomyelin, it remains the largest phospholipid fraction, in contrast to findings in a-β-lipoproteinemia. Plasma triglyceride levels were high normal or slightly elevated in all six cases.

Serum Lipoproteins

Analysis of lipoproteins with a variety of methods reveals the earmark of TD, namely almost complete absence in plasma of HDL. The cholesterol content of the density 1.063—1.21 fraction was in all cases below 2 mg per 100 ml as compared to 40—50 mg in normals (see table 3).

Table 3. *Plasma lipoproteins in Tangier disease (in mg/100 ml plasma)*

Patient	Sex	Age, years	Whole plasma		D 1.019		D 1.019–1.063		D 1.063–1.21		D >1.21	
			C	PL	C	PL	C	PL	C	PL	C	PL
E. L.	F	7	84	113	53	55	31	42	1	5	1	11
Pe. Lo.	F	8	107	137	14	33	92	91	1	2	1	11
Pa. Lo.	F	12	67	69	12	37	54	44	1	3	1	12
Controls	F	23—29	187	237	19	24	108	78	54	134	2	21
T. L.	M	6	93	127	35	57	56	56	2	2	1	12
C. N.	M	45	30	68	19	44	11	15	1	2	1	7
L. N.	M	48	50	104	33	70	13	23	1	3	1	8
Controls	M	21—28	171	215	26	31	97	69	43	111	2	21

C = cholesterol.
PL = phospholipids.
D = density.
Source: Fredrickson (1966); data for controls from Havel et al. (1955).

After paper-electrophoretic separation no lipid stainable material is found in the α_1 area. Upon preparative ultracentrifugation, the fraction with d 1.063—1.21 is absent.

When the plasma of a patient is treated with rabbit antibodies against HDL, only a faint precipitation line is visible on the agar (see fig. 3). Accordingly, immunoelectrophoresis with a variety of antisera fails to show precipitation lines for α-lipoproteins. These findings are the same whether the subjects are fasting or have recently eaten a fatty meal; furthermore, the late rise in plasma phospholipids which is observed after fat absorption in normals, is not seen in TD. The findings show that the lipid as well as the protein moiety of HDL are missing or markedly diminished in patients with TD.

In some plasmas (cases from Tangier and from Missouri) which were concentrated five-fold, Levy (1966) was able to identify small amounts of a high density lipoprotein which behaved antigenically like the normal HDL. Semiquantitative determination according to the method of Preer (1956) showed a level which was approximately 2% of normal.

The behavior of low density lipoproteins (LDL) is of interest. In all six patients the concentration of lipoproteins of density 1.019 to 1.063 was lowered while that of lipoproteins of d < 1.019 was elevated in some cases. In both LDL subgroups the cholesterol : phospholipid ratio was lowered. The decreased levels of lecithin

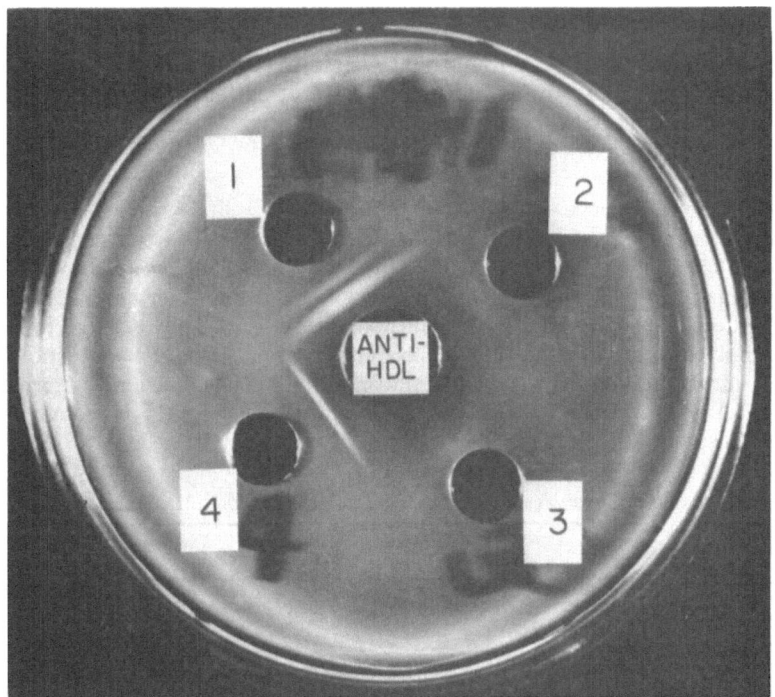

Fig. 4a. Precipitation lines formed by Ouchterlony agar diffusion technic with serum from normal subject (1), patients with Tangier disease (2, 3) and patient with a-β-lipoproteinemia (4) against rabbit antibodies prepared against human lipoproteins of density 1.063—1.21 ("anti-HDL"). Both precipitation lines at (1) are attributed to HDL

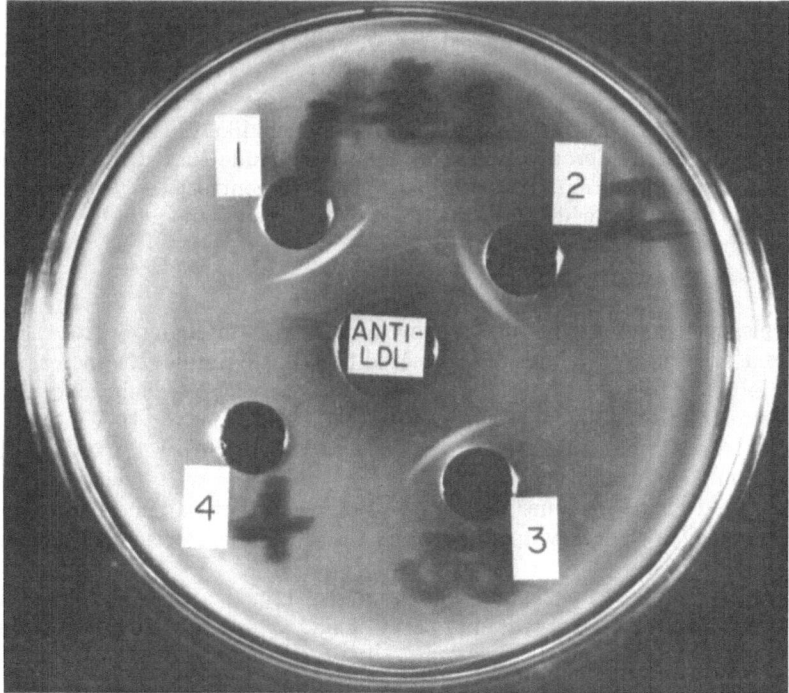

Fig. 4b. Arrangement same as in fig. 4a, except rabbit antibodies were prepared against human lipoproteins of density <1.063 ("anti-LDL"). Here both patients with Tangier disease demonstrated LDL, which was further shown by immunoelectrophoresis. Plates prepared by Dr. R. I. Levy. Source: HOFFMAN and FREDRICKSON (1965). (Reproduced with kind permission of The American Journal of Medicine and the authors)

and sphingomyelin which are found upon analysis of a total lipid extract, mirror the findings in the LDL. Immunologically, LDL of patients with TD are identical with those of normal controls.

Chylomicrons

Chylomicrons deserve particular attention in TD since their protein moiety normally contains peptides identical with those of HDL (RODBELL and FREDRICKSON 1959; SCANU and PAGE 1959; FREDRICKSON 1965). Fat absorption procedes normally in TD, and TD-chylomicrons behave like "normal" chylomicrons upon ultracentrifugation and phase contrast microscopy. They are dissimilar from the normal particles in that their cholesterol content is only about one quarter that of normal chylomicrons, while phospholipid concentration is normal (see table 4). A slight delay in chylomicron removal was found in some patients (FREDRICKSON 1966).

Table 4. *Chylomicron lipid composition (in μM/100 μM glyceride)*

	Phospho-lipid	Esterified cholesterol	Free cholesterol
Control	6.1	12.8	7.2
Control	6.8	8.7	7.5
Tangier disease:			
L. N.	8.3	3.2	1.8
E. L. + T. L.	7.0	2.0	1.1

Chylomicrons were obtained from plasma after fat feeding (RODBELL, M., and D. S. FREDRICKSON 1959). The controls were patients with familial fat-induced hyperglyceridemia. It is noteworthy that portions of the chylomicrons of controls were also incubated for 18 h at 2°C with chylomicron-free plasma from the other subjects. This produced no difference in the lipid content of their chylomicrons. Source: FREDRICKSON (1966).

It has not been established whether the HDL peptide is present or absent in the chylomicrons of patients with TD. If, as seems very likely, the HDL peptide is missing in the chylomicrons of TD, one has to conclude that it is not necessary for chylomicron formation (FREDRICKSON 1966), in contrast to the β-lipoprotein peptide, the absence of which (a-β-lipoproteinemia) results in an inability of chylomicron formation or release.

Tissue Lipids

Tonsils, spleen and lymph nodes show rather uniform changes with regard to their lipid pattern. Total lipids are increased two- to three-fold, the increase being due mainly to excessive accumulation of cholesterol esters. Their concentration may range from 20 to over 100 times normal (see table 5). In contrast, free cholesterol which makes up most of the total tissue cholesterol in normals is increased only slightly or not at all in TD.

Other lipid classes are insignificantly altered. Both total phospholipids and glycerides were low in a lymph node, but the glyceride fraction was increased in a spleen.

No atypical lipids were found in the organs examined, and in particular glycolipids were absent. The organ lipid fatty acid pattern in TD reflects that of cholesterol esters (see table 6). Even normally organ cholesterol esters do not have the high (50—60%) linoleic acid content of plasma cholesterol esters. In TD, oleic acid is the main fatty acid (over 50% in some cases). This finding, the significance of which is not known, is in analogy to findings in other disorders associated with

Table 5. *Tissue lipids in Tangier disease (In mg/gm dry weight of tissue)*

Source	Tissue	Total lipid	Chole-sterol esters	Free chole-sterol	Total phospho-lipid	Leci-thin	Sphin-gomye-lin	Gly-ceride	Lipid-bound hexose
C. N.	Spleen (fresh)	244	75	21	74	23	11	14	1
Control A	Spleen (fresh)	79	5	15	40	8	8	2	1
Control B	Spleen (fresh)	103	2	15	68	19	9	2	—
T. L.	Tonsil (formalin-fixed)	210	136	13	32	—	—	—	—
Pe. Lo.	Tonsil (formalin-fixed)	145	90	11	36	—	—	—	—
E. L.	Tonsil (fresh)	162	89	20	63	—	—	—	—
Controls (8)	Tonsils (fresh)	69	1	11	49	—	—	—	—
T. L.	Lymph node (fresh)	386	284	36	38	13	2	31	—
Controls (2)	Lymph nodes (fresh)	131	2	9	66	34	9	54	—

Source: FREDRICKSON (1966).

cholesterol storage such as Hand-Schüller-Christian disease (FREDRICKSON 1966) or atherosclerotic plaques (BÖTTCHER et al. 1960, 1961). There is no evidence for the occurrence of atypical fatty acids among total organ fatty acids. A fraction which makes up about 6% of splenic fatty acids may correspond to long chain poly-unsaturated fatty acids such as docosa-pentaenoic or docosahexaenoic acids.

Table 6. *Fatty acid composition of spleen total lipids (in per cent of total fatty acids)*

Fatty acid	Tangier disease (case C. N.)	Control
$C_{14:0}$	0.5	0.5
$C_{15:0}$	1.0	1.4
$C_{16:0}$	21.5	22.3
$C_{16:1}$	—	0.8
$C_{17:0}$	0.6	1.1
$C_{18:0}$	12.3	16.9
$C_{18:1}$	28.2	15.3
$C_{18:2}$	9.2	6.4
$C_{18:3}$	1.1	—
$C_{20:0}$	0.1	—
$C_{20:4}$	13.3	12.7
$C_{22:0}$	1.9	3.4
x	6.2	—
$C_{24:1}$	4.0	7.0
x^1	—	8.3

Source: FREDRICKSON (1966).

Pathogenetic Aspects

In TD, pathogenetic discussions center around the abnormality of plasma HDL and the deposition of cholesterol esters in reticuloendothelial tissues. Other changes, such as a low plasma level of carotenes in adult cases, apparently result from the decreased concentration of LDL and are, in contrast to those of a-β-lipoproteinemia, without clinical consequences in TD. Of interest is the existence in the Kentucky kindred of cases with pigmentary retinitis (see fig. 5); such subjects had low or normal plasma HDL, and a relation between the retinopathy and TD is improbable. On the other hand, splenic bone marrow inhibition in one subject is most probably a result of the underlying disease. This has not been established for the occurrence of coronary thrombosis in one patient, in whom an autopsy was not performed and the condition of the vasculature is not known. A predisposition in TD toward the development of atherosclerotic lesions cannot be excluded.

It is not yet known whether lack of plasma HDL is the primary disturbance or whether an intracellular lesion leads to the deposition of cholesterol esters in TD. It is likely that deposition in tissues of cholesterol esters results, at least in part, from synthesis in loco, since most body tissues can synthesize cholesterol esters (SRERE et al. 1948).

Preliminary studies on cholesterol synthesis by tonsillar tissues of a TD patient based on the incorporation of labeled precursors, have not yielded evidence of altered synthesis rates (Fredrickson 1966).

In addition to synthesis in loco, potential sources of cholesterol and other lipids in tissues where red cell destruction occurs, are lipids of erythrocytes (Fredrickson 1966), but the quantitative aspects of this process are not known.

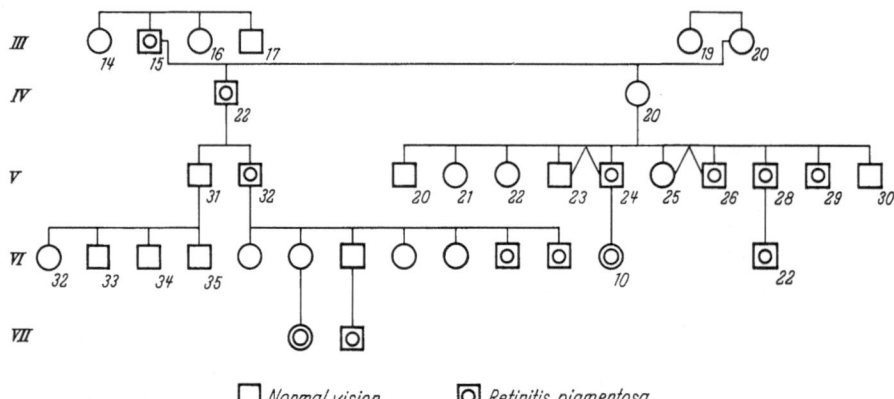

Fig. 5. Predigree of Kentucky propositi, showing distribution of retinitis pigmentosa. Numbers are same as in fig. 1. Source: Hoffman and Fredrickson (1965). (Reproduced with kind permission of *The American Journal of Medicine* and the authors)

Degradation of cholesterol to bile acids is limited to the liver. There is no evidence of cholesterol degradation by storing tissues nor of an elevated serum bile acid level in TD. It is likely that cholesterol transport is normally associated with HDL, and cannot be accomplished by LDL. The accumulation of cholesterol in the tissues in TD may therefore be due to impaired transport from storing organs to the liver. In this regard, the lack of HDL in TD, like the absence of LDL in a-β-lipoproteinemia, presents an interesting model for the study of the functional role of lipoproteins, and the impaired transport of cholesterol esters from tissues in TD may in some way correspond to hampered movement of triglycerides from their sites of synthesis, namely small bowel mucosa and liver, in a-β-lipoproteinemia. Both diseases are likely to be due to deficient synthesis of certain proteins; that of HDL in the former and that of LDL in the latter.

Since Fredrickson's group could show with immunological methods that there are traces of HDL in TD, it appears that the genetic information for the synthesis of the HDL protein is actually present, but that for some reason protein synthesis is insufficient.

It can be speculated that the formation of a structurally similar protein may inhibit the synthesis of the normal HDL protein in TD. If this is the case the hypothetical abnormal protein must lack lipid binding since an atypical lipoprotein is not found in the plasma of TD patients. It remains for future studies to establish the normal function of HDL and to clarify the cause of this interesting hereditary disorder.

Diagnosis

Clinical signs and symptoms are discrete and largely non-specific. The typical discoloration of the tonsils with a translucent orange ring surrounding the mucosal tags may provide the only diagnostic clue for someone who has had occasion to observe this change before. Splenomegaly, hepatomegaly and lymph node enlargement are uncharacteristic findings, and present also in more common lipidoses such as Niemann-Pick disease and Gaucher's disease, while leukemia can be excluded with relative ease. Differentiation from Gaucher's disease is possible by the increase of acid serum phosphatase and the appearance of Gaucher cells in the bone marrow in this disorder. Foam cells, however, may be similar in TD, Gaucher's disease and Niemann-Pick disease. Evidence for disease progression as observed in Niemann-Pick disease is not seen in TD. Hepatosplenomegaly of essential hyperlipemia is frequently associated with serum turbidity and, in about 30% of patients, with xanthomas; both are absent in TD. When cholesterol levels are below 100 mg per 100 ml, a-β-lipoproteinemia has to be considered, but values between 100 and 130 mg per 100 ml are normal in some populations, and are found in disorders like malabsorption syndromes and hyperthyroidism. While cholesterol storage in tissues occurs in the Refsum syndrome, here it is usually associated with an increase in all neutral lipids, and differentiation can be secured by the typical finding in plasma of large amounts of a branched chain fatty acid (3, 7, 11, 15-tetramethylhexadecanoic acid) in Refsum's disease.

Numerous tedious laboratory procedures can be avoided by the use of paper-electrophoresis for lipoproteins, where in analogy to missing LDL in the Bassen-Kornzweig syndrome, the lack of the HDL band is diagnostic for TD.

References

Böttcher, C. J. F., and C. M. van Gent: Changes in the composition of phospholipids and of phospholipid fatty acids associated with atherosclerosis in the human aortic wall. J. Atheroscler. Res. 1, 36 (1961).

— F. P. Woodford, C. Ch. ter Haar Romeny-Wachter, E. Boelsma-van Houte, and C. M. van Gent: Fatty acid distribution in lipids of the aortic wall. Lancet 1960/I, 1378.

Frantz jr., I. D., H. S. Schneider, and B. T. Hinkelman: Suppression of hepatic cholesterol synthesis in the rat by cholesterol feeding. J. biol. Chem. 206, 465 (1954).

Fredrickson, D. S.: The inheritance of high density lipoprotein deficiency (Tangier disease). J. clin. Invest. 43, 228 (1964).

— Symposium on pathophysiological and clinical aspects of lipid metabolism, Heidelberg 1965. Ed.: G. Schettler. Stuttgart: Thieme 1967.

— Familial high density lipoprotein deficiency: Tangier disease, in: The metabolic basis of inherited disease. Eds.: J. B. Stanbury, J. B. Wyngaarden, and D. S. Fredrickson. New York: McGraw-Hill Book Co. 1966.

— and P. H. Altrocchi: Tangier disease (familial cholesterolosis with high density lipoprotein deficiency) in: Cerebral sphingolipidoses. Eds. S. M. Aronson, and B. W. Volk, p. 343. New York: Academic Press 1962.

— — L. V. Avioli, DeW. S. Goodman, and H. C. Goodman: Tangier disease. Ann. intern. Med. 55, 1016 (1961).

— T. Shiratori, and O. M. Young: Genetic control of high density lipoprotein concentrations in man. Circulation 26, 653 (1962).

Havel, R. J., H. A. Eder, and J. H. Bragdon: The distribution and chemical composition of ultracentrifugally separated lipoproteins in human serum. J. clin. Invest. 34, 1345 (1955).

Hoffman, H. N., and D. S. Fredrickson: Tangier disease. (Familial high density lipoprotein deficiency) Clinical and genetic features in two adults. Amer. J. Med. 39, 582 (1965).

Levy, R. I.: in H. N. Hoffman, and D. S. Fredrickson (1965), and Fredrickson (1966).

Preer, J. R.: A quantitative study of a technique of double diffusion in agar. J. Immunol. 77, 52 (1956).

Rodbell, M., and D. S. Fredrickson: The nature of the proteins associated with dog and human chylomicrons. J. biol. Chem. 234, 562 (1959).

Scanu, A., and I. H. Page: Separation and characterization of human serum chylomicrons. J. exp. Med. 109, 239 (1959).

Srere, P. A., I. L. Chaikoff, and W. G. Dauben: The in vitro synthesis of cholesterol from acetate by surviving adrenal cortical tissue. J. biol. Chem. 176, 829 (1948).

Essential Hypercholesterolemia

By

G. Schettler, W. Kahlke, and G. Schlierf

Synonyms: Primary hypercholesterolemia, familial hypercholesterolemic xanthomatosis, hyperbetalipoproteinemia.

Definition and Introduction

Essential familial hypercholesterolemia (EFH) is an hereditary disorder of lipid metabolism which is characterized chemically by elevation of plasma cholesterol and phospholipids due to an increased concentration of beta-lipoproteins. The cholesterol to phospholipid ratio is greater than one. Typical clinical features are skin, fascial and tendon xanthomas, the incidence of which seems to depend on the plasma lipid level and increases with age. Xanthelasmas of the eyelids and arcus lipoides corneae are more frequent than in the general population. The prevalence of signs and symptoms of premature atherosclerosis is high. Since hypercholesterolemia in an individual is non-specific unless it is of very marked degree, the diagnosis of EFH frequently depends on the demonstration of one or more of these symptoms in several members of a kindred. Only rarely does a patient show all the symptoms of EFH; monosymptomatic (cholesterol elevation only) and heterosymptomatic forms are frequent.

Historical Review

The skin lesions of EFH were recognized well over 100 years ago. Following the description by RAYER (1836) of xanthelasmas ADDISON and GULL (1850) published a detailed report on xanthomatosis. The familial occurrence of xanthomas was observed for the first time in 1882 by STARTIN and independently by MACKENZIE (1882). A relationship between the development of xanthomas and plasma lipids was suspected as early as 1878 by QUINQUAUD and supported by analyses of xanthomas (PICK and PINKUS 1908). From observations in obstructive liver disease CHAUFFARD and LA ROCHE (1910) stated that the "xanthoma is for hypercholesterolemia what the tophus is for gout". In 1914, SCHMIDT first measured serum cholesterol levels in xanthomatosis with the method of AUTENRIETH and FUNK (1913); since then the connection between xanthomatosis and hypercholesterolemia was generally recognized.

In contrast to typical cases of EFH where the plasma is clear, numerous reports of plasma turbidity or its equivalent, significant elevation of triglycerides, in "EFH" were described during the last 15 years. These were discussed as "mixed" cases of EFH and essential hyperlipemia by BORRIE (1957) and others. Recent evidence (FREDRICKSON and LEES 1966) suggests that such cases belong to one or more separate categories, the relationship of which to endogenous hyperlipemias remains to be clarified (see page 452 and 460). For most patients reported as EFH, differentiation in retrospect is not possible, and the clinical material from which the following information is compiled, is not entirely homogenous. However, from studies in Fredrickson's and our own laboratories it appears that the sympto-matology in patients with this (these) separate form(s) is very similar to that of "pure" EFH with the exception of frequent occurrence of carbohydrate intolerance and a slightly different xanthomatosis in the former.

Incidence (Age, Sex, Race, Family)

Although cholesterol determinations are now being carried out almost routinely, the prevalence of EFH in the general population has not been established. Studying subjects with hypercholesterolemia SCHAEFER et al. (1958) found a prevalence of EFH of 12% among 250 males and 250 females in New York City. There was a frequency in hypercholesterolemic Jewish persons of 21% as compared to 9% in non-Jews. In contrast to the predisposition for EFH in the Jewish race the disease is rare in Negroes and orientals.

From studies of approximately 1500 cases from 150 families which have ap-peared during the past 10 years, it is apparent that marked hypercholesterolemia and xanthomatosis may be found in children, and death from coronary heart disease may occur before the age of 10 (see page 419). In the great majority of subjects who are to develop EFH, hypercholesterolemia is present by that age.

Variable figures have been given for the prevalence of EFH in affected families. Since such data rest on plasma cholesterol levels of examined members, which are not only the result of the genetic pattern exhibited by either parent but also of racial, geographic, nutritional and many other factors, and since, in addition, "hypercholesterolemia" was defined differently by different authors, the figures cannot be compared. Some examples follow: PIPER and ORRILD (1956) examined systematically almost all members of 12 families with EFH, previously described by KORNERUP (1948). Plasma cholesterol levels were found to be above 324 mg/100 ml in children or above 340 mg/100 ml in adults in 112 out of 425 cases (26%). Since the upper limits had already been used in the study of KOR-NERUP, they have also been employed in the follow-up study, although they are far higher than the upper limits of normal used by most authors. HARRIS-JONES et al. (1957) studied five families and found 38 subjects out of 150 with hyper-cholesterolemia (25%). A higher percentage is reported by GURAVICH and VENEGAS (1962) who found hypercholesterolemia in 38% of 123 members from 2 families. An even higher occurrence was reported by LEONARD (1956), with 36 subjects having plasma cholesterol levels above 300 mg/100 ml among 67 members of an affected family (54%).

The transmission of EFH is not sex-linked, and members of both sexes are equally affected. Of 48 hypercholesterolemic subjects (GURAVICH and VENEGAS 1962), 23 were males and 25 were females. The mode of genetic transmission is still controversial and hereditary problems of EFH are considered in detail by FUHRMANN in the chapter on genetics (see page 513).

Clinical Manifestations

Xanthomatosis

Whereas hypercholesterolemia is present in all patients according to definition, other signs or symptoms such as xanthomas may or may not occur in an individual with EFH, depending on at least two factors, the age of the patient and his plasma cholesterol level. This does not imply that the relation between plasma cholesterol and development of xanthomas is completely predictable. The importance of tissue factors should also be considered in their pathogenesis. One opinion (HIRSCHHORN and Wilkinson 1959) states that xanthomatosis is the expression of a double dose of the abnormal allele while hypercholesterolemia alone occurs already with the single dose. Although this matter has not yet been settled, an alternate explanation is more likely, namely that juvenile xanthomatosis indicates carriers of a double

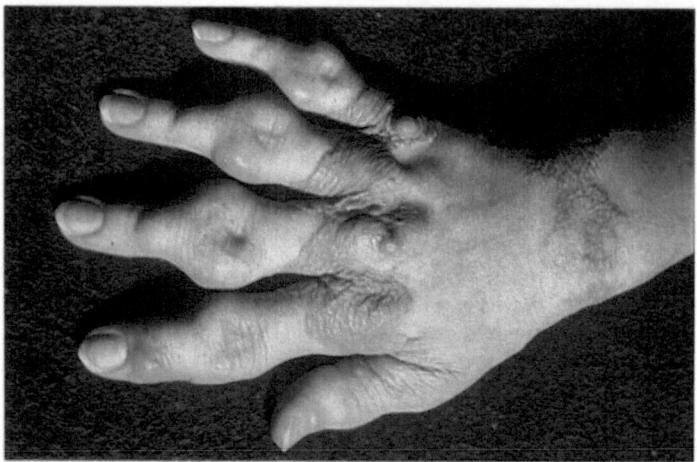

Fig. 1: Deformity of fingers resulting from deposition of xanthomatous material in joint capsules and tendons. Normal uric acid level. Tuberous and plane xanthomas overlying the dorsal aspect of the wrist and the metacarpal-phalangeal joints of fingers 2 to 5. Source: Schettler 1960. Reproduced with permission of *Urban and Schwarzenberg*, München-Berlin, Germany

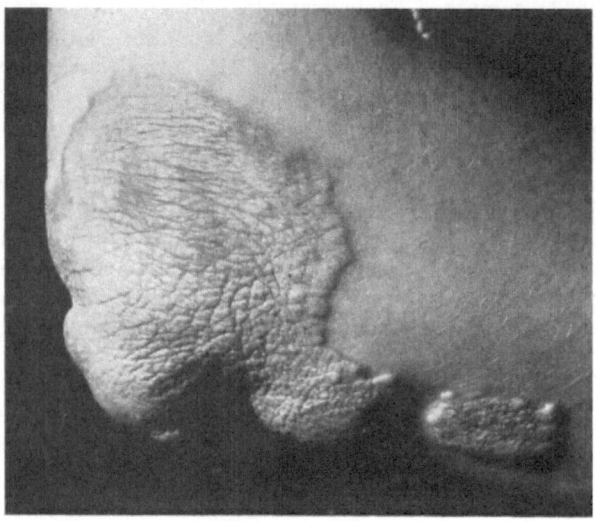

Fig. 2. Deposition of xanthomatous material in bursa of elbow, covered and surrounded by flat intra-cutaneous xanthomas. Source: Schettler 1960. Reproduced with permission of *Urban and Schwarzen-berg*, München-Berlin, Germany

dose of the abnormal gene, while xanthomatosis which occurs later in life may be due to only one abnormal gene (Khachadurian 1964).

Tendon xanthomas are characteristic of EFH and involve most frequently the Achilles tendons, less often the extensor tendons of fingers and toes, the patellar tendons, triceps tendons and rarely flexor tendons (see fig. 1 and 2). They are attached to the skin as well as to the underlying tissues, and form round or oval shaped nodes which occasionally reach the size of a small fist. Frequently their

distinction from xanthomas originating from periosteum or fascia is not possible
by palpation alone, and occasionally differentiation from tophi of gout is difficult.
Tendon xanthomas are least amenable to therapy of all types of xanthomas.

Almost as characteristic for EFH are *xanthomata plana*. They consist of flat,
yellow to red-brown plaques which have a velvety texture, may be confluent and

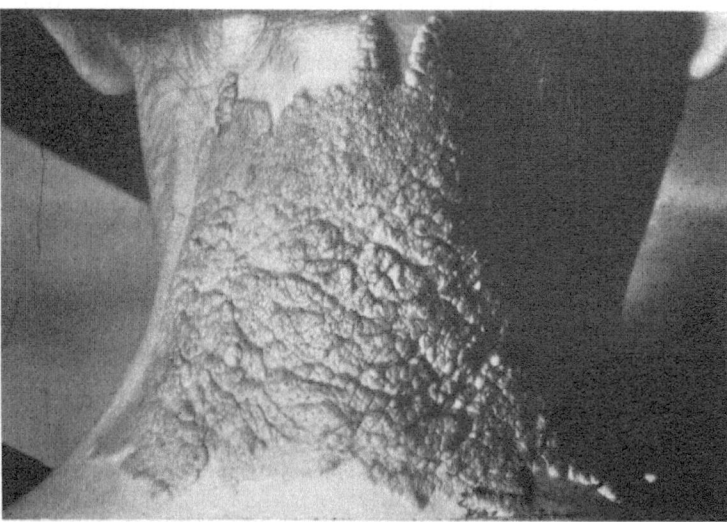

Fig. 3. Large, verrucous xanthomatous area on the back of the neck. Source: SCHETTLER 1960. Reproduced with permission of *Urban and Schwarzenberg*, München-Berlin, Germany

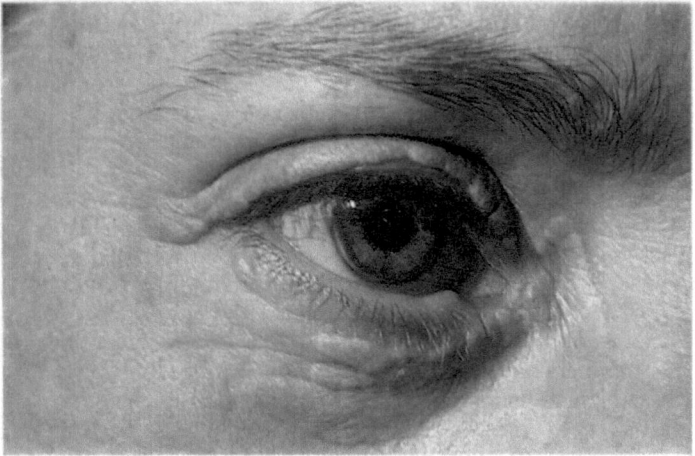

Fig. 4. Xanthelasmas and arcus lipoides corneae in EFH

can reach considerable size. They may be seen on the neck, shoulders, back and
extremities (see fig. 2 and 3). A particular type of plane xanthomas are xanthelasmas: flat, yellow lipid deposits in the upper and lower eyelids towards the
nasal corner of the eyes (see fig. 4). They, too, may become quite large (BLODI
and YARBROUGH 1962), and their occurrence is not restricted to patients with EFH.
Xanthelasmas are frequently found in the absence of hypercholesterolemia in older
people, especially postmenopausal women, and BLODI and YARBROUGH (1962)
consider venous congestion in the border of the medial part of the eyelids to be

a predisposing factor in the deposition of lipids. The incidence of xanthelasmas in EFH as given by various authors is as follows: ADLERSBERG et al. (1949) 35%, SCHETTLER and DIETRICH (1953) 25%, LEONARD (1956) 8%, and PIPER and ORRILD (1956) 18%. Elevated plasma lipid levels were found in 30—60% of patients with xanthelasmas by several groups of authors (POLANO 1936, 1940, CURTIS and BERGER 1945, FOWLKES and FORBES 1950, EPSTEIN et al. 1952, MONTGOMERY 1952, BLODI and YARBROUGH 1962). In the largest relevant series (PEDACE and WINKELMAN 1965) of 869 subjects with xanthelasmas, hypercholesterolemia was found only in 33% of the males and 40% of the females.

While, according to GOFMAN et al. (1954), tendon xanthomas correlate best with an increased content in plasma of Sf 0—12 lipoproteins, which is typical for EFH (see page 422), another type of xanthomas, *tuberous xanthomas* (see page 463), is found with elevated Sf 20—100 and to a lesser degree, Sf 100—400 lipoproteins. Since elevation of Sf 20—400 lipoproteins is associated with an increased plasma triglyceride as well as cholesterol level, cases with tuberous xanthomas seem to belong to a separate group which has been described in this volume as endogenous hyperlipemia with essential hypercholesterolemia on page 460 or as type III hyperlipoproteinemia (FREDRICKSON et al. 1966). Analyses of more cases with tuberous xanthomas will ultimately confirm or disprove this hypothesis, which cannot be supported from most reported cases, since triglyceride determinations and/or lipoprotein measurements were not performed in the majority of cases reported as EFH in the literature. Tuberous xanthomas also occur in essential hyperlipemias (FLEISCHMAJER 1965).

In reviewing 700 cases from the literature we find xanthomatosis in one-third to one-half of patients of all ages with hypercholesterolemia. The rate may approach 100% in some severely affected families. Thus in the F1 generation of kindred 1 branch A of GURAVICH and VENEGAS (1962) 7 out of 9 children suffered from skin or tendon xanthomas; for the total number of patients examined by this group, the prevalence of xanthomas was 62%. In 36 patients with hypercholesterolemia, LEONARD (1956) described 14 with tendon xanthomas and 4 with skin xanthomas. PIPER and ORRILD (1956) found 42 cases with xanthomas in 112 hypercholesterolemic patients, while in SCHETTLER's (1955) series of 24 cases with hypercholesterolemia, 11 exhibited xanthomas.

Although most xanthomas occur after age 20, earlier occurrence has been described. These include an unusually severe case of SCHETTLER et al. (1959) where xanthomas appeared during the first year of life; and a family of 6 children (EPSTEIN et al. 1959) who according to their mother exhibited the skin lesions by the age of 4 years. That such an occurrence is indicative of a very grave prognosis, is apparent from the fact that all 6 children expired at an early age (7, 13, 13, 15, 16 and 23 years old) from xanthomatosis of the coronary arteries, in two cases verified by autopsy (MAHER et al. 1958). Two brothers described by RIEDERER (1961) also exhibited skin and tendon xanthomas at an early age, and died with symptoms of cardiovascular xanthomatosis aged 10 and 15 years respectively. Finally DEBUCH and KAHLKE (1964) observed two unrelated boys with EFH, 10 and 12 years old, who had plasma cholesterol levels of 855 mg/100 ml and 912 mg/100 ml respectively; skin and tendon xanthomas were present in both cases.

The majority of xanthomas appear in the 4th decade, and the prevalence increases during the following decades. Some authors have discussed a lower rate of occurrence with further increase of age, but the early mortality of patients with xanthomas from coronary heart disease has to be considered here. The youngest patient with xanthomas in the study of PIPER and ORRILD (1956) was 19 years old; in the age group from 20—29, 3 out of 10 (30%) exhibited xanthomas. The corresponding figures for the 4th decade were 13 out of 25 (52%), and for the 5th decade 9 out of 13 (69%). The figures for the next 3 decades were 47%, 57% and 75% respectively, with the number of subjects decreasing. Hood and Angervall (1959) found only one subject with tendon xanthoma (21 years old) in a group of 45 patients below age 30. According to these authors the most marked xanthomatosis occurred in men up to age 50 and in women up to age 60, whereas persons above these age limits had less severe lesions. A higher incidence of xanthomatosis with advancing age is well documented in the material of Kornerup (1948) who found xanthomas in 50% of his cases, xanthelasmas in 28% and arcus senilis in 38% during the period from 1941 to 1943. Upon re-examination of the same patients by Piper and Orrild (1956) the values had increased to 68%, 50% and 48% respectively.

Repeated attempts have been made to relate the degree of hypercholesterolemia to the development of xanthomas (Leonard 1956, Piper and Orrild 1956, Harris-Jones 1957, Hood and Angervall 1959, Guravich 1959, Nitter-Hauge 1966). Although exact statements are difficult to make because the time of the first manifestation of xanthomas is not always known, the following can be summarized from the above mentioned studies: With plasma cholesterol levels between 300 and 350 mg per 100 ml, in 20 patients below age 50 only one subject exhibited xanthomas (in the 5th decade); the prevalence of xanthomas during the next two decades was 6 out of 11 and 4 out of 8 respectively. With cholesterol levels between 351 and 400 mg per 100 ml, xanthomas have been observed in the 4th decade, and the prevalence was higher in the higher age groups. With plasma cholesterol levels between 400 and 450 mg per 100 ml, 3 out of 5 patients in the 3rd decade and 5 out of 6 in the 4th decade exhibited xanthomas.

Adult patients without xanthomas therefore usually have lower cholesterol levels than younger patients with xanthomas. This is illustrated by adolescent patients of Epstein et al. (1959) (A 17; plasma cholesterol 1033 mg per 100 ml, died aged 13, xanthomas since age 5), of Schettler (1960) (two siblings with xanthomas at age 4 and 6, plasma cholesterol levels 860 and 940 mg per 100 ml respectively, sudden cardiac deaths at the ages of 6 and 8, respectively), of Debuch and Kahlke (1964) (plasma cholesterol levels 800—900 mg%, xanthomas when 10 and 12 years old), and of Piper and Orrild (1956) (xanthomas when 19 years old, cholesterol values between 601 and 650 mg per 100 ml).

Corneal Arcus

Arcus lipoides corneae or corneal arcus is an area of increased density at the corneal margin, initially arch-shaped but later annular in appearance (see fig. 4). This condition, like xanthelasma, is not necessarily secondary to a disturbance in lipid metabolism (Schettler 1955, Lindholm 1960, Rohrschneider 1962) and is not pathognomonic for EFH, although apparently more frequent in sufferers from this disease as compared to the incidence in the general population. Local factors in the area of the corneal margin predisposing to deposition of lipid are probably important in the development of corneal arcus (Finley et al. 1961). The lack of blood vessels favors the deposition of lipid-containing materials and metabolic waste in this area.

The finding of corneal arcus in adolescents and younger adults should always be considered suggestive of EFH or other disturbances of lipid metabolism. In higher age groups it is a frequent finding. Rohrschneider (1960) reported from biomicroscopic examinations of the cornea of 400 patients at the Munich Eye Clinic a prevalence of 80% in persons between 50 and 60 years, and of 90% in the 7th decade.

Guravich (1959) observed arcus senilis in 8 of his 22 cases below age 40, the youngest subject being 27 years old. Three years later Guravich and Venegas (1962) found corneal arcus in 24 out of 47 patients with hypercholesterolemia. Their 28 borderline cases (plasma cholesterol levels between 250 and 300 mg per 100 ml) included 4 persons with arcus (all in the 7th decade), whereas the incidence in 47 normocholesterolemic persons was two. The prevalence of corneal arcus in EFH as given by other authors is as follows: Adlersberg et al. (1949) 18% (material contains a number of normocholesterolemic relatives of affected subjects), Leonard (1956) 6%, Piper and Orrild (1956) 24%. Careful examination, preferably by an ophthalmologist, is indicated for the diagnosis of corneal arcus, especially in the early stages. Discrepancies in reported incidence or prevalence may be explained in part by inadequate search in some studies for this, admittedly very non-specific, clinical sign.

Cardiovascular Xanthomatosis

The term cardiovascular xanthomatosis will be used for the sum of valvular (see fig. 5) and arterial atheromatous lesions which are found in subjects with EFH. Although its use serves to emphasize some peculiarities of both kinds of lesions as compared to "general" atherosclerosis (age of victim, preponderance of foam cells) it does not imply that atherosclerosis in EFH can be reliably distinguished on morphological grounds from other atherosclerosis.

The incidence and prevalence of signs and symptoms of atherosclerosis is high in subjects with EFH. An early discussion relevant to this subject was published from Addison's school (Fagge 1872). Cardiovascular xanthomatosis has been found since in numerous cases at autopsy (Lehzen and Knauss 1889, Bross 1920, Hess 1934, Schildhaus 1934, Franz 1936, Siegmund 1938, Duchosal and Rutishauser 1943, Rigdon and Willeford 1950, Giampalmo 1951, 1953), while Leube (1889) diagnosed cardiovascular xanthomatosis for the first time in vivo.

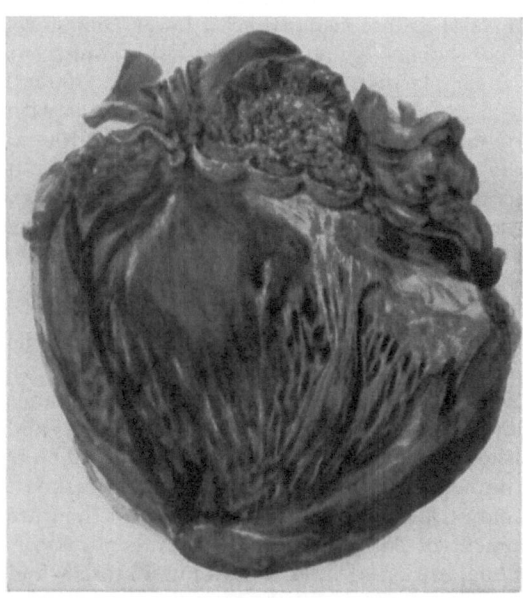

Fig. 5. Xanthomatous lesions of the endocardium. Case of Hess (1934)

Coronary heart disease as evidenced by angina pectoris and myocardial infarction (sudden cardiac death) below age 35 is very suggestive of EFH. Myocardial infarctions are often diagnosed only at autopsy. While data from the Framingham study (Dawber et al. 1957) and other epidemiologic investigations (see Epstein 1965) give the prevalence of coronary heart disease in the general population as 4.6 to about 8 per cent, data in patients with EFH are much higher. Adlersberg (1955) described 168 cases of angina pectoris in 390 cases from 77 kindreds. Of the 390 cases, 223 showed elevation of plasma cholesterol levels giving a 75% incidence of coronary heart disease among the hypercholesterolemic patients. The corresponding figure in KORNERUP's (1948) material was 22%, if calculated from the subjects with plasma cholesterol values above 325 and 340 mg per 100 ml respectively. At the time of re-examination by PIPER and ORRILD (1956) the percentage had increased to 40%, when 17 patients, who had died in the interval, were included. The mean age of 10 patients of this latter group (who had died from vascular occlusions) was 47.2 years; the average age of the remaining 7 who had died from other causes was 66 years. There were 14 out of 41 hypercholesterolemic patients with clinical symptoms of coronary heart disease in GURAVICH's (1959) subjects; in 4 cases coronary occlusion was confirmed at autopsy. Several years later (GURAVICH and VENEGAS 1962) the incidence of clinically manifest coronary artery disease was 18 out of 47 (38%); 9 of the 18 had already expired.

Disturbances of peripheral and cerebral circulation in EFH are much less common than coronary insufficiency (GURAVICH and VENEGAS 1962). One reason for this phenomenon is that patients may not survive until large vessels become occluded. Besides, the epidemiology of cerebrovascular disease differs in several aspects from that of coronary heart disease.

Sudden death in young persons with EFH seems to be more frequent in families exhibiting a high incidence of the disease and all the features of the syndrome. High plasma cholesterol levels in childhood, accompanied by early appearance of xanthomas, are of prognostic significance as regards cardiovascular complications and longevity. We found in the literature 36 reports of sudden cardiac deaths in adolescents and young adults below the age of 26; to this figure may be added 7 of our own observations in children up to age 12. All 43 cases had EFH, and, with the exception of 6, exhibited skin and tendon xanthomas. Included in this figure are 6 children (EPSTEIN et al. 1959) 4 of whom had died aged 7, 13, 15, and 23 respectively without subsequent autopsy. The clinical course and the pathologic anatomical findings of the remaining two (sudden death aged 13 and 16) are reported in detail by MAHER (1958). Autopsy data are unavailable for the two brothers described by RIEDERER (1961), who died aged 10 and 15 years. The clinical findings, however, were suggestive of xanthomatous valvular and coronary involvement. An impressive case is that of a 9 year-old boy with tuberous xanthomas and a plasma cholesterol level of 510 mg per 100 ml (PÜRSCHEL and RUST 1953). Heart disease was diagnosed when this patient was 1 year old; during the following years he complained of chest pain and finally developed congestive failure ending in death. At autopsy extensive arterial atheromatosis was observed, including the aortic valves, and in addition there were scars resulting from myocardial infarctions.

A diagnosis of valvular xanthomatosis may be made after exclusion of congenital and rheumatic heart disease by a search for skin and tendon xanthomas and determination of plasma lipid levels.

Auscultation of the heart in cases of xanthomatous lesions of the endocardium frequently reveals rough, loud systolic murmurs and soft, low-pitched diastolic murmurs over the mitral and aortic areas, depending on degree and localization of the atheromatous lesions. Clinically, valvular xanthomatosis may present as mitral insufficiency (LEUBE 1889, FISHER and KNOWLES 1921), mitral stenosis (LOW 1910, HUFFSCHMITT and NESSMAN 1931, GOLDSTEIN 1935) or occasionally as aortic stenosis (SCHETTLER et al. 1959). Valvular forms of xanthomatous heart disease usually lead to chronic congestive failure, as illustrated by SANSONE et al. (1960) who reported a 7 year-old child with hypercholesterolemia, left-sided congestive failure but no angina. The findings at autopsy were atheromatous lesions of the aorta and the aortic valves, and calcified xanthomatous stenosis of the mitral valves. Recently, Stanley et al. (1965) published the case of a 12 year-old patient with xanthomatous aortic stenosis, in whom the lesion was corrected surgically. This approach has now to be kept in mind, since cardiac surgery is becoming available in many centers; long-term prognosis nevertheless seems poor due to other xanthomatous involvement and the possibility of recurrences, since xanthomas have been shown to develop preferentially where tissue is altered. Other rare lesions include cases of xanthomatous stenosis of the pulmonary artery as described by Piper and Orrild (1957) and of xanthomatous pulmonary atherosclerosis in a 48 year-old woman (Schettler 1955).

Laboratory Findings

Cholesterol

The earmark of EFH and "conditio sine qua non" is elevation of the plasma cholesterol level. However, there are considerable difficulties in defining "normal" and "abnormal" values, since a bimodal distribution which might be expected to result from cholesterol levels of normal persons on the one hand and from those of patients with EFH on the other, has not been unequivocally demonstrated (Epstein et al. 1959). One possible reason why such bimodality is not apparent is the great number of exogenous factors which are known to modify plasma cholesterol levels in normals and, to a lesser degree, in patients with EFH. Figure 6 shows the result of one large study on the age dependence of the plasma cholesterol level in an unselected population. An approximation of normal cholesterol and phospholipid concentrations based on samples from 256 subjects as given by Fredrickson and Lees (1966) is as follows:

Age (years)	Cholesterol, mean and 90 % limits mg/100 ml	Phospholipid, mean and 90 % limits mg/100 ml
1—19	180 (115—240)	215 (155—265)
20—29	180 (125—240)	235 (175—300)
30—39	210 (150—280)	270 (205—340)
40—49	245 (160—325)	275 (185—355)
50—59	250 (140—340)	305 (225—380)

Review of the pertinent literature reveals a considerable lack of uniformity with regard to values thought to represent significant elevation of serum cholesterol levels. The data of Piper and Orrild (1956) have been mentioned; these authors used 324 mg per 100 ml in children and 340 mg per 100 ml in adults as the cut-off point for EFH. Lower values were used in the study of Epstein et al. (1959) with 280 mg per 100 ml. Fredrickson (1960) found for 20 patients with EFH an average value of 443 mg per 100 ml. As a working rule it has proved useful to consider values above 250—350 mg per 100 ml as suggestive of EFH when generally accepted methods are used, depending on age, sex and geographic situation of the proband. While EFH can never be diagnosed solely from cholesterol levels, in the "borderline" zone ancillary studies are particularly necessary to exclude or confirm EFH. Cholesterol levels above 800 mg% are rarely observed in EFH, while values in this range or higher are frequently seen with marked endogenous essential hyperlipemia (see page 468).

Phospholipids

There is significant elevation of phospholipids in EFH, although, as a rule, the levels of cholesterol are not reached, and therefore the cholesterol to phospholipid

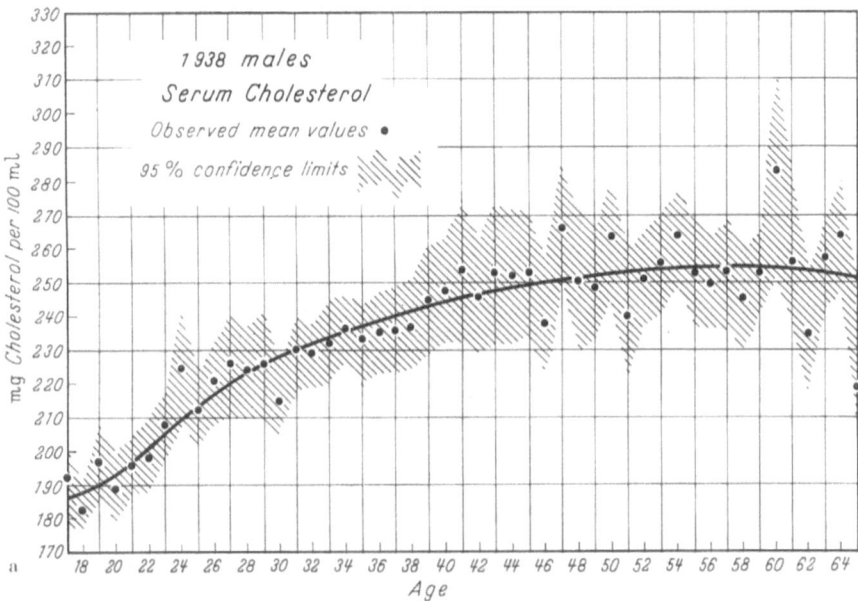

Fig. 6 a. Mean of single serum cholesterol determinations of male office personnel in Metropolitan New York City, stratified according to age. Each specific age category is comprised of a minimum of 18 and a maximum of 64 individuals.

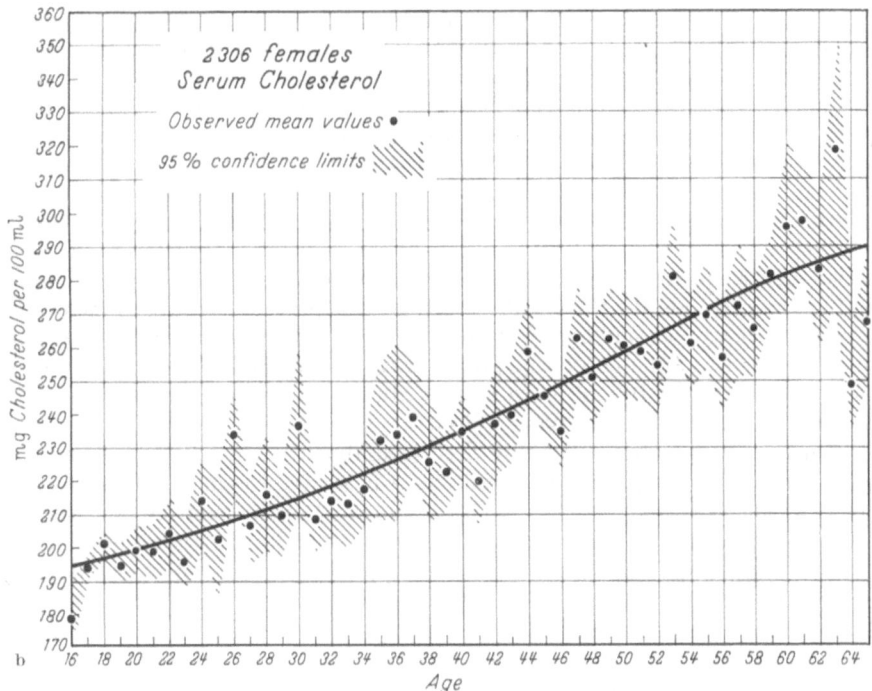

Fig. 6 b. Mean of single serum cholesterol determinations of female office personnel in Metropolitan New York City, stratified according to age. Each specific age category is comprised of a minimum of 15 and a maximum of 256 individuals. Source: SCHILLING et al. (1964). Reproduced with permission of *American Journal of Public Health* and the authors ratio is greater than 1. The average phospholipid level in 20 cases with EFH (Fredrickson 1960) was 402 mg per 100 ml.

As regards individual phospholipids, Nothman and Proger (1962, 1965) have reported a 2- to 3-fold increase of the absolute and relative concentration of phosphatidyl ethanolamine and phosphatidyl serine. A discussion of these findings has been given in the chapter on essential hyperlipemia on page 468 and will not be repeated here. Suffice it to say that a recent study by Wagener and Frosch (1964) did not confirm this finding.

Triglycerides

In pure EFH, plasma triglycerides are normal or only slightly elevated, in accordance with the low triglyceride concentration in beta-lipoproteins. When high triglyceride levels are observed associated with features of EFH rather than of essential hyperlipemia, one is probably dealing with a separate syndrome (see page 460).

Lipoproteins

A significant increase in beta-lipoprotein concentration has been established when using various methods.

Schettler and co-workers (1956, 1957) employing preparative ultracentrifugation, fractional precipitation modified from Cohn's procedure Nr. X (Schöll and Schettler 1961) and preparative starch electrophoresis (Schettler et al. 1957), have described a lipid and lipoprotein spectrum typical for EFH which is in accordance with data of Gofman et al. (1954) obtained by ultracentrifugation. The results obtained by starch electrophoresis show a slight increase in the cholesterol and phospholipid content of the alpha-1 fraction, while both lipids are normal in the alpha-2 zone; typically both cholesterol and phospholipids are markedly elevated in the beta-lipoprotein fraction. Lever and co-workers (1954, 1955) and Lever (1963), employing electrophoresis according to Tiselius also found consistently pathological increases of beta-lipoproteins. Godal et al. (1956) described 14 members of a family with EFH, aged 24 to 72 (mean age 48.1 years), and with a history of angina pectoris, all but one of whom averaged a 2-fold elevation of beta-lipoproteins; the alpha- to beta-lipoprotein ratio was decreased accordingly. Guravich (1959) found that lipoproteins of Sf 0—12 were increased consistently, frequently there was elevation of the Sf 12—20 fraction, and in about 50% of the cases, of the Sf 20—100 fraction. Lipoproteins with Sf values above 100 were normal and could be used to differentiate EFH from hyperlipemia. Lipoprotein fractions of the borderline group, with plasma cholesterol levels between 250 and 300 mg per 100 ml, were almost always normal on the basis of values given by Glazier and co-workers (1954).

Changes of plasma lipid classes as described above are in good agreement with those expected from the lipid composition of beta-lipoproteins (cholesterol 47%, phospholipids 23%, triglycerides 9%; Bragdon et al. 1956) and from the increased concentrations of this lipoprotein class, analogous to findings in the essential hyperlipemias, where other lipoprotein fractions prevail. Increase of the cholesterol-rich beta-lipoproteins also explains the findings of Hood and Angervall (1959) who examined the distribution of cholesterol between the Cohn fractions in hypercholesterolemic patients with different degrees of xanthomatosis. In patients with the most severe xanthomatosis (grade III according to these authors) and with high plasma cholesterol values (above 500 mg per 100 ml) they found 90% of the total cholesterol in the Cohn fractions I, II and III and 10% in IV, V and VI. With less severe xanthomatosis, usually accompanied by a milder hypercholesterolemia, and finally in cases without xanthomas, the above values changed gradually to 85% and 15%, respectively, in the males, and 79% and 21% in the females. The latter values correspond to figures found in survivors of myocardial infarctions.

The most recent contribution to the separation of lipoproteins and to the study of lipoprotein patterns in various forms of hyperlipidemias is that of FREDRICK-SON's (1966) group. Using a modified form of paper electrophoresis, FREDRICKSON and LEES (1966) described 5 different types of familial hyperlipoproteinemia, type II of which corresponds to EFH and is characterized by an intensely staining beta-band in their system.

They separate as a type III syndrome cases which, in addition to elevation of serum cholesterol, show also increased plasma triglyceride levels, occasionally with turbid plasma, and clinically, in addition to features of EFH, tubero-eruptive xanthomas and carbohydrate intolerance. Electrophoretically, these cases are characterized by either a broad beta-band with abnormal ultracentrifugal mobility (density less than 1.006) (more common) or a pre-beta-band in addition to a pronounced beta-band. As in endogenous hyperlipemias, triglyceride levels in such persons are easily carbohydrate induced, and lipid levels in general amenable to modification by diet and drugs. This syndrome probably includes cases which have been described as "mixed" (BORRIE 1957) or as EFH with secondary hyperlipemia (ZÖLLNER 1962a, b, KUO and BASSETT 1963).

Heparin, occasionally used for differentiation and treatment of different forms of hyperlipidemia, shows only a slight effect on lipoproteins in EFH which is of brief duration. Small decreases of phospholipids, cholesterol and glycerides have been observed, whereas in normals occasional lowering of glycerides only occurs. Analytical ultracentrifugation of plasma after heparin administration revealed no pattern of change specific for EFH but showed in all cases a slight shift of the beta-lipoproteins from higher to lower Sf classes (disappearance of beta-lipoproteins of Sf 30—70, decrease of Sf 12—20 and increase of Sf 0—10; LEVER et al. 1955). Visible changes are observed with electrophoresis after Tiselius or on paper strips (LEVER et al. 1955, HERBST et al. 1955, and HAENSCH 1957, 1958). Here injection of heparin effects a shift of lipoproteins from the beta-1 globulin area towards the alpha-2 globulins, but in contrast there is no change in migration of alpha-lipoproteins. These effects on beta-lipoproteins are not observed in normal plasmas.

Other Lipids

In addition to commonly determined lipids, the behaviour of plasma carotenoids has been studied by several authors. As early as 1929, STANNUS reported an increase of carotenoids in the blood of patients with xanthosis of the skin. More recently, studies by ZÖLLNER (1962b) revealed increases in carotenoids paralleling those in plasma cholesterol. Since carotenoids are of dietary origin, their elevation must be secondary to changes of other lipids or lipoproteins (beta-lipoproteins in particular) which illustrates the difficulties in deciding which changes found in EFH and other disorders of lipid metabolism represent an associated rather than a basic change. Finally, the studies of PELKONEN (1963) should be referred to, in which he reported on the metabolism of vitamin A and D in normal and hypercholesterolemic subjects, and on the distribution of these vitamins in the lipoprotein fractions.

Analysis of Xanthomas

Data about lipid content and composition of xanthomas are given by SCHETTLER (1960). Total lipids of *tendon xanthomas* from 6 analyses varied between 14 and

45 gm per 100 gm dry weight, with an average content of 28.7 gm per 100 gm (Epstein and Kreitner 1940, Favarger 1942, Schettler and Dietrich 1953). The contribution of cholesterol was approximately 50%, with 1—3% as ester, while phospholipids represented about 12% of the total lipids. Total lipid in normal tendon was reported by Schettler (1955) to average 7.5 gm per 100 gm in two cases (5.2 gm per 100 gm in a 16 year-old boy, 9.8 gm per 100 gm in a 64 year-old person); cholesterol constituted 18% of total lipid, and 20% of it was esterified.

Debuch and Kahlke (1964) studied a *tuberous xanthoma* in a 12 year-old boy with a plasma cholesterol level of 855—930 mg per 100 ml, and found the total lipid to be 32.5% of dry weight. Values obtained (percent of dry weight) after column chromatographic analysis of the total lipids were: phospholipids, 7.1%; cholesterol ester, 20.7%; and free cholesterol and triglyceride, each 2.2%. The high content of cholesterol esters in skin xanthomas was also found in other cases examined (Jepson et al. 1965); local factors responsible for the development of xanthomas and possibly the age of the lesion may play a role. Froehlich (1951) found more free than ester cholesterol in old xanthomas. It is noteworthy that a significantly higher proportion of oleic acid is found in all lipid fractions of xanthomas as compared to corresponding plasma lipid fractions. Oleic acid made up almost 50% of cholesterol ester fatty acids in 5 patients with tuberous xanthomas reported by Jepson et al. (1965).

The chemical composition of vascular and endocardial xanthomas has not yet been determined. The available analyses from different vessels, and from atherosclerotic lesions of different severity (Böttcher et al. 1960, 1961) have not been considered in relation to EFH.

Histopathology of Xanthomas

In contrast to eruptive xanthomas of essential hyperlipemia where extracellular lipid deposition and inflammatory reactions prevail, intracellular lipid deposition in foam cells are typical histologic features of tendon and plane xanthomas. They may be derived from reticuloendothelial cells, from histiocytes and, according to Froehlich (1951), possibly from connective tissue cells, by intracellular deposition of lipids. The morphogenesis of xanthomas has been treated repeatedly (Gottron 1932, 1942, Montgomery 1938, Sugg and Stetson 1937, Nödl 1951, Schirren 1952, Letterer 1959, and Fischer and Nikolowski 1960). According to these studies the difference between xanthomas of hypercholesterolemia and of hyperglyceridemia is that in hyperlipemic xanthomatosis, papillar edema is followed by imbibition of lipid, whereas hypercholesterolemic xanthomas originate perivascularly in the corium and form flat accumulations of foam cells in the subepidermal layer. Apparently foam cell formation is provoked by cholesterol more rapidly than by triglycerides, as has been suggested from feeding studies in rabbits and other experimental animals.

Associated Diseases

Rheumatic Diseases. Sinner (1961) described two siblings with all features of EFH (plasma cholesterol of 720—1324 and 680 mg per 100 ml, respectively; tendon and tuberous xanthomas), who at age 9 and 11 experienced onset of severe rheumatic fever with heart disease, following a sore throat. After a few weeks the first skin eruptions appeared and their number and size increased with each recurrence of the rheumatic process; histologically they had the typical appearance of xanthomas. Observations on the association between EFH and rheumatic affections were also reported by Fletcher et al. (1946), Coste and co-workers (1959), and Rausen and ADLERSBERG (1961). Earlier, MÜLLER (1939) studied 76 members of 17 families with all features of EFH: out of 33 persons who were examined in detail, 5 had "rheumatism" in their history. HELLAND-HANSEN (1956) reported 22 patients with "rheumatism" among 125 persons with xanthomatous hypercholesterolemia, and gave the frequency of rheumatism occurring with EFH as 80:1 compared with the frequency among the normal population. The mortality from rheumatism with xanthomatosis is supposed to be 16%, and without xanthomatosis 6%.

For more precise consideration it is necessary to make a distinction between rheumatic fever and chronic rheumatoid arthritis. Cardiac valves which have been affected by rheumatic fever may be damaged additionally in EFH by deposition of lipid and foam cell formation. Fibrosis, calcification, or even ossification may be enhanced by these lipid deposits, and the occurrence of EFH with rheumatic fever and its sequelae should therefore be considered a serious condition. It is not yet known with certainty whether or not rheumatic changes can affect intimal areas in arteries, and therefore possibly initiate or accelerate the atherosclerotic process.

The frequent occurrence of *Dupuytren's contracture* with hypercholesterolemia is striking. We have found this lesion in 24 out of 82 cases with EFH. Conversely, elevation of plasma cholesterol is frequent in patients with Dupuytren's contracture in the absence of a family history of EFH. A genetic linkage between these two diseases has been considered (LÖHR and NEUFFER 1959).

Another interesting parallelism has been reported between *EFH and gout*, (WOLFSON and co-workers 1949, FULTON 1952, SCHETTLER et al. 1957). HARRIS-JONES (1957) found elevated uric acid levels (in the range of 6—7 mg per 100 ml) in the serum of 9 out of 22 patients with hypercholesterolemia, the highest values being observed with coexisting xanthomas and when cholesterol levels were above 400 mg per 100 ml; none of his cases exhibited clinical signs of gout. Clinical symptoms of gout were also absent in the cases of ADLERSBERG (1949) in spite of an association of hypercholesterolemia and hyperuricemia in $1/_3$ of his 37 patients with EFH. Even without EFH, the incidence of elevated serum uric acid levels is rather high in patients with atherosclerosis and myocardial infarctions, that is, conditions which are frequently associated with elevated plasma lipids (GERTLER and WHITE 1951, ZÖLLNER 1957). Conversely, ALBRIEUX et al. (1953) frequently observed hyperlipemia and hypercholesterolemia in their patients with gout and serum cholesterol levels may rise during an attack of gout (WOLFSON et al. 1949). While, on the one hand, hyperuricemia in EFH may be the indirect result of the disturbance in lipid metabolism, since uric acid excretion is decreased on a high fat diet, on the other hand the possibility of genetic linkage must also be considered. In contrast to the above-mentioned studies, BERKOWITZ (1964) failed to find an association between elevated plasma cholesterol levels and uric acid levels, but rather observed a striking correlation of plasma triglyceride levels with serum uric acid. Similarly, JENSEN et al. (1966) in a recent follow-up report on 185 members of KORNERUP's (1948) original 12 families with EFH found no significant increase in serum uric acid. Further relevant studies are obviously necessary, since the possibility exists that the hypercholesterolemia and uric acid relationship was actually observed in subjects with essential hyperlipemias and with hyperlipidemia which would now be classed as type III hyperlipoproteinemia (FREDRICKSON and LEES 1966) or group 3 endogenous hyperglyceridemia (see page 460).

Another frequent combination is *EFH and hypertension*. The literature on this interrelationship, and 7 relevant cases were compiled by NOBBE (1962, 1963, 1965). The fact that each disease per se represents a risk factor for coronary heart disease, makes the combination particularly unfavorable. The reader is referred to the results of the Albany and Framingham studies, in both of which an increased risk of coronary heart disease was associated with hypercholesterolemia and with hypertension. Presumably the populations used in their studies included persons from hypercholesterolemic families; but analysis of this aspect is not available.

Diagnosis

Clinically, a presumptive diagnosis of EFH can be made from the finding of tendon xanthomas. Plane xanthomas as depicted in figure 3 are pathognomonic, unless one is dealing with a case of long-lasting biliary cirrhosis. The diagnosis of EFH is suggested when arcus lipoides appears early in life, and when coronary heart disease and myocardial infarction occur during or before the third decade.

The diagnosis is confirmed by the finding of an elevated plasma cholesterol level in excess of that compatible with sex, age, and geographic situation of the proband. Since elevation of plasma cholesterol is associated with an increase of serum beta-lipoproteins, demonstration of the latter with the use of lipoprotein electrophoresis or more complicated methods such as ultracentrifugal separation of lipoproteins are another means to confirm the diagnosis. The cholesterol to phospholipid ratio is greater than one.

In pure EFH, normal or nearly normal plasma triglyceride levels are found, and this finding serves for distinction from essential hyperlipemias as well as from "mixed" hypercholesterolemia and hyperglyceridemia (group 3 endogenous hyperglyceridemia, see page 460, or type III hyperlipoproteinemia, Fredrickson and Lees 1966). In the latter form, carbohydrate intolerance exists, which is not a feature of pure EFH. In equivocal cases and preferably in all cases, family members should be examined and the diagnosis of EFH thus confirmed or disproved.

Of the secondary hyperlipidemias those of hypothyroidism and biliary cirrhosis deserve particular attention, since they may show considerable elevation of cholesterol without hyperglyceridemia. In addition, xanthomas may occur in both with long duration. While biliary cirrhosis is characterized by the presence of jaundice, a very low ester cholesterol to free cholesterol ratio, and significant elevation of the phospholipid level, the exclusion of hypothyroidism is not always as simple and may require appropriate thyroid function tests.

Treatment

As long as the pathogenesis of EFH has not been elucidated, there obviously cannot be any causal therapy of EFH. Therapeutic attempts are directed mainly toward lowering of the plasma cholesterol level with the purpose of preventing or treating cardiovascular xanthomatosis, but the cholesterol level in EFH is considerably less amenable to modification by diet and drugs than elevated plasma cholesterol levels in conditions other than EFH. Other therapeutic measures consist of prevention and treatment of complications, resulting from ischemia and thrombosis; occasionally, skin or tendon xanthomas require treatment for mechanical reasons.

With regard to altering the plasma cholesterol level, 3 main points of attack may be considered: decrease of intestinal absorption of cholesterol, inhibition of synthesis and acceleration of catabolism and excretion. When changes in the plasma levels of cholesterol and other lipids are produced under the influence of different agents, it is also important to consider the total cholesterol and lipid content of the organism, and the possibility of shifts from plasma into tissues.

At present there is no proof that institution of a hypocholesterolemic regimen in EFH decisively improves the prognosis of cardiovascular complications, although preliminary results of long-term studies with such a regimen in the general population are promising. Only rarely is it possible to eliminate skin and tendon xanthomas with diet or drug therapy. An improvement in prognosis may be expected through the discriminating use of anticoagulants as protection against thromboembolic complications. Although good long-term studies are not available to prove or disprove this point for EFH, the conclusion seems logical in view of the favorable effect of anticoagulants during the first two years after a myocardial infarction, and in view of the increased incidence of thromboembolic complications in EFH. We recommend treating each patient with EFH with anticoagulants when the first signs of cardiovascular complications are noted.

Diet

As is the case in essential hyperglyceridemias, dietary modification represents the basis of a serum cholesterol-lowering regimen in EFH. Since the observations of Schettler (1949) in mice and Kinsell et al. (1952) and Groen et al. (1952) in men, the hypocholesterolemic effect of polyunsaturated fatty acids has been established without doubt, although there is still considerable controversy as to the mechanisms of this effect. We do know that the effect of polyunsaturated fatty acids is a positive one, and does not reside merely in a diminished intake of saturated fat or dietary cholesterol, since addition of polyunsaturated fatty acids to a fat – and cholesterol – free diet does result in further decrease of the serum cholesterol level (Kinsell et al. 1958). There seems also to be general agreement now that "essential" fatty acids per se are not necessary for a hypocholesterolemic effect (Ahrens et al. 1959) and that it is rather a function of polyunsaturation. Similarly sitosterol does not seem to be essential in the hypocholesterolemic action of vegetable oils, because cholesterol lowering occurs in its absence as was shown in studies with purified or synthetic materials such as ethyl linoleate (Kinsell et al. 1959) or arachidonate.

It is beyond the scope of this presentation to discuss in detail the various theories of the hypocholesterolemic mechanism of polyunsaturated fatty acids and the controversial results of numerous studies (Beveridge et al. 1955—1960, Gordon and co-workers 1957 a, b, Malmros 1957, Ahrens et al. 1957, Haust and Beveridge 1958, Lewis 1958, Hashim et al. 1959, Bergström 1961, Roels and Hashim 1962, Wilkens et al. 1962, Favarger 1963, Intengan et al. 1963, Siperstein and Fagan 1964). While most authors consider decreased cholesterol synthesis with the use of polyunsaturated fatty acids to be unlikely, the question is still not settled whether there occurs increased fecal steroid excretion or altered distribution between plasma and tissues with such diets. In contrast to results of animal experiments showing increase in liver (Avigan and Steinberg 1958) and muscle (Bieberdorf and Wilson 1964) cholesterol with polyunsaturated fatty acids, it could be shown that in the human at least there is no alteration of the liver cholesterol concentration with ingestion of polyunsaturated fatty acids (Frantz and Carey 1961). Several recent balance studies (Spritz et al. 1965, Avigan and Steinberg 1965) failed to show a consistent increase in excretion of cholesterol and metabolites with polyunsaturated fatty acids, which has been the most likely hypothesis for their action for years (Lit. see Spritz et al. 1965, Avigan and Steinberg 1965). Although these authors studied subjects with hypercholesterolemia, they did not define them as to the exact type. Since, on the other hand, Wood et al. (1966) were able to account for all the cholesterol lost from the plasma during the transition from saturated to unsaturated fat diets in normals on the basis of similar excretion studies, the matter remains unsettled at the present time, unless the defect in essential hypercholesterolemia is actually related to this aspect.

Keys et al. (1965) have recently reviewed the evidence on the effect of dietary cholesterol on the plasma cholesterol level, which has been a controversial subject for many years. They came to the conclusion that there is a predictable effect of exogenous cholesterol on plasma cholesterol. This has to be considered in the dietary approach to the treatment of essential familial hypercholesterolemia.

Practically, dietary treatment of EFH should start with restriction of total calories in overweight patients. According to Kinsell and Schlierf (1965) the composition of a lipid-lowering diet should be such that in addition to generally recommended amounts of protein, dietary fat should make up 40 to 45% of total calories, of which at least 40% should be polyunsaturated and no more than 20% saturated fat. The composition of such a diet is indicated in table 1. A regimen as outlined may result in significant improvement of xanthomatosis (Jepson 1961, our own observations). Another approach (Schettler 1957, 1959, 1961) uses diets with the fat content not exceeding 25% of total calories, and with polyunsaturated acids predominating. An even lower fat content is neither practical nor useful since very low fat diets are high carbohydrate diets and are usually associated with elevation of triglyceride levels. This applies particularly to the dietary management of the group 3 syndrome, which is very sensitive to carbohydrate induction.

Nicotinic Acid

In 1955 Altschul et al. reported the cholesterol-lowering effect of nicotinic acid. Subsequently this material has been employed by many workers in the treatment of EFH, using an average daily dosage of 3—6 gm. The lowering of cholesterol levels observed by Achor and co-workers (1963) in 18 hypercholesterolemic patients, using a daily dose of 3 grams, was 13%; and with 4.3 grams daily was as much as 28%. Berge (1961) treated 66 patients (mean plasma cholesterol level 327 mg per 100 ml) with daily doses of 1.5—6 grams, and observed a decrease in cholesterol level to a mean of less than 250 mg per 100 ml. There was a simultaneous fall of plasma free fatty acids and a decrease of the cholesterol-phospholipid ratio. In spite of subjective improvement of symptoms of coronary and peripheral artery insufficiency, the favorable effect could not be verified clinically, and 11 patients died from atherosclerotic complications during or after treatment.

Studies of the mode of action of nicotinic acid revealed the interesting fact that the hypocholesterolemic action is restricted to pure nicotinic acid and its salts (sodium and aluminium nicotinate) and that nicotinamide, part of the molecule of the codehydrogenases DPN and TPN, does not show any cholesterol-lowering effect. The relevant literature on these drugs has been summarized by Sanwald (1966).

No increase in excretion of cholesterol and bile acids under the influence of nicotinic acid was observed by Goldsmith et al. (1959 and 1962). The formation of "oxycholesterols" was considered by Altschul et al. (1955) and Altschul and Hoffer (1958) as a possible mode of action of nicotinic acid; and they also discussed a stress effect. Others suspect a heparin-like effect acting on the lipoprotein lipase system (O'Reilly 1958). In addition, a decreased methylating capacity of the liver has been considered, but simultaneous administration of methionine is without influence on the hypocholesterolemic action of nicotinic acid (Miller and co-workers 1960, Chiu 1961). Finally, the suggestion of Failey and co-workers (1959) should be mentioned: according to these authors the glycine requirement of nicotinic acid during its conversion to nicotinylglycine would favor conjugation of bile acids with taurine, which in turn might lead to "consumption" of more cholesterol, due to the increased rate of excretion of these conjugates. The above-mentioned finding by Goldsmith et al. (1959) of unchanged excretion rates of cholesterol and bile acids with nicotinic acid treatment, is inconsistent with this explanation.

Table 1. *Diet, rich in polyunsaturated fatty acids and low in cholesterol, for management of hypercholesterolemia (with kind permission of L. W. Kinsell, Oakland, Calif.)*

Calories:	1200	1600	1800	2000	2500
Daily use:					
Nonfat milk solids	25	25	25	25	90 gm
or	or	or	or	or	or
Liquid skim milk	250	250	250	250	900 ml
Fish, fowl, liver or cottage cheese	90	90	90	120	120 gm
Lean meat — beef, lamb or veal	60	90	90	120	120 gm
Safflower oil, corn, cotton or soy	30	50	60	60	75 ml
Nuts — 50% walnuts (100% in					
lower cal. diets)	35	35	65	65	65 gm
Whole grain cereal	100	100	100	100	100 gm
(cooked) or	or	or	or	or	or
Dry or prepared	20	20	20	20	20 gm
Fruits 20%	none	none	none	200	200 gm
or 10%	300	300	300	400	400 gm
Vegetables 20%	none	100	100	100	100 gm
7% (or "B" list)*	200	200	200	200	200 gm
3% (or "A" list)*	ad lib	ad lib	ad lib	ad lib	ad lib
Low fat bread	25	50	50	50	75 gm
Approximate protein	57	68	74	88	117 gm
Approximate fat	68	93	116	123	139 gm
Approximate CHO	92	127	131	137	196 gm
Approx. linoleic acid (see note)	32	42	50	50	57 gm
Approximate sodium (see note)	350	375	400	400	700 mgm

* see ADA-diet.

Linoleic acid is calculated as if cotton, corn or soy oil is used (approximately 50% linoleic acid) and that 100% walnuts (62% linoleic acid) are used on all diets up to 1600 calorie. For 2000 calorie diets and above, walnuts should supply 50% of nuts.

Sodium content is estimated as if all foods are prepared without added salt, using:

a) Regular cooked cereal (quick-cooking types often have sodium added).

b) Salt free bread; if low fat s.f. bread not available, substitute 70 gm (⅓ cup) 20% salt free vegetable during day.

c) Regular low calorie cottage cheese; if curd is used, which is very low sodium, sodium content is reduced to 275 mgm/100 gm cheese.

d) Lower sodium vegetables, omit: beets, carrots, celery, chard, kale, turnip, turnip greens and spinach.

15 ml = 1 tablespoon	100 gm cooked fruit = ½ cup (approx.)
5 ml = 1 teaspoon	100 gm cooked vegetable = ½ cup (approx.)
15 gm nuts = ½ oz. or 5 halves walnuts	120 gm fish or meat = 4 oz. or ¼ lb. (cooked weight)
35 gm walnuts = ⅓ cup	100 gm cottage cheese = ½ cup (approx.)
30 gm peanuts = ¼ cup	100 gm cooked cereal = ½ cup
25 gm bread = 1 slice	20 gm dry (prepared) cereal = ¾ cup
250 ml liquid milk = 1 cup (approx.)	30 ml oil = 35 gm walnuts.

Fruits and Vegetables: Consider banana, red and white grapes and sweetened canned fruit as 20% fruits, and all other fruits, either fresh or canned without sugar, as 10% fruits. Consider potato, corn, cooked dried beans, macaroni, spaghetti, and rice as 20% vegetables.

Low Fat Breads include sweet or sour French bread, Milwaukee pumpernickel, English muffins and Rye Krisp.

Oils: Safflower, corn, cottonseed and soy oils may be used in cooking, as a salad dressing, added to cereals or combined with butter milk, made from skim milk.

Olive and peanut oil not allowed. Be sure that all oil is used and none is left in the bowl or on cooking utensils.

Nuts may be eaten as such, blended with milk, or added to prepare dishes. At least half the nuts eaten should be walnuts, which are particularly rich in linoleic acid. Commercially fried nuts not allowed; however, nuts may be fried at home in one of the recommended oils. Other nuts may be used except coconut and cashews.

Iron and vitamin supplements are suggested.

Several studies, in part contradictory, are available concerning the influence of nicotinic acid on cholesterol biosynthesis. Perry (1960) reported from work with rat liver slices a decreased incorporation of ^{14}C-acetate into cholesterol with high concentrations of nicotinic acid in the medium; Schade and Saltman (1959) had obtained similar results in rabbits fed with nicotinic acid. On the other hand, Merrill and Lemley-Stone (1957) found increased cholesterol synthesis in liver slices of rats fed nicotinic acid, while Duncan and Best (1960) reported that nicotinic acid has no effect on ^{14}C-acetate incorporation. Parsons (1961a) studied the effects of nicotinic acid and niacin on incorporation of ^{14}C-acetate in man, and stated that considerably less conversion into serum cholesterol (free and esterified) and into erythrocyte cholesterol occurred during nicotinic acid administration. The concept of inhibition of cholesterol synthesis is also held by Goldsmith (1962); the point of inhibition supposedly occurs before the formation of squalene, because sterol intermediates between squalene and cholesterol could not be detected in serum.

In addition to the cholesterol-lowering action of nicotinic acid, the disappearance of plane and tuberous skin xanthomas and xanthelasmas has been observed following its administration (Parsons 1961a, b). However, side effects accompanying the high doses required cannot be disregarded. Flushing of the skin may be bothersome, though it is usually harmless; recent reports about toxic effects of nicotinic acid on the liver are more significant. Among the findings were pathologically increased bromsulphalein retention, elevation of alkaline phosphatase, SGOT, SGPT, LDH, uric acid and less frequently of bilirubin; and occasionally abnormalities of flocculation tests (Lit. see Rivin 1959, Parsons 1961a, b, Pardue 1961, Hoffer 1961). The tests usually became normal even with continuation of treatment (Christensen et al. 1964) and organic liver damage, with the occasional exception of fatty liver, has not been noted. Of relevance because of the necessity for long-term treatment, are reports on abnormal glucose tolerance tests (Christensen et al. 1964) and manifestations of latent diabetes mellitus during administration of nicotinic acid.

Insufficient information is available with regard to the effect of nicotinic acid on cardiovascular complications. Favorable results of nicotinic acid in angina pectoris have been reported by Öst (1960) and Hunter (1960, 1962).

Zöllner (1966) has described favorable results from the use of a nicotinic acid derivative (β-pyridyl-carbinol) with prolonged action available in the U.S.A. as Roniacol time-span[1]. With this material only about $\frac{1}{4}$ of the dose of nicotinic acid is required for the desired effect on plasma cholesterol level, and the occurrence of side effects is substantially decreased.

Ethyl-p-chlorophenoxyisobutyrate

Experiments with various alpha-hydroxyisobutyric acid derivatives led to the finding of the striking effect on serum lipids produced by ethyl-p-chlorophenoxy-isobutyrate (CPIB). Initially, the material was used in combination with androsterone as Atromid[2] until it was shown by several authors (Hellman et al. 1963, and others) that the active ingredient was actually CPIB alone. Early reports were given by Hellman et al. (1962); as in many other studies concerned with the evaluation of hypocholesterolemic effects, the patients were not selected for symptomatic and idiopathic hypercholesterolemias, and only the plasma cholesterol levels were used as reference points.

Berkowitz (1963) found lowering of serum cholesterol in 75% of his 25 hyperlipidemic patients. Counihan and Keelan (1963) reported even better results with lowering of serum cholesterol in 16 out of 17 hypercholesterolemic patients, whereas in a person with normal cholesterol level the opposite reaction was observed. Green et al. (1963) found in 601 patients,

---

[1] Roche Laboratories, Nutley 10, N.J.
[2] Imperial Chemical Industries Ltd., Alderley Park, Cheshire, England.

including 42 diabetics and 37 patients with xanthomas, with initial cholesterol levels below 300 mg per 100 ml an average decrease in serum cholesterol of 26%; for patients with initial values above 350 mg per 100 ml the average decrease was 35%. The dose given was 15 to 35 mg per kg body weight, or 1 to 2.25 g Atromid per day. HELLMAN and co-workers (1963), using daily doses of 2 gm, found in females an average decrease in serum cholesterol of 25%, and in serum phospholipids of 17%; the corresponding figures for males were 12% and 9%. The finding of a 27% lowering of serum cholesterol level in 18 patients with coronary heart disease and plasma cholesterol values above 300 mg per 100 ml has been reported by SRIVASTAVA et al. (1963). Comparable results were obtained by FROM HANSEN (1963) who observed for 11 patients with EFH effects similar to those obtained in the remainder of his 38 patients. In addition to a decrease in serum cholesterol and phospholipids, a reduction of tendon xanthomas has been observed in one case by HOWARD et al. (1963) and, in spite of the serum cholesterol remaining elevated, in two cases by ROPER (1964). Little cholesterol-lowering was seen by JEPSON and JAMES (1963) who treated 8 patients with familial idiopathic xanthomatosis with daily doses of Atromid of 2.25 grams, with a mean decrease in serum cholesterol of 9%. Similarly FASOLI and CESANA (1963) observed the smallest effect in a case of EFH. Finally CRAMER reported that from 9 hyperlipidemic patients treated with Atromid, 2 out of 3 persons with EFH showed no effect on their serum cholesterol level.

Several authors studied serum lipoproteins during administration of ethyl-p-chlorophenoxyisobutyrate. A decrease in the low density lipoproteins and a slight increase in the high density lipoproteins has been observed by FASOLI and CESANA (1963), CARLSON et al. (1963). In contrast, KOUTTINEN and PALOHEIMO (1963) found no change for alpha-lipoprotein cholesterol. The significant fall of the beta-lipoprotein concentration results in an increase of the alpha/beta lipoprotein ratio (KERNOHAN and NEELY 1963) and a decrease of the total serum cholesterol to phospholipid ratio (HOWARD and co-workers 1963). The lipid-lowering effect and a decreased beta-lipoprotein level were also found to run parallel by CRAMER (1963) and by DELCOURT and VASTESAEGER (1963).

Comparative studies in patients with EFH and essential hyperlipemia, on the effect of CPIB and dextrothyroxine on low and very low density lipoproteins respectively, were performed by STRISOWER and STRISOWER (1964). CPIB lowered very low density lipoproteins (and thus triglycerides) more than dextrothyroxine, but the latter drug was superior to CPIB as regards the depressing effect on serum beta-lipoproteins and thus on cholesterol (see also page 434).

The mode of action of the drug has not been clarified. Some relevant theories have been discussed in the chapter on essential hyperlipemias.

Among side effects not mentioned in that chapter are a decrease of linoleic acid in cholesterol esters and triglycerides in favor of palmitoleic and oleic acids as observed by BERRY et al. (1963) and JURAND and OLIVER (1963). There was a simultaneous increase in glyceryl arachidonate. The proportion of cholesterol linoleate generally found in total cholesterol esters (50%) was decreased to 33% after 4 weeks of treatment, and returned to the initial value only after discontinuation of the drug. While the significance of these observations is difficult to evaluate, the effect is the opposite of that produced by the use of dietary fats rich in linoleic acid. Weight gain with Atromid has been frequently observed. In OLIVER's 93 cases with ischemic heart disease, weight gain was registered in 55%, the maximum increase being 10 kg; and in 4 patients concomitant worsening of dyspnea, or onset of left-sided congestive failure occurred. One of 8 EFH cases treated by JEPSON and JAMES (1963) had to be dropped from the study because of increased angina pectoris. Of the 601 persons under study by GREEN et al. (1963) one-fifth suffered side effects usually in the form of mild gastrointestinal disturbances. The simultaneous administration of anticoagulants caused bleeding in 26 patients of this group, two of whom died. Other authors (HAYWARD and co-workers 1963, COUNIHAN et al. 1963, KOUTTINEN and PALOHEIMO 1963, ROBERTS and PANTRIDGE 1963) also noted a decreased requirement for anticoagulants during the administration of Atromid which was of the order of 30%. OWEN WILLIAMS et al. (1963) observed fluctuations in hemoglobin concentration which they were unable to explain, but hoped to pursue further.

Of particular interest is the observation of many authors of an increase in fibrinolytic activity accompanying the hypocholesterolemia produced by Atromid, whereas this activity is not infrequently decreased in hypercholesterolemia. As regards other parameters of blood clotting, Jepson and James (1963) did not find changes in clotting time, but reported reduction in plasma fibrinogen. The latter finding has also been observed by Cotton et al. (1963), but fibrinogen level tended to become normal as treatment continued. Gilbert and Mustard (1963) described a decrease in aggregation of thrombocytes; kinetic studies were suggestive of increased life span and decreased turnover rate. Finally, another observation should be mentioned. In studies on the toxicity of Atromid, with particular reference to changes in the subcellular structure of the liver, Paget (1963) found an increase in number and size of mitochondria and lysosomes. As an experimental procedure, administration of CPIB to patients with EFH appears to be of value in some but not all cases.

Cholestyramine

Favorable results have been reported by Hashim and van Itallie (1965) with the use of cholestyramine in EFH. This material, an anion exchange resin, as the chloride salt exchanges Cl^- for bile acids and thus promotes their excretion. Its hypocholesterolemic effect appears to rest on both induction of increased catabolism of cholesterol and its decreased reabsorption. The above authors treated 9 persons with EFH with daily doses averaging 13.3 gm/day for 1 month to 4 years and observed a decrease of the serum cholesterol levels to 80—50 per cent of the average control values. Xanthomas became softer and smaller.

Side effects with the doses used have been few and consist mainly of a tendency to constipation. Since with higher doses steatorrhea has been observed and long-term administration may result in deficiencies of various fat soluble vitamins, the recommended daily amounts of 12—15 gm should not be exceeded.

Sitosterol

Sitosterol is not used widely in the treatment of EFH and of hypercholesterolemic cardiovascular disease, since the therapeutic potential of this material is limited by the high dosage required (30 gm/day), the transitory effect and the high cost. Administration of sitosterol in EFH may lead to a significant decrease of plasma cholesterol levels, although normal values are rarely reached. Xanthomas generally remain unaffected as is the case with most attempts at therapy. This point is illustrated by Breslaw (1958), who observed in a young man a decrease in cholesterol level from 624 to 486 mg per 100 ml with the use of sitosterol with concomitant reduction of phospholipids, neutral fats and alpha$_2$-, beta- and gamma-globulins; there was no effect on the extensive xanthomatosis.

The influence of sitosterol on cholesterol absorption, on the cholesterol content of plasma and different organs and on experimental atheromatosis has been the subject of numerous studies (Peterson 1952, Pollak 1953, Diller and co-workers 1958, Best and Duncan 1956, 1958, 1959). The effect on existing atheromatous vascular lesions has been studied by Betzien et al. (1961); they observed in hens a significant decrease in cholesterol content of the atherosclerotic plaques, of the liver, and to a lesser degree, of the serum. The same group reported from a clinical trial in the inhabitants of a nursing home (aged 60—80) a depression of plasma cholesterol level, with the greatest decrease occurring when initial levels were high. Farquhar and Sokolow (1958) observed in ambulatory patients treated for six to twelve months with beta-sitosterol a decrease predominantly in the Sf 0—10 beta-lipoprotein fraction, the cholesterol content of which decreased by 22%. With use of a combination of sitosterol and safflower oil, the decrease was 34%. They concluded from this additional effect, and from the different time course of changes in cholesterol levels during and after treatment, that the decrease of plasma cholesterol level produced by safflower oil was not secondary to its sitosterol content.

The mode of action of sitosterol, which differs in structure from cholesterol by possession of an ethyl group on C-24, has not been established. In contrast to cholesterol, intestinal absorption of sitosterol has been shown to take place in only very small quantities (SCHOENHEIMER 1929, 1932, BEST 1956, SCHETTLER 1961) and amounts to about 5% of administered sitosterol, (GOULD 1955). According to one theory sitosterol interferes with the absorption of cholesterol. If cholesterol and sitosterol are administered simultaneously, the absorption of the former is markedly decreased (HERNANDEZ et al. 1953); only one-third of the cholesterol is absorbed if both substances are administered in equal parts, while cholesterol absorption is nil when cholesterol and sitosterol are fed in the proportion of 1:7 (POLLAK 1953). Mixed crystal formation may be responsible for this effect, as suggested by the in vivo and in vitro studies of DAVIS (1955) and of HUDSON and co-workers (1959), who found crystals with an X-ray diffraction pattern different from either cholesterol or sitosterol, and suspected the presence of a less-dispersible compound. The assumption of SWELL et al. (1954) that there is competitive inhibition of esterification of cholesterol by sitosterol, has been refuted by BLOMSTRAND and AHRENS (1958), and the suggestion of GLOVER et al. (1957) of competition for acceptor lipoproteins is unproved. GERSON and SHORLAND (1963), on the basis of isotopic studies in rats, considered the effect of beta-sitosterol on cholesterol absorption to be less important, and discussed the effects of the sterol on cholesterol metabolism and on the cholesterol content of different tissues.

Hormones

The use of *estrogens* in the prophylaxis of myocardial infarction is based on the fact that myocardial infarction is rare in normally menstruating women, whereas the incidence increases after the menopause. Furthermore, myocardial infarctions are not rare in young females after ovarectomy (Lit. see SCHETTLER 1961). We are not aware of any controlled studies on the use of these agents in EFH only, but there have been long-term investigations with groups of high-risk subjects or patients with coronary heart disease, which very likely contained a number of subjects with EFH.

Three relevant studies are available. STAMLER et al. in 1959 initiated a double blind study with Premarin[1] (conjugated equine estrogens), in which were included 275 males with coronary heart disease, all below age 50 at the beginning of the study. During 5 years the Premarin-treated group (10 mg daily) showed an increasingly favorable course compared with the control group, the main benefit being derived by high-risk patients with previous severe infarctions or recurrent infarctions. However, there was an increased mortality during the first 3 months of treatment with the 10 mg dose. Similarly favorable results were reported by MARMORSTON and co-workers (1960) from a study with 432 males, over a two year period and with a Premarin dosage of 0.625 to 2.5 mg/day. The coronary death rate was 5% in the treated group as compared to 11% in the control group. Ethinyl estradiol had no significant effect on the survival rate, although the expected estrogen effect on plasma lipids and lipoproteins, and on general well-being was observed. These results show that clinical success does not necessarily parallel changes in plasma lipids and lipoproteins. OLIVER and BOYD (1959), using ethinyl estradiol, also saw no improvement in survival rate in 50 treated males during 2 years as compared to 50 control subjects. Significant side-effects, particularly related to the gonads, are usually observed with estrogen therapy; biopsies of testicular tissue in these cases show severe lesions. Feminizing effects were less with the lower dose of Premarin (MARMORSTON et al. 1960.) It should also be mentioned that a metastasizing adenocarcinoma of the breast has been observed in a patient, who had been treated with estrogens for a period of 9 years after a myocardial infarction at age 36.

In summary, it may be said that estrogen treatment of patients with myocardial infarction and coronary insufficiency, including subjects with EFH, according to present knowledge, cannot be considered a routine method of treatment because of the marked side-effects. Premarin treatment might be considered in post-myocardial infarction patients who have a particularly poor prognosis, when all other therapy fails, and feminizing effects then weigh less heavily.

Reports on the effect of *ACTH and adrenocortical steroids* on blood lipids are controversial. While ADLERSBERG (1959) reported elevation of various plasma

---

[1] Ayerst Laboratories, New York.

lipid fractions with these hormones in experimental animals and man, daily doses of cortisone of 100—200 mg have been shown by Oliver and Boyd (1958) to lower plasma cholesterol in hypercholesterolemic patients but, as was emphasized by the authors, the dosage is far too high for long-term treatment.

Since hypercholesterolemia of hypothyroidism will disappear upon treatment with *thyroid*, thyroxin and its analogs have been of particular interest in the search for cholesterol lowering drugs.

It is possible to lower plasma cholesterol levels in euthyroid hypercholesterolemic persons with doses which affect the BMR insignificantly, or not at all (Chiu 1961). Studies on cholesterol synthesis, absorption and distribution in hyperthyroidism have been performed by Gould et al. (1955), Kritchevsky (1960) and Chiu (1961); hypercholesterolemia in hypothyroidism was investigated by Schettler (1950), Kritchevsky et al. (1962) (see also page 73). From these reports it is apparent that cholesterol synthesis is in fact increased in hyperthyroidism and decreased in hypothyroidism. It appears that the effect of thyroxin and its analogs consists of an increase in catabolism and excretion of cholesterol and bile acids which exceeds the increased synthesis rate. Studies by Cutting (1934) and Stamler and co-workers (1950) with 2,4-dinitrophenol suggested that the increased basal metabolism per se is not responsible for the hypocholesterolemia, because the elevation of basal metabolic rate in animals by di-nitrophenol was not accompanied by changes in plasma cholesterol level. While, with the use of thyroxin, production or aggravation of angina pectoris was an almost predictable compli-cation even with careful regulation of dosage (Bansi 1960, Oliver and Boyd 1958, Schettler 1950) and, on the other hand, angina pectoris can be treated by making the patients clearly hypothyroid with radioactive iodine (Blumgart et al. 1951, 1955), the complication of angina may be less frequent with the use of dextrorotatory isomers.

Studies with *dextrothyroxine* in patients with hyperlipidemias including EFH were performed by Kuo and Bassett (1963), by Strisower and Strisower (1964), by Duncan and Best (1964) and others, with a good hypocholesterolemic effect. Lowering of Sf 0—20 (beta) lipoproteins in the study of Strisower and Strisower averaged 21% and exceeded the effect of Atromid (see page 431). Decrease in size of xanthomas or their disappearance with dextrothyroxine therapy has been reported by Owen et al. (1962), Bernheim et al. (1963) and others.

Among other hormones which have been examined for their usefulness in therapy of EFH, is *glucagon*. Amatuzio et al. (1962) examined the lipid-lowering effect of glucagon in hypercholesterolemia and found that it reduced serum cholesterol in 3 females, but not in 2 males. The hormone has not been used on a large scale in the treatment of hypercholesterolemia.

Heparin and Heparinoid Drugs

Heparin, shown to be useful in some hyperlipemic conditions, is of only limited value in EFH. Polymanuronide sulfate, a mucopolysaccharide similar to heparin in chemical composition, has been used by Constantinides et al. (1960) in hypercholesterolemia. A rapid decrease of total lipids was observed during the first 24 hours of treatment; lowering of cholesterol, however, required 72 hours in two-thirds of the cases and an even longer period in the remaining one-third. With a dosage of 2.5 mg per kg body weight, side effects or an anticoagulant action were not observed. The activity of this sulfated polymanuronide far sur-passes the effect of heparin, and its mode of action is considered by Constan-tinides and Saunders (1958) to be activation of lipoprotein lipase with ad-ditional stimulation of the reticulo-endothelial system, whereas heparin supposedly has only the former effect.

Other Drugs

P-aminosalicylic acid was shown in several studies to have a cholesterol-lowering action. With doses of 12 grams per day, which were more efficient when given by mouth as compared to i.v., Tygstrup et al. (1961) achieved an average decrease of serum cholesterol levels of 30%. The side effects with this high dosage make this drug unsuitable as a cholesterol-lowering agent.

SAVITZKY (1962) found a decrease in serum cholesterol level after a single injection of a hetero-logous *desoxyribonucleic acid* preparation from 5 mammal species. Neither species specifity nor dependence on the cholesterol level of the donor animals were observed. This excludes the assumption of a transfer of specific genetic information as the mechanism of the observed change in regulation of serum cholesterol by heterologous, homologous and autologous DNS.

Although the effectiveness of all these drugs as regards the prevention of atheromatous vascular lesions remains to be proved, possibly therapeutic trials may contribute to clarification of the pathogenesis of EFH. This potentially important aspect seems to justify the extensive consideration that has been given to these materials.

Pathogenetic Aspects

The metabolic error which causes EFH has not yet been elucidated. Only a few of a great number of possible mechanisms have been studied and will be men-tioned briefly. Areas where research is particularly needed will be pointed out.

In spite of the emphasis which has been put on the cholesterol moiety, it is possible that the cause for the increase in plasma beta-lipoproteins actually resides with the protein moiety or with abnormal binding of protein to cholesterol. Alternatively, the phospholipid moiety may be involved primarily, while chol-esterol elevation may only be secondary. Here is a particularly interesting field for future investigation.

There is no evidence that any constituent of the beta-lipoproteins in "pure" EFH is abnormal with regard to chemical structure. In particular, no abnormal lipid component has been found in patients with EFH. The lipid composition and ratios of lipid to protein of the beta-lipoproteins are very similar to those found in normals (FREDRICKSON and LEES 1966). In contrast, an atypical lipoprotein with beta-mobility and the ultracentrifugal properties of very low density lipo-proteins has been found in the type III hyperlipoproteinemia (FREDRICKSON et al. 1966).

As regards the cholesterol moiety, a variety of mechanisms could cause its increase in the plasma, none of which could yet be identified as responsible for the disease. Since dietary cholesterol does contribute to the plasma cholesterol level in men, its unchecked absorption could result in hypercholesterolemia. Such a mechanism would affect the reabsorption of endogenous cholesterol as well as that of exogenous cholesterol, and the hypothesis cannot be tested solely with ad-ministration of cholesterol-free diets, which have been shown not to eliminate the hypercholesterolemia in patients with EFH. Another possibility, namely increased production of endogenous cholesterol in EFH, cannot be excluded. We know that in men, as in experimental animals, a feedback mechanism located at the step from beta-hydroxy-beta-methylglutaric acid to mevalonic acid checks the synthesis of cholesterol (SIPERSTEIN and FAGAN 1964). Deletion of this feedback mechanism or a defect located at any of the 24 known steps of cholesterol biosynthesis could be involved in the pathogenesis of EFH. Experimental studies of this aspect have given contradictory results (HELLMAN et al. 1955, GEE et al. 1959).

Another subject which remains to be clarified is whether or not decreased catabolism of cholesterol with decreased excretion of cholesterol and/or bile acids leads to hypercholesterolemia in EFH. Considerable methodological difficulties are now being overcome in this field. Data in two subjects with EFH do not show any significant difference in cholic acid turnover and half life as compared to normals (LINDSTEDT et al. 1965). Reported data on cholesterol and bile acid excretion in hypercholesterolemic subjects (EFH ?) are of similar magnitude to those of normals (SPRITZ et al. 1965, AVIGAN and STEINBERG 1965). In view of the great variability of such values in different individuals, and of the great differences found by different groups of workers, final judgement has to be withheld in this matter. Neither an abnormal free cholesterol to ester cholesterol ratio (Thannhauser 1958), nor significant abnormalities of the cholesterol ester fatty acid pattern have been found in EFH (Zöllner 1963) which eliminates potential causes for impaired cholesterol catabolism.

The development of the various types of xanthomas seems to be associated with elevation of certain plasma lipid fractions rather than with the (unknown) specific defect in EFH, since xanthomas do occur in secondary hyperlipidemias. Their localization may be determined by local factors and exogenous influences. Since lipoproteins are precipitated by chondroitin sulfate in vitro, and mesenchymal tissues do contain significant amounts of chondroitin sulfate, it has been proposed (Greiling 1964) that this mechanism may play a role in the pathogenesis of xanthomas. Inflammation and other injury, by lowering the tissue pH, were thought to be additional factors. Predilection of xanthomas for areas exposed to chronic irritation (Schirren 1957, Guravich and Venegas 1962) might be similarly interpreted. In analogy to the lesions of "general" atherosclerosis, xanthomas show a lipid composition which is different from that of plasma (see page 423); for the pathogenesis of both kinds of lesions, factors other than mere lipid infiltration must play a significant role, such as synthesis in loco, exchange and degradation of certain components, etc.

Summary and Conclusions

EFH is an hereditary disorder of lipid metabolism. There is always hypercholesterolemia, hyperphospholipidemia and an elevated cholesterol to phospholipid ratio. Characteristic changes in lipoproteins consist of an increased concentration of beta-lipoproteins. One-third to one-half of all patients exhibit skin and/or tendon xanthomas.

Approximately 30 per cent of all cases have symptoms and signs referable to the cardiovascular system. Coronary heart disease occurs earlier and more frequently in EFH as compared with the general population.

Xanthelasmas and arcus corneae are non-specific signs of EFH and are not pathognomonic for the disease. The proportions of cholesterol and cholesterol esters in skin and tendon xanthomas are different and characteristic for each type of lesion. A combination of EFH with other disorders, such as rheumatic diseases or gout, is frequently observed. These accompanying diseases, and in addition hypertension, obesity, and diabetes mellitus, worsen the prognosis in EFH.

Causal treatment of this disorder, the pathogenesis of which is still unknown, does not exist. Lasting reduction of serum cholesterol level with its supposedly favorable effect on cardiovascular complications, is only rarely achieved by diet and drug treatment; and there is still no conclusive proof that success in lowering serum cholesterol levels will prolong life.

References

Achor, R. W. P., N. A. Christensen, K. G. Berge, and H. L. Mason: Treatment of hypercholesteremia with triparanol and comparison with nicotinic acid. Proc. Mayo Clin. 38, 32 (1963).

Addison, T., and W. Gull: On a certain affection of the skin, vitiligoidea. (a) plana, (b) tuberosa with remarks. Guy's Hosp. Rep. 7, 265 (1850).

Adlersberg, D.: Newer advances in gout. Bull. N.Y. Acad. Med. 25, 651 (1949).

— Hypercholesterolemia with predisposition to atherosclerosis: an inborn error of lipid metabolism. Amer. J. Med. 11, 600 (1951).

ADLERSBERG, D.: Inborn errors of lipid metabolism. Clinical, genetic, and chemical aspects. Arch. Path. (Chic.) **60**, 481 (1955).

— Adrenocortical hormones and experimental atherosclerosis. In: Hormones and atherosclerosis, G. Pincus (Ed.). New York: Academic Press 1959.

— A. D. PARETS, and E. P. BOAS: Genetics of atherosclerosis. J. Amer. med. Ass. **141**, 246 (1994).

AHRENS jr., E. H., D. HIRSCH, W. INSULL, T. TSALTAS, R. BLOMSTRAND, and M.-L. PETERSON: The influence of dietary fats on serum-lipid levels in man. Lancet 1957/I, 943.

— W. INSULL, J. HIRSCH, W. STOFFEL, M. L. PETERSON: The effect on human serum-lipids of a dietary fat, highly unsaturated, but poor in essential fatty acids. Lancet 1959/I, 115.

ALBRIEUX, A. S., Y. COSTA, and R. SARACHAGA: Cited after HARRIS-JONES (1957); An. Fac. Med. Montevideo **38**, 480 (1953).

ALTSCHUL, R., and A. HOFFER: Effect of nicotinic acid upon serum cholesterol and upon basal metabolic rate of young normal adults. Arch. Biochem. **73**, 420 (1958).

— and J. D. STEPHEN: Influence of nicotinic acid on serum cholesterol in man. Arch. Biochem. **54**, 558 (1955).

AMATUZIO, D. S., F. GRANDE, and S. WADE: Effect of glucagon on the serum lipids in essential hyperlipemia and in hypercholesterolemia. Metabolism **11**, 1240 (1962).

AUTENRIETH, W., u. A. FUNK: Über kolorimetrische Bestimmungsmethoden: Die Bestimmung des Gesamtcholesterins im Blut und in Organen. Münch. med. Wschr. **60**, 1243 (1913).

AVIGAN, J., and D. STEINBERG: Effect of saturated and unsaturated fat on cholesterol metabolism in the rat. Proc. Soc. exp. Biol. (N.Y.) **97**, 814 (1958).

— — Sterol and bile acid excretion in man and the effects of dietary fat. J. clin. Invest. **44**, 1845 (1965).

BANSI, H. W.: Hypothyreosen — Strumen — Thyreoiditiden. Verh. dtsch. Ges. inn. Med. **66**, 103 (1960).

BERGE, K. G., R. W. P. ACHOR, N. A. CHRISTENSEN, H. L. MASON, and N. W. BARKER: Hypercholesteremia and nicotinic acid. A long-term study. Amer. J. Med. **31**, 24 (1961).

BERGSTRÖM, S.: Metabolism of bile acids. Fed. Proc. **20**, Suppl. 7, 121 (1961).

BERKOWITZ, D.: The effects of Atromid on serum cholesterol, serum triglycerides, and radioactive fat tolerance in patients with hyperlipidemia. A preliminary report. J. Atheroscler. Res. **3**, 538 (1963).

— Blood lipid and uric acid interrelationships. J. Amer. med. Ass. **190**, 856 (1964).

BERNHEIM, C., G. FORSTER, E. LÜTHY u. F. v. PLANTA: Die Behandlung von Hypercholesterinämie, Hyperlipämie und tuberöser Xanthomatosis mit D-Thyroxin. Schweiz. med. Wschr. **93**, 238 (1963).

BERRY, C., A. MOXHAM, E. SMITH, A. E. KELLIE, and J. D. N. NABARRO: The effects of Atromid on the metabolism of adrenal steroids and on plasma lipid fractions. J. Atheroscler. Res. **3**, 380 (1963).

BEST, M. M., and C. H. DUNCAN: Effects of sitosterol on the cholesterol concentration in serum and liver in hypothyroidism. Circulation **14**, 344 (1956).

— — Effects of the esterification of supplemental cholesterol and sitosterol in the diet. J. Nutr. **65**, 169 (1958).

— — Effects of thiouracil and sitosterol on diet-induced hypercholesteremia and lipomatous arterial lesions in the rat. Amer. Heart J. **58**, 214 (1959).

— — Effects of cholesterol-lowering drugs on serum triglycerides. J. Amer. med. Ass. **187**, 37 (1964).

BETZIEN, G., H. BRACHARZ, P. B. DIEZEL, H. FRANKE, R. KUHN u. TH. SEIDL: Zur Wirkung des Sitosterins auf den Cholesterin-Stoffwechsel beim Warmblüter. Drug Research, Arzneimittel-Forsch. **11**, 751 (1961).

BEVERIDGE, J. M. R., W. F. CONNELL, and G. A. MAYER: Dietary factors affecting the level of plasma cholesterol in humans: The role of fat. Canad. J. Biochem. **34**, 441 (1956).

— — — The nature of the substances in dietary fat affecting the level of plasma cholesterol in humans. Canad. J. Biochem. **35**, 257 (1957).

— — — J. B. FIRSTBROOK, and M. S. DEWOLFE: The effects of certain vegetable and animal fats on the plasma lipids of humans. J. Nutr. **56**, 311 (1955).

— — H. L. HAUST, and G. A. MAYER: Dietary cholesterol and plasma cholesterol levels in man. Canad. J. Biochem. **37**, 575 (1959).

— — G. A. MAYER and H. L. HAUST: Plant sterols, degree of unsaturation, and hypocholesterolemic action of certain fats. Canad. J. Biochem. **36**, 825 (1958).

— — — — The response of man to dietary cholesterol. J. Nutr. **71**, 61 (1960).

BIEBERDORF, F. A., and J. D. WILSON: Influence of unsaturated fat on cholesterol C^{14} metabolism in the isotopic steady state in the rabbit (abstract). Clin. Res. **12**, 262 (1964).

BLODI, F. C., and J. C. YARBROUGH: Ocular manifestations of familial hypercholesterolemia. Amer. J. Ophthal. **60**, 304 (1962).

BLOMSTRAND, R., and E. H. AHRENS jr.: The absorption of fat studied in a patient with chyluria. II. Palmitic and oleic acids. J. biol. Chem. **233**, 321 (1958). — III. Cholesterol. J. biol. Chem. **233**, 327 (1958).

BLUMGART, H. L., A. S. FREEDBERG, and G. S. KURLAND: Treatment of incapacitated euthyroid patients by producing hypothyroidism with radioactive iodine. New Engl. J. Med. **245**, 83 (1951).

— — — Treatment of incapacitated euthyroid cardiac patients with radioactive iodine. Summary of results in treatment of 1070 patients with angina pectoris or congestive failure. J. Amer. med. Ass. **157**, 1 (1955).

BÖTTCHER, C. J. F.: Lipids of the human arterial wall. In: Proceedings of the Symposium (Milano 1960) on "Drugs affecting lipid metabolism", p. 54. Amsterdam: Elsevier 1961.

— and F. P. WOODFORD: Chemical changes in the arterial wall associated with atherosclerosis. Fed. Proc. **21**, Suppl. II, 15 (1962).

BORRIE, P.: Essential hyperlipaemia and idiopathic hypercholesterolemic xanthomatosis. Brit. med. J. **1957/II**, 911.

BRAGDON, J. H., R. J. HAVEL, and E. BOYLE: Human serum lipoproteins. I. Chemical composition of four fractions. J. Lab. clin. Med. **48**, 36 (1956).

BRESLAW, L.: Xanthoma tuberosum: a 6-month control study. Amer. J. Med. **25**, 487 (1958).

BROSS, K.: Beitrag zur Kenntnis der generalisierten Xanthomatose. Virchows Arch. path. Anat. **227**, 144 (1920).

BURNS, F. G.: Contribution to the study of xanthoma tuberosum multiplex. Arch. Derm. Syph. (Chic.) **2**, 415 (1920).

CARLSON, L. A., B. HÖGSTEDT, and L. ORÖ: Effect of Atromid on plasma lipids and lipoproteins in subjects with hyperlipoproteinemia. A preliminary report. J. Atheroscler. Res. **3**, 467 (1963).

CHAUFFARD, A., et G. LA ROCHE: Pathogénie du xanthélasma. Sem. méd. (Paris) **30**, 241 (1910).

CHIU, G. C.: Mode of action of cholesterol-lowering agents. A critique of facts and theories. Arch. intern. Med. **108**, 717 (1961).

— Unpublished data. Cited by CHIU (1961).

CHRISTENSEN, N. A., R. W. P. ACHOR, K. G. BERGE, and H. L. MASON: Hypercholesterolemia: Effects of treatment with nicotinic acid for three to seven years. Dis. Chest. **46**, 411 (1964).

CONSTANTINIDES, P., C. JOHNSON, B. M. FAHRINI, R. NAKASHIMA, and H. W. MCINTOSH: Human hyperlipemia. Rapid correction with a sulphated polymannuronide. Brit. med. J. **1960/I**, 535.

— and P. SAUNDERS: Effect of sulfated algenic acid (SAA) on preestablished rabbit atherosclerosis. II. Study in the absence of concomitant cholesterol feeding. Arch. Path. **65**, 360 (1958).

— — Atherosclerotic and lipophage-stimulating effects of mannuronate. Arch. Path. **65**, 499 (1958).

COSTE, F., J. CAYLA, F. BASSET et G. TSCHOBROUSKY: Cited after SINNER (1961). Rev. Rhum. **26**, 1 (1959).

COTTON, R. C., E. G. WADE, and G. W. SPILLER: The effect of Atromid on plasma fibrinogen and heparin resistance. J. Atheroscler. Res. **3**, 648 (1963).

COUNIHAN, T. B., and P. KEELAN: Atromid in high cholesterol states. J. Atheroscler. Res. **3**, 580 (1963).

CRAMER, K.: Action of Atromid on serum lipids and on β-lipoprotein lipids and protein. J. Atheroscler. Res. **3**, 500 (1963).

CURTIS, A. C., and J. P. BERGER: Effect of feeding a lipotropic substance to patients with xanthelasma. Arch. Derm. Syph. (Chic.) **52**, 252 (1945).

CUTTING, W. C., D. A. RYTAND, and M. L. TAINTER: Relationship between blood cholesterol and increased metabolism from dinitrophenol and thyroid. J. clin. Invest. **13**, 547 (1934).

DAVIS, W. W.: II. The physical chemistry of cholesterol and β-sitosterol related to the intestinal absorption of cholesterol. Trans. N.Y. Acad. Sci. **18**, 123 (1955).

DAWBER, T. R., W. B. KANNEL, and N. REVOTSKIE: Some factors associated with the development of coronary heart disease. Amer. J. publ. Hlth **49**, 1349 (1959).

— F. E. MOORE, and G. V. MANN: Coronary heart disease in the Framingham study. Amer. J. publ. Hlth **47**, 4 (1957).

DEBUCH, H., and W. KAHLKE: Unpublished results (1964).

DELCOURT, R., and M. VASTESAEGER: Action of Atromid on total and β-cholesterol. J. Atheroscler. Res. **3**, 533 (1963).

DILLER, E. R., B. L. WOODS, and O. A. HARVEY: Effect of β-sitosterol on regression of hypercholesterosis and atherosclerosis in chickens. Proc. Soc. exp. Biol. (N.Y.) **98**, 813 (1958).

DUCHOSAL, P. W., and E. RUTISHAUSER: Goutte lipoidique, cas familiaux et sporadiques. Helv. med. Acta **10**, 223 (1943).

DUNCAN, C. H., and M. M. BEST: Lack of nicotinic acid effect on cholesterol metabolism of the rat. J. Lipid Res. 1, 159 (1960).

EPSTEIN, E. u. H. KREITNER: Beitrag zu einer vergleichenden Pathologie und Pathochemie der allgemeinen Cholesterinlipoidosen. Virchows Arch. path. Anat. 306, 53 (1940).

EPSTEIN, F. H.: The epidemiology of coronary heart disease. A review. J. chron. Dis. 18, 735 (1965).

— W. D. BLOCK, E. H. HAND, and TH. FRANCIS: Familial hypercholesterolemia, xanthomatosis and coronary heart disease. Amer. J. Med. 26, 39 (1959).

EPSTEIN, N. M.. R. H. ROSENBAUM. and J. W. GOFMAN: Serum lipoproteins and cholesterol metabolism in xanthelasma. Arch. Derm. Suppl. 65, 70 (1952).

FAGGE, C. H.: General xanthelasma or vitiligoidea. Trans. Path. Soc. (London) 24, 242 (1872/73).

FAILEY jr., R. B., E. BROWN, and M. E. HODES: Effect of nicotinic acid on conjugation pattern of bile acids in man. Circulation 20, 984 (1959).

FARQUHAR, J. W., and M. SOKOLOW: Response of serum lipids and lipoproteins of man to β-sitosterol and safflower oil: a longterm study. Circulation 17, 890 (1958).

FASOLI, A., and A. CESANA: Serum lipid and lipoprotein changes after treatment with Atromid in patients with atherosclerosis. essential hyperlipaemia and familial hypercholesterolaemia. J. Atheroscler. Res. 3, 475 (1963).

FAVARGER, P.: Étude clinique de 3 cas de goutte lipoidique dout 2 cas familiaux et un apparaissant sporadique. Arch. int. Pharmacodyn. 86, 81 (1942).

— Mécanisme d'action des acides gras non saturés sur la cholestérolémie. Bull. Soc. clin. Biol. 45, 461 (1963).

FINLEY, J. K., D. BERKOWITZ, and M. N. CROLL: The physiologic significance of gerontoxon. Arch. Ophthal. 66, 211 (1961).

FISCHER, H., u. W. NIKOLOWSKI: Zur formalen Genese der hyperlipidämischen Xanthome. Arch. klin. exp. Derm. 210, 141 (1960).

FISHER, H. N., and F. C. KNOWLES: Xanthoma tuberosum in childhood with visceral and tendon sheath involvement. J. Amer. med. Ass. 77, 1557 (1921).

FLEISCHMAJER, R.: Dyslipidoses. Med. Clin. N. Amer. 49, 633 (1965).

FLETCHER, R. F., and J. GLOSTER: The lipids in xanthomata. J. clin. Invest. 43, 2104 (1964).

FOWLKES, R. W., and J. C. FORBES: Cholesterol fractionation studies of the serum of xanthelasma patients. Arch. Derm. Syph. (Chic.) 62, 681 (1950).

FRANTZ jr., I. D., and J. B. CAREY jr.: Cholesterol content of human liver after feeding of corn oil and hydrogenated coconut oil. Proc. Soc. exp. Biol. (N.Y.) 106, 800 (1961).

FRANZ, G.: Über Xanthomatose mit besonderer Beteiligung des Gefäßsystems. Frankfurt. Z. Path. 49, 41 (1936).

FREDRICKSON, D. S.: Essential familial hyperlipidemia. In: The metabolic basis of inherited disease. Eds.: J. B. Stanbury, J. B. Wyngaarden, and D. S. Fredrickson, p. 489. New York: McGraw-Hill Book Co. 1960.

— and R. S. LEES: Familial hyperlipoproteinemia. In: The metabolic basis of inherited disease. Eds.: J. B. Stanbury, J. B. Wyngaarden, D. S. Fredrickson. New York: McGraw-Hill Book Co. 1966.

— — and R. I. LEVY: Genetically determined abnormalities in lipid transport. In: Progress in Biochemical Pharmacology, vol II. Eds.: R. Paoletti, D. Kritschewsky, and D. Steinberg. Basel-New York: Karger 1966.

FROEHLICH, A. L.: Les xanthomatoses. Brussels: Acta medica belgica 1951.

FROM HANSEN, P.: The effect of diet, d-thyroxin and Atromid on serum cholesterol and triglycerides in man. J. Atheroscler. Res. 3, 584 (1963).

FULTON, J. K.: Essential lipemia, acute gout, peripheral neuritis and myocardial disease in a Negro man. Arch. intern. Med. 89, 303 (1952).

GEE, D. J., J. GOLDSTEIN, C. H. GRAY, and J. F. FOWLER: Biosynthesis of cholesterol in familial hypercholesterolemic xanthomatosis. Brit. med. J. 1959/II, 341.

GERSON, T., and F. B. SHORLAND: Effect of β-sitosterol on cholesterol and lipid metabolism in the rat. Nature (Lond.) 200, 579 (1963).

GERTLER, M. M., S. M. GARN, and S. A. LEVINE: Serum uric acid in relation to age and physique in health and in coronary heart disease. Ann. intern. Med. 34, 1421 (1951).

— — and P. D. WHITE: Young candidates for coronary heart disease. J. Amer. med. Ass. 147, 621 (1951).

GIAMPALMO, A.: Le tesaurosi lipidiche. Atti. Soc. ital. Pat. 29, 225 (1951).

— Les lipoidoses cholestérimiques du systéme nerveux. 5. Intern. Neurolog. Kongress, Lissabon 1953.

GILBERT, J. B., and J. F. MUSTARD: Some effects of Atromid on platelet economy and blood coagulation in man. J. Atheroscler. Res. 3, 623 (1963).

Glazier, F. W., A. Tamplin, B. Strisower, O. De Lalla, J. W. Gofman, T. Dewber, and E. Phillips: Human serum lipoprotein concentrations. J. Geront. 9, 395 (1954).

Glover, J., and C. Green: Sterol metabolism: III. The distribution and transport of sterols across the intestinal mucosa of the guinea pig. Biochem. J. 67, 308 (1957).

Godal, H. C., I. C. Lund, and E. Silvertsen: Lipids and lipoproteins in serum in cases of familial essential hypercholesteremia and xanthomatosis. Acta med. scand. 156, Suppl. 319, 125 (1956).

Gofman, J. W., L. Rubin, J. P. McGinley, and H. B. Jones: Hyperlipoproteinemia. Amer. J. Med. 17, 514 (1954).

Goldsmith, G. A.: Mechanism by which certain pharmacologic agents lower serum cholesterol. Fed. Proc. 21, Suppl. II, 81 (1962).

— J. G. Hamilton, and O. N. Miller: Investigation of mechanism by which unsaturated fats, nicotinic acid, and neomycin lower serum lipid concentrations: Excretion of sterols and bile acids. Trans. Ass. Amer. Phycns 72, 207 (1959).

Goldstein, D. W.: Xanthoma tuberosum. Sth. med. J. (Bgham., Ala.) 28, 902 (1935).

Gordon, H., B. Lewis, L. Aeles, and J. E. Brock: Effect of different dietary fats on the faecal end products of cholesterol metabolism. Nature (Lond.) 180, 923 (1957a).

— — — — Dietary fat and cholesterol metabolism. Faecal elimination of bile acids and other lipids. Lancet 1957/II (b), 1299.

Gottron, H.: Xanthoma tuberosum multiplex. Zbl. Haut- u. Geschl.-Kr. 40, 152 (1932).

— Familiäres Juvenilxanthom bei 2 Geschwistern. Zbl. Haut- u. Geschl.-Kr. 68, 76 (1942).

Gould, R. G.: Absorbability of β-sitosterol. Trans. N.Y. Acad. Sci. 18, 129 (1955).

— G. V. LeRoy, G. T. Okita, J. J. Kabara, P. Keegan, and D. M. Bergenstal: The use of C14 labeled acetate to study cholesterol metabolism in man. J. Lab. clin. Med. 46, 372 (1955).

Graham, G., and A. G. Stansfield: J. Path. Bact. 58, 543 (1946); cited after Sinner (1961).

Green, K. G., W. H. W. Inman, and J. M. Thorp: Multicentre trial in the United Kingdom and Ireland of a mixture of ethyl chlorophenoxyisobutyrate and androsterone (Atromid). A preliminary report. J. Atheroscler. Res. 3, 593 (1963).

Greiling, H., E. Peter u. B. Schuler: Zur Pathogenese der hypercholesterinämischen Xanthomatose. Dtsch. med. Wschr. 40, 1887 (1964).

Groen, J., B. K. Tjiong, C. E. Kamminga, and A. F. Willebrands: The influence of nutrition, individuality and some other factors, including various forms of stress, on the serum cholesterol: An experiment of 9 months' duration in 60 normal human volunteers. Voeding 13, 556 (1952).

Guravich, J. L.: Familial hypercholesteremic xanthomatosis: Prelim. report. I. Clinical, electrocardiographic and laboratory considerations. Amer. J. Med. 26, 8 (1959).

— and J. Venegas: Familial hypercholesterolemia. Fed. Proc. 21, Suppl. 7, 44 (1962).

Haensch, R.: Der Heparin-Effekt auf das Lipoidelectrophorese-Diagramm bei idiopathischer hyperlipidämischer Xanthomatose. Arch. klin. exp. Derm. 205, 413 (1957).

— Heparin-Therapie und Klinik der idiopathischen hyperlipidämischen Xanthomatose. Arch. klin. exp. Derm. 205, 512 (1958).

Harris-Jones, J. N.: Hyperuricaemia and essential hypercholesterolaemia. Lancet 1957/I, 857.

— E. G. Jones, and P. G. Wells: Xanthomatosis and essential hypercholesterolaemia. Lancet 1957/I, 855.

Hartmann, G., G. Creux, L. K. Widner u. H. Staub: Eine einfache Methode zur Erkennung von Hyperlipidämien. Helv. med. Acta 29, 515 (1962).

Hashim, S. A., and T. B. van Itallie: Cholestyramine resin therapy for hypercholesterolemia. J. Amer. med. Ass. 192, 289 (1965).

— R. E. Clancy, D. M. Hegsted, and F. Stare: Effect of mixed fat formula feeding on serum cholesterol-level in man. Amer. J. clin. Nutr. 7, 30 (1959).

Haust, H. L., and J. M. R. Beveridge: Effect of varying type and quantity of dietary fat on the fecal excretion of bile acids in humans subsisting on formula diets. Arch. Biochem. 78, 367 (1958).

Hayward, P. J., A. V. Davies, T. Deegan, and C. S. McKendrick: The effect of Atromid on serum lipids and coagulation activity. J. Atheroscler. Res. 3, 571 (1963).

Helland-Hansen, B. K.: Rheumatic fever in hereditary xanthomatosis. Acta med. scand. 156, Suppl. 319, 79 (1956).

Hellman, L., R. S. Rosenfeld, M. L. Eidinoff, D. K. Fukushima, T. F. Gallagher, C. Wang, and D. Adlersberg: Isotopic studies of plasma cholesterol of endogenous and exogenous origins. J. clin. Invest. 34, 48 (1955).

— B. Zumoff, G. Kessler, R. S. Rosenfeld, and T. F. Gallagher: Reduction of serum cholesterol in man by an oral androsterone preparation. J. clin. Invest. 41, 1364 (1962).

— — — E. Kara, I. L. Rubin, and R. S. Rosenfeld: Reduction of cholesterol and lipids in man by ethyl-p-chlorophenoxy-isobutyrate. Ann. intern. Med. 59, 477 (1963).

Herbst, F. S. M., W. F. Lever, and N. A. Hurley: Idiopathic hyperlipemia and primary hypercholesteremic xanthomatosis. VI. Studies of the serum proteins and lipoproteins by moving boundary electrophoresis and paper electrophoresis before and after administration of heparin. J. invest. Derm. 24, 507 (1955).

Hernandez, H. H., D. W. Peterson, I. L. Chaikoff, and W. G. Dauben: Absorption of cholesterol-4-C^{14} in rats fed mixed soy bean sterols and β-sitosterol. Proc. Soc. exp. Biol. (N. Y.) 83, 498 (1953).

Hess, F. O.: Herztod infolge schwerer allgemeiner Xanthomatose. Verh. dtsch. Ges. inn. Med. 46, 355 (1934).

Hirschhorn, K., and C. F. Wilkinson jr.: The mode of inheritance in essential familial hypercholesterolemia. Amer. J. Med. 26, 60 (1959).

Hoffer, A.: The relationship of nicotinic acid to cholesterol metabolism. J. clin. exp. Psychopath. 22, 165 (1961).

Hood, B., and G. Angervall: Studies in essential hypercholesterolemia and xanthomatosis. Relationship between age, sex, cholesterol concentrations in plasma fractions, and rise of tendinous deposits. Amer. J. Med. 26, 35 (1959).

Howard, R. P., P. Alaupovic, O. J. Brusco, and R. H. Furman: Effects of ethyl chlorophenoxyisobutyrate, alone or with androsterone (Atromid) on serum lipids, lipoproteins and related metabolic parameters in normal and hyperlipidemic subjects. J. Atheroscler. Res. 3, 482 (1963).

Hudson, J. L., E. R. Diller, R. R. Pfeiffer, and W. W. Davis: Formation of mixed cystals of cholesterol and sitosterol in vitro and in rabbit intestine. Proc. Soc. exp. Biol. (N. Y.) 102, 461 (1959).

Huffschmitt, G., et W. Nessman: Xanthomes familiaux. Bull. Soc. franç. Derm. Syph. 36, 1109 (1931).

Hunter, J. D.: Nicotinic acid therapy in patients with coronary disease. N. Z. med. J. 59, 280 (1960).

— Nicotinic acid therapy in coronary disease. Amer. Heart J. 63, 143 (1962).

Intengan, C.: Studies on coconut oil. II. Relation to bile acid excretion in man. Thesis, Columbia University 1961.

Intengan, C. L., S. A. Hashim, W. H. Sebrell, and T. B. van Itallie: Cited after van Itallie and S. A. Hashim. Clinical and experimental aspects of bile acid metabolism. Med. Clin. N. Amer. 47, 629 (1963).

Jensen, J., D. H. Blankenhorn, and V. Kornerup: Blood-uric-acid levels in familial hypercholesterolaemia. Lancet 1966/I, 298.

Jepson, E. M.: Hypercholesterolaemic xanthomatosis: Treatment with a corn oil diet. Brit. med. J. 1961/I, 847.

— J. D. Billimoria, and N. F. Maclagan: Serum and tissue lipids in patients with familial xanthomatosis. Clin. Sci. 29, 383 (1965).

— and D. C. O. James: The treatment of hypercholesterolaemic xanthomatosis with Atromid. J. Atheroscler. Res. 3, 554 (1963).

Jurand, J., and M. F. Oliver: The effects of ethyl chlorophenoxyisobutyrate on serum cholesteryl, triglyceride and phospholipid fatty acids. J. Atheroscler. Res. 3, 547 (1963).

Kernohan, R. J., and R. A. Neely: The effects of Atromid on the β-lipoprotein ratio in coronary disease. J. Atheroscler. Res. 3, 518 (1963).

Keys, A., J. T. Anderson, and F. Grande: Serum cholesterol response to changes in the diet. II. The effect of cholesterol in the diet. Metabolism 14, 759 (1965).

Khachadurian, A. K.: The inheritance of essential familial hypercholesterolemia. Amer. J. Med. 37, 402 (1964).

Kinsell, L. W., G. D. Michaels, G. Walker, P. Wheeler, S. Splitter, and P. Flynn: Dietary linoleic acid and linoleate. Effects in diabetic and nondiabetic subjects with and without vascular disease. Diabetes 8, 179 (1959).

— — R. W. Friskey, and S. Splitter: Essential fatty acids, lipid metabolism and vascular disease. In: Essential fatty acids, H. M. Sinclair (Ed.). London: Butterworths Sci. Publ. 1958.

— J. Partridge, L. Boling, S. Margen, and G. Michaels: Dietary modification of serum cholesterol and phospholipid levels. J. clin. Endocr. 12, 909 (1952).

— and G. Schlierf: Dietary fat in diabetes mellitus with particular reference to vascular disease. Excerpt med. Internat. Congr. Series No. 84, p. 430, 1965.

Kornerup, W.: Familiaer hypercholesterolaemi og xanthomatose. Kolding, Denmark, 1948.

Kouttinen, A., and J. Paloheimo: The effects of Atromid on serum lipids, proteins and some liver function tests in hypercholesterolaemic patients. J. Atheroscler. Res. 3, 525 (1963).

Kritchevsky, D.: Influence of thyroid hormones and related compounds on cholesterol biosynthesis and degradation: a review. Metabolism 9, 984 (1960).

Kuo, P. T., and D. R. Bassett: Primary hyperlipidemias and their management. Ann. intern. Med. 59, 495 (1963).

Lehzen, G., u. K. Knauss: Über Xanthoma multiplex, planum tuberosum mollusciforme. Virchows Arch. path. Anat. 116, 85 (1889).

Leonard, J. C.: Hereditary hypercholesterolaemic xanthomatosis. Lancet 1956/II, 1239.

Letterer, E.: In: Lehrbuch d. allgem. Pathologie. Stuttgart: Thieme 1959.

Leube: Xanthoma endocardii. In Lehzen u. Knauss (1889).

Lever, W. F.: Systemische Lipoidosen mit erhöhten Serumlipoidwerten. In: Handbuch der Haut- und Geschlechtskrankheiten, Ergänzungswerk, Bd. III/1, p. 87. Ed.: H. A. Gottron. Berlin-Göttingen-Heidelberg: Springer 1963.

— F. S. Herbst, and N. A. Hurley: Idiopathic hyperlipemia and primary hypercholesteremic xanthomatosis. IV. Effects of administration of heparin on serum lipids in idiopathic hyperlipemia. Arch. Derm. 71, 150 (1955).

— P. A. J. Smith, and N. A. Hurley: Idiopathic hyperlipemia and primary hypercholesteremic xanthomatosis. I. Clinical data and analysis of the plasma lipids. J. invest. Derm. 22, 33 (1954).

Lewis, B.: Effect of certain dietary oils on bile-acid secretion and serum-cholesterol. Lancet 1958/I, 1090.

Lindholm, H.: Arcus lipoides corneae and arteriosclerosis. Acta med. scand. 168, 45 (1960).

Lindstedt, S., J. Avigan, D. S. Goodman, J. Sjövall, and D. Steinberg: The effect of dietary fat on the turnover of cholic acid and on the composition of the biliary bile acids in man. J. clin. Invest. 44, 1754 (1965).

Löhr, K., u. P. Neuffer: Xanthomatöse Tendinopathien bei Stoffwechselstörungen. Verh. dtsch. Ges. inn. Med. 65, 414 (1959).

Low, R. C.: Xanthoma tuberosum multiplex with lesions in the heart and tendon sheaths. Brit. J. Derm. 22, 109 (1910).

Mackenzie, S.: Trans. path. Soc. Lond. 33, 370 (1882).

Maher, J. A., F. H. Epstein, and E. A. Hand: Xanthomatosis and coronary heart disease. Arch. intern. Med. 102, 437 (1958).

Malmros, H.: The effect on serum cholesterol of diets containing different fats. Lancet 1957/II, 1.

Marmorston, J., F. J. Moore, J. J. Lewis, O. Magidson, and O. Kuzma: Estrogen therapy in men with myocardial infarction: occurrence of lipid changes before feminization. Clin. Pharmacol. Ther. 1, 449 (1960).

Merrill, J. M., and J. Lemley-Stone: Effects of nicotinic acid on serum and tissue cholesterol in rabbits. Circulat. Res. 5, 617 (1957).

Miller, O. N., J. G. Hamilton, and G. A. Goldsmith: Investigation of the mechanism of action of nicotinic acid on serum lipid levels in man. Amer. J. clin. Nutr. 8, 480 (1960).

Montgomery, H.: Cutaneous xanthoma especially in relation to disease of the liver. J. invest. Derm. 1, 325 (1938).

— Discussion to Epstein et al. (1952).

Müller, C.: Xanthoma, Hypercholesterolemia, Angina pectoris. Acta med. scand. Suppl. 89, 75 (1938).

— Angina pectoris in hereditary xanthomatosis. Arch. intern. Med. 64, 675 (1939).

Nitter-Hauge, S.: Juvenile xanthomatosis — a recessive inherited disease ? Acta med. scand. 179, 71 (1966).

Nobbe, F.: Familiäre hypercholesterinämische Xanthomatose und Hypertonie. Beitr. path. Anat. 126, 256 (1962).

— Hypercholesterinämie und Coronarsklerose. Verh. dtsch. Ges. inn. Med. 69, 640 (1963).

— Familiäre Hypercholesterinämie und Hochdruck. Beitr. path. Anat. 131, 450 (1965).

Nödl, F.: Zur Histo-Pathogenese der Xanthomatose. Arch. Derm. Syph. (Berl.) 193, 176 (1951).

Nothman, M. M., and S. Proger: Cephalins in the blood. Patients with coronary heart disease and patients with hyperlipemia. J. Amer. Ass. Soc. 179, 40 (1962).

— — Kephaline im Blut Gesunder und an Atherosklerose der Kranzarterien Erkrankter. Med. Welt (Berl.) 1965, 190.

Oliver, M. F.: Further observations on the effects of Atromid and of ethyl chlorophenoxy-isobutyrate on serum lipid levels. J. Atheroscler. Res. 3, 427 (1963).

— and G. S. Boyd: The effect of estrogen on the plasma lipids in coronary artery disease. Amer. Heart J. 47, 348 (1954).

— — Hormonal aspects of coronary artery disease. In: Vitamins and Hormones, vol. 16, p. 147. New York: Academic Press 1958.

— — Thyroid and estrogen treatment of hypercholesterolemia in man. In: Hormones and atherosclerosis, G. Pinkus (ed.), p. 403. New York: Academic Press 1959.

O'Reilly, P. O.: Some clinical aspects of nicotinic acid therapy in hypercholesteremia. Canad. med. Ass. J. 78, 402 (1958).

Öst, C. R.: Nikotinsyrabehandling vid arterioskleros och blodlipidrubbningar. Nord. Med. **64**, 1380 (1960).

Owen, W. R., J. C. Owens, and W. B. Neely: Objective effects of dextrothyroxine therapy. Angiology **13**, 75 (1962).

Owen Williams, G. E., M. J. Meynell, and R. Gaddie: Atromid and anticoagulant therapy. J. Atheroscler. Res. **3**, 658 (1963).

Paget, G. E.: Experimental studies of the toxicity of Atromid with particular reference to fine structural changes in the liver of rodents. J. Atheroscler. Res. **3**, 729 (1963).

Pardue, W. D.: Severe liver dysfunction during nicotinic acid therapy. J. Amer. med. Ass. **175**, 137 (1961).

Parsons jr., W. B.: Treatment of hypercholesteremia by nicotinic acid. Progress report with review of studies regarding mechanism of action. Arch. intern. Med. **107**, 639 (1961a).

— Studies of nicotinic acid use in hypercholesteremia. Changes in hepatic functions, carbohydrate tolerance, and uric acid metabolism. Arch. intern. Med. **107**, 653 (1961b).

Pedace, F. J., and R. K. Winkelmann: Xanthelasma palpebrarum. J. Amer. med. Ass. **193**, 893 (1965).

Pelkonen, R.: Plasma vitamin A and E in the study of lipid and lipoprotein metabolism in coronary heart disease. Acta med. scand. **174**, Suppl. 399, 1 (1963).

Perry, W. F.: Effect of nicotinic acid and nicotinamide on incorporation of acetate into cholesterol, fatty acids and CO_2 by rat liver slices. Metabolism **9**, 686 (1960).

Peterson, D. W., C. W. Nichols jr., and E. A. Shneour: Some relationship among dietary sterols, plasma and liver cholesterol levels, and atherosclerosis in chicks. J. Nutr. **47**, 57 (1952).

Pick, L., u. F. Pinkus: Über doppelbrechende Substanz in Hauttumoren, ein Beitrag zur Kenntnis der Xanthomatose. Mschr. prakt. Dermat. **5**, 46 (1908).

Piper, J., and L. Orrild: Essential familial hypercholesterolemia and xanthomatosis. Follow-up study of twelve danish families. Amer. J. Med. **21**, 34 (1956).

— — Xanthomatosis of the pulmonary artery in a patient with essential familial hyper-cholesterolaemia. Acta med. scand. **157**, 103 (1957).

Polano, M. K.: Über die Pathogenese der Cholesterosen der Haut. Arch. Derm. Syph. (Berl.) **174**, 213 (1936).

— Die Xanthelasmatosen der Haut. Arch. Derm. Syph. (Berl.) **181**, 139 (1940).

Pollak, O. J.: Successful prevention of experimental hypercholesteremia and cholesterol atherosclerosis in the rabbit. Circulation **7**, 696 (1953).

Pürschel, W., u. S. Rust: Xanthomatöse Haut- und Organveränderungen bei Hypercholesterinämie. Z. Haut- u. Geschl.-Kr. **15**, 89 (1953).

Quinquaud, C.-E.: Recherches hémato-chimiques et dermato-chimiques. Rev. Soc. Clin. **2**, 259 (1878).

Rausen, A. R., and D. Adlersberg: Idiopathic (hereditary) hyperlipemia and hypercholesteremia in children. Pediatrics **28**, 276 (1961).

Rayer, P. F. O.: Traité des maladie de la peau. Paris 1836.

Riederer, J.: Kardiale Xanthomatose bei familiärer Hypercholesterinämie. Verh. dtsch. Ges. inn. Med. **67**, 441 (1961).

Rigdon, R. H., and G. Willeford: Sudden death during childhood with xanthoma tuberosum. J. Amer. med. Ass. **142**, 1268 (1950).

Rivin, A. U.: Jaundice occurring during nicotinic acid therapy for hypercholesteremia. J. Amer. med. Ass. **170**, 2088 (1959).

Roberts, S. D., and J. F. Pantridge: Effect of Atromid on requirements of warfarin. J. Atheroscler. Res. **3** 655 (1963).

Roels, O. A., and S. A. Hashim: Influence of fatty acids on serum cholesterol. Fed. Proc. **21**, Suppl. II, 71 (1962).

Rohrschneider, W.: Personal communication (1960).

— Die klinische Bedeutung des Arcus lipoides corneae senilis. Wien. med. Wschr. **112**, 845 (1962).

Roper, B. W.: Essential hypercholesteremic xanthomatosis. Brit. med. J. **1964/II**, 990.

Sansone, G., O. Baruffaldi, and C. Romano: Essential familial hypercholesteraemia with tendino-cutaneous and cardiovascular xanthomatosis. Clinical and pathological report. Ann. paediat. (Basel) **195**, 35 (1960).

Sanwald, R.: Nicotinic acid in the treatment of atherosclerosis. In: Atherosclerosis. Ed.: G. S. Boyd and G. Schettler. Amsterdam: Elsevier Publ. Co. 1966.

Savitsky, J. P.: Nongenetic prolonged serum cholesterol alteration induced by deoxyribonucleic acids. Amer. J. Physiol. **203**, 929 (1962).

Schade, H., and P. Saltman: Influence of nicotinic acid on hepatic cholesterol synthesis in rabbits. Proc. Soc. exp. Biol. (N. Y.) **102**, 265 (1959).

Schaefer, L. E., D. Adlersberg, and A. G. Steinberg: Heredity, environment and serum cholesterol. A study of 201 healthy families. Circulation **17**, 537 (1958).

Schettler, G.: I. Die Beeinflussung des Blut- und Organcholesterins durch verschiedene Fette und Öle ohne Cholesterinzusatz. Biochem. Z. **319**, 349 (1949).
— Schilddrüsenfunktion und Cholesterinstoffwechsel. Z. ges. exp. Med. **115**, 251 (1950).
— Essentielle familiäre xanthomatöse Hypercholesterinämie. In: Handb. d. inn. Med. VII/2, 4. Aufl., S. 680. Berlin-Göttingen-Heidelberg: Springer 1955.
— Erkrankungen durch Änderung des Lipoidstoffwechsels. Regensburg. Jb. ärztl. Fortbild. **5**, 493 (1957).
— Störungen des Fettstoffwechsels und die Grundsätze ihrer Behandlung. Regensburg. Jb. ärztl. Fortbild. **7**, 171 (1959).
— Erbliche Störungen des Fettstoffwechsels. Verh. dtsch. Ges. inn. Med. **64**, 287 (1959).
— Die essentielle familiäre xanthomatöse Hypercholesterinämie. Klin. d. Gegenwart Bd. IX, 573 (1960).
In: Arteriosklerose. Ätiologie, Pathologie, Klinik und Therapie. G. Schettler (Ed.). Stuttgart: Thieme 1961.
— u. F. Dietrich: Die Bedeutung von Xanthomen und Xanthelasmen für die Arteriosklerose. Klin. Wschr. **31**, 1040 (1953).
— H. Jobst, H. P. Käppler u. G. Körfgen: Familiäre Hypercholesterinämie. Dtsch. med. Wschr. **84**, 356 u. 368 (1959).
— G. W. Löhr u. E. Stein: Die Bedeutung der essentiellen Hyperlipämie und Hypercholesterinämie für die Entstehung von Herzinfarkten. Dtsch. med. Wschr. **82**, 610 (1957).
Schildhaus, J. M.: Xanthoma tuberosum. Münch. med. Wschr. **89**, 549 (1934).
Schilling, F. J., G. J. Christakis, N. J. Bennett, and J. F. Coyle: Studies of serum cholesterol in 4244 men and women: An epidemiological and pathogenetic interpretation. Amer. J. Publ. Hlth **54**, 461 (1964).
Schirren sen., C. G.: Über die Ursache der Lokalisation von Xanthelasmen bei einem Fall von idiopathischer Hyperlipämie. Hautarzt **3**, 552 (1952).
Schirren, C.: Hyperlipämische Xanthomatosen. Hautarzt **8**, 119 (1957).
Schmidt, E.: Über die Bedeutung des Cholesterins für die Xanthombildung. Dermat. Z. **21**, 137 (1914).
Schöll, H., u. G. Schettler: Die Lipoproteidlipase und ihre klinische Bedeutung. Ergebn. inn. Med. Kinderheilk. N. F. **16**, 245 (1961).
Schoenheimer, R.: Über die Bedeutung der Pflanzensterine für den tierischen Organismus. Z. physiol. Chem. **180**, 1 (1929).
— Die Spezifität der Cholesterinresorption und ihre biologische Bedeutung. Klin. Wschr. **11**, 1793 (1932).
Siegmund, H.: Kardiovaskuläre Xanthomatose als Todesursache beim Jugendlichen. Münch. med. Wschr. **85**, 1617 (1938).
Sinner, W.: Xanthomatose und Rheumatismus. Über zwei Fälle essentieller familiärer xanthomatöser Hypercholesterinämie mit chronischem Gelenkrheumatismus. Schweiz. med. Wschr. **91**, 1114 (1961).
Siperstein, M. D., and V. M. Fagan: Studies on the feedback regulation of cholesterol synthesis. Adv. Enzyme Regulation 2, 249. New York: Pergamon Press 1964.
— M. E. Jayko, I. L. Chaikoff, and W. G. Dauben: Nature of the metabolic products of C^{14} cholesterol excreted in bile and feces. Proc. Soc. exp. Biol. (N. Y.) **81**, 720 (1952).
Spritz, N., E. H. Ahrens jr., and S. Grundy: Sterol balance in man as plasma cholesterol concentrations are altered by exchanges of dietary fats. J. clin. Invest. **44**, 1482 (1965).
Srivastava, S. C., M. J. Smith, and H. A. Dewar: The effect of Atromid on fibrinolytic activity of patients with ischaemic heart disease and hypercholesterolaemia. J. Atheroscler. Res. **3**, 640 (1963).
Stamler, J., L. N. Katz, R. Pick, L. A. Lewis, I. H. Page, A. Pick, B. M. Kaplan, D. M. Berkson, and D. Century: Effects of long-term estrogen therapy on serum cholesterol-lipid-lipoprotein levels and on mortality in middle-aged men with previous myocardial infarction. In: Garattini, S., and R. Paoletti (Eds.): Proc. of the symposium on drugs effecting lipid metabolism, p. 432. Amsterdam: Elsevier 1961.
— R. Pick, L. N. Katz, A. Pick, and B. M. Kaplan: Interim report on clinical experiences with long-term estrogen administration to middle-aged men with coronary heart disease. Hormones and Atherosclerosis, p. 423. New York: Academic Press 1959.
— E. N. Silber, A. J. Miller, L. Akman, C. Bolene, and L. N. Katz: The effect of thyroid- and of dinitrophenol-induced hypermetabolism on plasma and tissue lipids and atherosclerosis in the cholesterol-fed chick. J. Lab. clin. Med. **35**, 351 (1950).
Stanley, P., C. Chartrand, and A. Davignon: Acquired aortic stenosis in a twelve-year-old girl with xanthomatosis. Successful surgical correction. New Engl. J. Med. **273**, 1378 (1965).
Stannus, H. S.: Hyperlipochromia (carotinaemia xanthosis cutis). Int. Clin. **39**, 146 (1929).
Startin, J.: Xanthelasma. Trans. path. Soc. Lond. **31**, 374 (1882).

STRISOWER, E. H., and B. STRISOWER: The separate hypolipoproteinemic effects of dextro-thyroxine and ethyl chlorophenoxy-isobutyrate. J. clin. Endocr. 24, 139 (1964).

SUGG, E. S., and D. D. STETSON: Xanthoma tuberosum associated with trauma and mild diabetes mellitus. J. Amer. med. Ass. 109, 414 (1937).

SWELL, L., T. A. BOITER, H. FIELD jr., and C. R. TREADWELL: Esterification of Soybean sterols in vitro and their influence on blood-cholesterol level. Proc. Soc. exp. Biol. (N. Y.) 86, 295 (1954).

— H. FIELD jr., and C. R. TREADWELL: Sterol specificity of pancreatic cholesterol esterase. Proc. Soc. exp. Biol. (N. Y.) 87, 216 (1954).

THANNHAUSER, S. J.: Cholesterol. In: Lipidoses. Diseases of the intracellular lipid metabolism, p. 32. Ed.: S. J. Thannhauser. New York: Grune and Stratton 1958.

TYGSTRUP, N., K. WINKLER u. K. JØRGENSEN: Behandlung von Hypercholesterinämie mit p-Aminosalicylsäure. Ugeskr. Laeg. 123, 255 (1961).

WAGENER, H., and B. FROSCH: Dünnschichtchromatographische Untersuchungen über die Phosphatide des Blutserums Gesunder und Arteriosklerosekranker. Z. ges. exp. Med. 138, 425 (1964).

WILKENS, J. A., H. DEWITT, and B. BRONTE-STEWART: A proposed mechanism for effect of different dietary fats on some aspects of cholesterol metabolism. Canad. J. Biochem. 40, 1091 (1962).

WOLFSON, W. Q., C. COLIN, R. LEVINE, E. F. ROSENBERG, and H. D. HUNT: Essential hyper-lipemia and gout. Ann. intern. Med. 30, 598 (1949).

WOOD, P., R. SHIODA, and L. KINSELL: Dietary regulation of cholesterol metabolism. Lancet 1966/II, 604.

ZÖLLNER, N.: Nukleinstoffwechsel. In: Thannhausers Lehrbuch des Stoffwechsels und der Stoffwechselkrankheiten, S. 511. Stuttgart: Thieme 1957.

— Idiopathische familiäre Hypercholesterinämie. In: Erbliche Stoffwechselkrankheiten, Linneweh (Ed.). München-Berlin: Urban & Schwarzenberg 1962a.

— Angeborene Störungen im Stoffwechsel der Lipoide. Gastroenterologia (Basel) 97, 247 (1962b).

— Untersuchungen über das Verhalten der Plasmalipoide bei idiopathischer Hypercholesterinämie, unter besonderer Berücksichtigung der Cholesterinester. Z. klin. Chem. 1, 18 (1963).

— Round-table discussion: Prophylaxis and treatment of atherosclerosis. In: Symposium on pathophysiological and clinical aspects of lipid metabolism. Heidelberg 1965. Ed.: G. Schettler. Stuttgart: Thieme 1966.

— and G. WERNEKKE: A comparative study of the hypocholesteremic effect of nicotinic acid and some compounds related to it. Pres. at the 6th intern. Congress for Gerontology, Copenhagen, 1963.

Essential Hyperlipemia

By

L. W. Kinsell, G. Schlierf*, W. Kahlke and G. Schettler

Synonyms: Essential (idiopathic, primary) hyperglyceridemia.

Definition and Introduction

"Milky" blood was observed frequently by physicians of the last century when blood letting was liberally employed. The fact that this turbid to creamy appearance of the blood serum was usually attributable to a high fat content had been clearly demonstrated by Hewson in 1774. However, numerous reports of serum turbidity prior to 1850 probably included conditions other than hyperlipemia (leukemias, etc.).

Lipemia in "uncontrolled" diabetes mellitus was well documented before 1900 (Tyson 1881). Other conditions which have been found associated with lipemia were hemorrhage as first described in rabbits by Boggs and Morris (1909) and reviewed by Feigl in 1921, experimental (Binet and Brocq 1929) and clinical (Brunner 1935) pancreatitis, pregnancy (lit. see Alvarez et al. 1959), nephrosis (lit. see Schettler 1955), alcoholism (Losowsky et al. 1963, Schapiro et al. 1965) and glycogen storage disease (see Field 1960). A detailed review of the older literature on lipemia has been given by Fischer (1903).

The plasma turbidity in these conditions results from the presence of increased amounts of emulsified fat particles which are of sufficient size (100 mμ) to cause scattering of light and which have a high glyceride content. The word "chylomicrons" was introduced by Gage and Fish (1924) and has replaced terms like blood dust or hemoconia.

The term „*essential hyperlipemia*" (EHL) describes a group of syndromes which are characterized by elevation of plasma triglycerides (TG) in excess of other serum lipids, which is not secondary to other recognized disease states. Turbidity of the serum is observed with plasma triglyceride levels above 400—800 mg per 100 ml (Albrink et al. 1955), and may depend to some degree on the origin of the particulate fat. The affected individuals may or may not exhibit clinical symptoms. Xanthomatosis is found frequently; enlargement of liver and spleen is occasionally observed and may be present intermittently. Severe colicky abdominal pain may occur with and without organomegaly. Such episodes are encountered only in the presence of marked hyperglyceridemia.

It has recently become possible to distinguish several major syndromes within EHL which exhibit slightly different clinical features, significantly different responses to dietary and other measures and probably quite different pathogeneses.

Historical Review

The first description of EHL as a separate clinical entity was given by Bürger and Grütz, who in 1932 described a case of "hepatosplenomegalic lipidosis with

---

* Work performed during tenure of a research fellowship at the Institute for Metabolic Research, Highland General Hospital, Oakland, Cal.

xanthomatosis of skin and mucous membranes" in a 12 year old boy with persistent lipemia throughout the 13 months period of observation. It seems probable that a number of cases which had been reported earlier as diabetic lipemia would now be considered EHL, particularly where the absence of ketone bodies has been emphasized (BEUMER and BÜRGER 1913). Likewise the case reported by WIJN-HAUSEN (1921) as recurrent pancreatitis with lipemia seems to have represented EHL since evidence of elevated blood lipids (eruptive xanthomas) preceded the first episodes of abdominal pain. The next patients with essential hyperlipemia were reported by OPITZ (1935), ABEGG (1937) and FRANKLIN (1937). The first detailed description of EHL in the English literature was given by HOLT et al. in 1939. They introduced the term "idiopathic familial hyperlipemia", and suggested that a defective removal mechanism for blood fat may be involved in the pathogenesis of the syndrome. The patient was an 11 year-old white girl who from age 4 had experienced recurrent colicky abdominal pains. The total serum lipids at the beginning of the observation period were as high as 7.37 gm per 100 ml resulting in grossly milky serum and the appearance of lipemia retinalis. Total cholesterol was 330 and phospholipids 430 mg per 100 ml. Total serum lipids of mother and sister were 1.43 gm per 100 ml and 1.14 gm per 100 ml, respectively; an asymptomatic brother exhibited lipid levels of 2.61 to 3.01 gm per 100 ml with hepatosplenomegaly and lipemia retinalis. Following their description, numerous case reports of the disease in children (BERNSTEIN et al. 1939, GOODMAN et al. 1940, LEVY 1946, HARSLÖF 1948, POULSEN 1950, BRUTON and KANTER 1951, CROCKER 1951, GASKINS et al. 1953) and adults appeared (see reviews by LEVER et al. 1954, MALMROS et al. 1954, and SCHETTLER 1955). ADLERSBERG in 1955 reported on studies in 25 cases of hyperlipemia and 64 members of the families of 20 of the hyperlipemic subjects.

By 1957 the non-homogeneity of cases reported as EHL had become quite apparent, and BORRIE, both by review of subjects described earlier by LEVER et al. and MALMROS et al. and from observations in cases of his own, called attention to the fact that a number of patients would exhibit symptoms and signs of both "essential familial hypercholesterolemia" (EFH) and EHL. In his opinion simultaneous occurrence of lipemia was insufficient cause to detract from the diagnosis of EFH if the clinical findings were appropriate, and he therefore classified such cases, as did THANNHAUSER one year later (1958), under the heading of essential familial hypercholesterolemia. For another group of patients exhibiting both signs of EFH and eruptive xanthomas, BORRIE introduced the term "mixed cases". ADLERSBERG in 1955 had already emphasized some relationship of EFH and EHL from his observations of an occurrence of both syndromes in the same pedigree.

Earlier, in 1950, THANNHAUSER had directed attention to the association of EHL with glycosuria, which he emphatically distinguished from hyperlipemia of uncontrolled diabetes, thus introducing another controversial subject into the consideration of EHL. A combination of essential hyperlipemia and hyperglycemia or "mild diabetes" has been described on many occasions since (JOYNER 1953, ADLERSBERG and WANG 1955, CHRISTENSEN et al. 1958, CARLSON and OLHAGEN 1959, FREDRICKSON 1960, HAVEL and GORDON 1960, FURMAN et al. 1961, KINSELL et al. 1962, SHIPP and MUNROE 1962), and the cases described by HAMWI et al. (1962) probably fall into the same category.

By 1961 it was generally assumed that EHL probably included several different syndromes (SCHETTLER 1955, FREDRICKSON 1960, HAVEL and GORDON 1960, KINSELL et al. 1961) and an abnormality of endogenous triglyceride metabolism was being seriously considered (SCHRADE et al. 1954, SCHETTLER et al. 1958, CARLSON and OLHAGEN 1959). At this time, AHRENS et al. (1961) presented the concept of the existence of two different forms of EHL with their studies of "carbohydrate-induced" and "fat-induced" hyperlipemia. This approach has proved a very fruitful and stimulating basis for subsequent research, particularly with the availability of methods (GORDIS 1962, LEES and HATCH 1963) which permit of distinction between alimentary and endogenous particulate fat as found under certain conditions in "fat-induced" and "carbohydrate-induced" hyperlipemia, respectively. Based on the latter authors' modified paper electrophoresis, FREDRICKSON and LEES (1965) have recently proposed a system of phenotyping hyperlipidemias according to certain lipoprotein patterns, which distinguishes four different forms of hyperglyceridemia in addition to hyper-β-lipoproteinemia (essential hypercholesterolemia). More detailed consideration of these aspects will be given in the section dealing with classification (see below).

Epidemiology and Incidence

The scarcity of epidemiologic data is to a great extent due to the lack of methods which are applicable for screening of larger population groups. Lipemia as detected by simple inspection is but the expression of severe hyperglyceridemia, and the determination of plasma triglyceride levels is still tedious and expensive. Even if both plasma glycerides and cholesterol are measured, information thus obtained permits only of undependable conclusions as to the prevailing lipoprotein pattern and thus hinders meaningful classification. Needless to say, controlled dietary studies are not feasible on a large scale.

HIRSCHHORN and coworkers in 1959 measured serum optical density following oral fat loading in Swedish students. From the number of hyperlipemic responses among their 998 subjects they estimated the incidence of hyperlipemia in the total population of Sweden to be of the order of 2—3%. Since no other clinical data are available and plasma triglycerides were not determined, this figure on the one hand probably includes secondary hyperlipemias, and on the other may have failed to detect mild forms of EHL. JAHNKE (1965) found an incidence of hyperlipemia in 3.7% of somewhat selected patients examined by his group between 1960 and 1964. In a group of 261 clinically healthy males between the ages of 45 and 54 included in the Oakland, California, portion of the National Diet-Heart Feasibility Study, 17 (ca. 7%) were found to be unequivocally hyperglyceridemic, i.e. to have fasting plasma triglyceride values in excess of 200 mg per 100 ml. The incidence of significant hyperglyceridemia is probably considerably higher since by the methods used most normal subjects have values below 160 mg per 100 ml (see page 467.).

The incidence of EHL is higher in males than in females. In ADLERSBERG's (1955) 25 cases the distribution was 72% and 28%, respectively. The corresponding figures in GADRAT's material (1958) were 37 males and 12 females, over 3 times more males than females, and the cases reported since do not significantly change this proportion.

The manifestation of EHL with regard to *age* is difficult to evaluate at the present time and may to some degree depend on the type of hyperlipemic syndrome. In general, hyperlipemia of the pure "fat-induced" variety appears to be detectable in early childhood and was diagnosed in one case during the immediate neonatal period (BIALKIN et al. 1962). The case reports during the 15 years following the original description by BÜRGER and GRÜTZ concerned only children up to 12 years of age, and the majority of subjects exhibited skin lesions during the first five years of life. A more intense response of the infant organism to hyperlipemia may have aided in early recognition during a period when routine blood tests were rather uncommon and the symptoms of abdominal pain, hepatosplenomegaly and xanthomatosis had resulted in hospitalization of the patients. Several reasons can be given why in many instances EHL is not diagnosed before adulthood. First, the finding of hyperlipemia may result from a routine blood examination or during evaluation of an affected family, thus establishing a diagnosis which may have gone unrecognized for years. Secondly, particularly in subjects with accompanying carbohydrate intolerance, hyperglyceridemia may be progressive and with methods generally available may not be detectable at an early age. In addition, data collected from the literature probably do not reflect true age incidence since until rather recently many cases with carbohydrate intolerance were considered to have diabetes mellitus and were therefore not reported as primary hyperglyceridemia.

According to BORRIE (1957), children below age 10 represent approximately one-third of all cases with EHL. The youngest patients were the infant described by GOODMAN et al. (1940) who expired at the age of 21 months, an 11 month-old female infant reported by CROCKER (1951), two siblings aged 4 and 9 months respectively at the time of diagnosis (RAUSEN and ADLERSBERG 1961), and one case of BIALKIN et al. (1962). In some patients, EHL was not detected before age 60 (LEVER and KLEIN 1958).

Considering all types of EHL, we found over 130 cases in the literature where clinical data in addition to lipid studies were *documented* (lit. see JOYNER 1953, LEVER et al. 1954, MALMROS et al. 1954, ADLERSBERG 1955, SCHETTLER 1955, CHRISTENSEN et al. 1958, GADRAT 1958, SCHETTLER et al. 1958, CARLSON and OLHAGEN 1959, FREDRICKSON 1960, HAVEL and GORDON 1960, SCHETTLER 1961, KINSELL et al. 1962, KNITTLE and AHRENS 1964, JUCHEMS et al. 1965, KUO et al. 1965, SIGSTAD 1965). In addition we know of over 200 cases which are presently being studied by several groups of investigators (SCHETTLER 1961, KNITTLE and AHRENS 1964, FREDRICKSON and LEES 1965, FURMAN 1965, JAHNKE 1965, KINSELL and SCHLIERF 1965). It is obvious that EHL is by no means a rare disease.

Occurrence of EHL is not limited to the Caucasian *race*, and detailed descriptions of the syndrome in Negros have been given (FULTON 1952, GASKINS et al. 1953, KUO and BASSETT 1963, KINSELL and SCHLIERF 1965).

Whereas FREDRICKSON in 1960 found *familial occurrence* in only 17 cases of 9 pedigrees, at least 18 publications (HOLT et al. 1939, LEVY 1946, HARSLÖF 1948, POULSEN 1950, BOHMAN 1951, BRUTON and KANTER 1951, KLATSKIN and GORDON 1952, GASKINS et al. 1953, MALMROS et al. 1954, SOFFER and MURRAY 1954, ADLERSBERG 1955, ADLERSBERG and WANG 1955, MARTT and CONNOR 1956, BOGGS et al. 1957, CHRISTENSEN et al. 1958, RAUSEN and ADLERSBERG 1961, BIALKIN et al. 1962, SIGSTAD 1965) describe familial cases by now. It appears from the literature and from observations in our own material that a hereditary predisposition exists in all forms of primary hyperglyceridemia. This will be discussed in detail in a separate chapter by FUHRMANN.

Basic Concepts of Triglyceride Transport

Before discussing the different forms of EHL and considering some pathogenetic factors involved in the production of different syndromes, a brief summary of present understanding of triglyceride transport may be in order. No attempt will be made at this time to discuss areas of controversy. For details we refer to reviews by FREDRICKSON and GORDON (1958), HAVEL (1958), JEANRENAUD (1961), and by

Dole and Hamlin (1962), as well as to other parts of this volume. Since human data are incomplete in many areas, findings from animal experiments will be included, with the full recognition that some of these data may be misleading because of species differences.

1. During digestion, *exogenous long chain triglycerides* are completely or partially hydrolyzed in the small intestine through the action of pancreatic and intestinal lipases in the presence of bile salts. They are absorbed and resynthesized within the intestinal mucosa and discharged into the thoracic duct via lymphatic channels as chylomicrons, which represent the lowest density lipoprotein fraction synthesized by body tissues (Isselbacher 1964). Data regarding their composition have been given recently by Wood et al. (1964) who found average figures of 2.5% protein, 9% phospholipids, 2.5% cholesterol and 86% triglycerides[1]. The protein moiety can apparently be synthesized by the mucosal cell from amino acids (Rodbell et al. 1959). The triglyceride fatty acids typically resemble the fed fat (Bragdon and Karmen 1960, Wood et al. 1964), whereas the fatty acids of cholesterol esters and phospholipids seem relatively unaffected by dietary fatty acid composition (Bierman 1965). The entry of dietary chylomicrons into the bloodstream results in postprandial lipemia, the intensity and duration of which varies greatly in different persons (Shah et al. 1963). As the actual chylomicron level at any time represents a balance between inflow and removal, its degree depends heavily on factors controlling absorption on one hand, and factors regulating utilization, such as the nutritional state of the individual, on the other. In normal subjects its peak may lie anywhere between 2 and 7 hours after a fat meal.

The fate of chylomicrons after their discharge into the blood is still incompletely understood (Dole and Hamlin 1962). A considerable portion of chylomicron triglyceride is hydrolyzed and taken up by extrahepatic tissues, particularly adipose tissue (Havel and Goldfien 1961, Nestel et al. 1962). Glucose (Albrink et al. 1958) and insulin (Rony and Ching 1930, Kessler 1962) appear to accelerate this process. The fatty acids are then reesterified within the adipose tissue cell for storage. Adequate carbohydrate metabolism in adipose tissue is required to supply α-glycerol-phosphate for such reesterification, since adipose tissue glycerokinase activity is very low and glycerol therefore cannot be used for esterification of fatty acids (Vaughan 1961).

To the liver has been attributed a significant role in initial removal of chylomicrons from plasma (Nestel et al. 1962), and evidence has been presented suggesting uptake of fat particles as units rather than fragments (Havel and Fredrickson 1956). Felts (1965), from careful studies with fresh chylomicrons, has recently questioned the quantitative importance of this process.

A portion of the chylomicronous fat may be oxidized for energy metabolism, either directly (Fredrickson et al. 1958) or following intra- and/or extravascular hydrolysis. Isotopic data suggest that a significant proportion of plasma free fatty acids (FFA) may be derived from chylomicrons (Havel and Fredrickson 1956, Nestel et al. 1962). The ratio of oxidized to stored chylomicron fatty acids depends on the nutritional state of the subject and is highest in the fasting state (Bragdon and Gordon 1958, Fredrickson et al. 1958).

Uptake of most of the chylomicron glycerides by adipose tissue is preceded by hydrolysis (Rodbell and Scow 1965), which is mediated, according to present concepts, by the enzyme(s) lipoprotein lipase located within the capillary wall (recently reviewed by Engelberg 1960).

---

[1] Undoubtedly some contamination of chylomicrons by endogenous very low density lipoprotein was present.

2. *Endogenous triglycerides* are discharged by the liver as constituents of lipoproteins (KAY and ENTENMAN 1961). The highest triglyceride content is found in lipoproteins of density less than 1.006 (VLDLP). The triglyceride fatty acids may be obtained from the following sources:

a) de novo synthesis from two-carbon fragments (WAKIL and BRESSLER 1962). The following sources have to be considered: dietary carbohydrate, protein, medium chain fatty acids (WALKER et al. 1953, UZAWA et al. 1964).

b) reesterification of free fatty acids originating from adipose tissue (HAVEL 1961).

c) chylomicron triglycerides, possibly after initial hydrolysis (DOLE and HAMLIN 1962).

Since excess concentration in plasma of free fatty acids would be undesirable, the liver functions as an important link in the energy cycle by transforming such free fatty acids, regardless of source, to the transport form of triglycerides, which then may return to the adipose tissue bank. Uptake of FFA by adipose tissue does occur (VAUGHAN 1961) although it may be of only minor significance in states associated with high FFA levels (starvation, diabetes mellitus) since it is dependent on a functioning carbohydrate metabolism.

There are no reliable data available regarding the exact proportion of dietary carbohydrate which is converted to triglycerides in the liver; lipogenesis in adipose tissue is probably quantitatively much more important under normal circumstances (SHAPIRO 1957). As far as is known, no lipoprotein glyceride is liberated from adipose tissue into the plasma.

With very high carbohydrate intake, VLDLP of Sf 20—400 (WALKER et al. 1953, HATCH et al. 1955, NICHOLS et al. 1957) and possibly under some circumstances, >400 are found in significant amounts in the plasma of most individuals leading to elevation of total triglycerides in the fasting plasma (HATCH et al. 1955, AHRENS 1957, KUO and CARSON 1959). Their triglyceride content is intermediate between chylomicrons and low density lipoproteins (GUSTAFSON 1965). This lipoprotein material migrates as pre-β-lipoprotein in the modified paper electrophoretic system of LEES and HATCH (1963), and can thus be conveniently differentiated from chylomicrons and β-lipoproteins. Endogenous lipoprotein triglyceride can be taken up by liver, muscle and adipose tissue (BEZMAN et al. 1962, FRIEDBERG and ESTES 1964).

There is some evidence to show that not only the amount but also the type of dietary carbohydrates influences the level and kind of lipids in serum. MACDONALD and BRAITHWAITE (1964) found higher plasma triglyceride levels in normal volunteers on high sucrose as compared to high starch diets, and of five preparations of carbohydrates used in a short term experiment (MACDONALD 1965), only the feeding of sucrose resulted in elevation of the plasma triglyceride level. It has been suggested that fructose may be the agent responsible for these observations.

As yet there is no evidence that the uptake of endogenously synthesized lipoprotein triglycerides by adipose tissue proceeds qualitatively differently from the uptake of chylomicron triglycerides. It is likewise accelerated by carbohydrate feeding (HAVEL 1957) and/or insulin administration (SCHLIERF and KINSELL 1965). No conclusive evidence has been presented as to whether endogenous and exogenous triglycerides differ as substrate for lipoprotein lipase as suggested by ENGELBERG (1962) for some cases of EHL.

The uptake of triglycerides by tissues other than adipose tissue possibly serves as an energy source in addition to the free fatty acid fraction and glucose (GOUSIOS et al. 1963, WOOD et al. 1965).

Classification and Pathologic Physiology of EHL

Ideally, diseases are classified on the basis of etiologic factors. It is the consensus of students in the field of lipid metabolism that such a goal has not been reached with regard to the various disorders of lipid metabolism; and the term „essential hyperlipemia" reflects this ignorance. However, significant advances from a purely

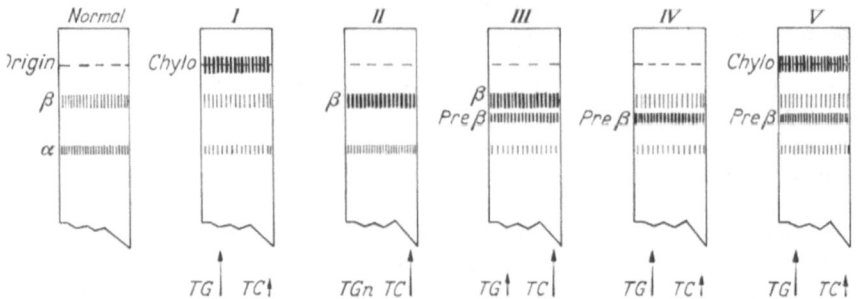

Fig. 1. As indicated: Chylomicrons remain at the origin. β-(low density, Sf 0—20) lipoproteins migrate least. Pre-β-(very low density, Sf 20—400) lipoproteins migrate ahead of β-lipoproteins. α-(high density) lipoproteins migrate more than other lipoproteins. Some material more dense than chylomicrons and less dense than Sf 20—400 may "trail". Modified from FREDRICKSON and LEES 1965

I. Familial fat-induced hyperlipemia. Plasma: creamy; Xanthomatosis: eruptive, tuberous; Hepatosplenomegaly; Chylomicrons on any fat intake; Post-heparin lipolytic activity: low; Glucose tolerance: normal.

II. Familial Hyper-β-Lipoproteinemia (Familial Hypercholesterolemia). Plasma: clear; Xanthomatosis: Tendon, tuberous, xanthelasmas; Arcus; Expression early; Severity increases with time; Post-heparin lipolytic activity: normal; Glucose tolerance: normal ? Atheromatosis.

III. Familial Hyper-β- and Pre-β-Lipoproteinemia ("Familial Hypercholesterolemia with Hyperglyceridemia"). Plasma: clear, cloudy or milky; Xanthomatosis: Tuberous, tendon, plane; Arcus; Post-heparin lipolytic activity: normal; Glucose tolerance: abnormal; Carbohydrate inducible; Atheromatosis.

IV. Familial Hyper-Pre-β-Lipoproteinemia. Plasma: clear, cloudy or milky; Xanthomatosis and hepatosplenomegaly as in type I; Post-heparin lipolytic activity: normal; Glucose tolerance: abnormal; Carbohydrate inducible.

V. Familial Hyperchylomicronemia and Hyper-Pre-β-Lipoproteinemia. Plasma: creamy; All manifestations seen in type I; Post-heparin lipolytic activity: low or normal; Glucose tolerance: abnormal; Fat and carbohydrate inducible.

descriptive use of the term have been made since the demonstration of the etiologic role of dietary carbohydrate in the production of very low density lipoproteins (see pg. 451), and the subsequent use of diets of specific composition to characterize subdivisions of EHL.

A classification of EHL, as proposed by THANNHAUSER (1950), into juvenile and adult forms — the latter frequently exhibiting mild glycosuria in addition to hyperglyceridemia — cannot be maintained in this strict sense. However, it still aids in consideration of differential diagnosis of EHL, since the endogenous hyperglyceridemias, to be described, are commonly diagnosed in adults.

Since hypertriglyceridemia is more specifically hyperlipoproteinemia, FREDRICKSON and LEES have recently (1965) used a simple modification of the standard paper electrophoresis procedure to classify patients with EHL into four more or less specific groups which they believe are associated with specific congenital defects. A schematic summary of their work is given in figure 1. This procedure represents a most helpful approach to the problem, since the concept of fat-induced or carbohydrate-induced EHL fails to account for the great number of hyperlipemic subjects who manifest marked hyperglyceridemia when fat or carbohydrate are present in the diet in sufficient amounts under appropriate conditions, as well as for cases bridging EHL and EFH. More data are required before one may adequately

evaluate the general applicability of this attractive method of phenotyping lipoprotein patterns in EHL.

For the purpose of this presentation a similar classification has been adopted,
which is sufficiently non-specific to permit of inclusion of most of the cases reported
and which to some degree is based upon our limited knowledge of pathogenetic
mechanisms. However, in view of the variety of factors affecting triglyceride
metabolism, it is to be expected that a number of subjects with hyperlipemia
cannot be included in any classification yet available. In addition, the pathogeneses
of some of the called "secondary" hyperlipemias are so poorly understood at the
present time as to make clear cut distinction difficult or impossible.

a) Exogenous Hyperglyceridemia

[Fat-induced hyperlipemia (FIHL), hyperchylomicronemia, type I of FRED-
RICKSON and LEES, alimentary hyperglyceridemia].

This is a relatively rare hereditary disorder, characterized by intolerance to
all types of dietary fat. On diets containing fat the serum shows various degrees of
turbidity and a characteristic "creaming" of the particulate fat after standing

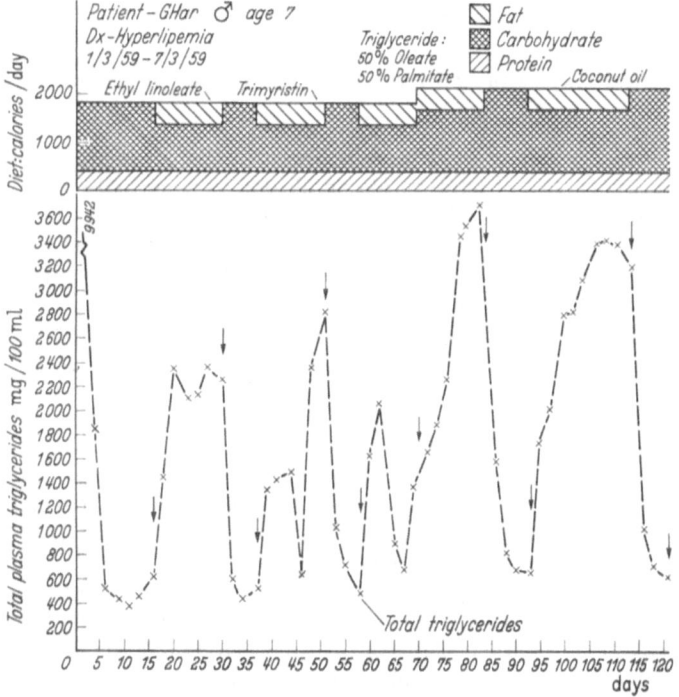

Fig. 2. Exogenous (fat-induced) hyperlipemia. Intake of any of a variety of fats in this boy resulted
in progressive hyperglyceridemia. Fat-free (high carbohydrate) diets were associated with rapid fall
of plasma glyceride levels toward normal. Glycerides in this study were determined by difference from
total lipids. Values are higher as compared with those of other figures

overnight. Fat-free diets produce clearing of the lipemia. Studies in a case of
exogenous hyperlipemia are shown in figure 2.

It is now generally agreed that in these subjects hyperlipemia is caused by
defective removal from the blood of dietary chylomicrons (HAVEL and GORDON
1960, FREDRICKSON and LEES 1965), the half life of which is usually markedly

prolonged, depending on the severity of hyperlipemia. Whereas in normal persons a single fat load is cleared from the circulation within 8 hours or less, fat loading in fat-induced hyperlipemia results in exaggerated and prolonged peak lipemia (Bürger and Grütz 1932) and clearing of a single fat load usually requires several days (Havel and Gordon 1960, Ahrens et al. 1961).

Table 1

Author	No. of subjects and diagnosis	Plasma Triglycerides mg/100 ml	Postheparin lipolytic activity Mean μEq FFA/min/ml	Range
Ahrens et al. (1961)	2 "FIHL"	—	—	0.04 — 0,06
	8 "CIHL"	—	—	0.26 — 0.49
Fredrickson et al. (1963)	9 "FIHL"	570 — 4200	0.16 ± 0.10	0.16 — 0.41*
	9 "CIHL"	211 — 2908	0.37 ± 0.09	0.26 — 0.50
	41 Normoglyceridemic			
	Males (17) and	30 — 152	0.38 ± 0.08	0.27 — 0.57
	Females (24)	32 — 193	0.37 ± 0.07	0.24 — 0.53
Kuo et al. (1965)	2 "FIHL"	2475 — 6800	0.10	0.09 — 0.11
	22 "mixed" HL	480 — 2840	0.42 ± 0.08	0.32 — 0.67
	30 normal controls	57 — 144	0.35 ± 0.06	0.28 — 0.41

FIHL = fat-induced hyperlipemia, CIHL = carbohydrate-induced hyperlipemia.
* Including one subject with FIHL whose postheparin lipolytic activity was 0.41 (mean of 5 tests).

Estimation of postheparin lipoprotein lipase in the plasma of these subjects using in vitro hydrolysis of triglyceride emulsions as a measurement has almost uniformly yielded very low values. This was first demonstrated by Havel and Gordon (1960) in three siblings of an affected family and in the meantime has been amply confirmed. Low activity of postheparin lipoprotein lipase was also found in nonhyperlipemic family members of affected patients (Fredrickson et al. 1963, Knittle and Ahrens 1964, Kuo et al. 1965). Data are given in Table 1.

Other factors which have been considered in the pathogenesis of hyperchylomicronemia are defective formation of chylomicrons in the small intestine during absorption of fat, and plasma or tissue inhibitors of lipoprotein lipase. No evidence has been presented to date to support the former mechanism. The "hyperlipemic" chylomicrons are presently indistinguishable from particulate fat which occurs in normal individuals after a fat meal with regard to composition (Ahrens et al. 1961) and are removed normally in control subjects (Havel and Gordon 1960). They are readily hydrolyzed by normal postheparin plasma (Ahrens et al. 1961, Furman and Robinson 1962). It remains to be determined whether their behavior differs from any of the characteristics of "normal" chylomicrons as summarized in Table 2. Most data from the literature were obtained in subjects other than pure "hyperchylomicronemics" and without controlled dietary conditions, where an array of various particles is usually present (Bierman et al. 1965). The presence of inhibitors of lipoprotein lipase has been suggested (Lever and Klein 1957, Engelberg 1962). Havel and Gordon (1960) were unable to demonstrate such inhibitors in their well studied patients.

There is some evidence that exogenous hyperglyceridemia includes more than one entity (Furman and Robinson 1962, Bialkin et al. 1962, Kinsell and Schlierf 1965). The latter have reported a remission in a boy with hyperchylomicronemia, which occurred about the time of onset of puberty, and after continuous daily administration of relatively large amounts of heparin for more than two years. Heparin was used in this patient because of the observation of rapid decrease in plasma glycerides during its administration, and despite the in vitro finding of low lipoprotein lipase activity. The case may be similar to the mother of the P family (HAVEL and GORDON 1960) who had normal plasma glycerides when examined then, but who had exhibited triglyceride values of 1600 mg per 100 ml

Table 2. *Properties of fat particles and very low density lipoproteins* (Modified from BIERMAN et al.: J. clin. Invest. *44*, 261 (1965))

| | Exogenous Particles (Chylomicrons) | | Endogenous particles "Hyperlipemic" Particles | VLDLP |
	"Primary"	"Secondary"		
Ultracentrifugation				
Sf.	>400	>400	$20-10^5$	20—400
Density	<1.006	<1.006	<1.006	<1.006
Electrophoresis				
Starch (Alb = 1)	.6 (α_2)	.23 (β)	.51 (α_2-β)	.57 (α_2)
Modified Paper Elect.	Origin	Origin	Pre-β with trail	Pre-β
PVP Flocculation	Top	Bottom	Diffuse spread from bottom	None or bottom
Lipid Composition (%) by weight				
TC	8	7	20	32
PL	6	3	10	18
TG	86	90	70	50
Protein	1	1	3	9

TC = total cholesterol.
PL = phospholipids.
TG = triglycerides.

when examined 7 years earlier by GASKINS et al. (1953). At any rate, it appears that a major abnormality in hyperchylomicronemia resides in the lipoprotein lipase system. Further studies will be necessary to establish the physiologic role of the enzyme(s) more firmly, particularly as regards its function in adipose tissue and liver.

Since it is frequently impossible to decide in retrospect whether a decrease in plasma lipids produced by dietary measures was caused by fat restriction rather than by the restriction in calories which is frequently associated with severely modified diets, a complete literature survey of FIHL has not been attempted. The majority of children with the syndrome of EHL probably belong to this category. Several well studied cases of exogenous hyperlipemia have been published during the last 6 years. Among those are the three siblings reported by GASKINS et al. in 1953 and later by HAVEL and GORDON (1960), three subjects studied by AHRENS et al. 1961 and by KNITTLE and AHRENS in 1964 (including the female patient initially reported by HOLT et al. 1939), three affected siblings described by FURMAN and ROBINSON (1962) and two individuals investigated by KUO et al. (1965), these being a 4 year old boy and a 17 year old negro girl. It has been estimated (FREDRICKSON 1965) that approximately 50 cases of FIHL have been or are being studied up to the present time.

b) Endogenous Hyperglyceridemias

[Carbohydrate-induced hyperlipemia (AHRENS et al. 1961), mixed hyperlipemia (KUO and BASSETT 1963), types III to V hyperlipoproteinemias (FREDRICKSON and LEES 1965), nonalimentary hyperlipemia (KINSELL and SCHLIERF 1965)].

When one departs from hyperchylomicronemia, the classification of EHL becomes much less simple. Since pure hyperchylomicronemia is a quite rare entity and since EHL is by no means rare, it is obvious that appropriate measuring sticks are necessary. Despite points of difference, it appears possible to concentrate upon certain features which most endogenous hyperlipemics have in common and come up with some clarification of the subject.

The term "endogenous" hyperglyceridemia as used here is not meant to imply that alimentary fat cannot contribute to the hypertriglyceridemia in such cases under appropriate conditions. However, it seems likely that a basic defect in all the syndromes to be discussed is associated with some type of abnormality of metabolism of endogenous very low density lipoprotein with regard either to formation (FARQUHAR et al. 1963) and/or clearing of these particles. Other mechanisms, secondary to this defect, seem to come into play particularly with more severe forms of the syndrome.

There is general agreement that the majority (perhaps all, when methods are sufficiently refined) of the nonhyperchylomicronemic, essential hyperlipemic patients have gross or occult *abnormality of carbohydrate metabolism*. Thus the association of overt carbohydrate intolerance and hyperlipemia has been noted for quite some time. Particularly during the last 16 years numerous reports have appeared in the literature describing essential hyperlipemia and accompanying glycosuria (THANNHAUSER 1950) or "mild diabetes" (ADLERSBERG and WANG 1955). These patients characteristically did not need insulin, and ketoacidosis — evidence of absolute lack of insulin — did not occur. The hyperlipemia therefore was considered to be of the essential type and not "secondary to diabetes mellitus."

Sporadic reports of abnormal glucose tolerance in EHL were given by MOVITT et al. (1951), CHRISTENSEN et al. (1958), CARLSON and OLHAGEN (1959), and HAVEL and GORDON (1960). WADDELL et al. (1958) were the first to examine systematically a group of hyperlipidemic subjects for signs of occult carbohydrate intolerance and observed a high incidence of abnormal glucose tolerance tests. Recent studies of carbohydrate metabolism in hyperlipemic subjects with syndromes other than pure hyperchylomicronemia have almost invariably resulted in the demonstration of abnormal carbohydrate tolerance (lit. see SCHLIERF and KINSELL 1965). Frequently this abnormality was evident with the oral glucose tolerance test (DAVIDSON and ALBRINK 1963, KANE et al. 1965). In other cases abnormal responses to the cortisone glucose tolerance test (KINSELL and SCHLIERF 1965) or an altered disappearance rate of intravenously injected glucose loads (BIERMAN et al. 1965) was demonstrated. Although AHRENS et al. (1961) originally found no evidence of "diabetes or hyperinsulinism" in carbohydrate-induced hyperlipemia, they have subsequently altered their position (KNITTLE and AHRENS 1964) when an abnormal response of blood sugar level and plasma insulin-like activity to tolbutamide was almost uniformly observed. An 80% incidence of carbohydrate intolerance of varying degrees has been reported in 100 subjects with EHL by JAHNKE (1965). A high frequency of "diabetes" in families with EHL as reported by CHRISTENSEN et al. (1958) is in accord with our own observations.

In spite of evidence suggesting some basic common denominator in most endogenous hyperglyceridemics, it seems reasonable at the present time to divide subjects with these syndromes into three major groups so as to not obscure existing differences and to stimulate further analysis and evaluation.

1. "Pure" Carbohydrate-induced Hyperglyceridemia

Following reports of triglyceride elevation in normal subjects on high carbohydrate diets, AHRENS et al. (1961) proposed that essential hyperlipemia may be divided into "fat-induced" and "carbohydrate-induced" forms, when they had noted that the majority of their hyperglyceridemic patients had higher plasma triglyceride values if carbohydrate was isocalorically substituted for fat in a formula diet. They suggested that this phenomenon represented an exaggerated form of the normal biochemical process which occurs in all people on high carbohydrate diets and felt that the latter category represented the great majority of essential hyperlipemics.

On the basis of our own experience and to some degree that of others, it seems probable that "pure" carbohydrate-induced hyperglyceridemia is a relatively rare entity, although by no means as rare as "pure" fat-induced hyperlipemia (hyperchylomicronemia). The condition corresponds to type IV hyperlipoproteinemia described by FREDRICKSON and LEES (1965). To qualify for membership in this group, it is necessary that the individual have major and maintained elevation of plasma glycerides on a high carbohydrate, low fat (or fat-free) diet and that the plasma glycerides reach normal or nearly normal levels when a large portion of the carbohydrate is replaced by fat, regardless of the type of fat. From studies in a limited number of normal subjects, LEES and FREDRICKSON (1965) have proposed tentatively that the elevation of glycerides induced by carbohydrate must exceed 400 to 500 mg per 100 ml in order to be considered pathologic. Fig. 3 demonstrates such a case.

Data have now become available with regard to physical and chemical characteristics of the lipemic particles of carbohydrate-induced hyperlipemia (AHRENS et al. 1961, BIERMAN et al. 1965). The particulate fat which, on a

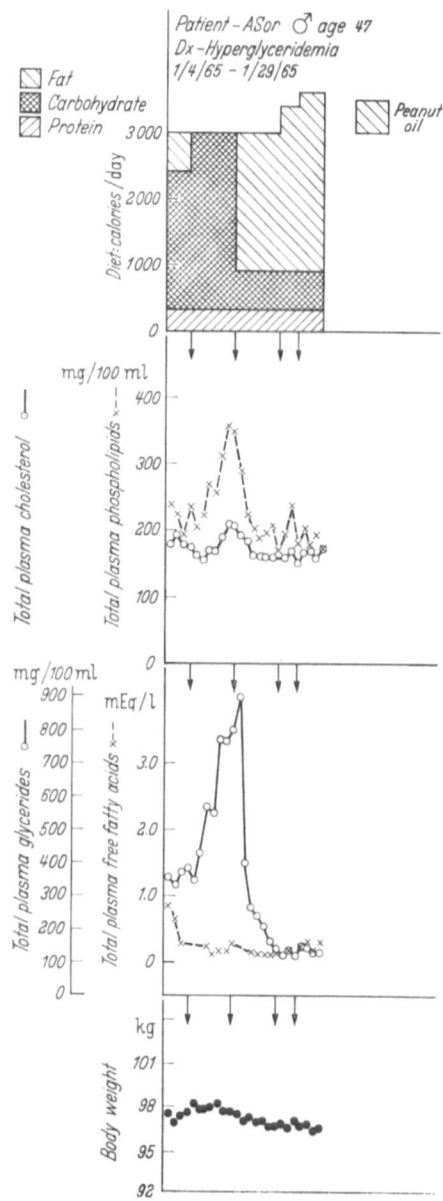

Fig. 3. "Pure" carbohydrate-induced hyperglyceridemia (endogenous hyperglyceridemia group 1). Significant hyperglyceridemia was observed in this 47 year old male subject on a high carbohydrate, fat-free diet. Substitution of most of the carbohydrate by fat resulted in progressive fall in plasma glycerides to normal

fat-free diet, is obviously of endogenous origin, differs from alimentary particles in lipid composition (higher cholesterol/triglyceride ratio) and triglyceride fatty acid pattern (predominately palmitic, palmitoleic and oleic acids) as well as in protein content and physical characteristics. With the paper electrophoretic technic of LEES and HATCH (1963), carbohydrate-induced hyperlipemics appear to be characterized by the appearance of excessive amounts of material which is present in the pre-β position and which is probably hepatic in origin. A synoptic view of some of the properties of "carbohydrate-induced" particles is presented in Table 2.

Recently, Kuo and BASSETT (1965) have compared the effect of starch with that of sucrose in five patients with "carbohydrate-induced" hyperlipemia and observed significantly higher plasma triglyceride levels on the latter diet (see also page 451).

2. Endogenous, Carbohydrate and Fat Inducible Hyperglyceridemia

This grouping is possibly not homogenous and may subsequently be subdivided. It includes subjects who have been described as having "mixed" hyperlipemia by Kuo and BASSET (1963), "calorie" induced hyperlipemia by KINSELL and SCHLIERF (1965) and probably type V of FREDRICKSON's and LEES' classification (1965). Whatever the homogeneity, it appears that these individuals accumulate very low density lipoproteins in plasma under essentially all dietary conditions except absolutely or relatively low calorie intake, and in some except during the administration of insulin.

That a number of subjects with "carbohydrate-induced" hyperlipemia will exhibit significant hyperglyceridemia even on low carbohydrate, high fat diets, is already evident from Fig. 6 given by AHRENS et al. in 1961 and from Table 1 of KNITTLE and AHRENS (1964). Other authors therefore have used the term "carbohydrate-accentuated" rather than "induced" to describe such patients.

It is particularly in this group that a relationship between the tendency to hyperglyceridemia and the level of calorie intake appears to be a significantly constant finding. These subjects exhibit hyperglyceridemia on both high carbohydrate and high fat diets with appropriate calorie intake. However, the absolute calorie level in relation to energy output which is associated with hyperglyceridemia varies appreciably from one individual to another, and may depend on the severity of the metabolic defect. In some, the calorie intake must be sufficient to result in significant weight gain. In others, reduction of hyperglyceridemia will occur only under conditions of significant weight loss. Fig. 4 shows the result of a controlled study in a subject who falls in this category.

The role of calorie intake in hyperlipemia has been repeatedly emphasized (ALBRINK 1962, CROFFORD 1962, Kuo and BASSET 1963, Kuo et al. 1965) and seems to apply particularly to this group, whereas in pure fat-induced hyperlipemia the absolute level of fat, and in the pure carbohydrate-induced form the absolute level of carbohydrate (LEES and FREDRICKSON 1965), appear to be the determining factors. A meaningful relationship to "carbohydrate-induced" hyperlipemia is suggested by the finding that in some subjects hyperglyceridemia may be induced by high carbohydrate intake at a lower calorie level than is required to induce hyperlipemia by fat.

Several mechanisms appear to be operating in this group of subjects. On the one hand, chylomicrons may accumulate with high fat diets. Evidence has been presented that in man the removal capacity for lipoprotein triglycerides can be rate limiting (FARQUHAR et al. 1964, 1965), and clearing mechanisms are easily saturated (DOLE and HAMLIN 1962). The rate of removal of chylomicrons was found to be inversely related to the fasting triglyceride level (NESTEL 1964). It is therefore reasonable to assume that hypercaloric intake with its increased demand for triglyceride transport and storage in many subjects may exceed the removal capacity of tissues for plasma triglycerides and that an expanded endogenous triglyceride pool may lead to deficient clearing of endogenous as well as exogenous triglycerides under appropriate conditions. That different kinds of fat in these patients may be handled differently is suggested by observations of FURMAN et al. (1961), HAMWI et al. (1962), and KINSELL et al. (1962) who in some subjects observed better control of hyperglyceridemia with unsaturated fats as compared to saturated fat intake. Lipemia after fat loading was less marked with unsaturated fat in such a subject (KINSELL et al. 1962).

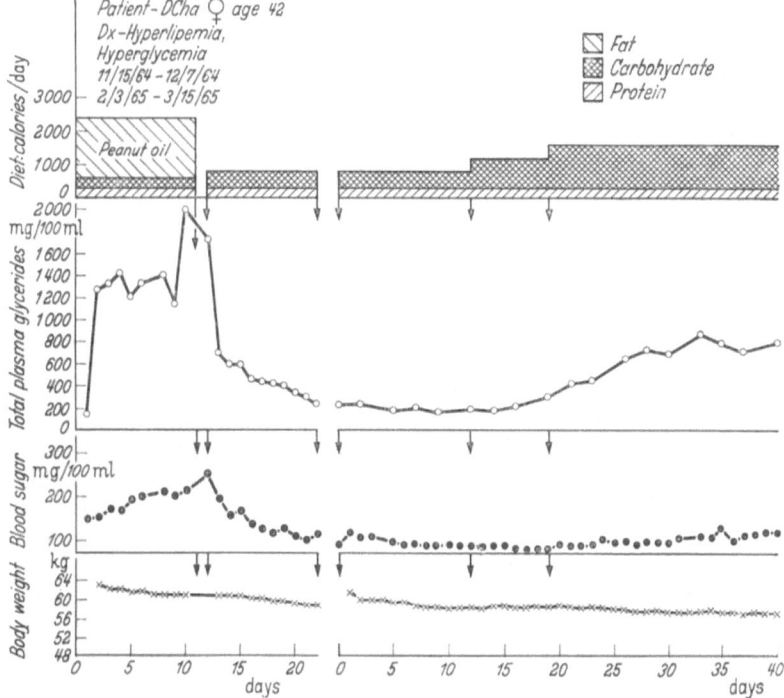

Fig. 4. Carbohydrate- and fat-inducible hyperglyceridemia (endogenous hyperglyceridemia group 2). Major "fat-induced" hyperglyceridemia and hyperglycemia developed in this 42 year old female patient on a high fat high calorie diet. Low calorie intake was associated with rapid fall in plasma glycerides and blood sugar towards normal. Stepwise increase in carbohydrate calories resulted in progressive "carbohydrate-induced" hyperglyceridemia

On the other hand, very low density lipoprotein (VLDLP, pre-β-lipoprotein) is present in increased amounts with both fat and carbohydrate induction. The very low density lipoprotein triglyceride fatty acids (fatty acids of pre-β triglycerides) in these subjects on fat free diets correspond to the pattern as described by AHRENS and his coworkers for carbohydrate-induced hyperlipemia. If however hyperglyceridemia is induced by high fat intake, the fatty acid composition of the pre-β glycerides bears a close resemblance to the ingested fat. Whether under these conditions the very low density lipoproteins are formed in the liver directly from chylomicrons, or from fatty acids which have resulted from intravascular hydrolysis of the circulating chylomicronous triglycerides is unknown at the present time. Likewise the role of lipoprotein interconversion, as discussed in detail by FREDRICKSON and GORDON (1958) and NICHOLS and SMITH (1965) remains to be evaluated, particularly since the simultaneous presence in plasma of increased amounts of particles with different origins and a decreased fractional turnover rate of these particles may favor such processes. As regards the contribution to VLDLP of free fatty acids (FFA), we have found that the plasma FFA composition in hyperlipemia can be profoundly and persistently altered on a short term basis by the kind of dietary fat, implying that a major source of FFA under these conditions is ingested fat, and endogenous triglyceride manufactured from such FFA would reflect dietary fat. The significance and quantitative contribution of FFA to elevated VLDLP in endogenous hyperglyceridemia is therefore another important matter which remains to be clarified. KINSELL et al. (1962) reported persistent marked elevation of FFA levels in one of their essential hyperlipemics. Repeated measurements with different methods gave values of the order of 2.5 mEq/l.

In reviewing the literature, it seems probable that the majority of cases of essential hyperlipemia which have been reported fall into this category. It should again be emphasized that this group probably is not homogeneous and may eventually be separated into several subsyndromes.

3. Endogenous Hyperglyceridemia with Essential Hypercholesterolemia

FREDRICKSON and LEES (1965) have described as their type III hyperlipoproteinemia, individuals who, in addition to clinical and laboratory evidence of essential hypercholesterolemia, show elevation of VLDLP (pre-β-lipoproteins) and are markedly susceptible to carbohydrate induction. In common with other endogenous hyperlipidemics, they manifest carbohydrate intolerance.

It is likely that cases who have been described in the past as essential hyperlipemia on the basis of lipemic plasma and who exhibited tendon xanthomas belong in this group. Cases of essential hypercholesterolemia with and without plasma turbidity, whose plasma triglycerides exceed the levels expected from increased β-lipoproteins, would qualify for membership. Such cases can be found in reports by LEVER et al. (1954), ADLERSBERG (1955), FURMAN et al. (1961), KUO and BASSET (1963) and others.

Recent findings from FREDRICKSON's laboratory (FREDRICKSON and LEES 1966) suggest that this group, too, is not homogenous. Its more common prototype is distinguished by the presence of large quantities of a β-lipoprotein which floats at density 1.006 and which may represent an abnormal lipoprotein with increased affinity for both cholesterol and triglycerides.

Role of Insulin

The usual occurrence of gross or occult *carbohydrate intolerance in endogenous hyperlipemia* has stimulated a discussion of possible *abnormalities in insulin secretion and/or action*. Such abnormalities were suggested by KNITTLE and AHRENS (1964) and SANBAR et al. (1964) when ILA was measured during tolbutamide administration and glucose tolerance tests, respectively. Data obtained with the insulin immunoassay, although scarce and inconclusive, seem to show that there is no deficiency in immuno-reactive insulin in EHL (SANBAR 1964, KANE et al. 1965, REAVEN et al. 1965) and suggest the presence of insulin antagonism or inhibition, or possibly of a modified insulin. Mechanisms by which a deficiency of insulin action could result in increased triglyceride synthesis and/or impairment of removal of endogenous and exogenous lipoprotein triglyceride have been discussed by KNITTLE and AHRENS (1964), FREDRICKSON and LEES (1965) and SCHLIERF and KINSELL (1965).

In support of a causative or accentuating role of abnormal insulin action in EHL are findings of SCHLIERF and KINSELL (1965) who have shown that intravenous infusion of small amounts of insulin will result in decreased levels of plasma glycerides as compared to the same subject during control infusion with saline solution. Coadministration of protamine, an inhibitor of heparin-induced lipoprotein lipase (BRAGDON and HAVEL 1954) with the insulin inhibits this effect, suggesting that at least a portion of the insulin effect is on the basis of stimulation of glyceride removal from the plasma. Contrary to previous views (THANNHAUSER 1950) it was also found (CHRISTENSEN et al. 1958, HAMWI et al. 1962, KINSELL and SCHLIERF 1965) that therapeutic administration of insulin to some patients with hyperglyceridemia and glycosuria results in major improvement and occasionally normalization of hypertriglyceridemia. It is frequently necessary to administer rather large amounts of insulin since resistance, particularly with very high triglyceride levels, may be marked. Inhibition of carbohydrate induction of hyperlipemia with administration of sulfonylurea has been reported by REAVEN et al. (1964); so far we have been unable to confirm this observation in pure carbohydrate-induced hyperlipemia. However, hyperglyceridemia has been controlled for several months with sulfonylurea in one subject with the category 2 syndrome. It is possible that in some patients the relative proportion of insulin reaching liver and extrahepatic tissues plays a role in control of triglyceride metabolism.

At this point it must be emphasized that the hypothesis of abnormal insulin activity as a basis for the pathogenesis of endogenous hyperlipemia, although attractive, is as yet far from established. Conceivably, both carbohydrate intolerance and hyperglyceridemia could be the result of such mechanisms as those proposed by HALES and RANDLE (1963) for the pathogenesis of diabetes mellitus. A primary elevation of free fatty acids might result in both elevated triglyceride levels and impaired uptake and oxidation of glucose by the cells, manifested as abnormal carbohydrate intolerance. FELBER and VANNOTTI (1964) could demonstrate glucose intolerance in humans when FFA levels were raised with infusion of a lipid emulsion. It is furthermore possible that the effects of insulin on hyperglyceridemia as described may represent a pharmacologic rather than a physiologic effect, although this appears unlikely in view of the small amounts of intravenously infused insulin which are effective.

Although some elevation of plasma triglycerides is frequently observed in diabetes mellitus, particularly in middle aged subjects with the disease (NEW et al. 1963), and hyperglyceridemia can be easily induced with high carbohydrate intake (BIERMAN and HAMLIN 1961), the average maturity onset diabetic behaves differently when studied under identical conditions with an endogenous hyperglyceridemic person (KINSELL and SCHLIERF 1965). Further studies of carbohydrate metabolism in hyperlipemia on one hand, and handling of lipids by the diabetic on the other hand may ultimately clarify the relationship of diabetes mellitus and essential endogenous hyperlipemias.

Clinical Manifestations

In spite of differences in pathogenesis of the various forms of EHL it is possible to consider their clinical manifestations together since the majority of signs and symptoms seem to vary only in a quantitative manner between syndromes. This, as well as the frequency of asymptomatic cases of EHL, indicates that at least the manifestations of lipemia retinalis, xanthomatosis and probably hepatosplenomegaly and abdominal crises are the results of the lipid elevation rather than primary expressions of the underlying pathogenetic mechanisms. Other evidence for the non-specificity of eruptive xanthomas and lipemia retinalis is their occurrence in secondary hyperlipemias (e.g. diabetic ketoacidosis).

Xanthomatosis

was first described by ADDISON and GULL (1850) and a detailed description of various forms has been given by THANNHAUSER and MAGENDANTZ (1938).

An excellent review of the subject is that of Crocker (1951). Xanthomatosis is the most common and in many instances the first readily recognizable sign of severe EHL. Thannhauser (1957) has emphasized the early and quite consistent appearance of xanthomas in children with hyperlipemia, whereas in adults they occur in only about 50% of cases. The same figure was given by Borrie (1957) and a similar incidence one year later by Gadrat (xanthomas in 25 out of 49 patients with EHL). A correlation between the prevailing lipoprotein pattern and the different forms of xanthomas has been attempted by Gofman et al. (1954)

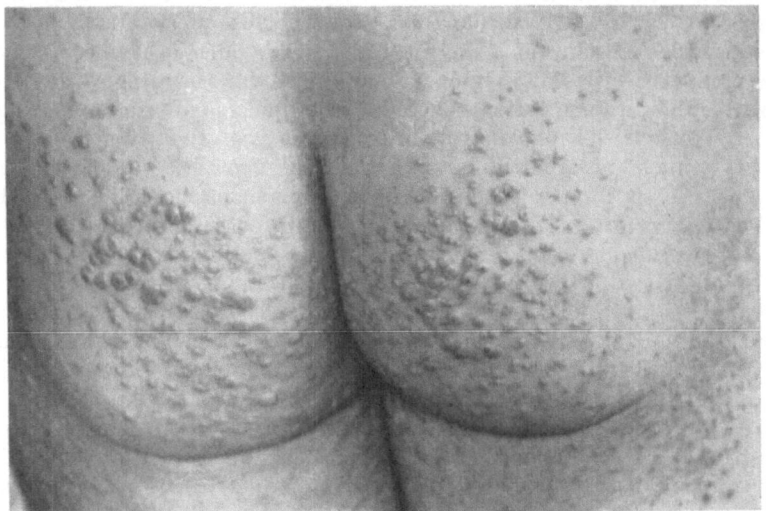

Fig. 5. Eruptive xanthomas in essential hyperlipemia

and was illustrated by Fredrickson (1960). Tuberous xanthomas are thus observed with predominant elevation of Sf 20—100, while eruptive xanthomas occur with the main lipoprotein elevation being in the Sf 100—400 class. Tendon xanthomas, characteristic for EFH, correlate best with elevated Sf 0—12 lipoproteins.

Data about lipid composition of skin xanthomas have been summarized by Schettler (1955, Handbuch, pg. 696); a recent study on xanthoma tuberosum was published by Fletcher and Gloster (1964). In spite of a significant elevation of plasma triglycerides in some of their cases, cholesterol was the prevailing lipid of the lesions.

Eruptive xanthomas (Fig. 5) are characteristic for hyperglyceridemia and do not occur in essential familial hypercholesterolemia. They consist of orange to light-yellow nodules occurring singly or in crops, varying in size and form, and particularly the recent ones are frequently surrounded by a bright red inflammatory halo. Cordlike infiltrations between xanthomas were observed in a case by Thannhauser (1957). Occasionally vesicular lesions were described which ruptured with discharge of a milky fluid. Disappearing eruptive xanthomas not infrequently leave areas of hyperpigmentation (Bürger and Grütz 1932, Holt and coworkers 1939, Bernstein and coworkers 1939, Thannhauser 1950). Commonly affected areas are the buttocks, the posterior aspects of the thighs, back, neck, and the extensor surface of extremities. On occasion xanthomas have been found diffusely distributed over the whole body. Instances where cheeks and ears were affected (Schettler 1955) and of xanthomas on lips and oral mucosa (Bürger and Grütz 1932, Thannhauser and Magendantz 1938, Schirren 1957) have been reported.

Tuberous xanthomas (Fig. 6 a and b) have been described in EHL with a predilection for elbows, knees, hands and feet. They may occasionally assume bizzare proportions. In other instances differentiation from eruptive xanthomas may be difficult, and has frequently been neglected. Thus ADLERSBERG (1955) only used the term tuberous xanthomas which he found in 14% of his patients with EHL and

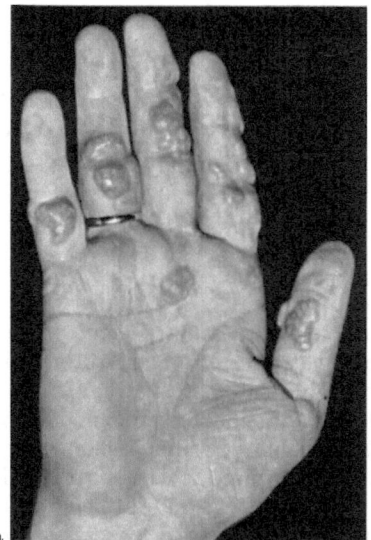 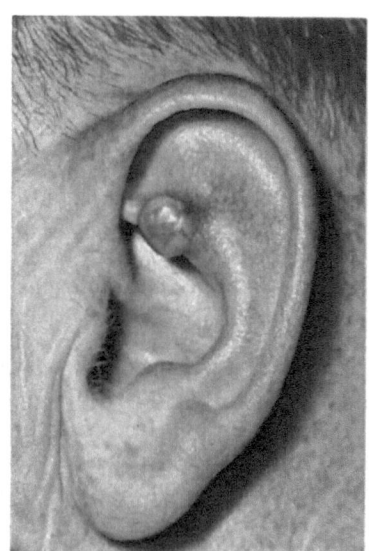

Fig. 6 a and b. Tuberous xanthomas in essential hyperlipemia

their family members as compared to 2% in EFH. LEVER (1954) similarly found tuberous xanthomas more frequently in EHL than in EFH, while eruptive xanthomas were not observed at all in the latter disease. It is likely that a number of cases of EFH exhibiting tuberous xanthomas represent "mixed forms" of essential hypercholesterolemia and hyperlipemia (endogenous hyperglyceridemia group 3, FREDRICKSON and LEES' type III).

Tendon xanthomas are rarely if ever observed in pure EHL: when they were described (LEVER et al. 1954, ADLERSBERG 1955, FREDRICKSON 1960), features of EFH were usually present suggesting again the presence of a group 3 syndrome.

Xanthomata plana (xanthelasmas) are not considered characteristic of hyperlipemia; their occurrence however has been described by MALMROS and coworkers (1954), ADLERSBERG (1955), SCHETTLER (1955), MATRAS (1956), SCHIRREN (1957) and HAENSCH (1958). The presence of xanthelasmas in EHL seem either to indicate that one is dealing with a combination with essential hypercholesterolemia or that they are unrelated to the disease since they do occur in a significant percentage of normolipemic subjects.

Little is known about the factors responsible for the development of xanthomas in an individual case of xanthomatosis. A rough correlation between the total serum lipids and individual lipid fractions on the one hand, and the fluctuations of eruptive xanthomas on the other, exists without doubt, and a critical value for their development with 2.5 to 3 gm triglycerides per 100 ml plasma can be derived statistically. Such data are of no value for the individual case. Thus FREDRICKSON (1960) reported the rapid appearance of xanthomas with a serum triglyceride level of 2000 mg per 100 ml in one case, whereas another patient did not exhibit any xanthomas with average triglyceride levels of 4000 mg per 100 ml over a period of 6 years. Similarly the patient described by HARSLÖF (1948) did not have any skin changes with a plasma lipid level of over 7 gm per 100 ml.

Hepatosplenomegaly

This sign was present in the first case of BÜRGER and GRÜTZ (1932) as evidenced by their definition of the disease. The liver was enlarged four finger breadths, the spleen three finger breadths below the costal margin. Hepatosplenomegaly of different degree was present in all the juvenile patients who were subsequently described by OPITZ (1935), FRANKLIN (1937), HOLT and coworkers (1939), BERNSTEIN and coworkers (1939), and in the case of GOODMAN and coworkers (1940). An 8 year-old boy in whom the spleen reached the umbilicus was reported by LEVY (1946). On the other hand, liver, gallbladder, pancreas and appendix were found to be normal at laparotomy in the case of BLOOMFIELD and SHENSON (1947) although the surgery was performed because of severe right upper quadrant pain. BORRIE (1957) gives an incidence of hepatosplenomegaly of 50%. Likewise in 49 cases collected by GADRAT (1958) hepatosplenomegaly was observed in 23, and occurred equally frequently in children and adults. Enlargement of the liver alone was observed in eight patients, splenomegaly without enlarged liver in four. Splenic enlargement appears to be more frequent and more marked in children with EFH. According to FREDRICKSON (1960) enlargement of one or both organs is observed in two thirds of patients who are diagnosed before their 6th year of life, and in one third in the rest of the cases. In reviewing 122 cases from the literature up to 1965, we found hepatomegaly reported in 54 and splenomegaly in 34 cases. That these figures are lower than the ones reported previously may be caused in part by greater emphasis on laboratory findings as compared to clinical symptoms in most of the recent studies.

The organomegaly appears to be caused by the accumulation of fat. A relationship between hepatomegaly and degree of hyperlipemia was discussed by HOLT et al. (1939) and is clearly demonstrated in the child described by RAUSEN and ADLERSBERG (1961). The regression of the organ enlargement with diets low in fat (ABEGG 1937, CHAPMAN and KINNEY 1941, LEVY 1946, KOSZALKA and LEVIN 1950) supports this thesis. THANNHAUSER (1958), referring to the child reported by CHAPMAN and KINNEY, where an increased fat content of the liver could not be demonstrated at autopsy, does not agree with this interpretation, at least with regard to the liver (THANNHAUSER and REINSTEIN 1942). The case in question might however have been a special one, since this child had died during the course of an infection and at the time of death was accordingly undernourished.

Abdominal Crises

Episodes of abdominal pain occur in approximately 30% of all cases with severe EHL, with great variability as regards intensity, frequency, duration and localization. Detailed description of such crises habe been given by HOLT et al. (1939) and BLOOMFIELD and SHENSON (1947). Often the pain is localized in the epigastrium or mid-abdomen; many patients complain of radiation to the back. Occasionally the attacks last several days (GADRAT 1958) and simulate in some cases surgical emergencies with nausea, vomiting, tachycardia and a shocklike picture. The bowel motility is usually unaffected and stools are normal. A case of urinary retention during such a crisis was described by HOLLISTER and KANTER (1955). Diffuse guarding throughout the abdomen is common, and fever up to 102° F and leucocytosis of 15,000 to 30,000 with polynuclear neutrophils prevailing were observed (BLOOMFIELD and SHENSON 1947, GADRAT 1958).

Several patients underwent laparotomy during the course of such crises and the findings at surgery have been described (HOLT and coworkers 1939, BLOOM-FIELD and SHENSON 1947, POULSEN 1950, HOLLISTER and KANTER 1955, GARU-NAS 1957, VAN ITTERBEEK and DELOBEL 1964). Aside from hepatosplenomegaly which had been noted before surgery, the organs, including the pancreas, were usually grossly normal. In a few cases small amounts of a sterile yellowish fluid were found in the abdominal cavity together with other signs of pancreatitis. AHRENS (1954) described a case where the findings at surgery were suggestive of temporary occlusion of the thoracic duct and where chylous infiltration of the retroperitoneal space and exudation into the abdominal cavity were thought possibly to have caused the abdominal symptoms. From a limited number of observations it appears that abdominal crises are more frequent in pure fat-induced hyperlipemia than in other forms of EHL (KNITTLE and AHRENS 1964) which corresponds with a higher incidence of such crises in younger individuals.

Several reasons for the occurrence of this symptom have been discussed. A rapid increase in size of liver and spleen precipitated by fatty meals or otherwise may be one possible cause of the abdominal colics resulting in stretching of the capsule of these organs. In HOLT's case, 8 gm per 100 ml appeared to be a critical level for serum lipids; with values above this level abdominal crises occurred frequently. An alternative explanation for these acute episodes would be the occurrence of recurrent pancreatitis as has been discussed repeatedly in the literature. This aspect will be considered below. A third possible cause in some cases may be impaired oxygen supply to the intestines as has been postulated by KUO et al. (1959) and others for the myocardium, resulting in a kind of "intermittent claudication" of the bowel.

Pancreatitis

There has been considerable dispute in the literature with regard to frequency of pancreatitis in EHL as well as with regard to the cause and effect relationship. A thorough review of the subject is that of KLATSKIN and GORDON (1952). The diagnosis of pancreatitis has been established in several well documented cases of EHL by the finding of elevated serum or urine amylase levels and was confirmed at surgery (POULSEN 1950, KLATSKIN and GORDON 1952). It has been proposed by the latter authors that emboli from agglutination of fat particles may be responsible for the development of this complication. Although experimental proof for this theory has not yet been supplied, the fact that in the case of the latter authors xanthomata preceded the abdominal crises, and that in both studies a positive family history for hyperlipemia was established, supports strongly the assumption of pancreatitis being secondary to hyperlipemia rather than its cause. Since skin lesions preceded pancreatitis also in the case of WIJNHAUSEN (1921) and COLLET and KENNEDY (1948), we follow KLATSKIN and GORDON in assuming that those authors apparently were dealing with EHL.

However, when transient lipemia occurs during the course of acute pancreatitis, as documented by BRUNNER (1935) and MARCUS (1937), and abdominal episodes far precede hyperlipemia (JOEL 1924), it appears proper to consider such hyperlipemia secondary to pancreatitis (THANNHAUSER 1950). This concept is supported by the animal experiments of BINET and BROCQ (1929) and others. For further discussion of experimental aspects of the subject we refer to SCHETTLER (1955, Handbuch pg. 724—725).

At present it appears best to evaluate both possibilities at the bedside of each case of hyperlipemia with abdominal symptoms, and support the diagnosis of either EHL or pancreatitis as the primary disease with data from personal history, family history and by observation of the course of hyperglyceridemia.

Lipemia Retinalis

This phenomenon was first observed in a case of diabetic acidosis by HEYL (1880) and quite certainly only reflects the degree of plasma turbidity resulting from increase in VLDLP and/or chylomicrons. The fundus in lipemia retinalis is characteristic and can only be imitated to some degree by leukemias. The retinal vessels appear flattened and show increased light reflexes; arteries and veins are difficult to distinguish on a salmon colored background. Vision is usually not impaired, and the case of DE ROSA (1952) with blindness of the left eye was due to other changes (atrophy of the left optic nerve with massive lipid deposits lateral to the optic disc.)

The finding of lipemia retinalis was mentioned in the first description of EHL by BÜRGER and GRÜTZ (1932) and appeared quite consistently in early reports of the syndrome (OPITZ 1935, HOLT and coworkers 1939, GOODMAN and coworkers 1940, LEVY 1946, BLOOMFIELD and SHENSON 1947, GROSSMANN and HITZ 1948, ROHN and coworkers 1948, THANNHAUSER 1950, BRUTON and KANTER 1951, HOFFMAN and GRAYSON 1952). In 122 cases of EHL where clinical descriptions were available to us, lipemia retinalis was documented in 18 cases.

According to LEPARD (1944), visible signs of lipemia retinalis appear with total serum lipids above 3.5 g per 100 ml and disappear if plasma lipid levels fall below 2.5 g per 100 ml. This is in agreement with the value given by HOLT et al. (1939) with 3 g per 100 ml and by DUNPHY (1950) who measured total serum fatty acids; the figures given by him for disappearance and recurrence of visible fundus changes were 2 gm and 2.5 gm per 100 ml respectively. Rapid disappearance of lipemia retinalis was observed by GROSSMAN and HITZ (1948) and many others, with a low fat diet.

Histopathology of Essential Hyperlipemia

The histologic picture of eruptive xanthomas according to THANNHAUSER (1957) is primarily not that of a typical fat-accumulating lesion. Spindle-shaped cells are embedded in a collagenous ground substance and foam cells are rarely found. Particularly at the border of the lesion extracellular lipid is deposited perivascularly, and inflammatory changes are seen. This description is in accord with the skin changes in hyperlipemia as reported earlier by GRÜTZ (1926) who emphasized the rarity of foam cells and absence of Touton giant cells in these lesions. Such observations are of value in the microscopic differential diagnosis of eruptive xanthomas and xanthomas of EFH (THANNHAUSER 1957); in the latter aggregations of foam cells prevail and are surrounded by granulomatous tissue containing giant cells. The significance of "sudanophilic granules" (GRÜTZ) surrounding the vessels of the upper and middle layers of the cutis for the development of stenosing lesions of bigger arteries is not known (SCHETTLER 1955).

When one departs from xanthomatosis, typical histologic abnormalities in EHL are scarce and inconsistently present. The finding of hepatosplenomegaly has frequently resulted in microscopic examination of these organs.

No abnormalities were observed in several autopsy specimens of the liver (CHAPMAN and KINNEY 1941, MARTT and CONNOR 1955, BOGGS et al. 1957) and in a biopsy specimen of JOYNER's case (1953) taken after regression of a distinctly enlarged liver. This is in contrast to the finding of lipid deposition in the RES cells of the liver by KOSZALKA and LEVIN (1950) and by BRUTON and KANTER (1951) with reversible parenchymal involvement in the latters' case. Intracellular and extracellular lipid infiltration of this organ was found by CAMELIN et al. (1955) and by MOVITT et al. (1951). Their 42 year old patient however suffered from progressive obesity in addition to hyperlipemia. GASKINS et al. (1953) described the occurrence in the liver of "coarsely granular cord cells, with a number of fat vacuoles and scattered multinuclear giant cells." The finding of simple fatty livers has been described by SCHETTLER et al. (1958) and recently in three cases of EHL by JUCHEMS et al. (1965).

Needle biopsies of the spleen were done only in a few cases. While FRANKLIN (1937) reported normal findings, CHAPMAN and KINNEY (1941) and SHORE and SCHRIRE (1947) were able to find foam cells in their specimens.

Numerous results of bone marrow biopsies have been published: a normal microscopic structure was reported by MOVITT et al (1951), GADRAT et al. (1952), HOLLISTER and KANTER (1955), and CETNAROWICZ et al. (1953), whereas HOLT et al. (1939), FRANKLIN (1937), CHAPMAN and KINNEY (1941), SHORE and SCHRIRE (1947), GROSSMANN and HITZ (1948), KOSZALKA and LEVIN (1950), POULSEN (1950), BRUTON and KANTER (1951), GASKINS et al. (1953), HAKIMI (1954), and GARUNAS (1957), described foam cells in their specimens, the percentage of which in HOLT's case was 1.6. A resemblance of these cells with Gaucher cells was pointed out by LOWGREN (1952). The negative Smith-Dietrich reaction of their lipid droplets serves to differentiate them from Nieman-Pick cells (FREDRICKSON 1960).

Scattered foam cells in lymph nodes were found in a case by CHAPMAN and KINNEY (1941).

Intracellular lipid droplets, mainly in cells of the RES, do occur in diabetics (SCHULTZE 1912, WARREN and ROOT 1926) and would not appear to be an expression of increased synthesis in vivo but rather the result of phagocytosis by histiocytes caused by the high serum lipid levels.

Laboratory Findings

The presence of plasma turbidity indicates marked increase of *plasma glycerides*. Cases with triglyceride values of 100 times normal and above have been reported and a serum glyceride content of 3 to 5% (similar to the fat content of milk) is not uncommon. It is reasonable to assume that for each case with marked elevation of plasma glycerides several individuals with mild forms of hyperglyceridemia will be found once this lipid fraction is determined routinely in a sufficiently large number of subjects and particularly among family members of grossly hyperlipemic persons. The upper limits for a "normal" fasting triglyceride level varies to some degree with different methods; values above 150—160 mg per 100 ml plasma are considered abnormal by most laboratories. The average fasting triglyceride level for a group of 46 normal young subjects (medical residents and dietetic interns) was 95 ± 22 (range 58—134) mg per 100 ml in our laboratory. The mean value derived from three triglyceride determinations on different occasions in each of 261 clinically healthy males aged 45 to 54 was 103 ± 48 (range 30 to 472) mg per 100 ml. Since this latter sample of the population includes several individuals with obvious hyperglyceridemia, it seems reasonable to exclude glyceride values exceeding this mean + 2SD (103 + 96 = 199 mg per 100 ml) from a calculation of the "normal" mean glyceride level. By so doing the corrected average fasting plasma glyceride level for 244 healthy middle aged men is 95 ± 33 mg per 100 ml plasma. This corrected mean + 2SD (= 161 mg%) agrees closely with the upper limits of normal given by ALBRINK and MAN (1959) with 5.4 mEq/l of triglyceride fatty acids (= 160 mg%).

Plasma total cholesterol is usually increased; the degree of elevation of this lipid fraction depends on both the kind and degree of hyperglyceridemia. Only mildly elevated levels (2—3 times normal) are frequently found in hyperchylomicronemia as would be expected from the lipid composition of chylomicrons. Subnormal levels may occur during treatment. Levels of more than 1000 mg per 100 ml plasma are not rare in other forms, and can again be roughly estimated from the lipid composition of the prevailing lipoprotein fraction. Usually free and ester cholesterol are proportionately elevated, but occasionally, in cases with marked hyperglyceridemia, the per cent contribution of ester cholesterol is diminished (BÜRGER and GRÜTZ 1932, HOPGOOD 1948). This phenomenon is probably not attributable to a disturbance in liver function, but rather to preponderance of very low density lipoproteins which contain much free cholesterol (BRAGDON et al. 1956). FURMAN, HOWARD, LAKSHMI and NORCIA (1961) found as much as 90% of the total serum cholesterol and phospholipid in fractions of density less than 1006 in some hyperglyceridemics. The data of ALBRINK (1961) are similar.

In spite of an absolute decrease in the phospholipid rich high density lipoprotein fraction, the *plasma total phospholipids* are also increased in essential hyperglyceridemia and values up to 1000 mg per 100 ml have been reported (BÜRGER and GRÜTZ 1932, BERNSTEIN and coworkers 1939, LEPARD 1944, THANNHAUSER 1950, DUNPHY 1950, CETNAROVICZ et al. 1953). Measurement of the individual phospholipid classes has been performed by several authors with conflicting results. Many of these differences may be attributable to methodologic difficulties, particularly with regard to results obtained before the era of thin-layer chromatography. According to THANNHAUSER (1950) the increase in plasma phospholipids is due almost exclusively to elevation of plasma lecithin, while MALMROS et al. (1954) also found increased sphingomyelin levels. NOTHMAN and PROGER (1962) studied the cephalins, phosphatidyl ethanolamine and phosphatidylserine, in a group of patients with hyperlipemia, xanthomatosis and elevated plasma cholesterol levels and found the percentage contributions of these two phosphatides to the total phospholipids to be 2—3 times the values in normal persons. Since these authors reported higher levels of phosphatidyl serine than phosphatidyl ethanolamine in normal plasma and this finding conflicts with data obtained by chromatography and autoradiography (TROUP et al. 1960) of phospholipids, the subject obviously requires further evaluation. Whatever the amount of phosphatidyl serine in hyperlipemic plasma, this phospholipid is present only in trace amounts or not at all in normal plasma (TROUP et al. 1960, SKIPSKI et al. 1962). A significant increase in plasmalogen in serum of patients with EHL has been reported by SECKFORT and BRAUN-FALCO (1957), with a level of 9.5 mg per 100 ml instead of 2—6.6 mg per 100 ml found normally.

Reports of *free fatty acid levels* in hyperlipemia have to be interpreted with similar reservations as regards the reliability of conventional methods in the presence of such extreme amounts of other lipids. In addition, the rapid turnover of this fraction and wide fluctuations of utilization and release within very brief periods of time would require optimal standardization of the conditions at the time of measurement. Normal values for fasting FFA in EHL were reported by DOLE (1956) and by FURMAN et al. (1961) except for hyperlipemic subjects with "mild diabetes". From more recent reports (SANBAR et al. 1964, JAHNKE 1965) it appears that elevation of FFA is a frequent finding in EHL. Levels tend to be lower in exogenous hyperlipemia as compared to endogenous hyperlipemia (CARLSON and OLHAGEN 1959, HAVEL and GORDON 1960). Particularly in the presence of overt carbohydrate intolerance significant elevation of FFA may be observed (KINSELL et al. 1962). It is not known at the present time whether this elevation in such cases occurs as the result of carbohydrate intolerance or represents a basic abnormality of the disease (see page 460).

Characterization of the *plasma lipoproteins* in EHL, in addition to or in conjunction with controlled dietary studies is increasingly recognized as being of key importance in diagnosis and differentiation of the various hyperlipemic syndromes. Since levels and ratios of the different plasma lipid classes are determined by the prevailing lipoprotein pattern, methods for quantitative and qualitative evaluation of lipoproteins confirm and refine impressions obtained by measuring plasma glycerides, cholesterol and phospholipids.

Separation of lipoproteins according to density by established *ultracentrifugation* procedures (GOFMAN et al. 1949, HAVEL et al. 1955) shows the greatest increase in the fractions of d < 1.006 (Sf 20 to 10^5). Lipoproteins of d 1.019—1.006 (Sf 12—20) are usually slightly increased, while the quantities of d 1.063—1.019 (Sf 0—12) are decreased (GOFMAN et al. 1954, HAVEL and GORDON 1960, CORNWELL et al. 1961) except in syndromes of group 3. A significant decrease is observed in the α-lipoprotein (HDLP) fraction of d 1.063—1.21 (CORNWELL et al. 1961, ALBRINK 1961, FURMAN et al. 1964) which tends to be reversible with control of hyperlipemia. ZÖLLNER (1962) discussed a possible lack of acceptor protein as a cause; an alternate possibility is association of HDLP with VLDLP and/or chylomicrons as proposed by FURMAN et al. (1961, 1962, 1964).

A method for ultracentrifugal subfractionation of VLDLP (d < 1.006) has recently been published by GUSTAFSON et al. (1965). This procedure allows separation of 5 lipoprotein subfractions A—E with Sf rates from 20 to > 5000. Their lipid composition is in good agreement with corresponding fractions obtained by BIERMAN et al. (1965) (see below) with different methods. Its application to plasmas of hyperlipemic subjects should aid in differentiation and analysis of the various syndromes.

Interaction of lipoproteins with various media and the electrical charge of the molecular complex are the main determining factors for separation of lipoproteins by *electrophoresis*. The significance of the protein moieties in such separation supplements ultracentrifugal methods and allows distinctions not possible with fractionation according to density alone.

SWAHN (1953) and CARLSON and OLHAGEN (1954) found that lipemic plasma subjected to free and starch electrophoresis respectively, contained two turbidity peaks. Increases in lipids migrating as β-lipoproteins on starch have been reported by DIETRICH (1955) and by SCHETTLER et al. (1958), who also observed a significant decrease of this fraction after preliminary ultracentrifugation and separation of the "chylomicron" fraction. PARONETTO et al. (1957) described increases in α₂-lipoproteins on starch electrophoresis. SCHETTLER et al. (1958) described disappearance of "chylomicrons" in this area on low fat diets.

We know now that depending on pathogenesis and dietary conditions, a variety of lipoproteins with d < 1.006 may accumulate in EHL. Thus BIERMAN et al. (1965) have recently characterized the migration characteristics of three classes of lipoproteins with d < 1.006 on *starch block electrophoresis* during controlled dietary periods in subjects with endogenous hyperlipemia. Alimentary particles (primary and secondary particles) migrate in this system to the α₂- and β-area respectively, and appear to be identical with particles occurring in normal subjects after a fat load (BIERMAN et al. 1962). In addition, endogenous (hyperlipemic) particles (on fat free diets) can be recovered from the α₂-β-area, where they are mixed with fresh chylomicrons ("primary particles") if the latter are present. They can be separated from "primary" particles by polyvinylpyrrolidone (PVP) flocculation (see below). Hyperlipemic particles (endogenous particles) closely resemble α₂-lipoproteins (Sf 20—400) which are present normally in small quantities in fasting plasma. On lipid analysis they are found to have a significantly higher cholesterol and lower triglyceride content than chylomicrons, and, if present in large quantities, account for the cholesterol-rich lowest density lipoprotein fraction reported in hyperlipemic subjects of the endogenous variety by

SCHETTLER et al. (1958), HAVEL and GORDON (1960), ALBRINK (1961) and FURMAN et al. (1961). The existence of these particles would provide an alternative interpretation to the suggestion of ALBRINK (1961) that chylomicrons persisting in the circulation from exogenous fat intake may take up cholesterol and phospholipid.

Conventional *paper electrophoresis* for separation of lipoproteins has been employed in normals and subjects with coronary heart disease (CHD) (SMITH 1957); a pre-β-band was indicative of increased amounts of Sf 20—100 lipoproteins. In hyperlipemia, very low density lipoproteins and chylomicrons usually failed to separate and appeared in form of an intensive trail extending from the origin to the β-lipoproteins (HERBST et al. 1955) and occasionally to the front of the β-area (SCHETTLER et al. 1958). The modification of this technique by LEES and HATCH (1963) by addition of albumin to the buffer permits of better separation of alimentary and endogenous particles in hyperlipemia. According to FREDRICKSON and LEES (1965) a band at the origin indicates the presence of chylomicrons ("primary" and „secondary" particles); this is found in exogenous hyperlipemia (hyperchylomicronemia). Endogenous hyperlipemias are characterized by the appearance of a pre-β-band (see Fig. 7), occasionally with trailing as observed in pure carbohydrate-induced hyperlipemia (FREDRICKSON and LEES' type IV). Both a chylomicron band and a pre-β-band are usually present in fat and carbohydrate inducible hyperlipemia (type V of FREDRICKSON and LEES) and an increased pre-β-band in addition to a large β-band in essential hypercholesterolemia with hyperlipemia (see Fig. 1).

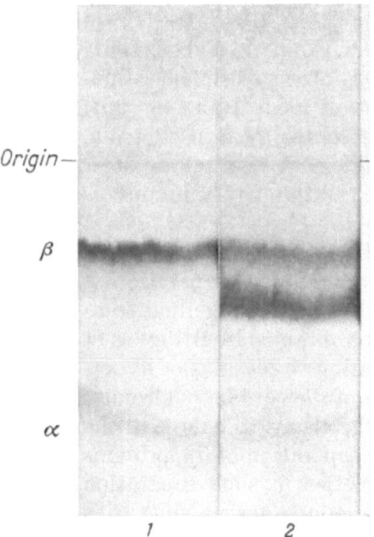

Fig. 7. Paper electrophoresis with albumin-containing buffer of a normal plasma (*1*) and plasma of a subject with endogenous hyperglyceridemia (*2*). Lipid stain with oil red O. A clearly separated pre-β-band is present in endogenous hyperglyceridemia. The α-lipoprotein band is stained faintly in the normal control, but hardly visible in the hyperlipemic subject

The separation of lipoproteins with d <1.006 on a *PVP gradient column* has been described by GORDIS (1962) and BIERMAN et al. (1962, 1965) and the flocculation characteristics of exogenous and endogenous particles in this system are given in Table 2.

Lipoprotein lipase (post-heparin lipolytic activity): The enzyme(s), extracted by KORN (1955) from a variety of tissues, particularly adipose tissue, and probably identical with the heparin-induced clearing principle (HAHN 1943), is thought to play a significant role in removal of triglyceride from the circulation. Its release by human liver has only recently been demonstrated (CONDON et al. 1965).

The lipolytic activity of post-heparin plasma is usually assessed by in vitro hydrolysis of a fat emulsion and conveniently expressed as μEq FFA released per ml per minute (FREDRICKSON et al. 1963). Low values are, as mentioned, quite consistently found in exogenous hyperlipemia and normal levels in endogenous hyperlipemias. Table 1 presents such data from the literature. If the test is performed during periods of fat restriction, low values may be found in normal individuals as well as in endogenous hyperlipemia (FREDRICKSON et al. 1963, KUO et al. 1965).

Liver function in EHL is typically normal when determined by measurement of serum bilirubin and galactose utilization. Lipemia makes flocculation tests unreliable. The sedimentation rate may be increased.

Diagnosis

Once the presence of fasting lipemia has been established, *differentiation between primary and secondary hyperlipemias* can usually be made on the basis of presence or absence of clinical and laboratory findings characteristic of an underlying disease. Plasma lipid and lipoprotein patterns as determined by lipid analyses, ultracentrifugation and electrophoresis are not necessarily diagnostic since similar findings are present in EHL and hyperlipemia of diabetic ketoacidosis, acute pancreatitis, alcoholism, etc. (SCHETTLER 1955, LEES and FREDRICKSON 1964, JAHNKE 1965).

If EHL is suspected in the presence of clear plasma, measurement of triglyceride and cholesterol levels will uncover the defect.

Further classification can usually be achieved by a combination of the laboratory methods described. Assuming that dietary and other conditions are well defined, one may proceed as follows:

a) *Inspection* of a plasma sample which has been allowed to stand over night will show some creaming if chylomicrons are present, while endogenous particles will not float by gravity alone during this period. In the presence of significant amounts of both chylomicrons and VLDLP (endogenous particles) two layers of particulate fat can be observed after standing overnight (BORRIE 1957) or brief ultracentrifugation. These have been decribed as "light" and "heavy" chylomicrons by ALBRINK et al. (1961) and as "a less turbid saline layer immediately below a cream layer" by KUO et al. (1961). Suggestive of the different origin of these fractions is a different fatty acid composition as reported by these workers.

b) *Paper electrophoresis* using albumin-buffer in most cases will provide sufficient information with regard to the presence of exogenous and endogenous particles. It is necessary that it be performed while the subject is consuming an "average" diet since dietary alterations may significantly modify the tracing. Difficulties may be encountered in the presence of marked lipemia when intensive trailing of the pre-β-fraction occurs.

c) Separation of particulate fat in plasma with the use of *PVP columns* will be helpful in these instances and can be used to confirm the patterns found on paper electrophoresis in others.

d) In vitro *assay of lipoprotein lipase* must be performed while the subject is on a diet containing normal amounts of fat for reasons already mentioned.

e) If at this point a satisfactory classification has not been achieved, two *periods of controlled diets* with isocaloric high fat and high carbohydrate intake respectively will in most cases permit of the proper diagnosis. Formula diets have been used to good advantage for this purpose; a minimum of two weeks should be allowed for each period, during which serial lipid determinations and other studies may be carried out.

f) *Ancillary studies* should include search for evidence of carbohydrate intolerance (glucose tolerance test, cortisone glucose tolerance test, tolbutamide test); and a thorough examination for signs and symptoms of premature atherosclerosis. The presence of carbohydrate intolerance and evidence of atheromatosis would favor the diagnosis of endogenous hyperlipemia (see below).

g) *Other findings* such as organomegaly, xanthomatosis and abdominal crises appear to be more frequent in exogenous hyperlipemia. The presence of corneal arcus and particularly tendon xanthomas in combination with hyperlipemia suggests that one is dealing with combined hypercholesterolemia and hyperglyceridemia.

h) *Familial occurrence* of hyperlipemia should be searched for; finding of elevated plasma glycerides in other members of a pedigree may on occasion aid in the differentiation from secondary hyperlipemias. A family history of "diabetes mellitus" will frequently be elicited in endogenous hyperlipemia.

In summary, a combination of personal and family history, plasma lipid determination, paper electrophoresis, lipoprotein lipase assay and evaluation of carbohydrate tolerance will in most cases be sufficient to identify different hyperlipemic syndromes. Occasionally controlled dietary studies will be necessary and ultracentrifugation studies may aid in further differentiation of subsyndromes.

Fat Loading

A variety of fat loading procedures have been employed in the evaluation of families with EHL and reports of abnormal tests in relatives without fasting hyperlipemia have been given and were interpreted as a means of identifying asymptomatic carriers of the trait(s) (BIALKIN et al. 1962). Although delayed clearing of a single fat load in a subject with exogenous hyperlipemia when studied during normoglyceridemia is striking, mild abnormalities in fat tolerance are nonspecific and have been described in other disease states, particularly in subjects with coronary heart disease (BROWN et al. 1961, HARLAN and BEISCHER 1963).

The use of radioisotopes as a diagnostic tool in evaluation of triglyceride turnover has not been introduced into the clinic. Pool size artefacts have to be considered in the interpretation of such data.

Complications
Coronary Heart Disease (CHD)

Hyperglyceridemia has been reported to correlate better with CHD than hypercholesterolemia (ALBRINK and MAN 1959), and subjects with CHD exhibit marked and prolonged postprandial lipemia (BROWN et al. 1961). However, while there is wide agreement on a strong correlation between essential hypercholesterolemia and the premature occurrence of CHD, evidence for an increased incidence of atherosclerotic complications in essential hyperlipemias is controversial.

In the literature up to 1950, an association of EHL and atherosclerosis was never mentioned and the reviews of POULSEN (1950), MOVITT et al. (1951), and JOYNER (1953) do not contain any cases with unequivocal affection of the cardiovascular system. Similarly the collection of 49 cases from the literature by GADRAT (1958) contained only one case with angina pectoris which had been described by LEVER and KLEIN (1958). Thus it was stated by several authors that, although in EHL the degree of lipemia obviously far exceeds levels usually found in CHD (DOLE et al. 1963), EHL would not seem to predispose to the development of early or particularly severe atheromatous vascular lesions (THANNHAUSER 1958, ZÖLLNER 1962).

Numerous case reports with symptoms and signs of vascular lesions have been given since (BOHMAN 1951, FULTON 1952, LEVER et al. 1954, MALMROS et al. 1954, SCHETTLER et al. 1957, 1958, 1961, SOFFER and MURRAY 1954, MARTT and CONNOR 1956, and JUCHEMS et al. 1965). A particularly high incidence of CHD has been reported by ADLERSBERG (1955) where out of a total number of 89 subjects (25 patients with EHL and 64 family members of 20 patients) 30 showed evidence of CHD. 56% of his 25 patients with EHL and 25% of the family members were affected. 5 out of 6 patients with EHL described by KUO et al. (1959) suffered from CDH, the sixth had intermittent claudication and one subject showed signs of both. FLEISCHMAJER (1960) reviewing 82 cases of EHL found 21 subjects with angina pectoris, myocardial infarction or other evidence of arteriosclerosis and BIALKIN et al. (1962) suggested that the age in which signs and symptoms of

CHD make their appearance, may depend on whether the subject is homozygous or heterozygous for the hyperlipemic trait. An increased incidence of atherosclerosis at relatively young age in the families of hyperlipemic students has been reported by HIRSCHHORN et al. (1959). Familial occurrence of CHD in EHL has also been described by SCHETTLER (1961).

It seems possible that the incidence of atherosclerotic complications differs for the various hyperlipemic syndromes and that contradictory findings could at least in part be explained if the type of hyperlipemia had been further classified at the time. BORRIE (1957) has discussed this aspect for a number of the cases reported by LEVER et al. (1954) and MALMROS et al. (1954) and has added five examples of his own. The occurrence of xanthelasmas and tendon xanthomas with hyperlipemia indicated to him that one was actually dealing with EFH. For other patients, who in addition exhibited eruptive xanthomas, he coined the term "mixed cases". In retrospect it appears that these cases probably represented examples of essential hypercholesterolemia and essential hyperlipemia as described on page 460. The case of a child who died at the age of ten from myocardial infarction (BOGGS et al. 1957) quite certainly represented such an occurrence. The findings at autopsy were characteristic of EFH. The four subjects reported by SOFFER and MURRAY (1954) who between the ages of 35 and 56 exhibited symptoms of atherosclerosis, angina pectoris and intermittent claudication might have fallen into a similar category as suggested by their response to heparin administration.

Significant differences in lipoprotein patterns of exogenous and endogenous hyperlipemias with particular reference to the particles of d <1006, resulting in higher elevation of total cholesterol levels in the latter as compared to the former type may play a role in the development of vascular lesions. It has been emphasized recently that premature atherosclerosis has not been observed in pure fat-induced hyperlipemia (HAVEL and GORDON 1960, KNITTLE and AHRENS 1964, FREDRICKSON and LEES 1965). If time bears out this impression, the lack of reports on an association of hyperlipemia and CHD during the time when only severe forms of exogenous hyperlipemia were recognized would find a satisfactory explanation. KUO et al. (1965) recently proposed the interesting theory that deficiency of lipoprotein lipase in fat-induced hyperlipemia may actually protect such individuals from increased susceptibility to atherosclerosis. Another fact to be born in mind is that most exogenous hyperlipemia was described in children or young adults, whereas reports on endogenous hyperlipemia generally dealt with a much more atherosclerosis-prone group.

The possible relationship between overt and occult carbohydrate intolerance in endogenous hyperlipemias and the development of premature atherosclerosis remains to be evaluated.

Of interest are observations in lipemia with regard to blood clotting and oxygen supply to the myocardium (lit. see SCHETTLER 1961). Hyperlipemia, regardless of cause, can be accompanied by a state of hypercoagulability as shown in studies by O'BRIEN (1957) and by LASCH et al. (1960). There may be simultaneous decrease in fibrinolysis (GREIG 1956). Increased aggregation of erythrocytes has been observed by SWANK et al. (1956). The explanation for this phenomenon given by PECHAR et al. (1960) is formation of a lipid film around erythrocytes, which could also result in impairment of oxygen exchange between red cells and tissues. Decreased arterial oxygen saturation during the peak of lipemia has been observed by KUO and coworkers (1959) in arteriosclerotic patients with angina pectoris. With drug induced clearing of lipemia the arterial oxygen saturation in two patients increased from 92.1 and 92.16 to 95.8 and 96.1%, respectively. HELLEMS and REGAN (1960) observed impaired myocardial blood flow in postprandial lipemia. All these findings are of significance in the discussion of factors which may trigger or accelerate the development of coronary artery insufficiency in the presence of hyperlipemia.

Interstitial Keratitis Lipemica

Dunphy (1949) observed in several cases of EHL a severe form of nonspecific keratitis (occasionally accompanying lipemia retinalis) with yellowish discoloration and opalescense of distinctly outlined corneal areas and proposed the term "keratide interstitielle lipidique". Examination of his cases with the aid of a slit lamp showed small areas with fine granular radial streaks. Refractive properties suggested the presence of cholesterol crystals in these lesions. The cause of this condition is unknown. It is possible that transudation of lipemic lymph fluid into canals of the cornea is responsible.

Associated Disorders

Association of essential hyperlipemia with *hyperuricemia and gout* has been reported (Wolfson et al. 1959, Fulton 1952, Schettler et al. 1957) and, in our experience, is quite frequently encountered. Conversely, Berkowitz and Glassman (1965), emphasizing the relationship of gout, hyperlipidemia and diabetes, found elevated glyceride levels in 24 out of 25 subjects with gout.

An unusual case of hyperlipemia with xanthomatosis and *plasmacellular* bone tumors was described by Brehmer and Lübbers (1950), where the marrow, in addition to xanthomatous areas, showed foci with the typical appearance of multiple myeloma. The autopsy findings of the arterial system were quite unusual: In addition to generalized atherosclerosis of moderate degree as a morphological basis of this patient's coronary and cerebral ischemia, there was proliferation of lipid-containing cells in the thoracic aorta and in several arteries of the lungs and spleen, and some xanthomatous thyroid adenomas. Furthermore, there was lymphangiomatosis xanthomatosa of the pharynx, the trachea and the bronchi as well as of lungs, liver, and spleen. Other xanthomatous areas were found in the kidneys, the mucosa of the esophagus, small bowel and urinary bladder, and the central nervous system. There was concomitant lipuria up to 11 gm daily without proteinuria. (Lipuria in hyperlipemia has also been described by Roesch and Riecke, cit. after B. Fischer.)

A similar patient was observed by Schettler (1961). Typical findings of multiple myeloma as evidenced by protein electrophoresis and x-ray signs of bone lesions were associated with eruptive xanthomas and a total lipid level of 1.6 gm per 100 ml. A hemorrhagic diathesis existed in spite of normal platelet count and function. The patient expired from progressive uremia one year after the first symptoms were noted. At autopsy there was only a moderate degree of atherosclerosis compatible with the patient's age, but no findings of xanthomatous atherosclerosis. This seems particularly interesting in view of the striking similarity of this case to the one described above and suggests once more that hyperlipemia, even when complicated by a nephrotic syndrome, does not necessarily favour the development of atheromatous vascular lesions.

Management

Lowering of plasma lipid levels in EHL is obviously desirable even though the incidence of atherosclerotic complications still remains to be established. Incapacity resulting from abdominal episodes and the occurrence of xanthomatosis would be sufficient reason to institute an effective therapeutic regimen in any case.

A conscientiously executed *dietary program* represents the cornerstone of therapy in essential hyperlipemias. That such treatment will be quite different for the various hyperlipemic syndromes is evident from the considerations on the pathogenesis of each form. In general a diet has to be devised which will establish or maintain ideal body weight and contain sufficient amounts of proteins, essential vitamins and minerals.

Limitation of fat intake represents the most effective tool in exogenous hyperlipemia. The amount of fat tolerated will vary in different individuals, but probably should never exceed 15% of total calories. The kind of fat seems to be of minor importance with regard to control of exogenous hyperlipemia but in view of the fat restriction a sufficient intake of linoleate should be assured. WILKINSON (1956), because of the delayed clearing of alimentary fat, has recommended a program of spaced fat feeding (one fat meal per day). Medium chain triglyceride has been recommended by AHRENS and SPRITZ (1963) and FURMAN et al. (1963) because of its absorption into the portal circulation (BLOOM et al. 1951) and consequent lack of contribution to chylomicron formation (JOBST and SCHETTLER 1956).

In pure carbohydrate-induced hyperlipemia, restriction of carbohydrate compatible with acceptability of the diet and prevention of ketosis is recommended. Thus 50—70% of calories may be given as fat with a carbohydrate content below 25%. If a significant amount of the fat comes from unsaturated sources, it may be cleared from plasma faster than saturated fats (ENGELBERG 1964) and hypercholesterolemia may be further reduced. Such a regimen should also be optimal in the combination of essential hypercholesterolemia and hyperlipemia.

The importance of the calorie level in "carbohydrate and fat inducible" hyperlipemia (group 2) has been emphasized. In this group the lowest feasible calorie intake will result in lowest plasma lipid levels. Unsaturated at the expense of saturated fat should be emphasized.

Although dietary manipulation in EHL will produce most striking results if it is adhered to (as opposed to the state of affairs in essential hypercholesterolemia, where dietary treatment is frequently ineffective), in many cases such a dietary regimen fails to achieve complete control of hyperlipemia. Also patient cooperation may be poor if a quite restricted diet is prescribed for an indefinite period.

Treatment with a variety of agents has therefore been tried, usually without overwhelming sucess.

If hyperlipemia is associated with hyperglycemia, we have found, contrary to THANNHAUSER (1950), that *insulin* can be effective in reducing plasma triglycerides to levels below those achievable by diet alone. A similar observation was reported by CHRISTENSEN et al. (1958). Reports of the effectiveness of oral antidiabetic agents have also been given (FURMAN et al. 1961, SHIPP and MUNROE 1962, REAVEN et al. 1964) although here too results are contradictory.

Administration of *heparin* has frequently been tried in EHL. Whereas no significant effect on plasma lipids was reported by KUO et al. (1959) and in a "heparin unresponsive subject" with "fat-induced" hyperlipemia by FURMAN et al. (1961), the latter authors demonstrated significant improvement in plasma lipid levels of two other patients with "carbohydrate-induced" hyperlipemia. One might anticipate unresponsiveness to long term heparin administration with low postheparin lipolytic activity found with the in vitro assay of FREDRICKSON et al. (1963) (see Table 1). Such a correlation is not necessarily present as evidenced by the response in a child with the "fat-induced" variety, whom we have observed (KINSELL and SCHLIERF 1965).

Response to administration of heparin and/or heparinoid drugs as evidenced by persistent lowering of plasma triglycerides and simultaneous regression of xanthomas is impressively illustrated in the following case (SCHETTLER 1961). A. K., a 58 year old male patient with familial EHL, has been followed by us since 1951. His xanthomas had increased up to this time despite administration of various drugs (Fig. 8 a—c). He suffered from abdominal colics and had severe episodes of angina pectoris. Therapeutic trials with nicotinic acid, choline, pyridoxine, vitamins A and E, lipocaic factor, ACTH, prednisolone and hyaluronidase were without effect on hyperlipemia and xanthomatosis. The decision for long term treatment with heparin drugs was made when the skin xanthomas of his hands impaired the patient's capacity to work. A preliminary acute test had shown a prompt fall in glycerides. Starting January 1958, heparin was administered intravenously or intramuscularly in a dose of 4 × 5000 units per week. After two weeks the treatment had to be stopped transiently because epistaxis occurred. From March to December 1958 treatment was resumed, this time with Depot-Thrombocid[1],

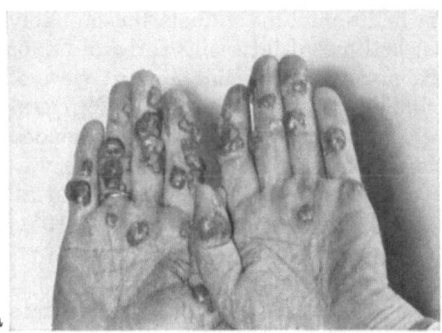

a

Fig. 8 a—c. Effect of heparin-like drugs (pentosan polysulfate sodium) on xanthomas in essential hyperlipemia; a before treatment, b after four months, c after twelve months of treatment (from: G. Schettler: Arteriosklerose. Stuttgart: Thieme (1961), with kind permission of the publisher)

3× and later 2× per week intramuscularly. No diet was followed by the patient during this period. With normalization of plasma lipids the tumor-like

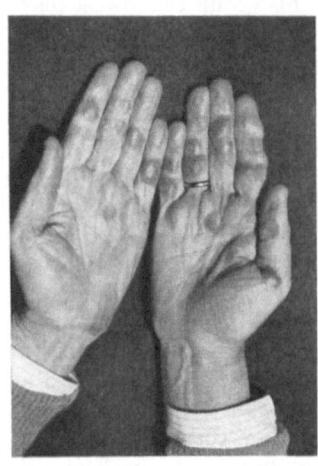

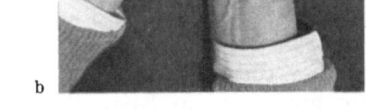

b

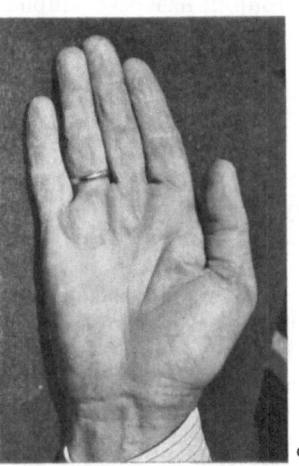

c

xanthomas regressed; abdominal symptoms and angina pectoris disappeared. The ECG, initially diagnostic of myocardial ischemia with WPW syndrome, showed partial reversal of the abnormal pattern. At the present time this patient feels well and does not have any signs of his disease while receiving 300 mg Depot-Thrombocid weekly. One of two sisters who also suffered from EHL with xanthoma and CHD was successfully treated in a similar manner. The other sister unfortunately rejected any therapy. Comparably favorable results were observed in a 58 year old female patient, where abdominal attacks, hepatomegaly and angina pectoris subsided completely and neutral lipids fell from 4—5 gm per

---

[1] Pentosan Polysulfate Sodium (Mw approx. 3000). Bene-Chemie GmbH., München-Solln, Germany.

100 ml to 65—150 mg per 100 ml. A loss of hair was reversible and did not recur with a lower dosage of Depot-Liquemin[1].

A similarly interesting case is that of a 68 year old male patient who was first seen in 1958 with symptoms of marked myocardial ischemia and electrocardiographic evidence of an old inferior myocardial infarction. Insulin dependent diabetes mellitus had been present since 1932. In spite of diabetic control with diet and insulin in this subject, lipemia (approximately 2 gm neutral fat per 100 ml plasma) persisted and abdominal colics recurred. With heparin and later Depot-Thrombocid his neutral lipids ranged between 300—500 mg per 100 ml and clinical symptoms (angina pectoris and episodes of abdominal pain) improved considerably. An additional feature in this patient was gout with uric acid levels above 9 mg per 100 ml and attacks of acute gouty arthritis on several occasions between 1958 and 1959.

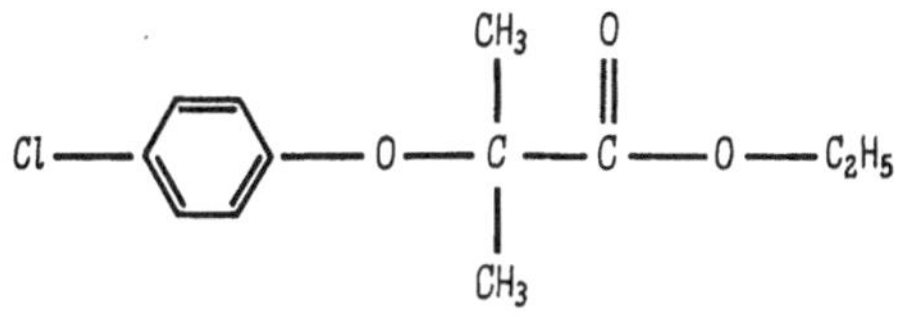

Fig. 9. Chlorophenoxyisobutyrate

These observations and many others (ROSENMAN and FRIEDMAN 1954, HOLLISTER and KANTER 1955, PFLEGER and TIRSCHEK 1956, MATRAS 1956, EGGSTEIN 1960, TRENCKMANN 1956, LEVER et al. 1955) demonstrate the favorable effect of long term heparin administration in EHL with regard to decrease in serum lipids, improvement of arterial vascular insufficiency and regression of xanthomas. It is mandatory that the patients treated in this way be followed closely during the regulatory period, until a minimal effective dose is found. Interestingly enough it may then be possible to omit injections for months and still maintain good control. We have not had success with local injections of heparin with regard to regression of xanthomas as has been reported by CORNBLEET (1955) and by CARTEAUD and MAMOU (1956).

Other effects of heparin on signs and symptoms of atherosclerotic complications are discussed by SCHETTLER (1961).

Chlorophenoxyisobutyrate (CPIB), an organic ester (formula see Fig. 9) is rapidly split in the body, and the anion of the acid has been shown to exhibit a significant hypolipidemic effect in experimental animals (THORP and WARING 1962). The compound has been studied in humans since 1962, originally in combination with a small amount of androsterone (Atromid[2], OLIVER 1962), until it was demonstrated (BEST and DUNCAN 1963, HELLMAN et al. 1963, HOWARD et al. 1963, OLIVER 1963, KNÜCHEL 1964) that the omission of the androgen (Atromid-S) at least in man, is without influence, qualitatively and quantitatively, on the hypolipidemic action of CPIB. During administration of the material lowering of both plasma cholesterol and triglyceride level is observed; the response differs from that of dextrothyroxine in that the hypoglyceridemic effect in most studies exceeded the decrease in cholesterol (BEST and DUNCAN 1964, STRISOWER and STRISOWER 1964). Accordingly, decrease of plasma lipoproteins is more marked in the Sf 20—400 fraction than in the Sf 0—20 fraction (CARLSON et al. 1963, HOWARD et al. 1963, WALTON et al. 1963, STRISOWER and STRISOWER 1964).

---

[1] 1 ml = 40000 I. U. heparin + 20 mg ephedrine hydrochloride. Deutsche Hoffmann-Laroche AG, Grenzach, Baden, Germany.

[2] Imperial Chemical Industries Ltd., Alderley Park, Cheshire, England.

Most clinical trials which have been reported were in patients selected for either evidence of coronary heart disease (DELCOURT and VASTESAEGER 1963, FASOLI and CESANA 1963, KN ÜCHEL 1964) or elevated plasma cholesterol levels (GREEN et al. 1963, KONTTINEN and PALOHEIMO 1963) rather than hyperglyceridemia per se. A detailed discussion of these results can be found in the proceedings of the 1963 Atromid symposium published in J. Atheroscler. Res. v 3 Sept/Dec 1963.

Findings on the effect of CPIB in EHL were in general particularly favorable (CARLSON et al. 1963, CRAMER 1963, FASOLI and CESANA 1963, HOWARD et al. 1963, WALTON et al. 1963). HARRISON and GOLDBERG (1963) described a 15 year old girl suffering from EHL, in whom severe fat restriction had led to some improvement. Administration of Atromid and later CPIB alone resulted in sustained normalization of all lipid fractions and disappearance of xanthomas. In another case of EHL (HELLMAN et al. 1963) plasma triglycerides fell from 1202 mg per 100 ml to 675 mg per 100 ml with administration of CPIB. KN ÜCHEL (1964) reported on two subjects with EHL where triglyceride levels became normal from values of around 1500 mg per 100 ml in each case. Xanthomas in 10 out of 11 patients with either EHL or essential familial hypercholesteremia who were treated with Atromid for periods of 18 to 24 months resolved completely (BORRIE 1964). It remains to be evaluated whether the drug is more effective in some forms of EHL than in others.

At least in man, the mode of action is still unknown. It has been proposed (THORP 1963) that a main site of action of CPIB is located at anion binding sites of plasma proteins, and that the mechanism of action is secondary to altered distribution of endogenous hormones, coenzymes etc. A major role in the effect of the material may be played by the liver, where CPIB inhibits cholesterol synthesis (GOULD et al 1964) and triglyceride secretion (DUNCAN et al. 1964), in the rat. In addition, an activating effect on lipoprotein lipase has been suggested (THORP, unpublished observations). The study of these aspects is hampered by the fact that a variety of effects of CPIB vary greatly in different species. Thus DUNCAN and BEST (1965) found that inhibition of catecholamine induced release of fatty acids from adipose tissue, as reported for the rat and dog (THORP 1963), cannot be demonstrated in the human and therefore is unlikely to be responsible for the lowering of blood lipids by CPIB.

The recommended dose, 25 mg per kg body weight per day or less (= 1—2,5 gm per day) should not be exceeded since in experimental animals and man a decrease or even reversal of the effect of the drug has been observed (GREEN et al. 1963). Furthermore, signs of pyridoxine deficiency could be produced in dogs treated with long-term administration of high doses of CPIB.

Side effects with recommended doses are rare and consist mainly of mild gastrointestinal symptoms (GREEN et al. 1963) or pruritus (FROM HANSEN 1963). Transient rises of SGOT were occasionally observed (OLIVER 1962, CARLSON et al. 1963, COUNIHAN and KEELAN 1963, STRISOWER 1963, WALTON et al. 1963) in the absence of other evidence of liver dysfunction. Serum alkaline phosphatase may be lowered (HELLMAN et al. 1963). A potentiation of anticoagulant drugs (warfarin sodium, phenindione) appears to be the rule (HELLMAN et al. 1963, OLIVER et al. 1963) and needs to be taken into account when anticoagulants and CPIB are administered simultaneously. A reduction of $^1/_3$ in the dose of warfarin sodium, as found necessary in 13 cases thus treated by COUNIHAN and KEELAN (1963) may serve as a guideline. In the absence of exogenous administration of anticoagulant drugs, CPIB was without effects on generally employed tests of coagulation (HELLMAN et al. 1963, HOWARD et al. 1963), however, lowering of the plasma fibrinogen level (JEPSON and JAMES 1963, COTTON 1963) as well as decreased platelet adhesiveness (CARSON et al. 1963, GILBERT and MUSTARD 1963) have been reported. Lastly, indirect evidence suggests a need for caution, where plasma proteins are believed or known to be lowered.

Obviously further studies are needed to establish the place of CPIB in the treatment of hyperlipemias, with particular emphasis on controlled experiments in different forms of EHL and long-term observations with regard to effectiveness and safety. The drug is not yet available on prescription in the United States.

Dextrothyroxine (DT-4), in addition to its hypocholesterolemic effect, has also been found to lower plasma triglycerides. A decrease in glyceride levels up to 67% was observed by BERKOWITZ et al. (1962) in 24 out of 25 patients selected for plasma cholesterol values above 275 mg per 100 ml. Similar results were obtained by EISALO et al. (1963); in their study the decrease in plasma triglycerides was found to be correlated with the starting level and was not observed with a dose of 4 mg as compared to 8 mg per day. BEST and DUNCAN (1964) administered dextrothyroxine to 12 patients with CHD and found appreciable lowering of plasma triglycerides in 50% of their cases.

The relative effectiveness of dextrothyroxine and chlorophenoxyisobutyrate (CPIB) in 14 subjects with EFH and/or hyperlipemia was examined by STRISOWER and STRISOWER (1964). While the action of CPIB was mainly on Sf 20—400 lipoproteins, DT-4, as mentioned earlier, affected lipoproteins of Sf 0—20 to a greater degree. The mean decrease of Sf 20—400 lipoproteins with dextrothyroxine was 12%.

Side effects were rarely observed in the studies cited; the fact that they are higher in other series, and reports of progressive deterioration of control in diabetic subjects during administration of dextrothyroxine (ZINN et al. 1964), necessitate further critical evaluation.

A clearing of alimentary lipemia and of some cases of EHL with the use of *"essential phospholipids"* has been observed by SCHRADE and coworkers (1959) and SCHOEN et al. (1963). This material contains 3.15% phosphorus, 1.4% nitrogen (60% choline-N, 38% ethanolamine-N), 10.5% glycerol, 14.2% saturated fatty acids, 36.8% unsaturated fatty acids; fatty acid composition: C16 = 14.1%, C18 = 3.5%, C18:1 = 6.3%, C18:2 = 71.3%, C18:3 = 4.8%. (SCHETTLER 1952, BETZING 1965).

SCHRADE et al. (1959) found that the injection of 750 mg of the preparation results within hours in effects similar to those obtained during the course of weeks with administration of polyunsaturated fatty acids by mouth. There was a fall in total serum lipids of as much as 500 mg per 100 ml within a few hours, accompanied by a visible decrease in turbidity. The best response was observed with high initial lipid concentrations. Blood ketones were elevated during this period of time. JUCHEMS et al. (1965) reported similar results. We were unable to produce significant clearing with this material. Further studies will be necessary in the different hyperlipemic syndromes.

Summary and Conclusions

Essential hyperlipemia is a term used for various syndromes associated with elevation of plasma glycerides, usually well in excess of other plasma lipids and not secondary to other known disease. Hyperglyceridemia, if marked, results in turbid or milky appearance of the serum.

The clinical picture typically features the appearance of xanthomas (eruptive and/or tuberous) and occasionally abdominal crises which may be mistaken for acute surgical emergencies. On the other hand, asymptomatic cases are not rare.

It has become apparent that the syndrome consists of several entities with different pathogeneses. A familial occurrence has been reported for all of these. The diagnosis may be made by a variety of laboratory procedures; after differentiation of essential hyperlipemia from "secondary" hyperlipemias further classification is essential with particular regard to therapy. The basis of treatment are dietary measures which will be significantly different for the various forms. Drug therapy is still experimental.

It seems probable that better understanding of essential hyperlipemia, while attractive and stimulating in its own right, has broad implications in clinical medicine. There is general agreement that maintained elevation of plasma lipids predisposes to rapid progression of atherosclerosis. For every patient with gross hyperlipidemia, there are probably hundreds or thousands with mild or moderate derangements of this sort. Information leading to the understanding and control of the patients with severe degrees of abnormality may well be utilizable in the approach to understanding and control of "average" degenerative vascular disease.

References

ABEGG, W.: Ein Fall von hochgradiger alimentärer „hepatogener" Fettretention im Blut bei einem 11jährigen Kinde. Jb. Kinderheilk. **149**, 94 (1937).

ADDISON, T., and W. GULL: On a certain affection of the skin, vitiligoidea (a) plana, (b) tuberosa with remarks. Guy's Hosp. Rep. **7**, 265 (1850).

ADLERSBERG, D.: Inborn errors of lipid metabolism. Clinical, genetic, and chemical aspects. Arch. Path. **60**, 48 (1955).

— and C. WANG: Syndrome of idiopathic hyperlipemia, mild diabetes mellitus and severe vascular damage. Diabetes **4**, 210 (1955).

AHRENS jr., E. H.: Essential Hyperlipemia, in: "Fat metabolism", p. 61. Baltimore: Johns Hopkins Press 1954.

— Nutritional factors and serum lipid levels. Amer. J. Med. **23**, 928 (1957).

— Symposium on pathophysiological and clinical aspects of lipid metabolism. Heidelberg 1965. G. Schettler (ed.). Stuttgart: Thieme 1966.

— J. HIRSCH, W. INSULL jr., T. T. TSALTAS, R. BLOMSTRAND, and M. L. PETERSON: The influence of dietary fats on serum-lipid levels in man. Lancet **1957/I**, 943.

— — K. OETTE, J. W. FARQUHAR, and Y. STEIN: Carbohydrate-induced and fat-induced lipemia. Trans. Ass. Amer. Phycns. **74**, 134 (1961).

— and N. SPRITZ: Further studies on fat- and carbohydrate-induced lipemia in man. Reduction of lipemia by feeding fat; in: Biochemical problems of lipids, A. C. Frazer (ed.), p. 304. Amsterdam: Elsevier Publ. Co. 1963.

ALBRINK, M. J.: Lipoprotein pattern as a function of total triglyceride concentration of serum. J. clin. Invest. **40**, 536 (1961).

— Triglycerides, lipoproteins and coronary artery disease. Arch. intern. Med. **109**, 345 (1962).

— J. R. FITZGERALD, and E. B. MAN: Reduction of alimentary lipemia by glucose. Metabolism **7**, 162 (1958).

— and E. B. MAN: Serum triglycerides in coronary artery disease. Arch. intern. Med. **103**, 4 (1959).

— — and J. P. PETERS: The relation of neutral fat to lactescence of serum. J. clin. Invest. **34**, 147 (1955).

— J. W. MEIGS, and M. A. GRANOFF: Weight gain and serum triglycerides in normal men. New Engl. J. Med. **266**, 484 (1965).

— — and E. B. MAN: Serum lipids, hypertension and coronary artery disease. Amer. J. Med. **31**, 4 (1961).

ALVAREZ, R. R., D. F. GAISER, D. M. SIMKINS, E. K. SMITH, and G. E. BRATVOLD: Serial studies of serum lipids in normal human pregnancy. Amer. J. Obstet. Gynec. **77**, 743 (1959).

ANGERVALL, G., P. BJÖRNTORP, and B. HOOD: Studies on the clearing phenomenon in essential hyperlipemia. Acta med. scand. **172**, 5 (1962).

BERKOWITZ, D., and S. GLASSMAN: Gout, hyperlipidemia, and diabetes inter-relationships. Clin. Res. **13**, 318 (1965).

— J. J. SPITZER, and W. LIKOFF: Practical significance of serum triglycerides and radioactive fat tolerance. Their relation to current therapy for hypercholesterolemia. Amer. J. Cardiol. **10**, 198 (1962).

BERNHARD, E.: Über einen Fall von Lipämie. Schweiz. med. Wschr. **66**, 261 (1936).

BERNSTEIN, S. S., H. H. WILLIAMS, F. C. HUMMEL, M. L. SHEPHERD, and B. N. ERICKSON: Metabolic observations on a child with essential hyperlipemia. J. Pediat. **14**, 570 (1939).

BEST, M. M., and C. H. DUNCAN: Hypoglyceridemic effect of ethyl-alpha-p-chlorophenoxy-isobutyrate with and without androsterone. Circulation **28**, 690 (1963).

— — Effects of cholesterol-lowering drugs on serum triglycerides. J. Amer. med. Ass. **187**, 37 (1964).

BETZING, H.: Personal communication (1965).

BEUMER, H., und M. BÜRGER: Beiträge zur Chemie des Blutes in Krankheiten mit besonderer Berücksichtigung der Lipoide. IV. Mitteilung: Diabetes und Lipämie. Z. exp. Path. Ther. **13**, 362 (1913).

BEZMAN, A., J. M. FELTS, and R. J. HAVEL: Relationship between incorporation of triglyceride fatty acids and heparin-released lipoprotein lipase from adipose tissue slices. J. Lipid Res. **3**, 427 (1962).

BIALKIN, G., S. ZUCKER, B. S. SKLARIN, K. HIRSCHHORN, and M. DAVIDSON: A genetic and metabolic study of a family with hyperlipemia. Pediatrics **29**, 566 (1962).

BIERMAN, E. L.: Particulate lipid components in plasma. In: Handbook of Physiology. Section 5: Adipose tissue. A. E. Renold and G. F. Cahill jr. (ed.), p. 511. Baltimore: Williams and Wilkins 1965.

— E. GORDIS, and J. T. HAMLIN III: Heterogeneity of fat particles in plasma during alimentary lipemia. J. clin. Invest. **41**, 2254 (1962).

— and J. T. HAMLIN: The hyperlipemic effect of a low fat, high carbohydrate diet in diabetic subjects. Diabetes **10**, 432 (1961).

— D. PORTE jr., D. D. O'HARA, M. SCHWARTZ, and F. C. WOOD jr.: Characterization of fat particles in plasma of hyperlipemic subjects maintained on fat-free, highcarbohydrate diets. J. clin. Invest. **44**, 261 (1965).

BINET, L., et P. BROCQ: La lactescence du sérum sanguin au cours de la pancréatite hémorrhagique. Paris med. **71**, 489 (1929).

BLOOM, B., I. L. CHAIKOFF, and W. O. REINHARDT: Intestinal lymph as pathway of transport of absorbed fatty acids of different chain length. Amer. J. Physiol. **166**, 451 (1951).

BLOOMFIELD, A. L., and B. SHENSON: The syndrome of idiopathic hyperlipemia with crises of violent abdominal pain. Stanf. med. Bull. **5**, 185 (1947).

BOGGS, J. D., D. Y. Y. HSIA, R. F. MAIS, and J. A. BIGLER: The genetic mechanism of idiopathic hyperlipemia. New Engl. J. Med. **257**, 1101 (1957).

BOGGS, T., and R. MORRIS: Experimental lipemia in rabbits J. exp. Med. **11**, 553 (1909).

BOHMAN, A. M.: Hyperlipemi av okaend genes. (2 fall). Nord. Med. **46**, 1076 (1951).

BORRIE, P.: Essential hyperlipemia and idiopathic hypercholesterolemic xanthomatosis. Brit. med. J. 1957/II, 911.

— The treatment of xanthomatosis with Atromid. Brit. J. Derm. **76**, 53 (1964).

— Treatment of xanthomatosis. Brit. med. J. 1964/II, 1135.

BRAGDON, J. H., and R. S. GORDON: Tissue distribution of C-14 after the intravenous injection of labeled chylomicrons and unesterified fatty acids in the rat. J. clin. Invest. **37**, 574 (1958).

— and R. J. HAVEL: In vivo effect of anti-heparin agents on serum lipids and lipoproteins. Amer. J. Physiol. **177**, 128 (1954).

— and E. BOYLE: Human serum lipoproteins. I. Chemical composition of four fractions. J. Lab. clin. Med. **48**, 36 (1956).

— and A. KARMEN: The fatty acid composition of chylomicrons of chyle and serum following the ingestion of different oils. J. Lipid. Res. **1**, 167 (1960).

BREHMER, W., u. P. LÜBBERS: Über eine generalisierte Xanthomatose mit Knochenbefall und diffuser Plasmazellwucherung im Knochenmark bei essentieller Hyperlipämie. Virchows Arch. Path. Anat. **318**, 394 (1950).

BROWN, D. F., A. S. HESLIN, and J. T. DOYLE: Postprandial lipemia in health and in ischemic heart diesase. New Engl. J. Med. **264**, 733 (1961).

BRUNNER, W.: Beitrag zur pankreatogenen Lipämie. Klin. Wschr. **14**, 1853 (1935).

BRUTON, O. C., and A. J. KANTER: Idiopathic familial hyperlipemia Amer. J. Dis. Child. **82**, 153 (1951).

BÜRGER, M., u. O. GRÜTZ: Über hepatosplenomegale Lipidose mit xanthomatösen Veränderungen in Haut und Schleimhaut. Arch. Derm. Syph. (Berl.) **166**, 542 (1932).

CAMELIN, A., P. ACCOYER, L. DUTEL, et G. GAURON: Hyperlipémie essentielle de l'adulte. Incidences et accidents thérapeutiques. Bull. Mém. Soc. Med. Hôp. Paris **4**, 1116 (1955).

CARLSON, L. A., and B. OLHAGEN: The electrophoretic mobility of chylomicrons in a case of essential hyperlipemia. Scand. J. clin. Lab. Invest. **6**, 70 (1954).

— — Studies on a case of essential hyperlipemia. Blood lipids, with special reference to the composition and metabolism of the serum triglycerides before, during and after the course of a viral hepatitis. J. clin. Invest. **38**, 854 (1959).

CARLSON, L. A., B. HÖGSTEDT, and L. ÖRÖ: Effect of Atromid on plasma lipids and lipoproteins in subjects with hyperlipoproteinemia. J. Atheroscler. Res. 3, 467 (1963).
CARSON, P., L. McDONALD, S. PICKARD, T. PILKINGTON, B. DAVIES, and F. LOVE: Effect of Atromid on platelet stickiness. J. Atheroscler. Res. 3, 619 (1963).
CARTEAUD, A., et H. MAMOU: Sur deux cas de xanthomatoses. Hyperlipémie essentielle et xanthomatose familiale. Action de l'heparine locale. Sem. Hôp. (Paris) 26, 1501 (1956).
CETNAROWICZ, H., M. KOPEC, J. ZAJACZKOWSKI, and E. KOWALSKI: Samoistne Zwiekszenie sie zawartosci tluszczu we Krwi (hyperlipaemia essentialis). Pol. Tyg. lek. 8, 713 (1953).
CHAPMAN, F. D., and T. D. KINNEY: Hyperlipemia, "idiopathic hyperlipemia". Amer. J. Dis. Child. 62, 1014 (1941).
CHRISTENSEN, S., E. DOLLERUP, and S. E. JENSEN: Idiopathic hyperlipemia, latent diabetes mellitus, and severe neuropathy. Acta med. scand. 161, 57 (1958).
COLLETT, R. W., and R. L. J. KENNEDY: Chronic relapsing pancreatitis associated with hyperlipemia in an eight year old boy. Proc. Mayo Clin. 23, 158 (1948).
CONDON, R. E., H. TOBIAS, and D. V. DATTA: The liver and postheparin plasma lipolytic activity in dog and man. J. clin. Invest. 44, 860 (1965).
CORNBLEET, T.: Local action of heparin on xanthomas. Arch. Derm. 71, 172 (1955).
CORNWELL, D. G., F. A. KRUGER, G. J. HAMWI, and J. B. BROWN: Studies on the characterization of human serum lipoproteins separated by ultracentrifugation in a density gradient. II. Serum lipoproteins in hyperlipemic subjects. Amer. J. clin. Nutr. 9, 41 (1961).
COTTON, R. C., E. G. WADE, and G. W. SPILLER: The effect of Atromid on plasma fibrinogen and heparin resistance. J. Atheroscler. Res. 3, 648 (1963).
COUNIHAN, T. B., and P. KEELAN: Atromid in high cholesterol states. J. Atheroscler. Res. 3, 580 (1963).
CRAMER, K.: Action of Atromid on serum lipids and on beta-lipoprotein lipids and protein. J. Atheroscler. Res. 3, 500 (1963).
CROCKER, A. C.: Skin xanthomas in childhood. Pediatrics 8, 573 (1951).
CROFFORD, O. B.: Studies on the mechanism of idiopathic hyperlipemia with hyperglycemia. Metabolism 11, 1194 (1962).
DAVIDSON, P., and M. J. ALBRINK: Hypertriglyceridemia and impaired glucose tolerance. Clin. Res. 11, 216 (1963).
DELCOURT, R., and H. VASTESAEGER: Action of Atromid on total and beta-cholesterol. J. Atheroscler. Res. 3, 533 (1963).
DE ROSA, L.: Su di un caso di infiltrazione lipoidea della retina. Boll. Oculist. 31, 677 (1952).
DIETRICH, F.: Zur Differenzierung der Lipoproteide des Serums mittels präparativer Elektrophoresemethoden. Hoppe-Seylers Z. physiol. Chem. 302, 227 (1955).
DOLE, V. P.: A relationship between non-esterified fatty acids in plasma and the metabolism of glucose. J. clin. Invest. 35, 150 (1956).
— E. GORDIS, and E. L. BIERMAN: Hyperlipemia and arteriosclerosis. New Engl. J. Med. 269, 686 (1963).
— and J. T. HAMLIN III: Particulate fat in lymph and blood. Physiol. Rev. 42, 674 (1962).
DUNCAN, C. H., and M. M. BEST: Inhibition of hepatic secretion of triglycerides by chlorophenoxyisobutyrate. Circulation 30, suppl. III, 7 (1964).
— — A comparison of the effects of ethyl chlorophenoxyisobutyrate and nicotinic acid on plasma free fatty acids. Lancet 1965/I, 191.
DUNPHY, E. B.: Ocular conditions associated with idiopathic hyperlipemia. Amer. J. Ophthal. 33, 1579 (1950).
EGGSTEIN, M.: Die essentielle Hyperlipämie. Klinik der Gegenwart 9, 637 (1960).
EISALO, A., P. AHRENBERG, and E. A. NIKKILÄ: Treatment of hyperlipidemia with dextrothyroxine. Acta med. scand. 173, 639 (1963).
ENGELBERG, H.: Heparin lipemia clearing reaction and fat transport in man. Summary of available knowledge. Amer. J. clin. Nutr. 8, 21 (1960).
— Lipid metabolic studies in patients with essential hypertriglyceridemia. Metabolism 11, 1250 (1962).
— Effect of highly unsaturated fat upon the rate of lipolysis of fasting triglycerides by postheparin lipoprotein lipase. Circulation 30, suppl. III, 9 (1964).
FARQUHAR, J. W., R. C. GROSS, R. M. WAGNER, and G. M. REAVEN: Validation of an incompletely coupled two-compartment nonrecycling catenary model for turnover of liver and plasma triglyceride in man. J. Lipid Res. 6, 119 (1965).
— G. M. REAVEN, R. C. GROSS, and R. M. WAGNER: Rate of plasma triglyceride synthesis in carbohydrate-induced lipemia. J. clin. Invest. 42, 930 (1963).
— — R. M. WAGNER, and R. C. GROSS: Studies of hepatic and plasma triglyceride turnover in man. J. clin. Invest. 43, 1299 (1964).

FASOLI, A., and A. CESANA: Serum lipid and lipoprotein changes after treatment with Atromid in patients with atherosclerosis, essential hyperlipemia and familial hypercholesterolemia. J. Atheroscler. Res. 3, 475 (1963).

FEIGL, J.: Über das Verhalten und die Verteilung von Fetten und Lipoiden im Blute nach Blutentziehung. Chemischer Beitrag zur Kenntnis des Lipämiegebietes VII. Biochem. Z. 115, 63 (1921).

FELBER, J. P., et A. VANNOTTI: Effet du taux des acides gras libres (NEFA) plasmatiques sur la glycémie et l'insulinémie. Helv. physiol. pharmacol. Acta 22, 13 (1964).

FELTS, J. M.: The metabolism of chylomicron triglycerides by perfused rat livers and by intact rats. Ann. N.Y. Acad. Sci. 131, 24 (1965).

FIELD, R. A.: Glycogen deposition diseases, in: The Metabolic Basis of Inherited Disease, p. 178. Ed. Stanbury, Wyngaarden, Fredrickson. New York: McGraw-Hill Book Co. 1960.

FISCHER, B.: Über Lipämie und Cholesterinämie sowie über Veränderungen des Pankreas und der Leber bei Diabetes mellitus. Virchows Arch. Path. Anat. 172, 30 u. 218 (1903).

FLEISCHMAJER, R.: The Dyslipidoses. Springfield (Ill.): Thomas 1960.

FLETCHER, R. F., and J. GLOSTER: The lipids in xanthomata. J. clin. Invest. 43, 2104 (1964).

FRANK, I., and L. M. LEVITT: Idiopathic hyperlipemia with secondary xanthomatosis. Arch. Derm. Syph. (Chic.) 64, 434 (1951).

FRANKLIN, S. N.: Splenomegaly with lipemia. Proc. roy. Soc. Med. 30, 711 (1937).

FREDRICKSON, D. S. in: The Metabolic Basis of Inherited Disease. Ed.: Stanbury, Wyngaarden, Fredrickson. New York: McGraw-Hill Book Co. 1960.

— Symposium on pathophysiological and clinical aspects of lipid metabolism, Heidelberg 1965. G. Schettler (ed.). Stuttgart: Thieme 1966.

— and R. S. GORDON: Transport of fatty acids. Physiol. Rev. 38, 585 (1958).

— and R. S. LEES: A system for phenotyping hyperlipoproteinemia. Circulation 31, 321 (1965).

— — in: The Metabolic Basis of Inherited Disease. Ed.: Stanbury, Wyngaarden, Fredrickson. New York: McGraw-Hill Book Co. 1966.

— D. L. McCOLLESTER and K. ONO: The role of unesterified fatty acid transport in chylomicron metabolism. J. clin. Invest. 37, 1333 (1958).

— K. ONO, and L. L. DAVIS: Lipolytic activity of post-heparin plasma in hyperglyceridemia. J. Lipid. Res. 4, 24 (1963).

FRIEDBERG, S. J., and E. H. ESTES, jr.: Tissue distribution and uptake of endogenous lipoprotein triglycerides in the rat. J. clin. Invest. 43, 129 (1964).

FROM HANSEN, P.: The effect of diet, D-thyroxin and Atromid on serum cholesterol and triglycerides in man. J. Atheroscler. Res. 3, 584 (1963).

FULTON, J. K.: Essential lipemia, acute gout, peripheral neuritis, and myocardial disease in a Negro man. Arch. intern. Med. 89, 303 (1952).

FURMAN, R. H., R. P. HOWARD, and P. ALAUPOVIC: Effect of chronic heparin administration on serum lipids, lipoproteins, nitrogen and electrolyte balance in normal and heparin-responsive and heparin-unresponsive hyperglyceridemic subjects. Metabolism 11, 879 (1962).

— — O. J. BRUSCO, and P. ALAUPOVIC: Effects of medium chain-length triglycerides in hyperchylomicronemia (dietary fat-induced hyperglyceridemia), a type of familial hyperlipemia. J. Lab. clin. Med. 62, 876 (1963).

— — K. LAKSHMI, and L. N. NORCIA: The serum lipids and lipoproteins in normal and hyperlipidemic subjects as determined by preparative ultracentrifugation. Effects of dietary and therapeutic measures. Changes induced by in vitro exposure of serum to sonic forces. Amer. J. clin. Nutr. 9, 73 (1961).

— and C. W. ROBINSON jr. in: "Adipose tissue as an organ", p. 213—222. Ed.: L. W. Kinsell. Springfield (Ill.): Thomas 1962.

— S. S. SANBAR, P. ALAUPOVIC, R. H. BRADFORD, and R. P. HOWARD: Studies of the metabolism of radioiodinated human serum alpha-lipoprotein in normal and hyperlipemic subjects. J. Lab. clin. Med. 63, 193 (1964).

GADRAT, J.: L'hyperlipémie essentielle. Paris: Masson et Cie. 1958.

— A. BAZEX, A. DUPRÉ, et R. DOUSTE-BLAZY: Xanthomes miliaires et très forte hyperlipidémie évoluant enpoussées déclenchées par une alimentation hyperlipidique. "Hyperlipémie essentielle de l'adulte avec éruption secondaire de xanthomes". Bull. Soc. Franç. Derm. Syph. 59, 359 (1952).

GAGE, S. H., and P. A. FISH: Fat digestion, absorption, and assimilation in man and animals as determined by the dark-field microscope, and a fat-soluble dye. Amer. J. Anat. 34, 1 (1924).

GARUNAS, A.: Abdominal pain in essential hyperlipemia. J. Amer. med. Ass. 163, 1135 (1957).

GASKINS, A. L., R. B. SCOTT, and A. D. KESSLER: Report of three cases of idiopathic familial hyperlipemia: Use of ACTH and cortisone. Pediatrics 11, 480 (1953).

Gilbert, J. B., and J. F. Mustard: Some effects of Atromid on plateled economy and blood coagulation in man. J. Atheroscler. Res. 3, 623 (1963).

Gofman, J., F. T. Lindgren, and H. Elliot: Ultracentrifugal studies of lipoproteins of human serum. J. biol. Chem. 179, 973 (1949).

— L. Rubin, J. P. McGinley, and H. B. Jones: Hyperlipoproteinemia. Amer. J. Med. 17, 514 (1954).

Goodman, M., H. Shuman, and S. Goodman: Idiopathic lipemia with secondary xanthomatosis, hepatosplenomegaly, and lipemia retinalis. J. Pediat. 16, 598 (1940).

Gordis, E.: Demonstration of two kinds of fat particles in alimentary lipemia with polyvinylpyrrolidone gradient columns. Proc. Soc. exp. Biol. (N. Y.) 110, 657 (1962).

Gould, R. G., D. R. Avoy, and E. A. Swyryd: Effect of alpha-parachlorophenoxyisobutyrate on cholesterol. Circulation 30, suppl. III, 11 (1964).

Gousios, A., J. M. Felts, and R. J. Havel: The metabolism of serum triglycerides and free fatty acids by the myocardium. Metabolism 12, 75 (1963).

Green, K. G., W. H. W. Inman, and J. M. Thorp: Multi-centre trial of a mixture of ethyl chlorophenoxyisobutyrate and androsterone (Atromid) in the United Kingdom and Ireland: A preliminary report. J. Atheroscler. Res. 3, 593 (1963).

Greig, H. B. W.: Inhibition of fibrinolysis by alimentary lipemia. Lancet 1956/II, 16.

Grossmann, E. E., and J. B. Hitz: Lipemia retinalis associated with essential hyperlipemia. Arch. Ophthal. 40, 570 (1948).

Grütz, O.: Zur Klinik und Histologie des Xanthoms bzw. der anisotropen Verfettung der Haut, nebst Bemerkungen über das Speicherungsvermögen der sog. Xanthomzellen. Arch. Derm. Syph. (Berl.) 150, 137 (1926).

Gustafson, A., P. Alaupovic, and R. H. Furman: Studies of the composition and structure of serum lipoproteins: Isolation, purification, and characterization of very low density lipoproteins of human serum. Biochemistry 4, 596 (1965).

Haensch, R.: Heparin-Therapie und Klinik der idiopathischen hyperlipidämischen Xanthomatose. Arch. klin. exp. Derm. 205, 512 (1958).

Hahn, P. F.: Abolishment of alimentary lipemia following injection of heparin. Science 98, 19 (1943).

Hakimi, P.: Hyperlipémie essentielle. Thèse (Genève) 2287 (1954).

Hales, C. N., and P. J. Randle: Effects of low-carbohydrate diet and diabetes mellitus on plasma concentrations of glucose, nonesterified fatty acid, and insulin during oral glucose-tolerance tests. Lancet 1963/I, 790.

Hamwi, G. J., O. Garcia, F. A. Kruger, G. Gwinup, and D. G. Cornwell: Hyperlipidemia in uncontrolled diabetes. Metabolism 11, 850 (1962).

Harlan, W. R., and D. E. Beischer: Changes in serum lipoproteins after a large fat meal in normal individuals and in patients with ischemic heart disease. Amer. Heart J. 66, 61 (1963).

Harrison, M. T., and D. M. Goldberg: The effect of Atromid in essential hyperlipemia. J. Atheroscler. Res. 3, 561 (1963).

Harslöf, E.: Idiopathic familial hyperlipemia attended with hepatosplenomegaly. Acta med. scand. 130, 140 (1948).

Hatch, F. T., L. L. Abell, and F. E. Kendall: Effect of restriction of dietary fat and cholesterol upon serum lipids and lipoproteins in patients with hypertension. Amer. J. Med. 19, 48 (1955).

Havel, R. J.: Early effects of fasting and of carbohydrate ingestion on lipids and lipoproteins of serum in man. J. clin. Invest. 36, 855 (1957).

— Transport and metabolism of chylomicra. Amer. J. clin. Nutr. 6, 662 (1958).

— Conversion of plasma free fatty acids into triglycerides of plasma lipoprotein fractions in man. Metabolism 10, 1031 (1961).

— H. A. Eder, and J. H. Bragdon: The distribution and chemical composition of ultracentrifugally separated lipoproteins in human serum. J. clin. Invest. 34, 1345 (1955).

— J. M. Felts, and C. M. Van Duyne: Formation and fate of endogenous triglycerides in blood plasma of rabbits. J. Lipid Res. 3, 297 (1962).

— and D. S. Fredrickson: The metabolism of chylomicra. I. The removal of palmitic acid-1-C[14] labeled chylomicra from dog plasma. J. clin. Invest. 35, 1025 (1956).

— and A. Goldfien: The role of the liver and of extrahepatic tissues in the transport and metabolism of fatty acids and triglycerides in the dog. J. Lipid. Res. 2, 389 (1961).

— and R. S. Gordon: Idiopathic hyperlipemia: Metabolic studies in an affected family. J. clin. Invest. 39, 1777 (1960).

Hellems, H. K., and T. J. Regan: The influence of postprandial lipemia on myocardial blood flow and metabolism. Amer. Coll. Physiol. Proc. 41st Annual Session, April 1960 (cit. by Brown et. al. 1961).

HELLMAN, L., B. ZUMOFF, G. KESSLER, E. KARA, I. L. RUBIN, and R. S. ROSENFELD: Reduction of cholesterol and lipids in man by ethyl p-chlorophenoxyisobutyrate. Ann. intern. Med. **59**, 477 (1963).

HERBST, F. S. M., W. F. LEVER, and N. A. HURLEY: Idiopathic hyperlipemic and primary hypercholesteremic xanthomatosis. VI. Studies of the serum proteins and lipoproteins by moving boundary electrophoresis and paper electrophoresis before and after administration of heparin. J. invest. Derm. **24**, 507 (1955).

HEWSON, W.: cit. from S. H. GAGE, and P. A. FISH. Amer. J. Anat. **34**, 1 (1924).

HEYL, A. G.: Intraocular lipemia. Trans. Amer. Ophth. Soc. **3**, 54 (1880).

HIRSCHHORN, K., R. HIRSCHHORN, M. FRACCARO, and J. A. BÖÖK: Incidence of familial hyperlipemia. Science **129**, 716 (1959).

HOFFMAN, L., and R. GRAYSON: Primary hyperlipemia. US armed Forces med. J. **3**, 1667 (1952).

HOLLISTER, L. E., and S. L. KANTER: Essential hyperlipemia treated with heparin and with chlorpromazine. Gastroenterology **29**, 1069 (1955).

HOLT, L. E., F. X. AYLWARD, and H. G. TIMBRES: Idiopathic familial lipemia. Bull. John Hopk. Hosp. **64**, 279 (1939).

HOPGOOD, W. C.: Idiopathic hyperlipemia. New Engl. J. Med. **238**, 429 (1948).

HOWARD, R. P., P. ALAUPOVIC, O. J. BRUSCO, and R. H. FURMAN: Effects of ethyl chlorophenoxyisobutyrate, alone or with androsterone (Atromid), on serum lipids, lipoproteins and related metabolic parameters in normal and hyperlipidemic subjects. J. Atheroscler. Res. **3**, 482 (1963).

ISSELBACHER, K. J.: in "Fat as a Tissue", p. 7. Eds.: K. Rodahl, and B. Issekutz. New York: McGraw-Hill Book Co. 1964.

ITTERBEEK, H. E. A. VAN, and L. DELOBEL: Hyperlipemia familialis idiopathica. T. Gastro.-ent. **7**, 52 (1964).

JAHNKE, K.: Symposium on pathophysiological and clinical aspects of lipid metabolism. Heidelberg 1965. G. Schettler (ed.). Stuttgart: Thieme 1966.

JEANRENAUD, B.: Dynamic aspects of adipose tissue metabolism: A review. Metabolism **10**, 535 (1961).

JEPSON, E. M., and D. C. O. JAMES: The treatment of hypercholesterolemic xanthomatosis with Atromid. J. Atheroscler. Res. **3**, 554 (1963).

JOBST, H., u. G. SCHETTLER: Über die chemische Zusammensetzung der Chylomikronen. 3d Int. Conf. biochem. Probl. Lipids, Brüssels 1956.

JOEL, J.: Zur Klinik der Lipämie. Z. Klin. Med. **100**, 46 (1924).

JOYNER, C. L.: Essential hyperlipemia. Ann. intern. Med. **38**, 759 (1953).

JUCHEMS, R., W. GROSS, K. WIDOK, and H. KAFFARNIK: Zur Klinik der essentiellen Hyperlipämie. Münch. med. Wschr. **107**, 328 (1965).

KANE, J. P., C. LONGCOPE, F. C. PAVLATOS, and G. M. GRODSKY: Studies of carbohydrate metabolism in idiopathic hypertriglyceridemia. Metabolism **14**, 471 (1965).

KAY, R. E., and C. ENTENMAN: The synthesis of "chylomicron-like" bodies and maintenance of normal blood sugar levels by the isolated, perfused rat liver. J. biol. Chem. **236**, 1006 (1961).

KESSLER, J. I.: Effect of insulin on release of plasma lipolytic activity and clearing of emulsified fat intravenously administered to pancreatectomized and alloxanized dogs. J. Lab. clin. Med. **60**, 747 (1962).

KINSELL, L. W., G. D. MICHAELS, G. WALKER, S. SPLITTER, and G. FUKAYAMA: An approach to understanding of the gross hyperlipidemic states. Metabolism **11**, 863 (1962).

— and G. SCHLIERF: Alimentary and nonalimentary hyperglyceridemia. Ann. N. Y. Acad. Sci. **131**, 606 (1965).

— — — and R. E. VISINTINE: Studies of patients with hyperglyceridemia. Amer. J. clin. Nutr. **9**, 1 (1961).

KLATSKIN, G., and M. GORDON: Relationship between relapsing pancreatitis and essential hyperlipemia. Amer. J. Med. **12**, 3 (1952).

KNITTLE, J. L., and E. H. AHRENS jr.: Carbohydrate metabolism in two forms of hyperglyceridemia. J. clin. Invest. **43**, 485 (1964).

KNÜCHEL, F.: Das Verhalten der Serumlipide und -lipoproteine unter Verabreichung von Regelan (Äthyl-p-chlorphenoxyisobutyrat). Med. Welt (Berl.) **1964**, 2530.

KONTTINEN, A., and J. PALOHEIMO: The effects of Atromid on serum lipids, proteins, and some liver function reflecting tests in hypercholesteraemic patients. J. Atheroscler. Res. **3**, 525 (1963).

KORN, E. D.: Clearing factor, a heparin-activated lipoprotein lipase. I. Isolation and characterization of the enzyme from normal rat heart. J. biol. Chem. **215**, 1 (1955).

KOSZALKA, M. F., and J. J. LEVIN: Idiopathic hyperlipemia. Ann. intern. Med. **33**, 473 (1950).

Kuo, P. T., and D. R. Bassett: The fat tolerance curves of patients with hyperlipidemia and atherosclerosis. Amer. J. clin. Nutr. 12, 241 (1963).
— — Primary hyperlipidemias and their management. Ann. intern. Med. 59, 495 (1963).
— — Dietary sugar in the production of hyperglyceridemia. Ann. intern. Med. 62, 1199 (1965).
— — A. M. Digeorge, and G. G. Carpenter: Lipolytic activity of post-heparin plasma in hyperlipemia and hypolipemia. Circulat. Res. 16, 221 (1965).
— and J. C. Carson: Dietary factors and diurnal serum triglyceride levels in man. J. clin. Invest. 38, 1384 (1959).
— A. F. Whereat, D. R. Bassett, and E. Staple: Study of the mechanism of hyperlipemia. Serum chylomicron fatty acid patterns of hyperlipemic patients before and after the ingestion of different food fats. Circulation 24, 213 (1961).
— — and O. Horwitz: The effect of lipemia upon coronary and peripheral arterial circulation in patients with essential hyperlipemia. Amer. J. Med. 26, 68 (1959).
Lasch, H. G., W. Kahlke, H. H. Sessner u. K. Schimpf: Zum Wirkungsmechanismus von alimentärem Fett auf die Faktoren der Blutgerinnung, in: „Gefäßwand und Blutplasma", Symposion Magdeburg 1959, R. Emmrich u. E. Perlick (eds.). Jena: Fischer 1960.
Lees, R. S., and D. S. Fredrickson: Use of paper electrophoresis in the diagnosis and study of hyperglyceridemia. Circulation 30, suppl. III, 20 (1964).
— — Carbohydrate induction of hyperlipemia in normal man. Clin. Res. 13, 327 (1965).
— and F. T. Hatch: Sharper separation of lipoprotein species by paper electrophoreses in albumin-containing buffer. J. Lab. clin. Med. 61, 518 (1963).
Lepard, C. W.: Lipemia retinalis in the nondiabetic patient. Albrecht v. Graefes Arch. Ophthal. 32, 37 (1944).
Lever, W. F., F. S. M. Herbst, and N. A. Hurley: Idiopathic hyperlipemia and primary hypercholesteremic xanthomatosis. IV. Effect of prolonged administration of heparin on serum lipids in idiopathic hyperlipemia. Arch. Derm. 71, 150 (1955).
— and E. Klein: The inhibition of lipemia clearing by hyperlipemic serum. J. invest. Derm. 29, 465 (1957).
— — Idiopathic hyperlipemia and primary hypercholesteremic xanthomatosis: a group of four cases. Arch. Derm. 77, 461 (1958).
— P. A. J. Smith, and N. A. Hurley: Idiopathic hyperlipemic and primary hypercholesterolemic xanthomatosis. I. Clinical data and analysis of the plasma lipids. J. invest. Derm. 22, 33 (1954).
Levy, B. M.: Idiopathic lipemia. J. Pediat. 29, 376 (1946).
Losowsky, M. S., D. P. Jones, C. S. Davidson, and D. S. Lieber: Studies of alcoholic hyperlipemia and its mechanism. Amer. J. Med. 35, 794 (1963).
Lowgren, E.: Essential hyperlipemia with report of a case including observations before and during pregnancy. Acta med. scand. 142, 71 (1952).
Macdonald, I.: The effects of various dietary carbohydrates on the serum lipids during a five-day regimen. Clin. Sci. 29, 193 (1965).
— and D. M. Braithwaite: The influence of dietary carbohydrates on the lipid pattern in serum and in adipose tissue. Clin. Sci. 27, 23 (1964).
Malmros, H., B. Swahn, and E. Truedson: Essential hyperlipemia. Acta med. scand. 149, 91 (1954).
Marcus, M.: The pancreas and intermediate fat metabolism; observations on disturbance of the fat metabolism with temporary lipemia in acute pancreatic disease. Fol. clin. orient. (Tel-Aviv) 1, 127 (1937); cit. after Klatskin and Gordon (1952).
Martt, J. M., and W. E. Connor: Idiopathic hyperlipemia associated with coronary atherosclerosis. Arch. intern. Med. 97, 492 (1956).
Matras, A.: Hyperlipämische Xanthomatosen und ihre Behandlung mit Heparin. Arch. klin. exp. Derm. 203, 503 (1956).
Movitt, E. R., G. Gerstl, F. Sherwood, and C. C. Epstein: Essential hyperlipemia. Arch. intern. Med. 87, 79 (1951).
Nestel, P. J.: Relationship between plasma triglycerides and removal of chylomicrons. J. clin. Invest. 43, 943 (1964).
— R. J. Havel, and A. Bezman: Extrahepatic removal of chylomicron fatty acids in intact dogs. Fed. Proc. 21, 290 (1962).
— — — Sites of initial removal of chylomicron triglyceride fatty acids from the blood. J. clin. Invest. 41, 1915 (1962).
New, M. I., T. N. Roberts, E. L. Bierman, and G. G. Reader: The significance of blood lipid alterations in diabetes mellitus. Diabetes 12, 208 (1963).
Nichols, A. V., V. Dobbin, and J. W. Gofman: Influence of dietary factors upon human serum lipoprotein concentrations. Geriatrics 12, 7 (1957).
— and L. Smith: Effect of very low-density lipoproteins on lipid transfer in incubated serum. J. Lipid Res. 6, 286 (1965).

NOTHMAN, M. M., and S. PROGER: Cephalins in the blood. J. Amer. med. Ass. **179**, 40 (1962).

O'BRIEN, J. R.: Fat ingestion, blood coagulation and atherosclerosis. Amer. J. med. Sci. **234**, 373 (1957).

OLIVER, M. F.: Reduction of serum-lipid and uric acid levels by an orally active androsterone. Lancet **1962/I**, 1321.

— Further observation on the effect of Atromid and of ethyl chlorophenoxyisobutyrate on serum lipid levels. J. Atheroscler. Res. **3**, 427 (1963).

— S. D. ROBERTS, D. HAYES, J. F. PANTRIDGE, M. M. SUZMAN, and I. BERSOHN: Effect of Atromid and ethyl chlorophenoxyisobutyrate on anticoagulant requirements. Lancet **1963/I**, 143.

OPITZ, H.: Hochgradige Lipämie unklarer Genese bei einem 12jährigen Knaben. Dtsch. med. Wschr. **61**, 88 (1935).

PARONETTO, F., C. WANG, and D. ADLERSBERG: Lipoprotein patterns by starch electrophoresis in idiopathic hyperlipemia and hypercholesteremia. Circulat. Res. **5**, 288 (1957).

PECHAR, J., H. VAVŘINKOVÁ, E. SEGOVÁ u. E. KUHN: Über die Fettbindung der Erythrozyten während der postprandialen Lipämie. Folia haemat. (Lpz.) **77**, 360 (1960).

PFLEGER, L., u. H. TIRSCHEK: Xanthomatose bei idiopathischer Hyperlipämie und Pankreatitis. Wien. klin. Wschr. **68**, 435 (1956).

POULSEN, H. M.: Familial lipemia. A new form of lipidosis showing increase in neutral fats combined with attacks of acute pancreatitis. Acta med. scand. **138**, 413 (1950).

RANDLE, P. J., C. N. HALES, P. B. GARLAND, and E. A. NEWSHOLME: The glucose fatty-acid cycle. Its role in insulin sensitivity and the metabolic disturbances of diabetes mellitus. Lancet **1963/I**, 785.

RAUSEN, A. R., and D. ADLERSBERG: Idiopathic (hereditary) hyperlipemia and hypercholesterolemia in children. Pediatrics **28**, 276 (1961).

REAVEN, G. M., J. W. FARQUHAR, L. B. SALANS, R. C. GROSS, and R. M. WAGNER: Carbohydrate-induced lipemia. Clin. Res. **12**, 277 (1964).

— A. FRANK, R. GROSS, L. SALANS, and J. FARQUHAR: Glucose and insulin metabolism in carbohydrate-induced lipemia. Clin. Res. **13**, 332 (1965).

RODBELL, M., D. S. FREDRICKSON, and K. ONO: Metabolism of chylomicron proteins in the dog. J. biol. Chem. **234**, 576 (1959).

— and R. O. SCOW: Metabolism of chylomicrons and triglyceride emulsions by perfused rat adipose tissue. Amer. J. Physiol. **208**, 106 (1965).

ROHN, R., C. H. GANDEK, and M. BARTLEY: Severe hyperlipemia associated with non-diabetic pregnancy, report of case. Arch. intern. Med. **82**, 339 (1948).

RONY, H. R., and T. T. CHING: Studies on fat metabolism. II. The effect of certain hormones on fat transport. Endocrinology **14**, 355 (1930).

ROSENMAN, R. H., and M. FRIEDMAN: Effect of acute and chronic administration of heparin on plasma lipids in idiopathic hyperlipemia. Fed. Proc. **13**, 121 (1954).

SANBAR, S. S., A. J. ZWEIFLER, and F. J. CONWAY: Carbohydrate metabolism in essential hyperlipidemia. Circulation **30**, suppl. III, 27 (1964).

SCHAPIRO, R. H., R. L. SCHEIG, G. D. DRUMMEY, J. H. MENDELSON, and K. J. ISSELBACHER: Effect of prolonged ethanol ingestion on the transport and metabolism of lipids in man. New. Engl. J. Med. **272**, 610 (1965).

SCHETTLER, G.: Zur Wirkung der lipotropen Substanzen. Klin. Wschr. **1952**, 627.

— Lipidosen, in: Handbuch der Inneren Medizin, Bd. VII, Teil 2, p. 609—778. Berlin-Göttingen-Heidelberg: Springer 1955.

— Essentielle Hyperlipämie und Arteriosklerose. In: Arteriosklerose. Ed. G. Schettler. Stuttgart: Thieme 1961.

— M. EGGSTEIN u. H. JOBST: Die essentielle Hyperlipämie. Dtsch. med. Wschr. **83**, 1 (1958).

— G. W. LÖHR u. E. STEIN: Die Bedeutung der essentiellen Hyperlipämie und Hypercholesterinämie für die Entstehung von Herzinfarkten. Dtsch. med. Wschr. **82**, 610 (1957).

SCHIRREN, C.: Hyperlipidämische Xanthomatosen. Hautarzt **8**, 119 (1957).

SCHLIERF, G., and L. W. KINSELL: Effects of insulin in hyperglyceridemia. Proc. Soc. exp. Biol. (N. Y.) **120**, 272 (1965).

SCHÖN, H., G. BERG u. C. WIEDMANN: Untersuchungen über die medikamentöse Beeinflußbarkeit der hyperlipämischen Atherosklerose. Med. u. Ernähr. **4**, 233 (1963).

SCHRADE, W., G. BECKER u. E. BÖHLE: Das Krankheitsbild der idiopathischen Hyperlipämie. Dtsch. Arch. klin. Med. **201**, 344 (1954).

— R. BIEGLER u. E. BÖHLE: Die Veränderungen der essentiellen Fettsäuren des Blutes bei verschiedenen Krankheiten, ihre Bewertung und ihre Bedeutung für die Ernährung. Schweiz. med. Wschr. **89**, 117 (1959).

— E. BÖHLE, and R. BIEGLER: Humoral changes in arteriosclerosis. Investigation on lipids, fatty acids, ketone bodies, pyruvic acid, lactic acid, and glucose in the blood. Lancet **1960/II**, 1409.

488   L. W. KINSELL, G. SCHLIERF, W. KAHLKE and G. SCHETTLER:

SCHULTZE, W. H.: Über großzellige Hyperplasie der Milz bei Hyperlipoidämie. Verh. dtsch. path. Ges. 15, 47 (1912).

SECKFORT, H., u. O. BRAUN-FALCO: Acetalphosphatide bei xanthomatösen Erkrankungen. Klin. Wschr. 1957, 866.

SHAH, S., V. POMEROY, and L. W. KINSELL: Glyceride and fatty acid response to fat intake in normal and abnormal subjects. Metabolism 12, 887 (1963).

SHAPIRO, B.: Lipid dynamics in adipose tissue. In: "Progress in the chemistry of fats"; vol. 4. London: Pergamon Press 1957.

SHIPP, J. C., and J. F. MUNROE: Effects of sulfonurea compounds on hyperlipemia and hypercholesterolemia in patients with minimal impairment of glucose tolerance. Diabetes 11, 69 (1962).

SHORE, S. C., and V. SCHRIRE: A possible case of idiopathic hyperlipemia. Clin. Proc. 6, 139 (1947).

SIGSTAD, H.: A family with mild diabetes mellitus, hyperlipemia and atherosclerosis. Acta med. scand. 177, 465 (1965).

SKIPSKI, V. P., R. F. PETERSON, and M. BARCLAY: Separation of phosphatidyl ethanolamine, phosphatidyl serine, and other phospholipids by thin layer chromatography. J. Lipid Res. 3, 467 (1962).

SMITH, E. B.: Lipoprotein patterns in myocardial infarction. Relationship between the components identified by paper electrophoresis and in the ultracentrifuge. Lancet 1957/II, 910.

SOFFER, A., and M. MURRAY: Relationship of essential hyperlipemia to premature atherosclerosis. Circulation 10, 611 (1954).

STRISOWER, E. H.: The response of hyperlipoproteinemias to Atromid and ethyl chlorophenoxyisobutyrate. J. Atheroscler. Res. 3, 445 (1963).

— and B. STRISOWER: The separate hypolipoproteinemic effects of dextrothyroxine and ethyl chlorophenoxyisobutyrate. J. clin. Endocr. 24, 139 (1964).

SWAHN, B.: Studies on blood lipids. Scand. J. clin. Lab. Invest. 5, Suppl. 9 (1953).

SWANK, R. L.: Effects of fat on blood viscosity in dogs. Circulat. Res. 4, 579 (1956).

THANNHAUSER, S. J.: Lipidoses: Diseases of the cellular lipid metabolism. New York: Oxford Press 1950.

— Lehrbuch des Stoffwechsels und der Stoffwechselkrankheiten. 2. Aufl. N. Zöllner (ed.). Stuttgart: Thieme 1957.

— Lipidoses, Diseases of the Intracellular Lipid Metabolism. 3d edition. New York: Grune and Stratton 1958.

— and H. MAGENDANTZ: The different clinical groups of xanthomatous diseases; a clinical physiological study of 22 cases. Ann. intern. Med. 11, 1662 (1938).

— and H. REINSTEIN: Fatty changes in the liver from different causes. Arch. Path. 33, 646 (1942).

THORP, J. M.: An experimental approach to the problem of disordered lipid metabolism. J. Atheroscler. Res. 3, 351 (1963).

— and W. S. WARING: Modification of metabolism and distribution of lipids by ethyl chlorophenoxyisobutyrate. Nature (Lond.) 194, 948 (1962).

TRENCKMANN, H.: Idiopathische Hyperlipidämie mit coronaren und peripheren Durchblutungsstörungen. Ärztl. Wschr. 11, 423 (1956).

TROUP, S. B., C. F. REED, G. V. MARINETTI, and S. N. SWISHER: Thromboplastic factors in platelets and red blood cells: Observations on their chemical nature and function in in vitro coagulation. J. clin. Invest. 39, 342 (1960).

TYSON, J.: A treatise on Bright's disease and diabetes, p. 267. Philadelphia: Lindsay and Blakiston 1881.

UZAWA, H., G. SCHLIERF, S. CHIRMAN, G. MICHAELS, P. WOOD, and L. W. KINSELL: Hyperglyceridemia resulting from intake of medium chain triglycerides. Amer. J. clin. Nutr. 15, 365 (1964).

VAUGHAN, M.: The metabolism of adipose tissue in vitro. J. Lipid Res. 2, 293 (1961).

WADDELL, W. R., R. P. GEYER, N. HURLEY, and F. J. STARE: Abnormal carbohydrate metabolism in patients with hypercholesterolemia and hyperlipemia. Metabolism 7, 707 (1958).

WAKIL, S. J., and R. BRESSLER: Fatty acid metabolism and ketone body formation. Metabolism 11, 742 (1962).

WALKER, W. J., E. Y. LAWRY, D. E. LOVE, G. V. MANN, S. A. LEVINE, and F. J. STARE: Effect of weight reduction and caloric balance on serum lipoprotein and cholesterol levels. Amer. J. Med. 14, 654 (1953).

WALTON, K. W., P. J. SCOTT, J. V. JONES, R. F. FLETCHER, and T. WHITE-HEAD: Studies on low-density lipoprotein turnover in relation to Atromid therapy. J. Atheroscler. Res. 3, 396 (1963).

WARREN, S., and H. F. ROOT: Lipoid containing cells in the spleen in diabetes with lipemia. Amer. J. Path. **2**, 69 (1926).

WIJNHAUSEN, O. J.: Über Xanthomatose in einem Fall rezidivierender Pankreatitis. Klin. Wschr. **58**, 1268 (1921).

WILKINSON jr., C. F.: Spaced fat feeding: A régime of management for familial hyperlipemia. Ann. intern. Med. **45**, 674 (1956).

WOLFSON, W. Q., C. COHN, R. LEVINE, E. F. ROSENBERG, and H. D. HUNT: Liver function and serum protein structure in gout. Ann. intern. Med. **30**, 598 (1949).

WOOD, P., K. IMAICHI, J. KNOWLES, G. MICHAELS, and L. W. KINSELL: The lipid composition of human plasma chylomicrons. J. Lipid Res. **5**, 225 (1964).

— G. SCHLIERF, and L. W. KINSELL: Plasma free oleic and palmitic acid levels during vigorous exercise. Metabolism **14**, 1095 (1965).

ZINN, W. J., and L. A. SCHLEISSNER: The effects of dextrothyroxine in diabetes. Calif. Med. **101**, 240 (1964).

ZÖLLNER, N.: Angeborene Störungen im Stoffwechsel der Lipoide. Gastroenterologia (Basel) **97**, 247 (1962).

Genetic Aspects of Lipidoses

By

W. Fuhrmann

Introduction

The lipidoses, as covered by this book,are inborn errors of metabolism, although some of them may be rather strongly subjected to modification by exogenous influences. Their exact classification depends largely on clinical, morphological, and particularly biochemical criteria. A few years ago only, our knowledge of the biochemistry of this group of disesaes was so insufficient, that e.g. in 1959 HARRIS in his well known work on Human Biochemical Genetics did not include a discussion of disturbances of lipid metabolism. Even to-day, we must admit, our understanding of the basic processes involved is incomplete to the extent that in many of the diseases, which customarily are included among the hereditary disorders of lipid metabolism, because the most obvious abnormalities are to be found in the area of blood lipids or in lipid storage of the tissues, it is not even proved, whether the primary defect is not located in carbohydrate or protein metabolism rather than in lipid metabolism.

Principally two possible approaches can be taken for genetic analyses, the formal analysis of segregation of phenotypes and the study of the metabolic disturbance, trying to come as close as possible to an elucidation of the primary defect, in other words, to find out which primary gene product may be altered or rendered deficient. Neither of these two approaches alone can possibly give us a complete answer. They may only complement each other. The demonstration of the primary gene product alone will not give us any clue about the mode of inheritance of the gene involved, and the formal genetic analysis, on the other hand, will remain inconclusive and incomplete as long as the diagnosis of subgroups of a disease is not established, which specifically in the lipidoses cannot be done without refined biochemical methods.

To avoid tiring reiterations when discussing the various diseases some introductory remarks of more general nature may be permitted.

As every human being possesses a definite morphological individuality which enables us to recognize a person without difficulty he also has a biochemical individuality. This has been demonstrated clearly e.g. by WILLIAMS (1957)(Fig. 1). Studying a multitude of biochemical functions in human beings it can be seen that each may vary within certain limits. Viewed together these variations add up in each person to a typical pattern which can be used to characterize a person as unmistakably as fingerprints may do. As long as these variations do not lead to disturbance of function, they normally will not be noticed and will be considered to be physiological. If, however, a mutation, that is, an alteration of a genetic locus, leads to a definite alteration of the respective primary gene product, then this may cause a metabolic defect resulting in disease in the sense of an inborn error of metabolism.

According to present knowledge primary gene products are peptides which may be used as building stones of proteins which then may exert enzyme function, may serve as transport proteins, or may be used for formation of organ structure.

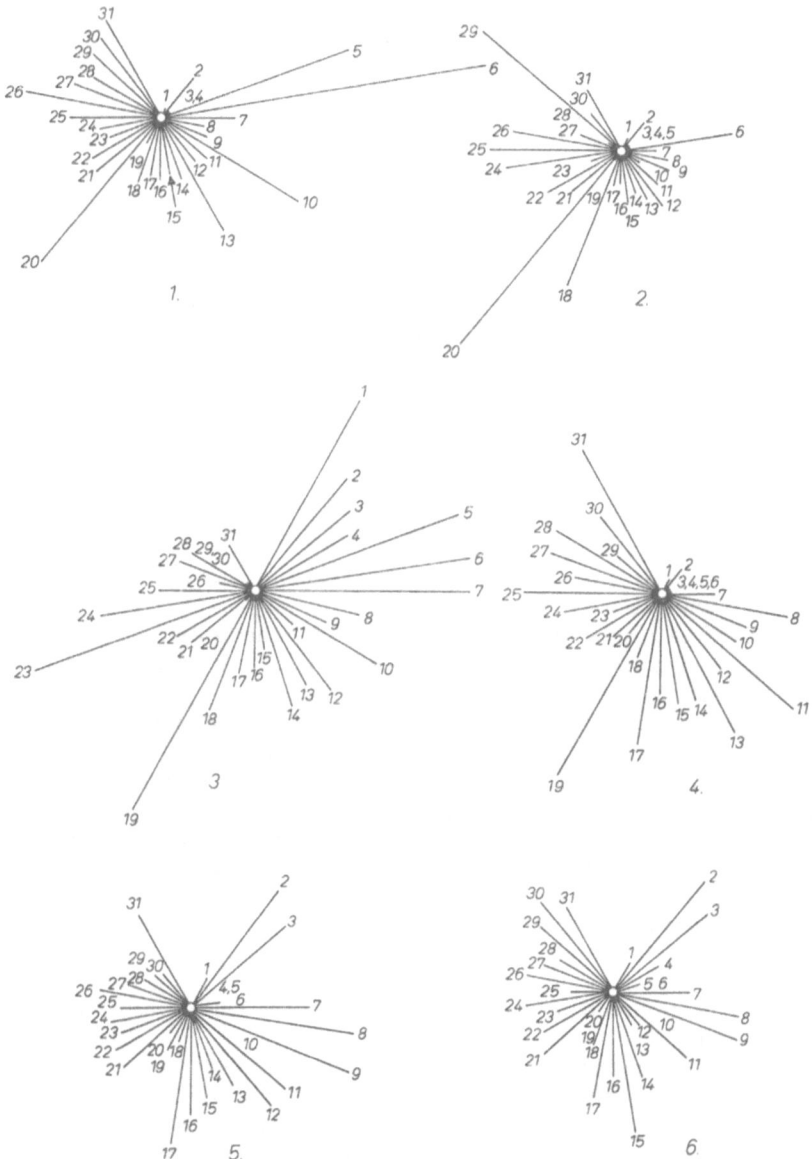

Fig. 1. Individual patterns for humans showing characteristics of taste sensitivities and concentrations of salivary and urinary constituents. The lengths of the polar coordinates indicate the relative amount of the various constituents for each individual. Notice the similarity of the patterns for individual numbers 5. and 6. who are identical twins. *Taste sensitivity:* 1, creatinine; 2, sucrose; 3, KCl; 4, NaCl; 5, HCl. *Salivary constituents:* 6, uric acid; 7, glucose; 8, leucine; 9, valine; 10, citrulline; 11, alanine; 12, lysine; 13, taurine; 14, glycine; 15, serine; 16, glutamic acid; 17, aspartic acid. *Urinary constituents:* 18, citrate; 19, base Rf 0.28; 20, acid Rf 0.32; 21, gonadotropin; 22, pH; 23, pigment/creatinine; 24, chloride/creatinine; 25, hippuric acid/creatinine; 26, creatinine; 27, taurine; 28, glycine; 29, serine; 30, citrulline; 31, alanine. (From WILLIAMS 1957)

While undoubtedly alteration of tissue and organ proteins may change their affinity to certain substances or may cause anomalies of metabolism by other mechanisms, most known examples of such disturbances are linked to altered transport proteins with diminished or lost functions or particularly to deficiencies of enzymes.

Reduced to its simplest model we can describe a metabolic process in the following manner (Fig. 2):

The deficiency of an enzyme may become deleterious by the excess of its substrate not being metabolized or by deficiency of one of the subsequent metabolic products of the pathway. In reality, of course, hardly any metabolic pathway will be as simple and linear. From branching and interrelation of pathways secondary disturbances may result or a block can be compensated for by use of an alternate pathway. A mutationally altered enzyme also could lead to a different product, which as such may cause metabolic trouble.

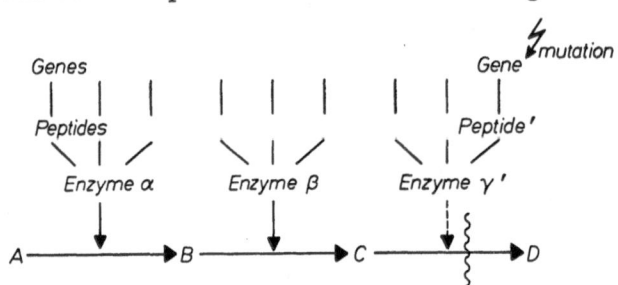

Fig. 2. Metabolic pathway and block, cf. text

Thus a mutation of a gene can act by

a) offsetting of production of an enzyme

b) leading to an enzyme, which possesses a diminished or increased activity due to alteration of one of its peptide chains

c) causing loss of substrate specificity or altering such specificity, and, finally,

d) by producing an altered enzyme which retaines its substrate specificity but catalyzes a different metabolic step.

Of highest practical importance, and by far the most probable results of mutation, are, of course, complete or partial loss of function.

In the sense described, an alteration may affect a gene which carries the information for enzyme structure respectively for a peptide chain, acting as a building stone for an enzyme, a so called structural gene. A mutation may, however, happen at a control gene locus as well (Jacob and Monod 1961), that is, a locus, controlling the activity of one or more structural genes and turning on and off the production of their primary gene products. Such a mutation does not cause the appearance of a qualitatively altered gene product, but only alters the rate of production of the normal gene product. The gene product may disappear or be produced in excess depending on the kind of control gene mutation involved.

Mutation of a structural gene usually will cause production of a qualitatively altered gene product which may or may not display altered enzyme function. Such an enzyme protein may have lost its catalyzing ability completely, but may have retained its immune-specificity, that is to say, it may still react with antibody formed against the intact enzyme and thus could be detected as a cross reacting material (CRM). Demonstration of CRM in the absence of detectable enzyme function may be considered proof of a mutation of a structural gene locus and definite disproof of a control gene mutation. If, however, CRM cannot be found, then one condition for acceptance of a control gene mutation is fullfilled, but no proof of a control gene mutation is furnished, for a structural gene mutation also can lead to complete absence of peptide formation or to an alteration, establishing loss of immune-specificity as well. Synchronous and coordinated forward- and back-mutation of several enzymes depending on one controller gene would be proof for mutation at a control gene locus and has been demonstrated in microorganisms. No such observations are available in humans. Extending the control gene hypothesis as developed in microbiology to biology of man should be done with great caution as long as specific proof is lacking and more conventional hypotheses offer acceptable explanations (CH. J. EPSTEIN 1964).

Another conceivable cause of metabolic disturbance could be formation of an inhibitor which also may be under genetic control.

A block of a metabolic pathway leading from a substrate A to a final product D in different individuals may depend on an identical mutation at the same specific gene locus. The disease then would be identical in those individuals, as for example usually would be the case, if we were dealing with cases of a dominant hereditary character appearing within the same family. Here we can expect that all pathological genes could be traced to one mutational event in the common ancestor. It could be, too, that in different individuals different mutations occur at the same gene locus. In other words, the same enzyme may be altered, but in different ways. Since genes at the same locus are called alleles, there then exist, the normal allele included, more than one allele for the same locus. This phenomenon usually is referred to as multiple allelism. The different alleles can be differentiated only if they alter the function of the enzyme as coded by the normal allele and if they do this in a different fashion. Depending on the specific mutational change, the (coincidental) combination of such differentially mutated genes may in some cases lead to distinguishable phenotypes.

Within the same pathway disturbances may occur in various metabolic steps. For example, the enzyme α or the enzyme β may be altered. The result then will depend on what determines the character of the disease, the lack of the endproduct or the accumulation of a specific metabolite respectively which one, and, furthermore, on whether there are alternate pathways available. The mutations thus may lead to clinically distinct pathology or to apparently the same disease. The latter case would represent an example of heterogeny. If an enzyme consists of two or more genetically determined peptide chains, which are coded independently by different gene loci, then heterogeny may be caused by mutations at any one of these loci.

Existence of heterogeny may be proved by detection of different primary biochemical defects in individuals stricken with the disease. In other cases it can be detected, if the disease can be shown to follow different modes of inheritance in various families. This is most obvious, if e.g. one type with sex-linked inheritance can be found, where location of the mutated gene on the X-chromosome is prerequisite, and for another type autosomal inheritance can be proved. (As examples Pelizaeus-Merzbacher's disease or the mucopolysaccharidoses may serve.)

Proof for heterogeny would be established, too, when two parents, being homozygously affected for a recessive character, produce normal and heterozygotic offspring, because they then obviously must be homozygous at different gene loci. Still another possibility to detect heterogeny is the detailed clinical analysis and demonstration of a clearly distinguishable variability in the course of the disease, showing the same pattern within certain families. Here, however, possible effects of modifyer genes, must be thought of these being genes which modify the effect of the studied genes, whose major effect, however, is not concerned with the character in question. Since, generally, we must assume an interaction of the various genes within the genome, such modifying effects are the rule rather than the exception. If larger sibships are available for analysis, however, the same modifying genes will not be present in all affected persons in the same manner. A high degree of constancy of a special clinical course within this sibship, therefore, will argue strongly in favor of heterogeny or multiple allelism.

With the exception of the sex chromosomes in the male, and disregarding chromosomal anomalies, each chromosome possesses an homologous partner. That is, each locus normally is represented twice. The genetic information of each locus, therefore, is present in each cell in double dose. If a mutation occurs in one chromosome, there still remains the unaltered genetic information available, being present in the other, the "normal" allele. If the effect of a given mutation consists in the defect of e.g. an enzyme, then the production of the normal enzyme will continue as determined by the matrix of the "healthy" allele. The pathological gene, therefore, in a single dose will not produce a recognizable defect and is called recessive. If, however, the mutated gene induces notable pathology e.g. by production of an altered gene product, which by itself exerts some detrimental effect, being manifest even in the presence of the normal allele, as may be effected by competitive inhibition or catalyzing of an abnormal metabolic pathway, it is considered dominant. Simplified in such a way, the effects of dominance and recessivity seem easy to explain. In reality things are not as simple. While in one group of heterozygotes the produced amount or activity of an enzyme corresponds to about half of that formed in the normal homozygote, in other hereditary defects of protein synthesis the concentration of the respective proteins in the heterozygotes approaches normal values. The regulatory mechanisms involved here are incompletely understood, particularly in higher organisms (Harris 1964, Markert 1964, Paigen 1964).

Complete dominance in its strictest definition is present only if the effects of a mutation are indistinguishable, whether the mutated gene is present in single dose or in double dose. If the phenotype of the heterozygote, possessing the mutated gene in single dose, displays less deviation from normal than the homozygote, then by this definition the mutation should be called incompletely dominant. In most rare dominant hereditary diseases we don't know the phenotype of homozygotes. It, therefore, has become customary to apply the term dominance, whenever the heterozygote deviates distinctly from the phenotype of the normal homozygotes. A gene is dominant or recessive only in respect to a certain allele in question. Moreover, the classification to a high degree depends on methods applied.

A gene producing disease only when present in double dose and, therefore, according to classical terminology classified as recessive, should logically be called incompletely recessive, if in heterozygous state it induces minor alterations, recognizable only by means of specific methods or (loading-) tests. A better term appears to be recessive with detectability of heterozygotes.

If the phenotype of heterozygotes is intermediate between both types of homozygotes, it would be equally justified to call the respective gene incompletely recessive as incompletely dominant and this has been done, depending whether the gene in question originally had been considered recessive or dominant. To avoid confusion, the uniform use of the term "incomplete dominant" for such genes is to be preferred.

Two other terms might need an explanation, too: incomplete penetrance refers to the phenomenon that genes which ordinarily behave as dominants occasionally may not manifest at all in a few known heterozygotes. Variable expressivity, on the other hand, implies that individuals heterozygous for the same gene, may display the phenotypical character to a variable degree.

It is not intended to recapitulate the features of the classical monogenic modes of inheritance as first analysed by Mendel. One point, however, may be emphasized, because even the most recent medical literature frequently contains erroneous ideas: The fact that many "sporadic" cases of a certain disease may be observed, among whose sibs or other relatives no similar pathology can be found, does not argue against causation of this disease by heredity in general and also not in the particular case. Assuming autosomal recessive transmission, as may be observed in most hereditary enzyme defects, and further assuming prevalence of small sibships, frequent occurrence of apparently isolated cases, indeed, must be expected. Affected individuals as a rule spring from the mating of two heterozygotes. The chance of any child of such parents being affected is 1/4, according to the segregation ratio of offspring of such parents (Fig. 3).

If we consider families with two children each, as commonly found nowadays, the combination of the probabilities permits the prediction that only $1/4 \times 1/4 = 1/16$ of such families with both parents heterozygous will produce two affected infants. In $2 \times 1/4 \times 3/4 = 6/16$ only one affected child will appear, and the remaining $3/4 \times 3/4 = 9/16$ of such families will have two healthy children alone and therefore, will not be recognized. Thus, of seven affected children only one could be expected to have an affected sib. Considering families with three children it can be calculated in the same fashion, using the general formula $(a + b)^n$, where n is the total number of children of

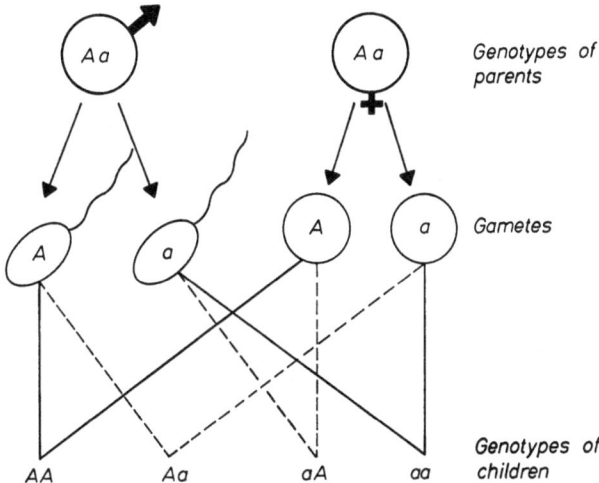

Fig. 3. Segregation of offspring of two heterozygotes

each family, that in 10 of 64 families 2 or 3 affected children are to be expected. 27 of 64 families of this size and with both parents heterozygous would have only one affected child. If the population would consist of two- and three-child-families in equal parts, two thirds of the observed cases would appear "sporadic", even though all of these cases were caused by homozygosity of the same recessive gene.

Particularly in the case of very rare diseases in such sporadic cases consanguinity of the parents may indicate autosomal recessive inheritance. This, of course, is based on the fact, that the rarer a mutation is, the smaller must be its chance of achieving homozygosity by random combination with another gene mutated in the same manner. Considering the extreme possibility that a specific mutation occurred only once in a population, it is clear that here homozygosity can occur only by consanguineous matings in the broadest sense. In completely dominant hereditary disease sporadic cases can be expected as the consequence of new mutations only. This must occur particularly frequently if the fertility of the affected individuals is severely impaired or even abolished.

Monogenic mendelian modes of inheritance in their classical forms will cause a distribution of the population in two or three alternative classes as, for example, affected and non-affected or affected, moderately affected, and non-affected corresponding to the two classes of homozygotes and, where distinguishable, the phenotype of the heterozygotes. If we are dealing with metric, quantitative characters, then each of these classes will be distributed around a mean value in a fashion somewhat similar to a Gaussian curve. When combined, the resulting distribution will be bimodal or trimodal. Bi- or trimodality will be recognizable, however, only if the sizes of the classes are big enough and the mean values of the respective

distributions are sufficiently different (Harris and Smith 1947/1949). A unimodal distribution thus does not exclude simple mendelian inheritance. Uni-
modality on the other hand is typical of the majority of all normal metric characters. It is to be expected always, when a character is determined not by a single
pair of genes, but by a few or even many cooperating genes. We then speak of
multifactorial inheritance. The analysis of this most common mode of transmission
is complicated further by the fact that the contributions of the single genes
are not necessarily equally important and simply additive (as would establish
polygenic inheritance in the strict sense according to Darlington and Mather)
and, moreover, their effect may vary towards the extremes of the distribution
curve. Within a multifactorial system a character may manifest itself only,
if a certain threshold is reached or surpassed (threshold effect). In special cases,
once a threshold is passed, a circulus vitiosus may start, leading to a self
enforcement of a character. Some genes acting in a multifactorial system may
exert a varying degree of dominance. If these become very powerful, then for
practical purposes the results may closely resemble the expected values for
simple dominant mendelian transmission. These facts will have to be kept in mind
e.g. when discussing the genetics of hypercholesterolemia.

In a large number of autosomal recessive inborn errors of metabolism it
depends on the methods used, whether heterozygotes can be recognized or not.
Using improved modern technique it sometimes is possible to directly measure a
diminished enzyme activity or demonstrate a pathologically altered enzyme function. More frequently heterozygotes can be differentiated from normal homozygotes by finding an increased concentration of some metabolic precursor or at times
by proving a diminished concentration of the products of the blocked metabolic
step. Sometimes a substance, not normally present, can be found as the result of an
altered enzyme function or use of an alternate pathway.

Particularly these indirect methods quite often do not permit suffcient differentiation between the heterozygotes and normals, unless some additional strain is
applied in the form of loading tests or the like, where the capacity of the studied
system is challenged to its limit.

Depending on their resolving power such studies can be of value in various ways.
Quite often the overlap between normals and heterozygotes is too big, to permit
a definite judgement in a single case. Such tests still may prove of high theoretical
importance when used in a statistical way.

If the separation of the particular groups is sufficiently complete to classify
single individuals reliably, such tests are of great value for the genetic analysis,
genetic counselling, early diagnosis of possible offspring of heterozygotes, and,
in as much as the heterozygotes may carry a certain morbidity risk themselves, for the commencement of preventive measures such as, for example, suitable
diet and so on. The example of hypercholesterolemia discussed later (chapter III b)
demonstrates the importance of distinguishing between heterozygous and homozygous affected individuals in a sibship.

Having recapitulated some basic genetic knowledge we now may turn to the
specific hereditary defects of lipid metabolism. The discussion of their genetics also
must be related to the basic biochemical defects of the various disorders. In this
section biochemical and clinical findings shall, however, be mentioned only insofar
as this is necessary to characterize certain subgroups and special forms. Their
detailed discussion will be reserved for the specific chapters.

For the discussion of their genetics the various diseases will be grouped in the
following order:

I. Sphingolipidoses
  a) Sphingomyelinoses (Niemann-Pick disease)
  b) Gangliosidoses (amaurotic family idiocies)
  c) Cerebrosidoses (Gaucher's disease)

II. Other rare lipidoses
  a) Leucodystrophies
  b) Familial cholesterolosis with defect of high density lipoproteins (Tangier disease)
  c) A-β-lipoproteinemia
  d) Heredopathia atactica polyneuritiformis (Refsum's syndrome)
  e) Further rare defects of lipid metabolism

III. Essential familial hyperlipidemias
  a) Essential familial hyperlipemias
  b) Essential familial hypercholesterolemia

IV. Other diseases commonly grouped with the lipidoses
  a) Mucopolysaccharidoses (lipochondrodystrophy, gargoylism)
  b) Hand-Schüller-Christian's disease.

I. The Sphingolipidoses

Sphingolipidoses are characterized by storage of specific sphingolipids. It seemed natural, to assume that each of the diseases included here derived from the mutation of one gene and in consequence the alteration of a specific enzyme. This original concept requires some enlargement, since it can be shown that each of these originally described classical diseases can be subgrouped by clinical, genetic or biochemical criteria. The recently developed refined preparative and analytical methods justify the expectation that subgrouping will be carried further, and particularly, that special disease entities which now are separated by clinical means only may eventually be based on proved biochemical differences.

a) Sphingomyelinoses

(Niemann-Pick Disease)

The analysis of the disease is complicated, since an absolutly certain differentiation from other similar storage diseases depends on biochemical and histological proof. In a large number of cases from the literature, therefore, the diagnosis is questionable. The early death of affected individuals and the rarity of the disease are further obstacles. There is general agreement among the authors that transmission is autosomal recessive. In other words the affected are homozygous for the pathological gene.

Available family data corroborate this statement (Fig. 4). Some 80 to 100 proven cases can be found in the literature. In about 30% affected siblings have

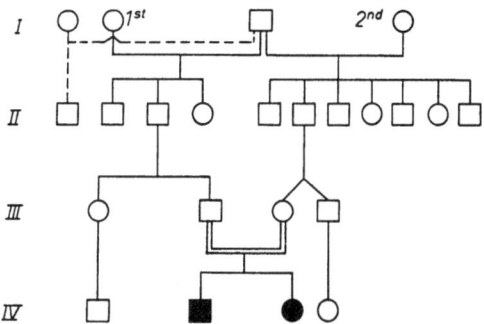

Fig. 4. Siblings with Niemann Pick disease as a result of a consanguineous marriage. (The parents are half-first cousins). (Observation of Ivemark)

been observed (Videbaek 1947). Freudenberg (1938) and Tourtelotte et al. (1962) each described one pair of monozygous twins concordant for the disease. Consanguinity of parents is not mentioned in the literature so frequently as would be expected in such a rare recessive disorder. Two explanations can be proposed. Reports are scattered widely in the literature, and many authors possibly did not pay enough attention to this specific question in the anamnesis of their patients. Moreover, the distribution of the mutant genes is not random and equal. The estimate of gene frequency, calculated from the above mentioned number of cases to be 0.001 to 0.01, therefore, does not describe the facts correctly. Of 91 cases collected from the literature Pfändler (1964) found 35 to be Jewish, 38 non-Jewish and 18 of unspecified origin. The corresponding accumulation of the gene for Niemann-Pick's disease in the Jewish population may, of course, facilitate the occurrence of homozygous children in non-consanguineous marriages.

Besides several variants of the classical infantile form of the disorder have been described which probably represent genetically distinct subgroups. Within the infantile form in a group of affected individuals the cherry-red spot of the macula may appear unusually late or may be missing. In these patients the disease manifests at a later age and their ethnic distribution seems different (Videbaek 1949, Crocker and Farber 1958). Another variant has been described in a genetic isolate of French catholics in Nova Scotia only. Here the typical biochemical and histological signs of the disease could be demonstrated, but the course of the disease was unusually protracted (Crocker and Farber 1958). In another subgroup the disease does not make its appearance before adult age. There is a notable lack of neurologic findings and prevalent parenchymatous infiltration of the lungs by lipid material. This particular type has been described by Pfändler (1946) in two brothers. A case of Terry (1954) probably belongs to the same variety.

The various forms of manifestation and clinical course strongly suggest heterogeny of Niemann-Pick's disease. To date, however, no biochemical differences in the stored lipid material could be detected (Dawson 1960, Ansell and Spanner 1961). This by itself is no argument against heterogeny, since in Niemann-Pick's disease no structurally abnormal lipids have been found anyhow, but all anomalies were quantitative in nature. The basic defect may rather lie in a faulty degeneration of sphingomyelin.

In these obviously still rarer subgroups consanguinity should be particularly frequent, but apparently has not been observed. If thus genetically described subforms of Niemann-Pick's disease may be discussed, heterogeny cannot be considered proved to-date.

Another insufficiently answered problem is posed by the obvious frequency of such a detrimental gene within the Jewish population. The discussion of this problem will be referred until the end of the chapter of amaurotic family idiocy, where the same phenomenon was observed to be even more pronounced.

Pfändler (1964) claims that heterozygotes can be diagnosed from "microsymptoms" or "rudimentary manifestation" in the serum. In two sibships observed by him he found in some of the clinically healthy relatives of affected individuals an increased concentration of total serum fatty acids and inorganic phosphorus. The appearance of vacuolated mononuclear cells in the peripheral blood of parents of affected children also has been claimed to be a manifestation in heterozygotes. This phenomenon, as mentioned by Ivemark (1963), referring to Rayner (1962), in Niemann-Pick's disease cannot be considered specific, and its causation by the pathologic gene in single dose is not proved. The latter findings have been discussed in detail by Spiegel-Adolf et al. (1962) and by Myrian-

THOPOULOS (1962). Large storage cells (15—45 μ) with coarse vacuolated plasma have been demonstrated in the bone-marrow of heterozygous parents by WIEDE-MANN et al. (1965).

b) Gangliosidoses

1. Infantile Amaurotic Family Idiocy

Differentiation of infantile amaurotic family idiocy (Tay-Sachs' disease), the late infantile and the juvenile form of the disease, and of Niemann-Pick's disease on clinical and morphological grounds alone may become difficult. Nevertheless, to-day, the infantile amaurotic family idiocy (Tay Sachs) constitutes a biochemically, clinically and genetically clearly defined entity. The disease is transmitted by an autosomal recessive gene. It regularly becomes manifest in the homozygotes and affects both sexes alike. There is general agreement in all statistics that infantile amaurotic idiocy is much more frequent among children of Jewish parents than among non-Jews. Among Jews it is to be found in a definitely higher rate among those of Eastern European descent (Ashkenazi) than among Jews of Western European extraction (Sephardi).

According to presently available studies (e.g. ARONSON et al. 1960) clinical, pathologic and biochemical findings are alike in patients of different racial background. It, therefore, can be inferred that in all of them a mutation at the same gene locus forms the basis of the disease. This is further corroborated by two cases recorded by MYRIANTHOPOULOS, which derived from matings of one Jewish and one non-Jewish parent. The same author states that in his series of 89 cases from 83 families in the USA about one third came from non-Jewish families. Among 219 cases from 189 sibships of ARONSON and VOLK, collected mainly from the area of New York City, only about 10% had no Jewish ancestors, three were Negroes.

Studies on the frequency of the disease, attempting to detect all cases that occurred in a given time interval within a certain geographic area, referable to a given population base, were undertaken in the USA. For New York City KOZINN et al. (1957) arrived at an estimate of 1 in 8300 Jewish and 1 in 450000 non-Jewish births. The corresponding estimates of frequency of heterozygotes was 0.022 or about 1:50 among Jews and about 1:300 in non-Jews. ARONSON and VOLK (1962) calculated from their results for the New York area the frequency of heterozygotes to be 0.031 or about 1:30 in Jews corresponding to the respective gene frequency of 0.016. They viewed their estimate to be conservative. MYRIANTHOPOULOS (1962) collecting all children born in the USA betwen 1954 and 1957 who died from Tay-Sachs' disease, found a disease frequency of 1:6000 in Jews and 1:500000 in non-Jews. The corresponding gene frequencies were 0.0126 in Jews and 0.00132 in non-Jews, the respective frequencies of heterozygotes 0.0248 or 1:40 in Jews and 0.00264 or 1:380 in persons of non-Jewish background. Studies conducted by GOLDSCHMIDT in Israel (1956) led to estimates of a disease frequency of 1:3000 for Jews of Eastern European descent (Ashkenazi), whereas the disease frequency for all other Jewish groups was much lower, probably in the range calculated for non-Jewish populations, the small number of cases precluded a definite statement for the latter groups.

Further information regarding geographic origin of the ancestors of their cases have been sought by ARONSON and VOLK. In 95.3% of their patients the grand-parents came from Eastern Europe as did 92% of the grandparents of a Jewish control group now living in the same area. In 4.3% of patients whose grandparents were said to come from Western Europe with one exception within the last two

generations ancestors on father's and mother's sides were derived from Eastern
Europe. Among the birthplaces of these ancestors the towns and provinces of
Lida, Grodno, Vilno, Kowno, Panevezys, and Kapsukas were quoted in a large
number of cases. These are neighbouring territories in the North-eastern parts of
Poland, the adjacent Southern part of Lithuania and Byelorussia. Whereas 44.7%
of the grandparents of patients with Tay-Sachs' disease came from these areas,
only 25.7% of the ancestors of the control group were traced to these territories,
the others being mainly from Southeastern and Central Poland or the Ukraine.
These data require confirmation. Further information can be hoped for, since
reliable methods for detection of heterozygotes have been developed in recent
years (see below). There is no way, however, of testing a relevant population at
the above mentioned areas of origin themselves, since Jews have been driven out
or killed and the original non-Jewish population of these areas has been scattered
widely.

All estimates of gene frequencies are subject to errors due to possible bias.
It must be considered, for example, that the ethnic composition of the basic population under study may play a role. Moreover the diagnostic acumen in regards
to a certain disease may vary between groups among which the disease is relatively
frequent and awareness, therefore, high, and others, where the disease seems to
be rare and may be missed or misclassified.

The data about consanguineous marriages among parents of patients are at
variance between the available series. A collection of such data from the literature
by ARONSON and VOLK arrived at an average figure of 28.9% for non-Jewish
parents of affected children of European descent and of 18.9% consanguinity up
to second cousins inclusive for Jewish parents. There were considerable discrepancies within the non-Jewish group when various geographic regions of origin were
differentiated. In the authors' own study which includes the largest number
of cases compiled in any single group, from 165 Jewish parents of affected children
in the USA only one marriage between first cousins and two marriages between
second cousins could be recorded, which would indicate a frequency of 1.8%, being
only slightly higher than the frequency in the general population.

As has been noted in the previous section on Niemann-Pick's disease the
pathologic gene appears to be disproportionally frequent among Jews. Compared
with non-Jews the gene causing Tay-Sachs' disease is found to be about 100 times
as frequent among the Jewish population. Within the Jewish population it again
is disproportionally frequent among certain groups which can be defined by their
geographic origin. Such a high frequency of a gene which constitutes a lethal factor
can be maintained only if the constant loss of genes caused by the early death
of homozygotes is compensated for by other factors favoring the existence of the
particular gene. The simplest explanation coming to mind would be a high mutation rate of the particular gene locus. Since the mutation rate would have to be
high enough to compensate for the loss of genes in the homozygotes a differential
mutation rate between Jews and non-Jews and probably between Ashkenazi and
Sephardi Jews as well would have to be claimed of the same magnitude as the differential morbidity in Tay-Sachs' disease. There is no acceptable example of such
a differential mutation rate for any locus in human populations. In experimental
genetics it also appears that the mutation rate of specific loci remains fairly constant within a given species. Viewed in absolute terms the mutation rate for
Tay-Sachs' disease in the Jewish population would have to be of a magnitude
hardly acceptable on theoretical grounds.

The second possible explanation for a continuously high frequency of a gene
in spite of constant and complete loss of homozygotes would be the postulation

of some advantage of the heterozygotes over the normal homozygotes. Examples for such a balanced polymorphism in man are well known in G-6-PD-deficiency, the sickle cell gene and others. In the quoted cases the heterozygotes have a better chance of survival than normal homozygotes, when stricken by malaria falciparum, which was endemic and accounted for a high proportion of infant mortality in the geographic areas where the respective genes are frequent. The extermination of malaria will remove the advantage of these heterozygotes and thus induce a decrease of the genes in question, hence the balance will be disturbed.

Up to date no such advantage can be demonstrated for the heterozygotes in Tay-Sachs' disease, and no such explanation can be found in Niemann-Pick's disease. Specific studies have also failed to detect an increased fertility of heterozygotes. Under to-day's circumstances considering psychological and social factors an increased fertility could be expected to appear only in heterozygotes who were not aware of being carriers, in other words who had not produced sick children and had not experienced the disease in near relatives.

The negative results of the search for an increased fitness of heterozygotes cannot be taken to disprove this still most probable hypothesis, particularly since a very small advantage would be sufficient. Assuming a frequency of homozygotes in the order of $1:10000$ an increase of fitness of heterozygotes of 1 % would suffice to make up for the loss of genes with the affected homozygotes. This follows from Hardy Weinberg's law $p^2 + 2pq + q^2 = 1$, and $p + q = 1$. A frequency of homozygotes (p^2) of $1:10000$ corresponds to a gene frequency p of 0.01. For each homozygous individual there would exist $\dfrac{2pq}{p^2}$ or 198 heterozygotes. Since with each homozygote, who does not reproduce, 2 genes are eliminated, an increased fitness of 1 % on the part of the heterozygotes would balance the loss. Furthermore, this advantage which once led to accumulation of the pathologic gene need not be effective any more under present circumstances. In this case we would not be dealing with a genetic equilibrium in regards to the studied gene, but its frequency would be decreasing slowly over many generations to a value sustained by new mutations. The theory of increased fitness of heterozygotes under certain local conditions in previous generations is supported to a certain degree by the observation that the ancestors of many affected persons can be traced to the same contiguous restricted area in Eastern Europe. These questions probably will be studied again using new methods which have become available for reliable detection of heterozygotes. The previously mentioned finding of vacuolized lymphocytes in patients and in some of the parents and siblings, which proved useful in juvenile amaurotic family idiocy (RAYNER 1952, 1962), was found unreliable or even useless in infantile amaurotic family idiocy of Tay-Sachs' type (cf. MYRIANTHOPOULOS 1962). Recently, however, VOLK, ARONSON and SAIFER (1964) claimed that they could demonstrate with great constancy a lack of fructose-1-phosphate-aldolase in children affected with Tay-Sachs' disease and in all their parents. The reliability and importance of these results for the elucidation of the pathogenesis of Tay-Sachs' disease is not entirely clear at present. BALINT et al. (1963, 1964) described a diminution of cephalin and sphingomyelin in the lipids of erythrocytes in heterozygotes.

2. Juvenile Amaurotic Family Idiocy

(Batten's Disease, Morbus Spielmeyer-Vogt)

This type does not usually manifest itself before the age of 5 to 7 years. It is clearly separated from the infantile variety on clinical, pathological and genetic grounds. Here, too, the transmission is autosomal recessive (SJÖGREN 1931). The disease has never been proved in Jewish individuals. There exists, however, an increased gene frequency in Northern Europe and particularly in certain isolates in Sweden. SJÖGREN (1931) calculated from 39 cases he himself examined and 76 kat-amnestically identified cases a frequency of homozygotes of 0.0038%, corresponding to a gene frequency of 0.6% and a frequency of heterozygotes of 1.2%. 30 years later, RAYNER (1962) studied a series of 37 proved cases and their relatives in Sweden and arrived at estimates of 0.0023% or 1:50000 for the frequency of affected individuals, corresponding to a gene frequency of 0.48% and a frequency of heterozygotes of 1.0%. The frequency of consanguineous matings (first cousins) among the parents of affected children was in SJÖGRENS material 15% and 9.1% in that of RAYNER. Strictly comparable data about the frequency of consanguineous marriages in the general population in Sweden are not available. BÖÖK (1948) arrived at values between 1% and 8% for various communities in Sweden.

In 1948 BAGH and HORTLING first described the appearance of vacuolized lymphocytes in various percentages in patients with juvenile amaurotic family idiocy representing a useful diagnostic sign. RAYNER 1952 corroborated these findings in affected individuals and emphasized the usefulness of the same sign for detection of heterozygotes.

The detection of biochemical differences between infantile amaurotic family idiocy and the juvenile form clearly demonstrated heterogeny.

In patients suffering from juvenile amaurotic family idiocy and apparently in symptomfree heterozygotes, too, BESSMAN and BALDWIN (1962) found generalized imidazolaminaciduria. Since the aminoacids concerned did not appear to be increased in the serum of these persons, their excretion probably is caused not by a primary defect of an enzyme but by disturbed tubular function.

3. Further Amaurotic Idiocies

Further varieties of amaurotic idiocy have been described, presenting special clinical or, as claimed in a few, biochemical features (JATZKEWITZ et al. 1965). Some of these cases eventually may be shown to belong to one of the two forms discussed. Others, however, may represent special genetic variants. This holds true in particular for the so-called congenital amaurotic idiocy (NORMAN and WOOD), the late infantile variety (BIELSCHOWSKY) and the adult type (MEYER, KUFS), the pigment variant of the amaurotic idiocy (SEITELBERGER and SIMMA 1962) and others. Often only single case reports are available, so that no critical judgement of the genetics can be made. Autosomal recessive inheritance is most likely. The special ophthalmological features of the various types have been discussed extensively by DANIS et al. (1957). A special variant has been described in 1959 by NORMAN et al. as "TAY SACHS disease with visceral involvement". Further examples of apparently the same disease entity were reported by CRAIG et al. (1959) and LANDING and RUBINSTEIN (1962) and termed "pseudo-HURLER disease" by the latter authors. A detailed study of eight infants suffering from this disease was presented by LANDING et al. in 1964. When O'BRIEN and coworkers added a ninth case (1965), they proposed the name of "generalized gangliosidosis". Since siblings have been affected in several instances and patients are evenly distributed among both sexes, autosomal recessive inheritance can be assumed.

Some resemblances of "generalized gangliosidosis" with another glycolipid thesaurismosis, Fabry's disease, angiokeratoma corporis diffusum, have been pointed out. In the latter, however, the evidence from family and linkage data is strongly in favor of X-chromosomal inheritance (OPITZ et al. 1965).

c) Cerebrosidoses

(Morbus Gaucher)

These rare hereditary diseases were described in 1882, but even to date the basic biochemical defect can not be isolated. We, therefore, cannot decide on biochemical grounds whether we are dealing with a single disease entity resulting from a mutation of one locus with the variation in clinical symptoms and course being differentiated in a quantitative fashion only, or whether two or more genetically independent subgroups exist. Clinical and genetic observations definitely speak for the existence of two or more independent groups.

Reliable estimates of the disease frequency apparently are lacking. As in the previously discussed sphingolipidoses the classical form of Gaucher's disease also was found to be particularly frequent in Jews.

The first manifestation of the disease might occur at any age; as a rule the patients will live to adulthood. Long remissions have been observed. Familial occurence is seen frequently. Affected siblings mostly display a very similar course of the disease. The parents of patients almost invariably are free of symptoms. Segregation ratios in these families are in good agreement with the assumption of autosomal recessive inheritance (HSIA et al. 1962, KNUDSON and KAPLAN 1962).

Clear-cut evidence for autosomal recessive transmission also was presented by HERNDON and BENDER (1950), who published the pedigree of a Negro family in which 5 children in 5 closely related sibships were affected with Gaucher's disease. In 4 of these families the parents were second cousins (Fig. 5). This, however, probably was of decisive importance in only three of them.

Reliable data about the frequency of consanguineous marriages among parents of affected individuals are not available.

HSIA and coworkers presented evidence pointing to a second form of Gaucher's disease with the same clinical course but autosomal dominant transmission. Of the published families supposedly showing manifestation of the disease in two generations only the family of FARBER and the one of HSIA and coworkers presented the full clinical manifestation and morphological proof of Gaucher's disease in both generations. This opens the possibility that some of the published observations on disease in parents of affected children indeed have to be viewed as being micromanifestations in heterozygous carriers of the recessive gene. Quite convincing in this respect appear to be the findings of GERKEN and WIEDEMANN (1964) who in a non-Jewish family observed 2 infants with the full clinical and morphological picture of Gaucher's disease and in the 5 year old apparently healthy sister of the children as well as in both healthy appearing parents found typical Gaucher cells in the bone marrow (cf. also GERKEN 1965). The extremely rare cases with full manifestations in 2 generations then could be judged to be rare occasions of pseudodominance produced by mating of a homozygous affected and a heterozygous parent. Only the observation of a clear-cut case in the third generation or the forthcoming of reliable tests for detection of heterozygotes can clarify this situation. Meanwhile it appears justified to consider the possible existence of a special autosomal dominant variety.

A rare subgroup, definitely to be separated by its different clinical course and its different ethnic distribution, is constituted by the acute infantile type of Gaucher's disease. Following the onset in early infancy involvement of the central nervous system soon becomes apparent. The patients die before completing the second year of life. The differential diagnosis has to consider particularly Niemann-Pick's disease. KNUDSON and KAPLAN (1962) were able to collect 43 cases from 27 families. Segregation ratios agreed within the random sampling variation with the expec-

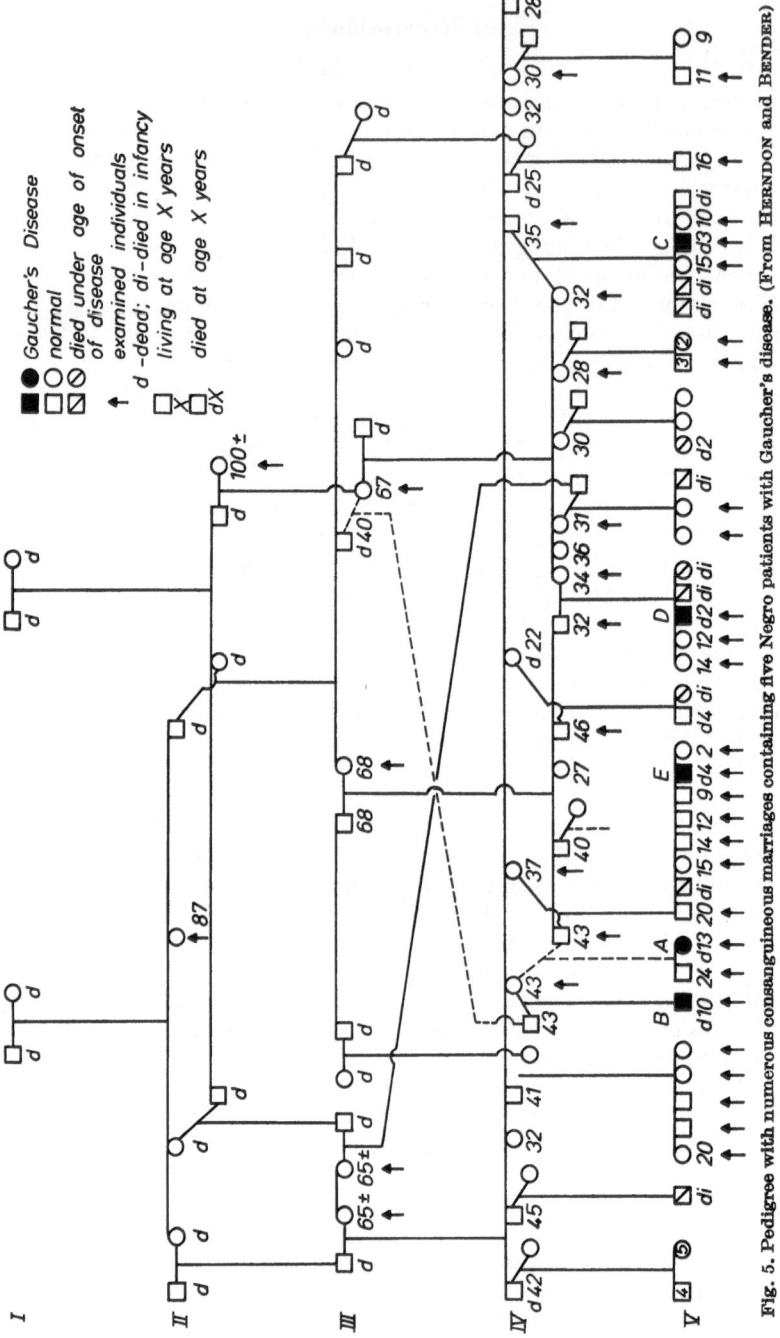

Fig. 5. Pedigree with numerous consanguineous marriages containing five Negro patients with Gaucher's disease. (From Herndon and Bender)

tation determined by autosomal recessive transmission. In no case were affected individuals found in more than one generation. Consanguinity was not mentioned. Only one of these cases was of Jewish extraction. RATH (1964) recently published the observation of one family in which two infants died from the acute form of Gaucher's disease with involvement of the central nervous system proved by autopsy. A third child was healthy. Nothing was stated about possible consanguinity or ethnic origin of the parents.

KNUDSON and KAPLAN (1962) distinguished a further variant, where central nervous system involvement is the principal manifestation. The affected, however, were older children or adults. Proper evaluation of these single observations taken mainly from the older literature is very difficult.

In summary then, we can consider two genetic variants proved: the autosomal recessive classical form and the most probably also autosomal recessive acute infantile variety with central nervous system involvement. There possibly exists a further subgroup with autosomal dominant inheritance resembling the classical type in its clinical course. Finally a special form with central nervous system involvement and onset late in childhood or in adult age may be considered. A statement as to whether multiple alleles or rather mutations at different loci are involved will have to await the demonstration of the primary biochemical defect. Some clues to the location of the primary metabolic defect and to possible biochemical heterogeny of Gaucher's disease have been given by the results of PHILIPPART and MENKES (1964).

II. Further Rare Lipidoses

a) The Leucodystrophies

The leucodystrophies represent a group of rare disorders of the central nervous system characterized by the widespread severe involvement of the myelin sheath. Various attempts have been made to group them according to clinical or morphological findings. Extensive discussions of these problems have recently been published by POSER (1962) and KOCH (1965), where also a very detailed review and documentation of the literature can be found. Our knowledge of the basic biochemistry involved is insufficient to devise any order on biochemical grounds. Because of some relations to lipidoses and particularly to the sphingolipidoses this group has to be mentioned in this connection.

The number of reported cases is too small to permit a definite statement on the genetics of the special varieties of this undoubtedly heterogeneous group. All of them have been observed in sibships and occasionally in other relatives. Consanguinity of parents has been reported repeatedly. The prevailing impression is that a primary enzyme defect is involved, and that, therefore, the leucodystrophies belong to the inborn errors of metabolism. Most observations point to autosomal recessive inheritance.

We possess better information about the inheritance of the also very rare Pelizaeus Merzbacher disease, which belongs to the orthochromatic leucodystrophies. The available observations recently have been reviewed by ZERBIN-RÜDIN and PEIFFER (1964), who added a further large kindred. These authors distinguish three forms of the disease:

1. **The classical type MERZBACHER** with onset at about one year of age and slow progression, in its final state being morphologically characterized by an extensive diffuse demyelination of the white matter of cerebrum and cerebellum with irregularly distributed isles of preserved myelin.

2. **The type SEITELBERGER,** where the demyelination or insufficient formation of myelin sheath starts before birth and where consequently a very extensive demyelination frequently without the typical isles of myelin is observed.

3. **The late form** (CAMP and LÖWENBERG 1941) with onset in the 3rd or 4th decade.

The subgroups 1 and 2 generally are thought to be due to an X-chromosomal recessive gene. The small number of affected females has been explained as rare instances of clinical manifestation in heterozygotes. Zerbin-Rüdin and Peiffer, however, feel that too many affected females have been reported to be accounted for by such a mechanism. This along with the observation |of consanguinity of parents in a few families indicates to them the existence of a further subgroup with autosomal recessive inheritance.

Zeman et al. (1964), however, who observed in one pedigree within five generations 21 males affected with the infantile form of Pelizaeus-Merzbacher disease and three female patients with somewhat different neurologic symptoms, believe in uniformly sex-linked recessive inheritance and try to explain the occasional manifestation in females by invoking the Lyon hypothesis. According to Mary Lyon's well-founded and generally accepted hypothesis, of the two X-chromosomes contained in each normal cell of a female one is inactivated early in embryonic development, inactivation taking place randomly. In a female, heterozygous for a pathologic gene at the X-chromosome, consequently, half of the cells on the average would be rendered hemizygous for the pathologic gene by inactivation of the X-chromosome carrying the normal allele. Depending on chance distribution, however, more or less than 50% of cells may become "affected" and thus a, generally milder, clinical manifestation of disease may occur in some individuals, in whom a critical threshold is surpassed. Similar observations could convincingly be demonstrated in X-chromosomal recessive muscular dystrophy (Pearson 1963, Emery 1965).

The late form of Pelizaeus-Merzbacher's disease which follows autosomal dominant single gene inheritance as established by Camp and Löwenberg (1941) and confirmed by Zerbin-Rüdin and Peiffer (1964) is not accepted by Zeman et al. (1964) to belong to the disease entity described by Pelizaeus and Merzbacher.

Summarizing, Pelizaeus-Merzbacher's disease must be viewed as a heterogeneous group involving at least three different gene loci corresponding to the classical X-chromosomal recessive type, the also X-chromosomal recessive type Seitelberger, the late form with autosomal dominant inheritance, and possibly a fourth autosomal recessive sub-group.

b) Familial Cholesterolosis with High-Density Lipoprotein Deficiency

Tangier Disease, Hypo-α-lipoproteinemia

The disease has been named after the isle of Tangier off the coast of Virginia where the first cases have been observed. It is characterized by the almost complete absence of high-density lipoproteins and storage of cholesterol and its esters in various tissues. The first observation concerned a five year old boy and his six year old sister. They had no further siblings. Further inquiries revealed that the parents were distantly related. Meanwhile two more affected families have been found in Missouri and Kentucky. The affected families are unrelated (Fredrickson et al. 1962, 1964).

The available data strongly suggest autosomal recessive inheritance. In the serum of presumed heterozygotes high-density lipoproteins have been shown to be diminished. In homozygous affected individuals this fraction is almost completely lacking, and cholesterol esters are stored in tissues. The plasma cholesterol concentration is diminished, and triglycerides are increased.

Recent studies demonstrated the presence of an atypical lipoprotein that immunologically corresponded to the α-lipoprotein, a so-called cross reacting material

(CRM). This has been found in diminished amount in patients. In presumed heterozygotes presence of two proteins could be shown: the normal α-lipoprotein and a small fraction of the atypical lipoprotein (LEVY and FREDRICKSON 1965, FREDRICKSON personal communication). These observations prove that a mutation at a structural gene locus and not a control gene mutation is responsible for the abnormality.

c) A-β-Lipoproteinemia

This is one of the hereditary defects in humans for which the causation by a control gene mutation has been suggested by various authors (BEARN 1963, PARKER and BEARN 1963, FREZAL 1964). It appears justified to view the lack of β-lipoproteins as the primary gene effect. All other symptoms may be related to the defect of these transport proteins. No cross reacting material has been found. A true absence of the primary gene product, therefore, can be assumed. As discussed in the opening paragraphs, absence of the primary gene product can be expected in a control gene mutation. It also may be caused, however, by some structural gene mutations.

Observation of manifest disease in siblings and consanguinity in at least three of the few known families indicate autosomal recessive inheritance. The parents of one of the patients of LAMY et al. (1963) were halfsibs. This disease, too, seems to be more frequent among Jews.

SALT et al. (1960) noted in one family a decreased plasma concentration of β-lipoproteins, cholesterol and phospholipids in assumed heterozygotes (parents and paternal grandfather). These observations have not been confirmed in other families. The possibility to recognize heterozygotes, therefore, remains questionable.

d) Heredopathia Atactica Polyneuritiformis (Refsum's Syndrome)

From the time of his first description of the disease in 1944/45 up to 1960 REFSUM could collect from the literature 29 patients from 15 families. In all 15 families the parents were free of symptoms. In 8 they were related, mostly first cousins. A number of new cases has been reported since. RICHTERICH et al. up to 1964 could find reports on 37 cases from 23 families. Four were excluded because of unproved diagnosis. Among 18 families where a statement regarding consanguinity had been made the parents were related in nine. Consanguinity was noted in the greatest frequency in 6 out of 7 Scandinavian families. Among a total of 81 children 31 were affected. Taking into regard the mode of ascertainment the segregation ratio was in accord with expected values for autosomal recessive inheritance. Both sexes were affected alike. A pedigree observed by REFSUM (1957) is shown in Fig. 6. This further corroborates the autosomal recessive mode of transmission.

More cases probably will be found in the near future, since a clearcut biochemical diagnosis now has become available

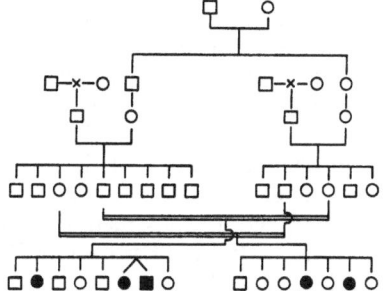

Fig. 6. Heredopathia atactica polyneuritiformis (REFSUM) in two sibships resulting from second cousin marriages. (From REFSUM 1957)

(KAHLKE 1964). The 3,7,11,15-tetramethylhexadecanoic acid, which is found in affected individuals, also could be demonstrated in small amounts in the serum of normals and heterozygotes studied (KAHLKE 1965).

e) Further Rare Anomalies of Lipid Metabolism

A number of diseases apparently due to anomalies in lipid metabolism has been seen in only a few cases or even in single families. Affected sibs here frequently point to autosomal recessive inheritance, but the small number of observations does not permit a definite statement.

Here the syndrome of *familial hypolipidemia* observed in two sisters by Hooft et al. (1962) has to be mentioned, which is characterized by extreme low concentrations of all plasma lipid fractions, retarded development, atypical retinitis pigmentosa, erythemato-squamous skin lesions and aminoaciduria.

The pathogenetically poorly understood group of *lipodystrophies* recently has been reviewed by Senior and Gellis (1964). The authors distinguished a generalized and a partial lipodystrophy. Both frequently are associated with increased plasma lipid concentration. The generalized form of the disease with onset in the newborn period has been described at least twice in siblings, in three or possibly four of the families the parents were related. Both sexes are affected with the same frequency. The available data strongly support the assumption of autosomal recessive inheritance. Senior and Gellis do not feel that the later manifesting forms of the disease are based on the same genetic defect. The partial form of the lipodystrophy also is thought to be a separate disease entity. Familial occurence of this form appears to be rare.

A special type of *lipodystrophy with gigantism and associated endocrine dysfunction* has been described for the first time by Donohue (1948/1954) under the name of "dysendocrinism". It now commonly is referred to as "Leprechaunism". The disease probably is identical to the syndrome described by Berardinelli (1953). It is characterized by missing of subcutaneous fat particularly in the face, acromegalic gigantism, muscular hypertrophy, hepatosplenomegaly and fatty degeneration of the liver, enlargement of the clitoris or the male genitals without other signs of pubertas praecox, a hyperlipemia concerning particularly the neutral fat fraction, and disturbance in blood glucose regulation. The ovaries of the girls contained follicular cysts. In the skin commonly a darkish-brown spotty pigmentation is obvious. Affected siblings and consanguinity of parents have been observed several times. Hence autosomal recessive inheritance is most probable. The limited number of cases precludes a definite decision. In heterozygotes Seip (1959) observed increase of neutral fats in the serum.

Morbus Whipple (lipodystrophia intestinalis, intestinal lipodystrophy) is another rare disease which according to Puite and Tesluk up to 1955 has been described in 59 cases. The disease has been observed in whites and highly preferentially in the male sex. With few exceptions manifestation does not take place before adult age. Clinical symptoms resemble the combination of malabsorption syndrome and polyserositis. The anatomical lesions as defined by Whipple (1907) consist of storage of neutral fats and fatty acids in the intestinal wall and in lymphnodes. The biochemical nature of the stored substances is not entirely clear. Most characteristic elements are conglomerates of sudan negative macrophages in lymphnodes and the mucous membrane of the small intestine. According to Black-Schaffer (1949) and Upton (1952) these cells contain a glycoprotein. Newer observations favor bacterial genesis or an important influence of a bacterial factor in the causation of the disease (Ashworth et al. 1964). Its interpretation as a primary disturbance of lipid metabolism, therefore, becomes very doubtful. The few reports of familial occurrence almost exclusively concern affected siblings. In one family the mother of two affected brothers might have had the disease. These observations could easily be related to exogenous factors rather than to inheritance.

Morbus Whipple occasionally has been referred to in the literature as *Lipogranulomatosis*. The same name was given in 1957 to another disease by FARBER, COHEN and UZMAN. Here first clinical symptoms appear shortly after birth. Prominent features are swelling of extremities with chronic, progressive, severe and generalized affection of the joints, nodular infiltration of periarticular and subcutaneous tissues, finally dysphonia due to fixation of laryngeal cartilages and dyspnoea caused by infiltration of the lungs. There is no hepatomegaly, but lymphnodes are invaded. Periodic episodes of fever are noted. The stored material mainly consists of lipoglycoproteins. Of three reported cases two were siblings. The third came from an unrelated family. Heredity is suggested by the observation of affected siblings. The disease is not related to Whipple's disease. The description, however, somewhat resembles the characteristic features of the *Lipoidosis cutis et mucosae* first described by SIEBENMANN (1908) and defined by URBACH and WIETHE (1929). A recent report has been published by BURNETT and MARCY (1963) under the title "Lipoid proteinosis". The disease becomes manifest later. Most obvious symptoms are pearly papules and nodules in the skin of face, neck and hands. On elbows and knees the lesions become hyperkeratotic. Similar papules and nodules can be observed on the mucous membranes. Affection of the larynx causes dysphonia and hoarseness particularly in early infancy. Tongue, frenulum, esophagus and sometimes rectum and vagina may be infiltrated. Eight out of 26 cases had intracranial calcifications. Alopecia has been described several times. The stored substance has been characterized as being hyalinelike, sudan- and Schiff (PAS)-positive. According to WOOD et al. (1956) it consists mainly of galactolipids. Alterations in serum proteins and lipids have been described, but reports are inconsistent. BURNETT and MARCY collected more than 100 cases from the literature. In 7 of 33 cases analysed further affected persons were known in the family. In no family were parents and child affected. Consanguinity of the parents has been noted several times. Diabetes mellitus was found to be more frequent in the affected families than in the general population.

Finally the *Lipocalcinogranulomatosis* (Calcinosis lipogranulomatosis progrediens) should be considered here, which originally has been described by TEUTSCHLÄNDER in 1935. A most recent case report and review has been given by TRACA et al. This rare disease is characterized by often symmetrically distributed tumors in subcutaneous tissues, which may infiltrate underlying muscles. They usually appear within the first or second decade of life and are located mainly in the region of large joints and bursae. There is storage of lipoid substances in the granulomatous tissue. Necrosis and calcification are essential features of the disease. We recently were able to restudy the original family of TEUTSCHLÄNDER, where meanwhile 3 of 6 siblings have become affected. The parents could be shown to be first cousins. Autosomal recessive inheritance thus appears most likely.

III. Essential Familial Hyperlipidemias

These diseases are characterized by gross alterations of plasma lipids. Because of their relatively high incidence in European and North American populations their diagnostic importance, their relationship to certain forms of atherosclerosis, and last but not least their response to diet and therapy they are of particular interest.

a) Essential Familial Hyperlipemias

In 1932 BÜRGER and GRÜTZ reported the classic triad of hepatomegaly, xanthomatosis and opaque serum and established the disease entity of hyperlipemia.

The classic clinical description of the disease has been given by HOLT et al. in 1939. Up to 1958 some 130 reliably documented cases could be found in the literature. The increased interest of recent years has led to a great number of further reports on well analysed cases. Biochemical and clinical studies disclosed differences between various patients in the pathogenetic mechanisms involved and thus forced the establishment of independent subgroups of the disease. In none of these subgroups could the primary defect be shown conclusively. Relationships between apparent subgroups, therefore, are not fully clarified. Distinction of subgroups depends entirely on clinical and particularly on biochemical criteria. It is difficult to discuss the justification of making such distinctions without discussing the biochemistry| of the disease extensively. Such discussion, however, will be left to the respective special chapter.

At least two groups of hyperlipemias are recognized and have been generally acknowledged, the fat-induced or fat-inducible hyperlipemia which apparently is caused by a defect of lipoproteinlipase activity (HAVEL and GORDON 1960, FREDRICKSON et al. 1963) and the carbohydrate-induced or carbohydrate inducible variety, where an increased lipogenesis from carbohydrate has been thought to occur (AHRENS et al. 1961). In the case of the fat-induced type a normal resorption of fat can be demonstrated being followed by an impaired removal of neutral fat particles from the serum, which may be explained by a variety of mechanisms. Based on the response to intravenous injections of heparin, i.e. whether lipolytic activity will be stimulated and clearing induced or not, a heparin sensitive and a heparin insensitive form can be differentiated. In the latter the disturbance is thought to lie in a primary defect of the enzyme itself (BIALKIN et al. 1962, and others).

Contrary to the long held opinion that the fat-induced type were the most common form of the disease more recent observations show the carbohydrate-induced variety to be more common (FREDRICKSON et al. 1963). Under discussion is the existence of further separate subgroups (KUO and BASSETT 1963, KINSELL et al. 1962, and others). From the genetic point of view it is to be emphasized that, whenever familial occurrence has been reported, all the affected individuals with rare exceptions had the same type of disease in that they displayed very similar reactions to the various tests.

Older observations on familial occurrence of essential hyperlipemia cannot in most cases definitely be attributed to any of the now acknowledged subgroups. Not uncommonly even the separation from hypercholesterolemia is uncertain.

Identical twins concordant for essential hyperlipemia have been described by JOBST et al. (1963). Siblings have been found to suffer from proven fat-induced hyperlipemia by, among others, HAVEL and GORDON and FREDRICKSON et al. In one family reported by BIALKIN et al. male identical twins were concordant for fat-induced, heparine sensitive hyperglyceridemia (hyperlipemia). A sister of the twins also had the full clinical picture. Another sister and a half-sister as well as the parents were classified as heterozygotes. The father of the half-sister could be studied only incompletely and on a single serum determination had normal values. Consanguinity of the parents could be excluded. Consanguineous matings in parents of children suffering from fat-induced hyperlipemia have been reported by BERGER et al. (1962) (Figure 7). These authors quoted consanguinity of parents observed by GRASSO and NEGRI (1951) and BOGGS (1957), but the first mentioned observation dates back to a time when distinction of subgroups was not yet made and the second, as confirmed and restudied by JAKOVCIC et al. (1964), concerned familial hypercholesterolemia.

In heterozygotes of fat-induced hyperlipemia the statistical mean of plasma neutral fat concentration is increased as compared with controls. Clearing after fat load (1,5 gm/kg body weight) is delayed and following intravenous application of heparin activation of lipolytic activity does not reach norm values (FREDRICKSON et al. 1963). Family studies generally conform to expectations of single gene autosomal recessive inheritance, which, when dealing with an hereditary enzyme defect, a priori is the most probable assumption.

The problems in explaining the basic pathogenetic mechanism are well demonstrated by an observation of FREDRICKSON et al. (1963). In one family with fat-inducible hyperlipemia these authors found an affected girl who in the heparin test showed the expected markedly diminished lipolytic activity, and an equally

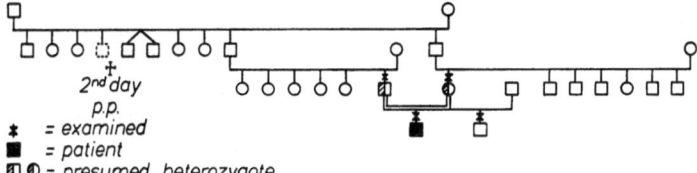

Fig. 7. Essential familial hyperlipemia of "retention type". The parents of the patient are first cousins.
(From BERGER et al.)

severely affected brother who in five repeated determinations always displayed a lipolytic activity well in the range of normal. Values of both parents and one further sister of the patients were, as usually in heterozygotes, near the lower limit of normal values.

Initially it was suggested that the carbohydrate-induced variety of hyperlipemia were an acquired metabolic disturbance (AHRENS et al., KUO and BASSETT). Presently most authors accept this form to be another genetic entity.

The large family, however, first published by BIGLER et al. and restudied by JAKOVCIC et al. (1964) and thought to suffer from carbohydrate-induced hyperlipemia had to be reclassified, since initially performed biopsy studies proved to be erroneous. Reevaluation confirmed the diagnosis of glycogen storage disease type I (v. GIERKE).

SPRITZ (1964) reported occurence of "carbohydrate-induced lipemia" in father and son. Evaluation of this observation, however, is difficult, because the father was an overt diabetic.

A familial history of diabetes has been reported several times in carbohydrate inducible hyperlipemia as well as in the later discussed "familial hypercholesterolemia with hypertriglyceridemia". The relationships of abnormal carbohydrate metabolism in these diseases and of the defect in diabetes mellitus are not clear.

FREDRICKSON and LEES recently suggested,, a system for phenotyping of hyperlipoproteinemias" based on a rapid and simple method utilizing paper electrophoresis performed on the serum after a 12 to 16 hours fast while the patient is on a "normal American diet". The classification is based on the distribution of the readily distinguishable major bands of lipoproteins, the chylomicrons, found at the origin, the β-lipoproteins, the pre-β-lipoproteins (corresponding to the α_2-lipoproteins of starch block electrophoresis), and the α-lipoproteins. Five different phenotypes can be distinguished and are designated arbitrarily as types I-V, a short and necessarily incomplete summary of which is given in table 1. Types II and III of this classification are discussed in the following chapter. This system, too, probably will prove to be insufficient for classification of all observed variants. It certainly, however, provides a useful base for diagnosis and is a valuable tool particularly for screening purposes. It appears quite probable that each of the various types represents a different genotype.

A peculiar disease entity has been described by HAGBERG et al. (1964) under the name of "malignant hyperlipemia in infancy". While essential familial hyper-

Table 1: *Classification of phenotypes of hyperlipoproteinemia according to* FREDRICKSON *and* LESS

Type	Name	Lipoproteindistribution				Plasma	Cholesterol	Triglyc.	PHLA*	Glucose-tolerance	
		Chylomicron	β	pre-β	α						
I	familial fat induced hyperlipemia	+++	—	(+)	—	creamy	+	+++	low	normal	fat inducible
II	fam. hyper-β-lipoproteinemia (fam. hypercholesterolemia)	n	++	—	n	clear	++	normal	normal	normal ?	
III	fam. hyper-β- and pre-β-lipoproteinemia-hypercholesterolemia and hypertriglyceridemia	n	+	++	n or (—)	clear, cloudy or milky	++	+	normal	ab-normal	carbohydrate inducible
IV	fam. hyperpre-β-lipoproteinemia (carbohydrate induced hyperlipemia)	n	—	++	n or (—)	clear, cloudy or milky	normal or (+)	++	normal	ab-normal	carbohydrate inducible
V	fam. hyperchylomicronemia and hyperpre-β-lipoproteinemia	++	n	++	n or (—)	creamy	+	++	low or normal	ab-normal	fat- and carbohydrate inducible

* PHLA = Postheparin Lipolytic activity

lipemia almost invariably took a relatively benign course in childhood, this particular form led to death in infancy. The total lipids in the serum were determined to be 1440 mg/100 ml, the triglycerides 782 mg/100 ml. Clinical signs were similar to those of acute reticuloendotheliosis with progressive pancytopenia, hepatosplenomegaly and infiltration of various organs with granuloma like cells. The lipoproteinlipase activity has not been measured. A sister of the proband had died in infancy with obviously the same clinical symptoms. A repeat study of the preserved microscopic material showed apparently the same histologic picture as in the patient. The parents and a healthy brother were clinically and biochemically normal and responded normally to fat loading. The observation suggests a genetically independent disease with autosomal mode of transmission.

The presently available data can be summarized to indicate that *essential familial hyperlipemia* describes a heterogeneous group of diseases which includes at least 2, most probably, however, more, according to KINSELL et al. (1962) at least 5, independent genetically determined diseases.

Where sufficient numbers of cases could be studied, single gene autosomal recessive inheritance could be demonstrated. Heterozygotes sometimes can be recognized. Our knowledge of the disease frequency in various populations is insufficient. Since the milky serum can easily be recognized, in this time of frequent routine blood studies the diagnosis should hardly be missed, once the physicians have become familiar with the disease.

HIRSCHHORN et al. (1959) attempted an estimate of the frequency of essential hyperlipemia in Sweden based on routine blood studies on students. They derived figures of 2 to 3% for heterozygotes. This study has met severe criticism in regard to methods applied and conclusions drawn. Certainly most individuals then classified as hyperlipemic don't belong to the group of the essential familial hyperlipemias discussed here. BIALKIN et al. partly on the base of HIRSCHHORN's data estimated the disease frequency as 1:5000 to 1:10000. The high estimate of heterozygote frequency in Sweden is difficult to reconcile with the fact, that no proved clear-cut case of essential familial hyperlipemia has been reported from this population.

YAMAMOTO et al. (1963) studying plasma lipid concentration in mice could show genetically determined variation. Without offering definite proof these observations could be explained best by assuming multifactorial inheritance with additive polygeny, that is, a system, where a greater number of genes is involved, each exerting about equal influence. The results of the twin studies of JENSEN et al. (1965) also are in good agreement with expectations under the hypothesis of polygenic control of plasma glyceride glycerol in man. It could be shown that intrapair variance was significantly greater in dizygotic twins than in monozygotic twins, the difference being significant at the 5% level. Interpair variance was greater than intrapair variance. Twins living apart had greater variance than twins living together.

Plasma concentration of lipids is the result of a multitude of interlocked metabolic events such as absorption from the intestines, transport, speed of clearing as measured by removal of chylomicrons, mobilization of depot fats, utilization of fats and fatty acids, and so on. Since each of these may be subject to genetically determined variation, the multifactorial model a priori appears most probable as it is in other metric characters of man. The interpretation has to proceed with caution, however, because secondary regulatory mechanisms certainly exist which cannot fully be taken into account and may mask an underlying discontinuous variation. The pathologic forms of essential hyperlipemia in man certainly have to be attributed to mutation and homozygosity of single important genes within the multifactorial system.

b) Essential Familial Hypercholesterolemia

This disease is characterized by abnormally increased plasma concentration of cholesterol, phospholipids and to a lesser degree triglycerides. In the severe forms of the disease frequently cutaneous and tendon xanthomata and arcus corneae are to be found. Distinction of primary familial hypercholesterolemia from secondary elevation of plasma cholesterols and sometimes from essential hyperlipemia may be difficult. The differential diagnosis is discussed in the respective chapters. There also the relationships to early coronary heart disease and artherosclerosis will be considered. Here the discussion will be restricted to genetic aspects of essential familial hypercholesterolemia clearly distinguished from primary hyperlipemia and from secondary forms of hypercholesterolemia. Some attention, however, will be given to diagnostic criteria.

Concentration of serum cholesterol is a metric character with continuous distribution in the population. As has been observed repeatedly in sample populations the distribution does not follow the normal (Gaussian) distribution faithfully, but has positive skewness, that is, it has too many values in the right hand or upper tail of the curve (SCHAEFER 1964, THOMAS et al. 1964). As THOMAS et al. pointed out the skewing is not pronounced enough to cause grave inaccuracy in tests on mean values but may be misleading in the calculation of the "95 percent range" using Gaussian parameters.

The level of serum cholesterol concentration of any given individual at a certain time obviously depends on a number of factors. Some exogenous influences on serum cholesterol are well recognized as e.g. age, sex, body weight, diet etc.

Others, particularly endogenous factors, which influence cholesterol synthesis and degradation are incompletely understood. It is not at all surprising, therefore, that the distribution of the serum cholesterol concentration in the population is continuous and generally unimodal as must be expected as a consequence of multi-factorial determination.

Several autors employed twin studies to estimate the relative importance of exogenous and hereditary factors for normal variation of serum cholesterol concentration. Osborne et al. (1959) for their analysis were able to use 82 examined pairs of twins of ages 18 to 55 years. Four pairs suffering from idiopathic hyper-cholesterolemia were excluded. By comparing identical twins and like-sexed binovu-lar twins as well as pairs living together or apart the influence of genetic as well as exogenous factors for the variation within the normal range could be demon-strated. No calculation of a "heretability ratio" or similar parameters of the quan-titive importance of hereditary influence was undertaken, because the number of cases was too small and available methods are of questionable value.

Unpublished data of Heuschert (1964) also demonstrated a high degree of concordance in a group of ten uniovular pairs of twins of older age (55—75 years of age) some living together and some apart.

Gedda and Poggi (1960) studied 50 pairs of identical twins and 50 pairs of binovular twins aged 6 to 19 years, all living together with their parents. Definite differences in variation of identical and nonidentical twins were considered evidence for the dependence of the cholesterol concentration on the genotype.

Similar conclusions were drawn by McDonaugh et al. (1962) from data of 56 twin pairs. In this study some hypercholesterolemic individuals were included. A recent study of Jensen et al. (1965) based on 31 monozygotic, 13 like-sexed dizygotic and 4 unlike-sexed twin pairs also found the intrapair variance for total cholesterol and free cholesterol as well as phospholipids significantly greater in dizygotic than in monozygotic twins. Differences in variance for free cholesterol and total phospholipids were significant at the 1% level, total cholesterol dif-ferences at the 5% level. Interpair variance was significantly greater than intra-pair variance, and twins living apart had greater variances than twins living to-gether. The strong influence of genetic as well as of environmental factors thus again could be proven. A precise partition of the relative contributions of these both factors still cannot be done.

The most important question then is whether individuals who qualify as hypercholesterolemic and normocholesterolemic individuals can be viewed as samples from a single population with near normal distribution of serum chol-esterol levels or whether hypercholesterolemic individuals are a qualitatively dif-ferent group. In other words, do hypercholesterolemics represent the upper tail of a more or less bell shaped distribution governed by a generally multifactorial system with relatively equal contribution of many factors, or is the character of hypercholesterolemia determined by a single, specific and rather powerful gene within the system? Epstein et al. (1959) studied the data of their large kinship with hypercholesterolemia for bimodality. Demonstration of bimodality or tri-modality could have supported the assumption of mendelian inheritance. Further-more, the finding and location of a minimum would have served to define an optimal cut-off point for the groups representing the different genotypes. When using age corrected cholesterol values the authors could demonstrate a suggestive bimodality in males, but failed to do so in women. No definite cut-off point between normo- and hypercholesterolemic individuals could be deduced.

Thomas et al. (1964) approached the question of distribution by studying 1018 white male medical students. They concluded that the observed distribution could be explained equally well by assuming a 2-parameter-log-normal model or by the alternate hypothesis that it was derived by the overlapping of two populations by the single gene hypothesis. Calculations based on the second model (Figure 8) characterized the two subpopulations as given in Table 2.

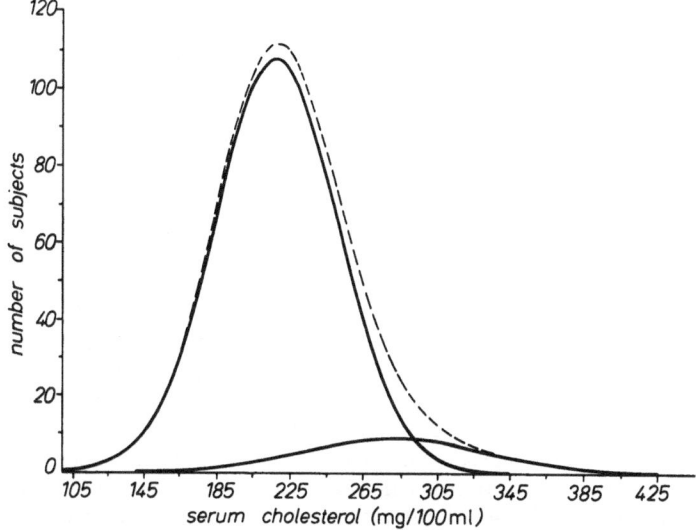

Fig. 8. Theoretical distribution curves of serum cholesterol values for the two constituent populations and the entire population of 1018 medical students, based on the maximum likelihood estimates. —— = two component curve; - - - = composite curve. (From THOMAS et al. 1964)

Assuming single gene inheritance and dominant mode of transmission the larger (left hand) population would represent the normal homozygotes. This, assuming a Hardy-Weinberg equilibrium, corresponds to p^2 in the formula $p^2 + 2pq + q^2 = 1$. The frequency of the normal gene then would be $p = 0,94$ and, since $p + q = 1$, the frequency of the pathologic gene q would be $q = 0,06$.

Mathematical analysis alone did not permit a decision between the two genetic models under discussion. Other criteria, therefore, have to be looked for.

For formal genetic analysis it is necessary first to define the character "hypercholesterolemia", that is to define the upper limit of normal. This has been done by various authors differently. Any definition will be somewhat arbitrary. A fixed cut-off point must disregard the age-trend. The attempt to correct for age on the other hand has no sound basis for the individual case. Definitions of the range of normal and the cut-off point, however, critically determine the result of the genetic analysis. In crucial observations, therefore, any single case must be evaluated carefully on its own merits.

Table 2

	left hand population	right hand population
Percentage of total	88,54	11,46
Mean	218,2 mg/100 ml	281,1 mg/100 ml
Standard deviation	33,6 mg/100 ml	50,9 mg/100 ml

The numerous pedigrees reported, have in most cases found either of two interpretations, single gene autosomal incompletely dominant inheritance or dominant inheritance with full penetrance but some variation in manifestation. Incomplete dominance has first been postulated by WILKINSON et al. (1948) and by ADLERSBERG et al. (1949). These authors assumed that the gene in single dose gives rise to moderate hypercholesterolemia, but in the homozygous state causes xantho-

33*

matosis, early atherosclerosis and death from myocardial infarction. In a more recent publication Hirschhorn and Wilkinson (1959) modified their interpretation in that, as they now regard as homozygotes also individuals without xanthomatosis, if the serum cholesterol concentration is 400 mg/100 ml or more. They insisted, however, that xanthomatosis is observed only in homozygotes.

Alternatively Müller (1938), Kornerup (1948), Stecher and Hersh (1949), and other authors regarded xanthomatosis and hypercholesterolemia as variable manifestation of a single dominant gene in heterozygous state.

Epstein et al. critically reviewed the literature up to 1959. The paper of Hirschhorn and Wilkinson (1959), which appeared at the same time, could not be included. Meanwhile additional family observations have become available.

The assumption that individuals with xanthomatosis generally represent heterozygotes for a single, fully penetrant autosomal dominant gene calls for a segregation ratio of 1:1 for affected and nonaffected among the offspring of matings with one parent with xanthomatosis and one parent being normocholesterolemic (according to the marriage type Aa × aa). Piper and Orrild (1956) found 82 % of such children to be hypercholesterolemic and Epstein et al. using the same data classified 88 % as being hypercholesterolemics. Thus the 1:1 ratio is not realized. Hypercholesterolemia, however, is not a very rare trait. Therefor, even when assuming that hypercholesterolemia with and without xanthomatosis represent phenotypic expressions of the same genotypes, there will be a proportion of homozygotes among the affected parents which is not negligable. Thus the ratio expected among the children is shifted slightly towards a higher proportion of affected. The alternative hypothesis, that all individuals with xanthomatosis were homozygotes for the pathologic gene would require 100 % hypercholesterolemic offspring from the same mating (then being regarded AA × aa), which again cannot easily be reconciled with the existing data. The exact segregation ratio determined depends as mentioned above on the definition of the cut-off point.

Recent publications supply more unquestionable observations of normocholesterolemic children of patients with xanthomatosis, though altogether such cases remain relatively rare. Such observations have been reported e.g. by Khacha-durian (1964) and Jakovcic et al. (1964).

Marriage of two hypercholesterolemic individuals with xanthomatosis, if these were heterozygotes, should yield 25% homozygotes for the normal allele, i.e. normocholesterolemic children. If, however, xanthomatosis generally indicates homozygosity for the pathologic gene, no normocholesterolemic children should be observed. According to the marriage type AA × AA all children would have to suffer from xanthomatosis or, when adopting the modified hypothesis of Hirsch-horn and Wilkinson (1959), at least should show serum cholesterol levels (corrected for age) above 400 mg/100 ml. Such matings of course are rare events. The pedigree of one such family as observed by Jakovcic et al. (1964) is reproduced in Figure 9. Two of the four children had xanthomatosis and arcus corneae, all had serum cholesterol concentrations well above 400 mg/100 ml. This family observation is in agreement with expectation under the assumption of homozygosity of both parents (I, 1; I, 2). No information was available about the mother of I, 2. The spouses I, 1 and I, 2 were unrelated.

If hypercholesterolemia without xanthomatosis results from heterozygosity and individuals with hypercholesterolemia and xanthomatosis generally are homozygotes for the pathologic gene, 25% of the offspring of matings between hypercholesterolemic patients without xanthomatosis should display hypercholesterolemia and xanthomatosis. Further 25% should be normocholesterolemic. The remaining 50% should be of the same phenotype as the heterozygous parents. Well documented families of this type again unfortunately are to be found rarely in the literature. Only those families, of course, qualify where heterozygosity of the parents is biochemically proven and not only deduced from the hypothesis adopted.

Out of the large kindred originally published by WILKINSON et al. and restudied by EPSTEIN et al. (1959) the latter authors quote the mating B_{10} and C_1 as a union between non-xanthomatous hypercholesterolemic individuals. According to the newer definition of HIRSCHHORN and WILKINSON (1959) because of serum cholesterol values of 485 and 460 mg/100 ml both spouses would have to

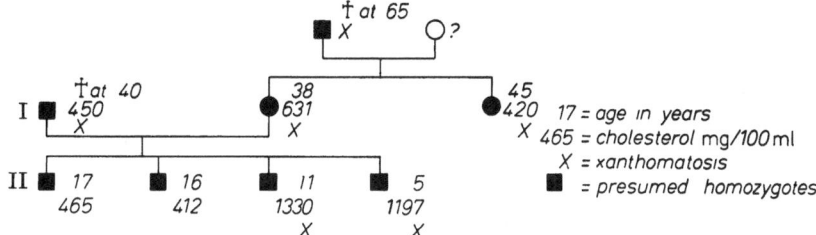

Fig. 9. Pedigree with marriage of homozygotes for hypercholesterolemia. (Observation of JAKOVCIC and HSIA)

be classified to be homozygotes. Appearance of two normocholesterolemic children having serum cholesterol concentrations of 186 and 193 mg/100 ml at age 28 and 17 years respectively, however, proved the parents to be heterozygotes. Among the children another 6 had xanthomatosis and cholesterol concentrations well above 400 mg/100 ml and 5 had cholesterol levels unquestionably within the range of heterozygote manifestation in the definition of HIRSCHHORN and WILKINSON. One more child had a cholesterol concentration of 267 mg/100 ml and must be considered probably heterozygous.

Two more well documented families of this type were reported by ADLERSBERG, PARETS and BOAS (1949) and PIPER and ORRILD (1956). The pedigree published by SCHETTLER et al. (1959) also comprises one marriage between two heterozygotes, where the mother had xanthomatous lesions, but at least one normocholesterolemic daughter was born. One such mating between non-xanthomatous hypercholesterolemic individuals can be found in the publication of MEILMAN et al. (1964) and this of KHACHADURIAN (1957) (Fig. 10a). Finally the family first reported by BOGGS et al. (1957) as hyperlipemic and shown to be hypercholesterolemic, when restudied by JAKOVCIC et al. (1964) must be mentioned. Here the parents were first cousins and with serum cholesterol concentrations of 319 mg/100 ml and 331 mg/100 ml respectively definitely had to be classified as heterozygotes. Of their 7 children 2 had xanthomatosis and one must be regarded to be homozygous, because of extreme hypercholesterolemia (621 mg/100 ml). Two children definitely were heterozygous and two normocholesterolemic (Figure 10b).

Added together the families of this particular mating type comprised 45 children. Of these 14 had to be classified as homozygotes, 19 qualified as heterozygotes and 12 were normocholesterolemic. These figures are in accord with the expected 1:2:1 ratio, particularly if one takes into consideration that at least a portion of these families had been ascertained via a child as the proband.

Summarizing the available information one has to conclude that the family observations definitely support the assumption of a single gene locus to be responsible for the disease entity of hypercholesterolemia. The claim for complete dominance of the pathologic gene over its normal allele, viewing the great majority of patients with most severe hypercholesterolemia and xanthomatosis as well as

patients with moderate hypercholesterolemia as heterozygotes, is not supported
by observed segregation ratios. The best established theory calls for incompletely
dominant inheritance leading to moderate hypercholesterolemia in heterozygotes
and severe hypercholesterolemia in homozygotes. The pathologic gene exerts its
influence within a system of interacting exogenous and endogenous factors which,
as shown, among others, by the study of Thomas et al. (1964), results in considerable
variation among each of the genotypically defined groups. Consequent overlapping is of such a degree that statistical analysis clearly shows differences of

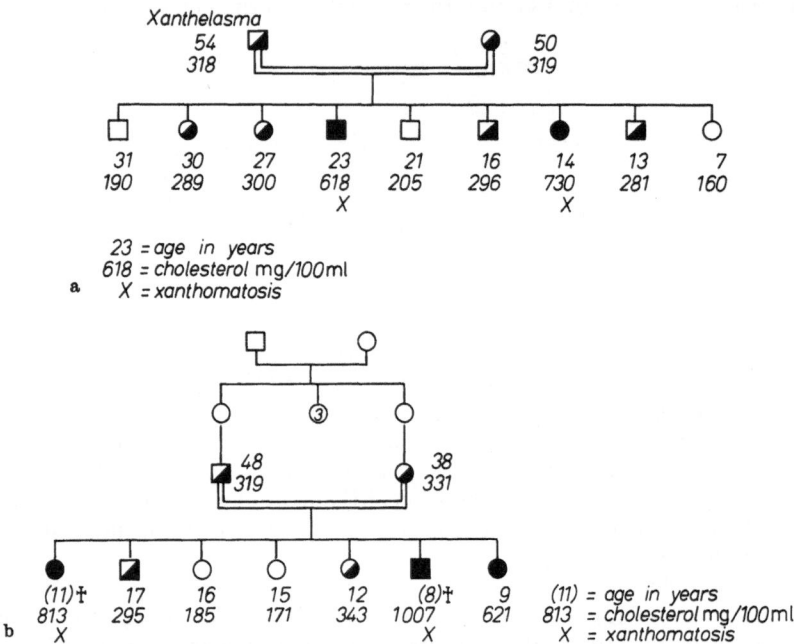

Fig. 10a and b. Pedigrees with marriage of heterozygotes for hypercholesterolemia. a) Observation of
Kachadurian; b) observation of Boggs et al., restudied by Jakovcic and Hsia

mean values, but as long as single cases have to be judged on serum cholesterol
concentration alone no definite classification of single individuals is possible and
in a great number of cases may lead to erroneous conclusions. This holds true
equally for the separation of homozygous normals from heterozygotes and of
heterozygotes and pathologic homozygotes. Heterozygotes may in the individual
case display cholesterol levels well within the range of normal, while some
individuals, homozygous for the normal allele, may reach serum cholesterol levels
in the range of heterozygotes. This also is supported by the theoretical distribution
curves in the sample population of Thomas et al. (1964). The cut-off point between
heterozygotes and individuals homozygously affected for analogous reasons cannot
be fixed at 400 mg/100 ml. One rather has to expect a range of uncertainty at
this borderline.

Formation of cutaneous and tendon xanthomata is secondary and depends on
several factors, mainly but not alone on the height of the cholesterol elevation
and the duration of this pathologic state. There may be a familial tendency
to develop xanthomatous lesions and/or arcus corneae, which points to importance
of modifying genetic factors (Figure 11a + b). The explanation of this familial
tendency does not require the assumption of various alleles of the gene for hypercholesterolemia although this may be a possibility.

Since generally early onset of hypercholesterolemia and high cholesterol levels
will lead to early and marked manifestation of xanthomata and arcus corneae
as well as to early atherosclerosis, this must be found closely correlated to homozygosity. The variability of serum cholesterol concentration in persons either homozygous for the pathologic gene or heterozygous explains why particularly in the

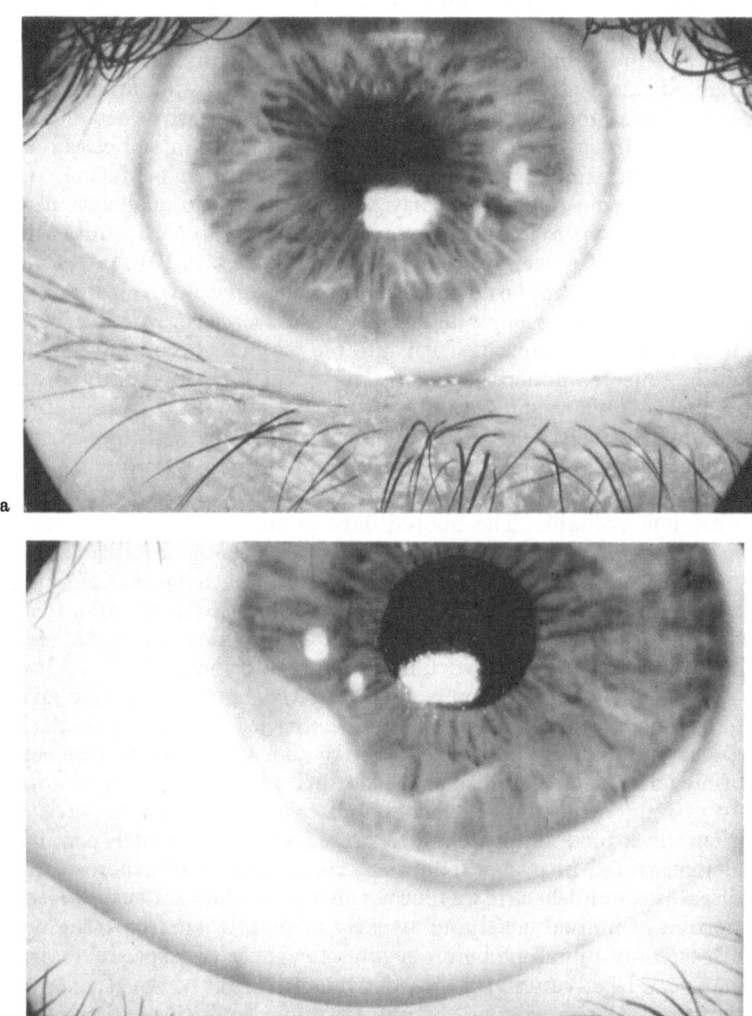

Fig. 11a and b. Arcus lipoides in father a) and son b) suffering from hypercholesterolemia. Father,
age: 56 years, tot. cholesterol: 420 mg/100 ml; Son, age: 11 years, tot. cholesterol: 340 mg/100 ml

range of the overlap some heterozygotes with manifest xanthomatous lesions will
be observed and why some homozygotes may not develop xanthomas. As KHACHA-
DURIAN emphasized, if heterozygotes develop xanthomas, they will do so at a
later age and to a milder degree. Thus, the concept of WILKINSON et al. (1948)
and HIRSCHHORN and WILKINSON (1959) postulating a single autosomal incompletely dominant gene which in single dose causes a moderate, in double dose,
however, severe elevation of cholesterol levels can be maintained but in its original
form requires two modifications: xanthomatosis is, as claimed, most often found

in homozygotes but homozygosity must not always lead to early xanthomatosis. Heterozygotes may occasionally develop xanthomas but in general will do so later and to a milder degree. The borders between homozygous normals and heterozygotes and between heterozygotes and homozygotes for the pathologic gene cannot be defined sharply by serum cholesterol levels alone.

The fact that repeatedly and sometimes in familial aggregation cases have been observed in which the increase of serum concentration of cholesterol and of trigly-cerides has been equally marked and which, therefore, cannot be safely attributed to either familial essential hypercholesterolemia or to essential familial hyperlipe-mia by means of available diagnostic methods does not justify the assumption of a common genetic basis of these two entities. The term "mixed cases" that has been introduced, therefore, appears unfortunate and rather confusing, this even more so, because these cases must clearly be separated from observations of coin-cidence of essential hypercholesterolemia and essential hyperlipemia within the same pedigree as this has been reported by HIRSCHHORN and WILKINSON (1959). At the present time it cannot be decided whether these special cases will have to be grouped later with one of the major disease entities discussed or whether further sub-groups will have to be recognized. Until suitable methods become available, these cases should be collected under the general, unspecified heading of hyperlipidemia or hyperlipoproteinemia as suggested by FREDRICKSON (1961) and FREDRICKSON and LEES, or descriptively be termed hypercholesterolemia with hypertriglycerid-emia. Careful collection and publication of such families is warranted.

As mentioned previously reliable estimates of the gene frequency for the hyper-lipidemias are not available. The quoted data point towards a frequency of the hyperlipemia genes of about 0.01 and even 0.06 for the gene of hypercholester-olemia. Again one may ask how pathologic genes could have reached and main-tained such a frequency, as known homozygotes frequently die at an early age or do not reproduce. To compensate for this loss of genes and establish genetic equilibrium by mutation alone, an unreasonably high mutation rate would be required. A more likely explanation is offered by the assumption of an advantage of the heterozygotes. The rapid increase of atherosclerotic cardiovascular disease in recent times undoubtedly is to be attributed to a variety of factors connected with life of modern western civilization. One such factor at least seems to be the rich supply of refined foods and the habit of overeating. In primitive cultures and in earlier times food supply has been restricted. Under such conditions, as has been demonstrated in post-war famine, manifestation of atherosclerosis and coronary disease is diminished. If we tentatively accept the view that at least a con-siderable portion of individuals dying at early or middle age from atherosclerotic vascular disease may represent heterozygotes for genes of hyperlipidemias, then the hypothesis can be advanced that the detrimental effect of these genes, which is obvious in times of plenty, may not be notable under conditions of restricted food supply. In fact, under these conditions the adverse influence may be converted to an advantage e.g. by conferring to heterozygotes the ability to withstand famine and deprivation better. A similar hypothesis has been advanced for diabetes mellitus by NEEL (1962) and discussed by McKUSICK (1963) for cardiovascular disease.

Myocardial infarction usually leads to death at an age beyond the reproductive period of most men, an age where on the other hand commonly a certain security for the family has been achieved. Sudden death of the father under such circum-stances may bring about a tendency to earlier marriage of the children and thus an earlier reproduction in those families, which in turn favors the spreading of such deleterious genes (EDWARDS 1963). In any case the observed gene frequencies will have to be explained by a complex interplay of various factors.

IV. Other Diseases Commonly Grouped with the Lipidoses

a) Mucopolysaccharidoses (Lipochondrodystrophy, Gargoylism)

These diseases at previous times generally have been viewed as primary disturbance of lipid metabolism. Today a disturbance of the metabolism of the mucopolysaccharides is thought to be the primary defect (BRANTE 1952). SEITELBERGER (1962) found the stored substance to be a complex of lipids and polysaccharides and feels that neither a pure lipidosis nor a pure defect in polysaccharide metabolism suffices as explanation.

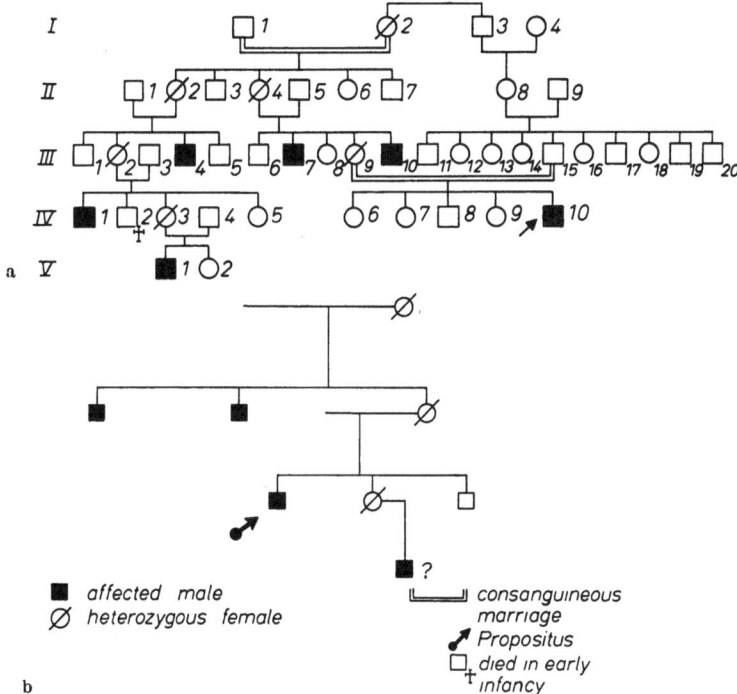

Fig. 12. Pedigrees with sex-linked type of mucopolysaccharidosis. a) From LAMY et al. 1957; b) from McKUSICK 1959

Genetically at least two forms must be separated (HERNDON 1954, LAMY et al. 1957), an autosomal recessive type, type PFAUNDLER-HURLER, and a sex-linked (X-chromosomal) recessive type, which following a suggestion of McKUSICK may be referred to as type HUNTER. Clinically and in the individual case these two genetically distinct forms cannot always be separated. In both chondroitinsulfate B and heparitinsulfate is excreted in the urine.

Among 269 cases collected by LAMY et al. (1957) 187 were males and 91 females. Clearcut pedigrees also prove the existence of an X-chromosomal recessive form of the disease in a number of cases (Figure 12a + b).

Since affected females undoubtedly belong to the autosomal recessive variety, LAMY and coworkers tested the fit of segregation ratios observed in families of female probands with values expected in autosomal recessive conditions. Giving due regard to the mode of ascertainment the observed value (determined according to Weinberg's method 31% of siblings affected) sufficiently agreed with the expected ratio (25%). Furthermore, in 16 of 49 families studied in this regard consanguinity of parents was noted. In 30 families no statement as to the question of consanguinity was available.

For clinical differentiation of the autosomal recessive and the sex-linked variety in affected males the corneal manifestations particularly can be used. While 90% of affected individuals belonging to the autosomal recessive type had corneal opacities, these were never found in the sex-linked form. Reilly-granules also had never been reported in the leucocytes of patients with the sex-linked form. It is not certain, however, whether the incomplete variety of this anomaly of the white cells has been searched for sufficiently. According to Rampini et al. (1964) the granulation of white cells is a constant feature of the autosomal recessive type, if the incomplete form is included. The latter is characterized by granules in lymphocytes only in the peripheral blood and in various celltypes in the bone marrow (Gasser 1950). In 16 cases of the children's hospital of Zurich the complete form of Reilly's anomaly was found twice and the incomplete type in the remaining 14.

Estimation of the proportion of cases belonging to the sex-linked variety can be based on the corneal manifestations or on the sex ratio observed in the total sample. Either method confirms that about one third of all observed patients is of the X-chromosomal type. These patients have a somewhat better prognosis but they, too, do not reproduce. Thus in each generation, with the affected males infertile, one third of all genes of this form will be eliminated, and, assuming equilibrium, will have to be replaced by mutation. As a result the high rate of mutation should lead to appearance of a corresponding excess of sporadic cases. The data of Lamy et al. seem to corroborate this assumption. This reasoning would not hold true, however, if generally mutations would occur more frequent in male gonads, as this has been demonstrated e.g. for hemophilia by Vogel (1965). Mutations in the X-chromosomes of men would lead exclusively to additional heterozygotes (carriers) among their daughters, in whose children affected patients would not be increased over randomly expected values. Two further variants may be recognized (cf. McKusick 1965): The Sanfilippo syndrome with urinary excretion of Heparitin-S, severe mental retardation and only mild somatic features. Clouding of the corneae is absent. The transmission is autosomal recessive.

In the Scheie-syndrome clouding of the corneae is present along with stiff joints, and coarse facial features as in the Hurler-Hunter and Sanfilippo syndromes, but the mental retardation is missing. In the urine chondroitin B-sulfate is found. The disease also appears to be autosomal recessively inherited.

Also grouped with the mucopolysaccharidoses can be the "true Morquio syndrome" with extraskeletal manifestations and keratosulfaturia present.

b) Hand-Schüller-Christian's Disease

The pathogenesis of this disease still awaits clarification. Little can be said for its explanation as a primary lipid storage disease. Most authors today place the disease in a line with eosinophilic granuloma and Abt-Letterer-Siwe's disease, grouping them together under the heading of histiocystosis — X. Some evidence points to an infectious genesis. Familial occurrence has been noted very rarely. Van Decken (1943) mentioned dizygotic twins concordant for an atypical form, and Jones (1939) observed identical twins discordant for the disease.

References

Adlersberg, D., A. D. Parets, and E. P. Boas: Genetics of atherosclerosis. J. Amer. med. Ass. 141, 246 (1949).
— Inborn errors of lipid-metabolism. Arch. Path. 60, 481 (1955).

ADLERSBERG, D., and L. E. SCHAEFER: The interplay of heredity and environment in the regulation of circulating lipids and in atherogenesis. Amer. J. Med. **26**, 1 (1959).

AHRENS jr., E. H., J. HIRSCH, K. OETTE, J. W. FARQUHAR, and Y. STEIN: Carbohydrate-induced and fat-induced lipemia. Trans. Ass. Amer. Phycns. **74**, 134 (1961).

ANSELL, G. B., and S. SPANNER: Studies on cerebral sphingomyelin. Biochem. J. **79**, 176 (1961).

ARONSON, S. M., B. E. ARONSON, and B. W. VOLK: A genetic profile of infantile amaurotic family idiocy. Amer. J. Dis. Child. **98**, 50 (1959).

— G. PERLE, A. SAIFER, and B. W. VOLK: Biochemical identification of the carrier state in Tay-Sach's disease. Proc. Soc. exp. Biol. (N. Y.) **111**, 664 (1962).

— M. P. VALSAMIS, and B. W. VOLK: Infantile amaurotic family idiocy (occurrence, genetic considerations and pathophysiology in the non-jewish infant). Pediatrics **26**, 229 (1960).

— and B. W. VOLK: Genetic and demographic considerations concerning Tay-Sachs' disease. In: Cerebral Sphingolipidoses. Ed. S. M. ARONSON and B. W. VOLK, p. 375. NewYork-London: Academic Press 1962.

ASHWORTH, C. T., F. C. DOUGLAS, R. C. REYNOLDS, and P. J. THOMAS: Bacillus-like bodies in Whipple's disease: disappaerance with clinical remission after antibotic therapy. Amer. J. Med. **37**, 481 (1964).

BAGH, K. V., and H. HORTLING: Blod fynd vid juvenil amaurotisk idioti. Nord. Med. **38**, 1072 (1948).

BALINT, J. A., H. L. SPITZER, and E. C. KYRIAKIDES: Studies of red cell stromal lipids in Tay-Sachs' disease and other lipidoses. J. clin. Invest. **42**, 1661 (1963).

— — — Further studies in Niemann-Pick disease. J. Lab. clin. Med. **63**, 1010 (1964).

BEARN, A. G.: Genetic variations in the serum proteins: studies on transferrin and the group specific components. 2nd Int. Cong. Congenital malformations, New York 1963, p. 125, Int. Med. Congr. Ltd, New York 1964.

BERARDINELLI, W.: Un nouveau syndrome endocrino-métabolique. Arch. bras. Endocr. **3**, 5 (1953).

BERGER, H., A. RICHTER, A. GILARDI, and H. WAGNER: Essential familial hyperlipaemia in a two-year-old child. Ann. paediat. (Basel) **199**, 455 (1962).

BESSMAN, S. P., and R. BALDWIN: Imidazole aminoaciduria in cerebromacular degeneration. Science **135**, 789 (1962).

BIALKIN, G., S. ZUCKER, B. S. SKLARIN, K. HIRSCHHORN, and M. DAVIDSON: A genetic and metabolic study of a family with hyperlipemia. Pediatrics **29**, 566 (1962).

BIGLER, J. A., R. F. MAIS, R. M. DOWBEN, and D. Y.-Y. HSIA: An inborn error of lipid metabolism. Pediatrics **23**, 644 (1959).

BLACK-SCHAFFER, B.: Tinctorial demonstration of glycoprotein in Whipple's disease. Proc. Soc. exp. Biol. (N.Y.) **72**, 225 (1949).

BLODI, F., and J. C. YARBROUGH: Ocular manifestations of familial hypercholesterolemia. Amer. J. Ophthal. **55**, 714 (1963).

BÖÖK, J. A.: The frequency of cousin marriages in three North Swedish parishes. Hereditas (Lund) **34**, 252 (1948).

BOGGS, J. D., D. Y.-Y. HSIA, R. F. MAIS, and J. A. BIGLER: The genetic mechanism of idiopathic hyperlipemia. New Engl. J. Med. **257**, 1101 (1957).

BRANTE, G.: Gargoylism — a mucopolysaccharidosis. Scand. J. clin. Lab. Invest. **4**, 43 (1952).

BÜRGER, M., u. O. GRÜTZ: Über hepatosplenomegale Lipoidose mit xanthomatösen Veränderungen an Haut und Schleimhaut. Arch. Derm. Syph. (Berl.) **166**, 542 (1932).

BURNETT, J. W., and S. M. MARCY: Lipoid proteinosis. Amer. J. Dis. Child. **105**, 81 (1963).

BURSTEIN, J., and C. W. MALM: Familial hypercholesterolaemic xanthomatosis and coronary disease. Acta med. scand. **175**, 569 (1964).

CAMP, C. D., and K. LÖWENBERG: An American family with Pelizaeus-Merzbacher disease. Arch. Neurol. Psychiat. **45**, 261 (1941).

CRAIG, J. M., J. T. CLARKE, and B. Q. BANKER: Metabolic neurovisceral disorder with accumulation of unidentified substance: Variant of Hurler's Syndrome. Amer. J. Dis. Child. **98**, 577 (1959).

CROCKER, A. C., and S. FARBER: Niemann-Pick disease. Medicine (Baltimore) **37**, 1 (1958).

DANIS, P., C. BEGAUX, et G. DECOCK: Bases ophthalmologiques d'une classification des idiotics amaurotiques. J. Génét. hum. **6**, 91 (1957).

DARLINGTON, C. D., and K. MATHER: The elements of genetics. London: Allan and Unwin 1949.

DAWSON, R. M. C.: A hydrolytic procedure for the identification and estimation of individual phospholipids in biological samples. Biochem. J. **75**, 45 (1960).

DECKEN, R. VAN: Hand-Schüller-Christian'sche Erkrankung bei zweieiigen Zwillingen. Arch. Kinderheilk. **128**, 50 (1943).

DEREUX, J.: La maladie de Refsum. Rev. neurol. **109**, 599 (1963).

Donohue, W. L.: Clinicopathologic conference at the Hospital for Sick Children: Sysendocrinism. J. Pediat. 32, 739 (1948).
— and I. Uchida: Leprechaunism; A euphemism for a rare familial disorder. J. Pediat.
45, 505 (1954).
Edwards, J. H.: The genetic basis of common disease. Amer. J. Med. 34, 627 (1963).
Emery, A. E. H.: Muscle histology in carriers of Duchenne Muscular Dystrophy. J. med.
Genet. 2, 1 (1965).
Epstein, Ch. J.: Structural and control gene defects in hereditary disease in man. Lancet
1964/II, 1066.
Epstein, F. H., W. D. Block, E. A. Hand, and T. Francis jr.: Familial hypercholesterolemia, Xanthomatosis, and coronary heart disease. Amer. J. Med. 26, 39 (1959).
Farber, S.: In "The child in health and disease: A textbook for students and practitioners
of medicine". C. G. Grulee, and R. C. Eley, eds., sec. ed., pp. 496, Baltimore: Williams &
Wilkins, 1952.
— J. Cohen, and L. L. Uzman: Lipogranulomatosis. J. Mt Sinai Hosp. 24, 816 (1957).
Fredrickson, D. S.: Essential familial hyperlipidemia. In Stanbury, J. B., J. B. Wyngaarden, and D. S. Fredrickson: The metabolic basis of inherited disease. New York-
Toronto-London: McGraw-Hill 1960.
— The inheritance of high density lipoprotein deficiency (Tangier disease). J. clin. Invest. 43,
228 (1964).
— and P. H. Altrocchi: Tangier disease (Familial cholesterolosis with high density lipoprotein deficiency). In Cerebral Sphingolipidoses, Ed. S. M. Aronson and B. W. Volk,
p. 343. New York-London: Academic Press 1962.
— and R. S. Lees: A system for phenotyping Hyperlipoproteinemia. Circulation 31, 321
(1965).
— K. Ono, and L. L. Davis: Lipolytic activity of post-heparin plasma in hyperglyceridemia.
J. Lipid. Res. 4, 24 (1963).
Freudenberg, E.: Klinische Beobachtungen und Untersuchungen an einem eineiigen
Zwillingspaar mit Niemann-Pick'scher Krankheit. Z. Kinderheilk. 59, 313 (1938).
Frezal, J.: Second Internat. Cong. longenital malformations. New York 1963, p. 153, Int
Med. Congr. Ltd., New York 1964.
Fuhrmann, W.: Untersuchungen über die Fettsäuren der Plasmalipide bei erbbedingter
kohlenhydratsensitiver Hyperlipidämie. Dtsch. med. Wschr. 89, 1293 (1964).
Gasser, C.: Diskussion zum Artikel von Alder. Schweiz. med. Wschr. 80, 1097 (1950).
Gedda, L., e D. Poggi: Sulla regolazione genetica del colesterolo ematico (uno studio su 50
coppie gemellar: MZ e 50 coppie DZ.). Acta Genet. med. (Roma) 9, 135 (1960).
Gerken, H.: Heterozygotennachweis bei Morbus Gaucher. Mschr. Kinderheilk. 113, 486 (1965).
— u. H. R. Wiedemann: Ein Beitrag zur Genetik des Morbus Gaucher. Ann. paediat.
(Basel) 203, 327 (1964).
Goldschmidt, E., R. Lenz, S. Merin, A. Ronen, and I. Ronen: (cited by Myrianthopoulos)
Abstr. 25th Ann. Meeting Genet. Soc. Amer. p. 1, 1956.
Grasso, E., and M. Negri: Méd. int. 59, 171 (1951); cited in Berger u. Mitarb. (1962).
Groen, J. J.: Gaucher's disease. Hereditary transmission and racial distribution. Arch.
intern. Med. 113, 453 (1964).
Hagberg, B., G. Hultquist, L. Svennerholm, and H. Voss: Malignant hyperlipemia in
infancy. Amer. J. Dis. Child. 107, 267 (1964).
Harris, H.: Human biochemical genetics. Cambridge: University Press 1959.
— The genetic control of enzyme formation in man. Congenital Malformations, Papers and
Discussions, presented at the second international conference on congenital malformation,
New York City, 1963, New York: Int. Med. Congr. Ltd., 1964.
— and C. A. B. Smith: The sib-sib age of onset correlation among individuals suffering from
a hereditary syndrome produced by more than one gene. Ann. Eugen. (Lond.) 14, 309 (1947
—1949).
Havel, R. J., and R. S. Gordon: Idiopathic hyperlipemia: metabolic studies in an affected
family. J. clin. Invest. 39, 1777 (1960).
Herndon, C. N.: Genetics of the lipidoses. Res. Publ. Ass. nerv. ment. Dis. 33, 239 (1954).
— and C. I. Bender: Gaucher's disease: Cases in five related negro-sibships. Amer. J. hum.
Genet. 2, 49 (1950).
Heuschert, D.: Unpublished data.
Hirschhorn, K., R. Hirschhorn, M. Fraccaro, and J. A. Böök: Incidence of familial
hyperlipemia. Science 129, 716 (1959).
— and Ch. Wilkinson jr.: The mode of inheritance in essential familial hypercholesterolemia. Amer. J. Med. 26, 60 (1959).
Holt jr., L. E., F. X. Aylword, H. C. Timbres: Idiopathic familial lipemia. Bull. Johns
Hopk. Hosp. 64, 279 (1939).

HOOFT, C., P. DE LAEY, J. HERPOL, F. DE LOORE, and J. VERBEEK: Familial hypolipidaemia and retarded development without steatorrhoea. Another inborn error of metabolism? Helv. paediat. Acta 17, 1 (1962).

HSIA, D. Y.-Y., J. NAYLOR, and J. A. BIGLER: The genetic mechanism of Gaucher's disease. In: Cerebral Sphingolipidoses Ed. S. M. ARONSON, and B. W. VOLK, p. 327. New York-London, Academic Press 1962.

IVEMARK, B., L. SVENNERHOLM, C. THORÉN, and R. TUNELL: Niemann-Pick disease in infancy. Report of two siblings with clinical, histologic, and chemical studies. Acta paediat. (Uppsala) 52, 391 (1963).

JACOB, F., and J. MONOD: Cellular regulatory mechanisms. On the regulation of gene activity. Cold. Spr. Harb. Symp. quant. Biol. 26, 193 (1961).

— — Genetic regulatory mechanisms in the synthesis of proteins. J. molec. Biol. 3, 318 (1961).

JAKOVCIC, S., J. C. CHRISTIAN, and D. Y.-Y. HSIA: Personal communication.

— W. FUHRMANN, and D. Y.-Y. HSIA: Essential familial hyperlipidemia in childhood. Pediatrics 34, 822 (1964).

JATZKEWITZ, H., H. PILZ, and K. SANDHOFF: Quantitative Bestimmungen von Gangliosiden und ihren neurominsäurefreien Derivaten bei infantilen, juvenilen und adulten Formen der amaurotischen Idiotie und einer spätinfantilen biochemischen Sonderform. The quantitative determination of gangliosides and their derivatives in different forms of amaurotic idiocy. J. Neurochem. 12, 135 (1956).

JENSEN, J., D. H. BLANKENHORN, H. P. CHIN, PH. STURGEON, and A. G. WARE: Serum lipids and serum uric acid in human twins. J. Lipid Res. 6, 193 (1965).

JERVIS, G. A., R. C. HARRIS, and J. H. MENKES: Cerebral lipidosis of unclear nature. In: Cerebral Sphingolipidosis, Ed. S. M. ARONSON, and B. W. VOLK, p. 101, New York-London: Academic Press 1962.

JOBST, H., H. HUBER u. G. SCHETTLER: Essentielle familiäre Hyperlipämie bei einem eineiigen Zwillingspaar. Med. Klin. 58, 710 (1963).

JONES, A. B.: Schüller-Christian disease. Report of case in one of identical twins. Arch. intern. Med. 13, 1068 (1939).

KAHLKE, W.: Refsum-Syndrom. — Lipoidchemische Untersuchungen bei 9 Fällen. Klin. Wschr. 42, 1011 (1964).

— Personal communication, 1965.

KHACHADURIAN, A. K.: The inheritance of essential familial hypercholesterolemia. Amer. J. Med. 37, 402 (1964).

KINSELL, L. W., G. D. MICHAELIS, G. WALKER, ST. SPLITTER, and G. FUKAYAMA: An approach to understanding of the gross hyperlipidemic states. Lipid Metabolism 11, 683(1962).

KNUDSON jr., A. G., and W. D. KAPLAN: Genetics of the sphingolipidoses. In: Cerebral Sphingolipidoses, Ed. S. M. ARONSON, and B. W. VOLK, p. 395. New York-London: Academic Press 1962.

KOCH, G.: Degenerative Entmarkungskrankheiten (Diffuse Sklerosen). In: Humangenetik. Ed. by P. E. BECKER. Bd. V. Stuttgart: Thieme (im Druck).

KORNERUP, V.: Familiaer hypercholesterolaemia og xanthomatose. Kolding, Denmark, 1948.

KOZINN, P. J., H. WIENER, and P. COHEN: Infantile amaurotic family idiocy. J. Pediat. 51, 58 (1957).

KUO, P. T., and D. R. BASSETT: Primary hyperlipidemias and their management. Ann. intern. Med. 59, 495 (1963).

— A. F. WHEREAT, D. R. BASSETT, and E. STAPLE: Study of mechanism of hyperlipemia. Circulation 24, 213 (1961).

LAMY, M., J. FREZAL, J. POLONOVSKI, G. DUREZ, and J. REY: Congenital absence of beta-lipo-proteins. Pediatrics 31, 277 (1963).

— P. MAROTEAUX et J.-P. BADER: Étude génétique du gargoylisme. Acta genet. (Basel) 7, 113 (1957).

— — Étude génétique du gargoylisme. J. Génét. hum. 6, 156 (1957).

LANDING, B. H., and J. H. RUBINSTEIN: Biopsy diagnosis of neurologic diseases in childhood with emphasis on lipidosis in "Cerebral Sphingolipidoses", p. 1—14. J. M. ARONSON and B. W. VOLK (Eds.). New York: Academic Press Inc. 1962.

— F. N. SILVERMAN, J. M. CRAIG, M. D. JACOBY, M. E. LAHEY, and D. I. CHADWICK: Familial neurovisceral lipidosis. Am. J. Dis. Child. 108, 503 (1964).

LEVY, R. J., and D. S. FREDICKSON: Heterogeneity of plasma high density liporoteins. J. clin. Invest 44, 426 (1965).

LYON, M. F.: Sex chromatin and gene action in the mammalian X-chromosome. Amer. J. hum. Genet. 14, 135 (1962).

MARKERT, C. L.: Cellular differentiation — an expression of differential gene function. In: Congenital Malformations. (Papers and discussions presented at the Second International Conference.) New York: International Medical Congress Ltd. 1964.

McDonaugh, J. R., G. G. Hames, and B. G. Greenberg: Observations on serum cholesterol levels in the twin population of Evans County Georgia. Circulation 25, 962 (1962).

McKusick, V. A.: Vererbbare Störungen des Bindegewebes. Stuttgart: Thieme 1959.
— Natural selection and contemporary cardiovascular disease. Circulation 27, 161 (1963).
— The genetic mucopolysaccharidoses. Circulation 31, 1 (1965).

Meilman, E., Ch. M. Holtzman, and P. Samuel: Familial hypercholesterolemia and xanthomatosis. Amer. J. Med. 36, 277 (1964).

Miescher, G.: Drei Fälle von familiärer Keratose der Haut und Schleimhäute, kombiniert mit Blasenbildung und kolloider, zu schweren Funktionsstörungen (Larynxstenose) führender Schleimhautdegeneration. Jb. Kinderheilk. 44, 189 (1925).

Müller, C.: Xanthomata, hypercholesterolaemia, angina pectoris. Acta med. scand. (supp.) 89, 75 (1938).

Myrianthopoulos, N. C.: Some epidemiologic and genetic aspects of Tay-Sachs' disease. In: Cerebral Sphingolipidoses, Ed. S. M. Aronson, and B. W. Volk, p. 359. New York-London: Academic Press 1962.

Neel, J. V.: The study of natural selection in primitive and civilized human populations. Hum. Biol. 30, 43 (1958).
— Diabetes Mellitus: A "Thrifty" genotype rendered detrimental by "Progress"? Amer. J. hum. Genet. 14, 353 (1962).

Neiman, N., J. Benrey, M. Tierson, P. Tridon, S. Sapelier, and P. Melin: Familial Urbach-Wiethe disease with indifference for pain. Bull. Soc. franç. Derm. Syph. 71, 292 (1964).

Norman, R. M., H. Urich, A. H. Tingey, and R. A. Goodbody: Tay-Sachs disease with visceral involvement and its relationship to Niemann-Pick's disease. J. Path. Bact. 78, 409 (1959).
— and N. Wood: Congenital form of amaurotic family idiocy. J. Neurol. Psychiat. 4, 175 (1941).

O'Brien, J. S., M. B. Stern, B. H. Landing, J. K. O'Brien, and G. N. Donnell: Generalized gangliosidosis. Amer. J. Dis. Child. 109, 338 (1965).

Opitz, J. M., F. C. Stiles, D. Wise, R. R. Race, R. Sanger, G. R. v. Gemmingen, R. R. Kierland, E. G. Cross, W. P. de Groot: The genetics of angiokeratoma corporis diffusum (Fabry's disease) and its linkage relation with the Xg-locus. Amer. J. hum. Genet. 17, 325 (1965).

Osborne, R. H., D. Adlersberg, F. V. DeGeorge, and Ch. Wang: Serum lipids, heredity, and environment. A study of adult twins. Amer. J. Med. 26, 54 (1959).

Paigen, K.: The genetic control of enzyme realization during differentiation. In: Congenital Malformations. (Papers and discussions presented at the Second International Conference). New York: International Medical Congress Ltd. 1964.

Parker, W. C., and A. G. Bearn: The application of genetic regulatory mechanisms to human genetics. Amer. J. Med. 34, 680 (1963).

Pearson, C. M.: Muscular dystrophy. Amer. J. Med. 35, 632 (1963).

Pfändler, U.: La maladie de Niemann-Pick dans le cadre des lipoidoses. Schweiz. med. Wschr. 76, 1128 (1946).
— Contribution au problème pathogénique de la maladie de Niemann-Pick. Schweiz. med. Wschr. 78, 250 (1948).
— Nouvelles conceptions sur l'hérédité et la pathogénie de la maladie de Niemann-Pick. Helv. med. Acta 20, 216 (1953).
— Stoffwechselkrankheiten. In: Humangenetik, P. E. Becker (ed.), Bd. 111/1, S. 1. Stuttgart: Thieme 1964.

Philippart, M., and J. Menkes: Isolation and characterization of the main splenic glycolysids in Gaucher's disease: evidence for the site of metabolic block. Biochem. biophys. Res. Commun. 15, 551 (1964).

Piper, J., and L. Orrild: Essential familial hypercholesterolemia and xanthomatosis. Amer. J. Med. 21, 34 (1956).

Poser, C. M.: Concepts of dysmyelination. In: Cerebral Sphingolipidoses. Ed. S. M. Aronson, and B. W. Volk, p. 141. New York-London: Academic Press 1962.

Puite, R. H., and H. Tesluk: Whipple's disease. Amer. J. Med. 19, 383 (1955).

Rampini, S., u. W. Adank: Hämatologische Befunde bei Patienten mit Gargoylismus u. heterozygoten Genträgern. Helv. paediat. Acta 19, 101 (1964).

Rath, F.: Akuter Morbus Gaucher bei einem Säugling. Mschr. Kinderheilk. 112, 355 (1964).

Rayner, S.: Juvenile amaurotic idiocy, diagnosis of heterozygotes. Acta genet. (Basel) 3, 1 (1952).
— Juvenile amaurotic idiocy in Sweden. Publ. Instit. Med. Genet. Univ. Uppsala, Lund 1962.

Refsum, S.: Heredopathia atactica polyneuritiformis. Acta genet. (Basel) 7, 344 (1957).
— Wld Neurol. 1, 334 (1960).

RICHTERICH, R., H. MOSER, and E. ROSSI: Refsum's disease (heredopathia atactica poly-neuritiformis); an inborn error of lipid metabolism with storage of 3,7,11,15-tetramethyl-hexadecanoic acid. III. Review of the literature: clinical findings. Humangenetik 1 (1965) (in print).

— S. ROSIN, and E. ROSSI: Refsum's disease (heredopathia atactica polyneuritiformis): an inborn error of lipid metabolism with storage of 3,7,11,15-tetramethylhexadecanoic acid. IV. Formal genetics. Humangenetik 1 (1965) (in print).

RÖSSLE, R.: Dystrophia pachydermica cutis et mucosae progressiva hereditaria. Arch. Sci. med. **50**, 155 (1927).

SALT, H. B., O. H. WOLFF, J. K. LLOYD, A. S. FORSBROOKE, A. H. CAMERON, and D. V. HUBBLE: On having no beta-lipoprotein: a syndrome comprising a-beta-lipoproteinemia acanthocytosis and steatorrhoea. Lancet **1960/II**, 325.

SCHAEFER, L. E.: Serum cholesterol-triglyceride-distribution in a "normal" New York City population. Amer. J. Med. **36**, 262 (1964).

SCHETTLER, G., H. JOBST, H. P. KÄPPLER u. G. KÖRFGEN: Familiäre Hypercholesterinämie. Dtsch. med. Wschr. **84**, 368 (1959).

SEIP, M.: Lipodystrophy and gigantism with associated endocrine manifestations. Acta paediat. (Uppsala) **48**, 555 (1959).

SEITELBERGER, F.: Die Pelizaeus Merzbacher'sche Krankheit. Klinisch-anatomische Unter-suchungen zum Problem ihrer Stellung unter den diffusen Sklerosen. Wien. Z. Nervenheilk. **9**, 229 (1954).

— Gargoylismus. In: FR. LINNEWEH (ed.): Erbliche Stoffwechselkrankheiten, S. 591. München-Berlin: Urban & Schwarzenberg 1962.

— and K. SIMMA: On the pigment variant of amaurotic idiocy. In: Cerebral Sphingolipi-doses, Ed. S. M. ARONSON, and B. W. VOLK, p. 29. New York-London: Academic Press 1962.

SENIOR, B., and S. S. GELLIS: The syndromes of total lipodystrophy and of partial lipo-dystrophy. Pediatrics **33**, 593 (1964).

SIEBENMANN, F.: Über Mitbeteiligung der Schleimhaut bei allgemeiner Hyperkeratose der Haut. Arch. int. Laryng. **20**, 101 (1908).

SJÖGREN, T.: Die juvenile amaurotische Idiotie. Hereditas (Lund) **14**, 197 (1931).

SPIEGEL-ADOLF, M., H. W. BAIRD, H. S. COLEMAN, and E. G. SZEKELY: Vacuolized blood lymphocytes in the lipidoses and other central nervous system diseases with special reference to histochemical studies. In: Cerebral Sphingolipidoses. Ed. S. M. ARONSON, and B. W. VOLK, p. 129. New York-London: Academic Press 1962.

SPRITZ, N.: Carbohydrate-induced lipemia. Report of a familial occurrence. New Engl. J. Med. **271**, 291 (1964).

STECHER, R. M., and A. H. HERSH: Note on genetics of hypercholesterolemia. Science **109**, 61 (1949).

TERRY, R. D., W. M. SPERRY, and B. BRODOFF: Adult lipidosis resembling Niemann-Pick disease. Amer. J. Path. **30**, 263 (1954).

TEUTSCHLÄNDER, O.: Über progressive Lipogranulomalose der Muskulatur. Klin. Wschr. **14**, 451 (1935).

THOMAS, C. B., and H. B. COHEN: Familial occurence of hypertension and coronary artery disease with observations concerning obesity and diabetes. Ann. intern. Med. **42**, 90 (1955).

— E. A. MURPHY, and D. R. BOLLING: The precursors of hypertension and coronary disease: Statistical consideration of distributions in a population of medical students. I. Total serum cholesterol. Bull. Johns Hopk. Hosp. **114**, 290 (1964).

TOURTELLOTTE, W. A., R. J. ALLEN, and R. N. DEJONG: A study of lipids in cerebrospinal fluid (and serum). VII. In several sphingolipidoses (Tay-Sachs' disease, metachromatic leucodystrophy, and Niemann-Pick disease). In: Cerebral Sphingolipidoses. Ed. S. M. ARONSON, and B. W. VOLK, p. 317. New York-London: Academic Press 1962.

TRACA, G., P. N. HENNEBERT, et A. MAZABRAUD: Considerations sur un cas de lipocalcino-granulomatose. Presse méd. **73**, 543 (1965).

UPTON, A. C.: Histochemical investigation of the mesenchymal lesions in Whipple's disease. Amer. J. clin. Path. **22**, 755 (1952).

URBACH, E., and C. WIETHE: Lipoidosis cutis et mucosae. Virchows Arch. path. Anat. **273**, 285 (1929).

VIDEBAEK, A.: Niemann Pick's disease. Acta paediat. (Uppsala) **37**, 95 (1949).

VOGEL, F.: Sind die Mutationsraten für die X-chromosomal recessiven Hämophilieformen in Keimzellen von Frauen niedriger als in Keimzellen von Männern? Humangenetik 1, 253 (1965).

VOLK, B. W., S. M. ARONSON, and A. SAIFER: Fructose-1-phosphate aldolase deficiency in Tay-Sachs' disease. Amer. J. Med. **36**, 481 (1964).

WHIPPLE, G. H.: A hitherto undescribed disease characterized anatomically by deposits of fat and fatty acids in the intestinal and mesenteric lymphatic tissues. Bull. Johns Hopk. Hosp. 18, 382 (1907).

WIEDEMANN, H.-R., H. GERKEN, E. GRAUCOB, and H. G. HANSEN: Recognition of heterozygosity in sphingolipoidoses. Lancet 1965/I, 1283.

WILKINSON jr., C. F., E. A. HAND, and M. T. FLIEGELMAN: Essential familial hypercholesterolemia. Ann. intern. Med. 29, 671 (1948).

WILLIAMS, R. J.: Biochemical genetics and its human implications. Acta genet. (Basel) 7, 163 (1957).

WOOD, M. G., F. URBACH, and H. BEERMAN: Histochemical study of a case of lipoid proteinosis. J. invest. Derm. 26, 263 (1956).

YAMAMOTO, R. S., L. B. CRITTENDEN, L. SOKOLOFF, and G. E. JAY: Genetic variations in plasma lipid content in mice. J. Lipid. Res. 4, 413 (1963).

ZEMAN, W., W. DEMYER, H. F. FALLS: Pelizaeus-Merzbacher disease. J. Neuropath. exp. Neurol. 23, 334 (1964).

ZERBIN-RÜDIN, E., u. J. PEIFFER: Ein genetischer Beitrag zur Frage der Spätform der Pelizaeus-Merzbacher'schen Krankheit. Humangenetik 1, 107 (1964).

Acknoledgement: The author wishes to thank Dr. GEORGE B. HUTCHISON, Boston, for valuable criticism and for proof reading the manuscript.

Author Index

Page numbers in *italics* refer to the bibliographies

Subject Index

Page numbers in bold face type: main discussion of topics

Page numbers in italics: figures and tables

The following abbreviations are used in the index: AAFI = adult amaurotic family idiocy; AβLP = abetalipoproteinemia; ACD = angiokeratoma corporis diffusum (Fabry's disease); AFI = amaurotic family idiocy; ATP = adenosine 5'-triphosphate; CAFI = congenital amaurotic family idiocy; CDP = cytidine 5'-diphosphate; CIHL = carbohydrate-induced hyperlipemia; CMP = cytidine 5'-monophosphate; CoA = coenzyme A; CTP = cytidine 5'-triphosphate; DD = differential diagnosis; EFH = essential familial hypercholesterolemia; EHL = essential hyperlipemia; FFA = free fatty acids; FIHL = fat-induced hyperlipemia; F-1-PA = fructose-1-phosphate aldolase; GD = Gaucher's disease; GOT = glutamic-oxalacetic transaminase; GPC = glycerolphosphorylcholine; HAP = heredopathia atactica polyneuritiformis (Refsum's disease); HD = Hurler's disease; JAFI = juvenile amaurotic family idiocy; LIAFI = late infantile amaurotic family idiocy; MCB = membranous cytoplasmic bodies; ML = metachromatic leucodystrophy; NANA = N-acetylneuraminic acid; NPD = Niemann-Pick disease; NVG = neurovisceral gangliosidoses; PAPS = phosphoadenosine phosphosulfate; RDE = receptor destroying enzyme; TSD = Tay-Sachs disease; TSH = thyroid stimulating hormone; UDP = uridine diphosphate.

AAFI, clinical manifestations of 241
—, definition of 241
—, differential diagnosis of 241
—, eyes in 241
—, ganglion cells in 241
—, gangliosides in 241
—, genetics of 502
—, histology of 242
—, lipid analyses in 241
—, neurologic signs in 241
—, pathology of 241
Abdominal crises in EHL 464
A-β-lipoproteinemia (AβLP), 382
—, anisocytosis in 387
—, apallesthesia in 386
—, asthma in 386
—, autopsy findings in 383, 384
—, bone marrow in 387, 388
—, case reports of 382, 384
—, central nervous system in 390
—, clinical manifestations of 395
—, congenital deformities in 387
—, definition of 382
—, diagnosis of 397
—, eyes in 387
—, gastrointestinal disturbances in 388
—, — tract, X-ray examination of 389
—, genetics of 507
—, growth impairment in 385

A-β-lipoproteinemia (AβLP) hematology in 387
—, heterozygotes 385
—, historical review in 382
—, hyperglycemia in 383
—, incidence of 383
—, kyphoscoliosis in 385, 386
—, lipid analyses in 390
—, lipids in intestinal mucosa 384, 394
—, lipids in serum 390, 391
—, — — —, fatty acids of 396
—, lipoproteins in 390, 392, 393
—, lipoproteins in heterozygotes 385
—, metabolic studies in 382, 383, 395, 396
—, muscle atrophy in 386
—, neurologic disturbances in 386
—, onset of 383
—, pathogenetic aspects of 394
—, pathology of 390
—, peripheral nerves in 390
—, pulmonary edema in 386
—, red cells, lipids in 393, 394
—, reflexes in 386
—, skeletal abnormalities in 387
—, skin atrophy in 385
—, small bowel biopsy 389
—, — intestine, lipids in 394
—, spino-cerebellar degeneration in 386
—, treatment of 398

Sphingoplasmalogens, nomenclature of 124
Sphingosine, acetylation of 137
—, biosynthesis of **124**
—, biosynthesis, isotope studies of **145**
— of brain, isotope studies 151
—, chemistry of 16
—, configuration of 128
—, configuration, determination of *137*
—, configuration, role for sphingomyelin
    synthesis 137
—, derivatives of 16
—, occurrence of 128
—, metabolism of 138
—, molecular model of 16
—, propionylation of 137
—, structure of 16
— in sulfatides in ML 324
—, synthesis of **124**
—, synthesis, kinetic studies of *127*
— in Tay-Sachs ganglioside 229, 231
18:sphingosine 123
— —, acylation of 155
— —, conversion to psychosine 155
C-20 sphingosine 123, 230, 231
— — in GD 277
Sphingosine-protein complex, antibodies to
    158
Spike potentials in electroencephalogram in
    TSD 220
Spinal cord, in AβLP 386
— —, in ACD 344
— —, cerebroside:sulfatide ratio, in ML 319
— — in GD 273
— — in HAP **365**
— —, in LIAFI 234
— — in NPD 299
— —, in TSD 224
— ganglia in ML 316
— roots in ML 315
Spleen, accessory in NPD 295
—, foam cells in, in NVG 242, 243, 244
—, ganglioside storage in, in NVG 243
—, gangliosides in, in NVG 244
— in GD 264, **269**
—, hexosamine in, in NVG 244
—, histology of, in ACD 344
— in LIAFI 236
—, lipid of, in ACD 344, 345
—, lipids of, in ML 322
—, lipids of, in normal infants 322
—, lipids of, in NVG 244
— in NPD **294**
—, rupture of, in GD 264
— in TD 404, 405
—, tubercles in GD 264
— biopsy in EHL 467
Splenectomy, bone changes after, in GD 272
— in GD 263, 265, 281

Splenectomy in NPD 291, 292, 305
— in TD 403
Splenomegaly in ACD 338
— in EHL 464
— in GD 262, 269
— in NPD 290, 291, 292, 294
— in NVG 243
— in TD 403
Spontaneous fractures in GD 272
Sprue, lipids in serum, fatty acids of 390, 392
Squalene, biosynthesis of *70*
— and cholesterol biosynthesis 69, 70
—, cyclization to lanosterol 71
—, formation from acetate 70
—, formation from dehydrosqualene 71
—, formation from farnesyl pyrophosphate
    70
— and phytanic acid biosynthesis 376
Scheie's disease see polydystrophic dwarfism
Schizophrenia in ML 313, 314
Stearic acid 23
— — in cerebrosides in GD 278
— — in sphingomyelin in brain in NPD 301,
    302
— — in Tay-Sachs ganglioside 230
Stearyl(-1-^{14}C)-sphingosine, incorporation
    into sphingolipids 152
N-stearyl-18:sphingosine and ceramide hy-
    drolase 129
Stearylamine and phospholipase B 110
Steatorrhea in AβLP 384, 388
— and medium chain fatty acids 45
Steroids, allo- and normal series *6*
—, allo-(trans-) series 5
—, biochemistry of **66**
—, biosynthesis of **66**
—, epi-configuration 5
—, normal-(cis)-series 5
—, α, β-orientation of substituents 5
—, spatial arrangement 5
Sterol oxidase of mitochondria 79
Sterols, biosynthesis of **75**
—, fecal 82, 83
—, neutral, in feces 82
Stigmasterol, formation from mevalonate 76
Stoke's law and estimation of particle size
    of lipoproteins 170
Strandin 22
Sudan black reaction of stored lipids in
    gargoylism 226
— — — of stored lipids in JAFI 226
— — — of stored lipids in ML 226
— — — of stored lipids in NPD 226
— — staining of lipids in ML 317, 318
Sudden death in EFH 418, 419
— — in HAP 357, 359, 368
Sugar containing lipids 122
Sulfatase in ML 325, 326